The Jossey-Bass Health Series brings together the most current information and ideas in health care from the leaders in the field. Titles from the Jossey-Bass Health Series include these essential health care resources:

At Risk in America: The Health and Health Care Needs of Vulnerable Populations, Second Edition, Lu Ann Aday

Collaborating to Improve Community Health: Workbook and Guide to Best Practices in Creating Healthier Communities and Populations, Kathryn Johnson, Wynne Grossman, Anne Cassidy, Editors

Creating Excellence in Crisis Care: A Guide to Effective Training and Program Designs, Lee Ann Hoff, Kazimiera Adamowski

Nutrition and HIV: A New Model for Treatment, Revised and Updated, Mary Romeyn, M.D.

PEOPLE IN CRISIS

PEOPLE IN CRISIS

Clinical and Public Health Perspectives

FIFTH EDITION

Lee Ann Hoff

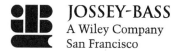

JOSSEY-BASS
A Wiley Company
San Francisco

Published by Jossey-Bass
A Wiley Imprint
989 Market Street, San Francisco, CA 94103-1741   www.josseybass.com

Jossey-Bass books and products are available through most bookstores. To contact Jossey-Bass directly call our Customer Care Department within the U.S. at 800-956-7739, outside the U.S. at 317-572-3986 or fax 317-572-4002.

Jossey-Bass also publishes its books in a variety of electronic formats. Some content that appears in print may not be available in electronic books.

Library of Congress Cataloging-in-Publication Data

Hoff, Lee Ann.
  People in crisis: clinical and public health perspectives /
Lee Ann Hoff.—5th ed.
        p. cm.—(Jossey-Bass health series)
    Includes bibliographical references and index.
    ISBN 0-7879-5421-7 (pbk.: alk. paper)
    1. Crisis intervention (Mental health services) I. Title. II.
Series. RC480.6 .H64 2001
    616.89'025—dc21   2001—001538

Printed in the United States of America
FIFTH EDITION
PB Printing   10 9 8 7 6 5 4 3

CONTENTS

2. UNDERSTANDING PEOPLE IN CRISIS   33

3. IDENTIFYING PEOPLE AT RISK   63

4. HELPING PEOPLE IN CRISIS   103

5. FAMILY AND SOCIAL NETWORK STRATEGIES DURING CRISIS   133

LIST OF TABLES, FIGURES, AND EXHIBITS

Tables

Figures

Exhibits

PREFACE

This book is about people in crisis and those who help them. As social beings, most of us need help to weather the storm of such events as sickness, divorce, sexual assault or other violence, disaster, or the death of a loved one. This book offers those who provide that help—health and social service professionals and others—a comprehensive yet concise view of how people feel, think, and act when navigating the storm of anxiety, emotional pain, or a full-blown crisis. *Understanding* the crisis experience lays the foundation for choosing the strategies and resources that we can use to help distressed people. Although mental health and other professionals traditionally have assisted upset and highly anxious people, this book situates emotional crisis within the *normal* range of human experience. At the same time, it shows how crisis intersects with serious health and mental health problems when necessary help is not available to people who are threatening suicide or violence or who are making other desperate responses to crisis.

Personal crises do not occur in a social or cultural vacuum. *People in Crisis: Clinical and Public Health Perspectives* is unique among contemporary texts in the extent to which it recognizes this fact. The inclusion of cross-cultural and social content, the clearly drawn relationship between crisis theory and practice, the emphasis on human development and resilience, the intersection between clinical and public health responses to events affecting a nation's health, the blending of individual, family, and group approaches to prevention and intervention, and the humanistic thrust of the book all reflect the commitment to viewing crisis in sociocultural context and with sensitivity to the unique experience of each person.

Audience

The comprehensiveness, global perspective, and interdisciplinarity of this book also reflect the fact that crisis care is *everybody's business* and not just the specialty of any one helping profession. All of us can grow in the knowledge and art of helping ourselves and others in crisis. *People in Crisis* was written to help readers in that learning process, in particular

- Frontline crisis workers—nurses (basic and advanced practice), social workers, physicians, police, clergy, teachers, and rescue workers
- Psychotherapists and specialized crisis workers, both volunteers and others
- Health and mental health educators who train physicians, nurses, social workers, psychologists, and counselors
- Human service administrators and program coordinators who must plan, develop, and supervise crisis services
- Social science teachers and researchers who are interested in the study and application of sociocultural theory in health and other human service practice
- The general reader who seeks a better understanding of personal crises

New in the Fifth Edition

Several areas have been expanded and updated for this edition:

1. A strengthened emphasis in this edition is the public recognition of the importance of primary health care in preventing illness, providing early treatment, and preserving a nation's health. The book's new subtitle, *Clinical and Public Health Perspectives,* reaffirms the traditional definition of crisis care in the prevention of serious mental and emotional disturbance through timely intervention as an integral aspect of all human service delivery systems. Yet primary care providers do not usually define themselves as "crisis workers," even though a high percentage of people in precrisis or acute crisis states are *first* seen by physicians and advanced practice nurses—often presenting themselves with requests for psychotropic drugs, symptoms that camouflage psychosocial problems, thoughts of suicide or violence toward others, or serious mental illness.

This edition addresses such real-world scenarios in an era of managed care and its implications for collaboration between frontline health professionals and paraprofessional crisis workers. For decades, these workers have fielded crisis calls from distressed people, including, recently, discharged mental patients—many of whom have little or no community support. Some late-night calls are from people whose primary care providers either were not confident about the basics of crisis care or could not respond to cries for help because of systemic or financial constraints.

2. Assuming crisis care as a *necessary* component of comprehensive health care, updated case examples illustrate the intersection between crisis and chronic problems. The examples underscore the principle that crisis intervention should not be misused as a stopgap cost containment measure to substitute for the longer-term mental health treatment that is required for some but that may be denied in a profit-driven health insurance industry.

3. Information from new research and clinical advances strengthens sections on sudden infant death, child witnesses to violence, workplace violence, and programs for violent men.

4. A revised Comprehensive Mental Health Assessment form (with new validity and reliability studies) is presented, with illustrations in Chapters Three, Four, Six, Eight, and Nine. In addition to its use in mental health settings, this tool—which emphasizes functional assessment rather than psychiatric labeling— is useful in primary care settings as an alternative or complement to the *Diagnostic and Statistical Manual of Mental Disorders* (DSM).

5. Since the earlier editions of *People in Crisis* were published in 1978, 1984, 1989, and 1995, national and global developments have underscored affirmation and strengthening of another of the book's key features: crisis work should be sensitive to the relationships between personal, family, sociocultural, public health, and human rights issues. Some of these issues include national and international initiatives to stem the tide of violence in public and domestic arenas; the continuing escalation of health care costs and the disparity in insurance coverage for mental health services; the disarray and crisis in the U.S. health care financing and governing system that often shortchange patients and exacerbate their stress levels; the continuing epidemics of alienation, suicide, and violence among youth; the persistence of homelessness for millions who are poor, lack community-based health care, or are refugees of political persecution and civil wars; the vulnerability of disadvantaged people to disasters linked with environmental threats, building code violations, and poverty; the widening gap between rich and poor and its impact on crisis vulnerability; health and safety hazards in the natural and work environment; and the continuing HIV-AIDS pandemic, especially in poor countries.

To meet the challenges posed by these developments, this fifth edition presents updated information along with an expanded theory and research foundation and public health perspective, as reflected in current references. The research-based Crisis Paradigm featured in earlier editions continues as this book's conceptual framework, with further clarification of the relationship between violence, victimization, and suicide. Reflecting current concerns, content has been revised or expanded in the following areas:

• Primary care and the interrelationship between violence, victim blaming, depression, and the negative sequelae of victimization, with new material on the role of advanced practice nurses and physicians (Chapters One through Four).

- A broadened global perspective on crisis, particularly in the care of victim-survivors. These additions draw on education and training experience in the United States and Canada, Russia, the Philippines, Portugal, and worldwide networking on this topic.
- Incorporation of the previous editions' chapter on the HIV-AIDS pandemic into Chapter Eleven, "Threats to Health Status and Self-Image." This change aims to highlight the pivotal role of primary care providers in prevention and the psychosocial care of these very vulnerable persons in a paradigm rooted in sociocultural and political context.
- A strengthening of the connection between primary prevention, crisis care, and mainstream psychiatric practice in an era when the interconnections between frontline crisis work and psychiatric treatment are sometimes overlooked or compromised because of the constraints of managed care and a profit-driven health care industry (especially in the United States).

Sources

As in previous editions, the examples are drawn from all major racial, ethnic, and socioeconomic groups in the United States and Canada, so that the variety of people seeking help during crisis can be accurately conveyed. In writing case examples, I have also used my experience and research in urban and rural settings, in this country and abroad, including volunteer work with abused women and people with AIDS. The cases are real but have been disguised to protect the identity of the people concerned.

While drawing on insights from several health and social sciences—among them nursing, psychology, social work, medicine, anthropology, and sociology—I have tried to avoid technical jargon. The book should therefore be understandable to student, professional, and lay readers alike, with additional references provided for those who wish to continue their study of a particular topic.

Organization

The book consists of three parts. Part One presents the basic concepts and strategies necessary to understand, identify, and provide skilled assistance to people in distress or crisis. It lays the foundation for considering major crisis experiences in greater depth in the book's later chapters. Part Two deals with violence, both as an *origin* of crisis (for example, victimization) and as a *response* to crisis (for example, suicide or homicide). Rather than the usual public-private categorization of violence, Chapters Eight and Nine focus respectively on the victim-survivor and the assailant-offender regarding prevention, crisis intervention, and follow-up care. The fearsome presence of violence, not only in U.S. society but throughout the world, necessitates the book's continued attention to topics such as routine assessment for victimization and assault-homicide danger, disasters originating from technological and human factors, and economic disparities between ethnic groups and nations. Part Three discusses those crisis states traditionally defined as situational and transitional, with an emphasis on the theme of passage, cultural context, and the need for "contemporary rites of passage" to assist individuals through these normal life events and the final passage to death.

Final Word

Crisis is intrinsic to life, but crisis intervention is not a panacea for all of life's problems. The Chinese symbol for *crisis* appears throughout this book. The symbol depicts crisis as a two-part character—*danger* and *opportunity*. We can determine for ourselves whether we come through a crisis enriched and stronger or stagnating and hopeless; whether we gain new awareness and coping ability or lose our emotional and physical health and the opportunity to die a peaceful death. It is my hope that this book will make a difference for all those who read it.

Appreciation

For over thirty years, I have worked with people in crisis, studied the dynamics and outcomes of this pivotal life experience, and shared what I have learned with students, colleagues, and others. This book is the result of that special opportunity to grow and learn from the pain and joy of people who live through life's crises. As this fifth edition goes to press, I remember with gratitude all those who have read and provided feedback to earlier editions of *People in Crisis*. These readers include thousands of students from various disciplines, colleagues, and workshop participants. You have affirmed the need to produce this edition and to keep people current with a comprehensive book on life crises.

Very special thanks go to the formal reviewers of this edition's first draft: Patricia Hanrahan, Eleanor Harder, and Karen Melillo. Your careful reading, affirmation, and detailed recommendations for revision were particularly helpful. I also thank Tmira Ring and Barbara Mawn for their recommendations based on use of the fourth edition with students in social work and nursing; Cynthia Medich for assistance with literature review; Jackie Dowling, Terry Lee Harrington, Heidi Kelleher, Elizabeth Moore, Lisa Love, and Sandra Quintal for suggestions and technical assistance with figures and exhibits.

Without affirmation of the earlier editions by faculty from a range of disciplines, in-service trainers, undergraduate and graduate students, and frontline crisis workers in the United States, Canada, and abroad, this fifth edition would never have seen the light of day. I thank you all and hope that this new edition will be helpful to you in your work with distressed people.

I especially thank Andrew Pasternack at Jossey-Bass for his constructive editorial suggestions in developing and launching this fifth edition. Amy Scott kept on top of the delicate dance between author, reviewers, and production manager. I also thank Marcy Marsh and Beverly Miller for their precise and sensitive copy-editing of the manuscript; Carolyn Uno for her constant support and direction and supervision of the production process; and Karen Warner, Alison Wong, and Justine Villanueva for managing the marketing program. Your friendly support, encouragement, and patience were a major boon in completing the work.

Last but not least, I thank my family and friends, who know what happens and what to expect and continue to stand by when another edition of *People in Crisis* takes center stage.

February 2001   Lee Ann Hoff
Boston, Massachusetts

THE AUTHOR

Lee Ann Hoff was born and raised in North Dakota, where she worked as a clinical specialist, teacher, and supervisor in psychiatric–mental health nursing, started one of the first twenty-four-hour crisis services, and pioneered in the community mental health movement of the 1960s. In 1969, she extended this work through a suicidology fellowship at Johns Hopkins University. Acting on her long-standing cross-cultural interests, she obtained a master's degree in social anthropology from the London School of Economics in 1978 and a doctorate from Boston University in 1984, specializing in women's health issues and a sociocultural analysis of violence. During her years as a clinician, teacher, consultant, and administrator, her special achievements include development of the first crisis outreach program and initiation of a program for the national certification of crisis programs. She also spearheaded a program for certifying individual crisis workers and an international consortium offering a graduate certificate in crisis, violence, and gender studies. In recognition of her work, she received the first service award from the American Association of Suicidology and the Honorary Recognition Award from the American Nurses Association.

Drawing on the holistic traditions of nursing and social anthropology, Hoff now focuses on building bridges between institutions, disciplines, and perspectives through her teaching, research, and writing—for example, between theory and practice regarding people at risk, academics and activists, feminist and mainstream analysis, cross-cultural distinctions and commonalities, and individual and social interventions.

Her teaching experience spans undergraduate, graduate, and continuing education programs in nursing, mental health disciplines, police departments, women's studies, and social sciences in U.S., Canadian, and Portuguese universities. She is also a frequent presenter at national and international conferences in women's health, nursing, anthropology, public health, psychiatry, suicidology, and victimology.

Hoff is founding director of the Life Crisis Institute, an international not-for-profit organization based in Boston and Ottawa (www. crisisprograms.com), and is professor at the University of Massachusetts Lowell, College of Health Professions, and adjunct professor at the University of Ottawa, Faculty of Health Sciences. Her current research is on the interface between violence, victimization, and suicide. Her other major publications include *Battered Women as Survivors* (1990), *Creating Excellence in Crisis Care* (with Kazimiera Adamowski, 1998), and *Violence Issues: An Interdisciplinary Curriculum Guide for Health Professionals* (1995).

Balancing her antiviolence and bridge-building efforts, she swims, hikes, enjoys the wonders of New England, Ontario, Quebec, and the Maritimes, and maintains her avid belief in human resilience and generosity through crisis and beyond.

To the memory of those whom we have lost in tragic deaths by murder, terrorism, the ravages of war, and other disasters

To the world's survivors of loved ones who died untimely deaths

To all who offer assistance, comfort, and care to people in crisis

and

To Epi, for his love, support, and affirmation of this book's message

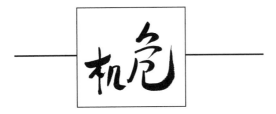

PART ONE

THE UNDERSTANDING AND PRACTICE OF CRISIS INTERVENTION

The concepts and strategies that form the nucleus of crisis theory and practice are fundamental to understanding and helping people in crisis. Chapter One sets the concepts in historical context, linking contemporary crisis intervention to the theories and practices that preceded it. A psychosociocultural perspective is highlighted in a Crisis Paradigm that is introduced in Chapter One, is discussed in detail in Chapter Two, and provides the theoretical framework for the entire book. In Chapter Three, the concepts are applied to the process of assessing individuals and familes for crisis risk. Chapter Four focuses on planning and implementing crisis care strategies, and Chapter Five extends the helping process to family, group, and community crisis situations. The concepts and strategies discussed in Part One constitute the foundation for all remaining chapters.

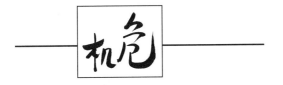

CHAPTER ONE

CRISIS THEORY AND PRACTICE: INTRODUCTION AND OVERVIEW

Deborah, age fifty, is married and the mother of two teenage children. One day at work, she has a heart attack and is taken to the hospital by an ambulance. This is clearly a medical emergency and a source of stress for Deborah and her family. However, a life-threatening event like this may also precipitate an emotional crisis for Deborah and for everyone involved. Chronic stress following Deborah's physical illness could lead to an emotionally troubled family or to the mental breakdown of individual family members, depending on the various psychological, social, and cultural factors involved in the crisis. Whether this hazardous situation results in growth and enrichment for Deborah and her loved ones or in a lower level of functioning for one or all of them depends largely on their problem-solving abilities, cultural values regarding illness and health, and current levels of social and economic support (Brown, 1993).

Deborah, it turns out, is a health care executive who has just received a promotion. She comes from a working-class family. One of her major life ambitions is to achieve professional success while also maintaining a stable family life. Deborah's husband and children are devoted to her, but she feels constant pressure to set an example of strength and to perform to an exacting standard. Being a responsible wife and mother and a successful professional are all-important to Deborah. These facts of Deborah's life and the lives of people like her signify the subjectivity of the crisis experience. This subjectivity contributes to the difficulty of scientific research and theory building about crisis (Antonvosky, 1987; Hoff 1990).

What Is Crisis and Crisis Intervention?

There are meaningful differences and relationships between the key terms *stress, predicament, emergency, crisis,* and *emotional* or *mental disturbance* or *breakdown.*[1] Stress is not crisis; stress is tension, strain, or pressure. Predicament is not crisis either; predicament is a condition or situation that is unpleasant, dangerous, or embarrassing. Emergency is not crisis; emergency is an unforeseen combination of circumstances that calls for immediate action, often with life-or-death implications. Finally, crisis is not emotional or mental illness. Crisis may be defined as a serious occasion or turning point presenting both danger and opportunity.

If Deborah or members of her family become extremely upset as a result of her heart attack and feel emotionally unable to handle the event, they are said to be in crisis. In this book, *crisis,* in clinical context, refers to *an acute emotional upset arising from situational, developmental, or sociocultural sources and resulting in a temporary inability to cope by means of one's usual problem-solving devices.* A crisis does not last long and is self-limiting. *Crisis management* refers to the entire process of working through the crisis to its end point of *crisis resolution,* a process that usually includes activities not only of the individual in crisis but also of various members of the person's natural and institutional social network. It is an integral facet of psychosocial health care. Whether the resolution of a crisis is positive or negative often depends on *crisis intervention,* that aspect of health service carried out by a crisis worker—nurse, social worker, police officer, physician, counselor, or minister. Crisis intervention is a short-term helping process. It focuses on resolution of the immediate problem through the use of personal, social, and environmental resources. Crisis intervention is related to but differs from psychotherapy. *Emergency psychiatry* is a branch of medicine that deals with acute behavioral disturbances related to severe mental or emotional instability. It may overlap with crisis intervention, but it also implies the need for distinct medical intervention such as medication or admission to an inpatient psychiatric service. The paradigm for this helping process and the theory supporting it constitute the *crisis model.* For related definitions, see Hoff & Adamowski (1998, chap. 3).

Predicaments, conflicts, and emergencies such as Deborah's lead to stress that can evolve into a crisis state. But stress is a common denominator in everyone's passage from infancy through childhood to adolescence, adulthood, and old age, and its effects vary. For example, your son finds himself in turmoil during adolescence; your son's friend does not. You face midlife as a normal part of human development; your friend becomes depressed; a neighbor becomes suicidal. Part of the beauty of life, though, is the rebirth of peace following turmoil and pain;

---

[1]The terms emotional or mental *breakdown, disturbance, illness,* and *disorder* are used interchangeably. This usage recognizes that the psychosocial, crisis, and psychiatric assessment processes are not exact science. See Chapter Three for elaboration and discussion of psychiatric labeling.

few escape the lows—and the subsequent highs—of living through stressful events or victimization by violence.

Although stressful events, emotional upsets, and emergency situations are parts of life that have a potential for crisis, a crisis does not necessarily follow a traumatic event. Nor does crisis imply or inevitably lead to emotional or mental breakdown. Something that is a crisis for me may not be for you. As long as we are able to handle stressful life events, we will not experience a crisis. But if stress overwhelms us, and we are unable to find a way out of our predicament, a crisis may result. Crises must be resolved constructively, or emotional or mental illness, addictions, suicide, or violence against others can be the unfortunate outcome. And once emotional breakdown occurs, a person is more vulnerable to other stressful life events, thus beginning an interacting cycle of stress, crisis, and destructive crisis outcomes. Crisis does not occur in isolation but is usually experienced in dynamic interplay with stress and illness in particular cultural contexts, as elaborated in Chapter Two.

Note that the events of our lives do not themselves activate crisis. Crisis occurs when our interpretation of these events, our coping ability, and the limitations of our social resources lead to stress so severe that we cannot find relief. Accordingly, understanding people in crisis and knowing how to help them involves attention not only to the emotional tension experienced but also to the social, cultural, and material factors that influence how people respond to stressful life events.

Key concepts and strategies necessary to understand and effectively assist people in crisis form the core of this text. They can be summarized broadly in the following aspects of crisis theory and practice:

1. The nature of the person in crisis (Chapter One)
2. The crisis experience (Chapter Two)
3. The environment and context of crisis care and resolution (Chapters One and Two)
4. The formal process of crisis care—assessment, planning, implementation, and follow-up (all remaining chapters)

Views and Myths About People in Crisis and How to Help Them

People have been experiencing stress, predicaments, and life crises from the beginning of time. They have also found a variety of ways to resolve predicaments and live through crises. People have always helped others cope with life events as well. Hansell (1976, pp. 15–19) cites the biblical Noah anticipating the great flood as an example of how our ancestors handled crises. Noah was warned of the serious predicament he and his family would be facing shortly. They prepared for the event, and through various clever maneuvers, they avoided being overwhelmed by the floodwaters.

Insights developed through the psychological and social sciences have helped people understand themselves and others in crisis. The advent of a more enlightened view of people in crisis has helped put to rest some old myths about "upset people." It is not so easy anymore to write off as "crazy" and institutionalize people who seem to be behaving strangely in the face of an upsetting event. However, the constraints of managed care in the United States and the continuing bias against those needing psychosocial care and residential psychiatric treatment can result in the social construction of suicidal crisis as a means of obtaining necessary treatment that might otherwise be denied (Hoff & Adamowski, 1998). Modern crisis theory has helped establish a new approach to people with problems.

Views about people in crisis and how to help them vary according to one's value system and the philosophical assumptions guiding practice. But whatever these values and assumptions are, they must be made explicit. People who are involved in crisis intervention—parents, spouses, social workers, nurses, counselors, teachers—can be most helpful if they recognize that everyone has vast potential for growth and that crisis is a point of *opportunity* as well as *danger*, as depicted by the Chinese symbol displayed in this book's chapter openers. For most of us, our healthiest human growth and greatest achievements can often be traced to the trust and hopeful expectations of significant others. Successful crisis intervention involves helping people take advantage of the opportunity and avoid the danger inherent in crisis. Our success in this task may hinge on our values and beliefs about the nature of the person experiencing crisis. In this book, the following values are assumed.

- People in crisis are basically *normal* from the standpoint of diagnosable illness, even though they are in a state of high tension and anxiety. However, the precrisis state for some persons in crisis may be that of emotional or mental disturbance. In these instances, the person can be viewed as ill while simultaneously experiencing a crisis. In some cases, emotional or mental breakdown is the result of a negative resolution of crisis, often because of inadequate social support. So even though crisis is related to emotional or mental disturbance, it is important to distinguish between crisis and diagnosable emotional and mental states—that is, *disorders* in the biomedical paradigm.
- People in crisis are social by nature and live in specific cultural communities by necessity. Their psychological response to hazardous events therefore cannot be properly understood apart from a sociocultural context. Cultural competence by crisis workers does not imply detailed knowledge of another's cultural system. But it does include withholding judgment about behaviors that may appear "strange" and instead inquiring sensitively about the meaning of customs and beliefs that inform one's interpretation of and response to life events.
- People in crisis generally want to and are capable of helping themselves, although this capacity may be impaired to varying degrees. Their need for self-mastery and their capacity for growth from the crisis experience are usually enhanced with timely help from friends, family, neighbors, and sometimes trained crisis workers. Conversely, failure to receive such help when needed can result

in diminished growth and disastrous crisis resolution in the form of addictions, suicide, assault on others, or mental breakdown. The strength of a person's desire for self-determination and growth, along with available help from others, will usually influence the outcome of crisis in a favorable direction.

- The prevention of burnout in human service workers is tied to their recognition of people's basic need for self-determination, even when in crisis. This implies resisting the tendency to rescue or "save" distressed people. Such tactics compromise the possibilities of a healthy crisis outcome. This is because actively fostering self-sufficiency contributes to the sense of control needed for positive crisis resolution. This is true especially when a fear of losing control is a major part of the crisis experience.

- The greatest economy and effectiveness of crisis care in terms of health promotion and the prevention of suffering occurs when practice with individuals is contextualized in a public health and human rights framework (see Farmer, 1999). Crisis intervention is recognized as the third of three revolutionary phases that have occurred since the turn of the century in the mental and public health fields: (1) Freud's discovery of the unconscious, (2) the discovery of psychotropic drugs in the 1950s, and (3) crisis intervention in the 1960s and after.

- Although crisis intervention is not merely a Band-Aid (as it was formerly deemed) or simply a necessary preliminary action trivial in comparison with real treatment carried out by professional psychotherapists, neither is it psychotherapy. The fact that some of the same techniques, such as listening, are used by both psychotherapists and crisis workers does not mean that psychotherapy and crisis intervention are equated, any more than either can be equated with friendship or consultation, which also employ listening. Psychotherapy is a helping process directed toward changing a person's feelings and patterns of thought and behavior. It involves uncovering unconscious conflict and relieving symptoms that cause distress to the person seeking treatment. In contrast, crisis intervention focuses on problem solving around hazardous life events and avoids probing into deep-seated psychological problems.

Growing numbers of counselors, family members, and others regard the stress and crises of human life as normal, as opportunities to advance from one level of maturity to another. Such was the case for the self-actualized individuals studied by Maslow (1970). His study, unique in its time for its focus on normal rather than disturbed people, revealed that people are capable of virtually limitless growth and development. Growth, rather than stagnation and emotional breakdown, occurred for these people in the midst of the pain and turmoil of events such as divorce and physical illness. This optimistic view of people and their problems is becoming a viable alternative to the popular view of life and human suffering in an illness paradigm. Interpreting crisis as illness implies treatment or tranquilization, whereas viewing it as opportunity invites a human, growth-promoting response to people in crisis.

The Evolution of Crisis Theory and Intervention Contexts

In the broadest sense, crisis and crisis intervention are as old as humankind. Helping distressed people is intrinsic to the nurturing side of human character. The capacity for creating a culture of caring and concern for those in emotional or physical pain is implicit in the social nature of humans. In a sense, then, crisis intervention is human action embedded in culture and in the process of learning how to live successfully through stressful life events among one's fellow human beings.

When considered in the context of professional human services, however, crisis intervention is very new—only a few decades old. As an organized body of knowledge and practice, crisis intervention is based on humanistic foundations. However, knowledge and experience from the social and health sciences enhance our ability to help others.

Today crisis intervention is accepted as an integral facet of health and human service delivery systems. In this text, the focus is on the interdisciplinary foundation of contemporary crisis theory and practice and on the distinctive contributions of each area or pioneer in the field, along with critiques of current issues and differences.

Freud and Psychoanalytic Theory

Decades ago, Freud made pioneering contributions to the study of human behavior and the treatment of emotional conflict. He laid the foundation for a view of people as complex beings capable of self-discovery and change. Through extensive case studies, he demonstrated the profound effect that early life experiences can have on later development and happiness. He also found that people can resolve conflicts stemming from traumatic events of childhood and thereby live fuller, happier lives. His conclusions, however, are based largely on the study of disturbed rather than normal individuals. Also, Freud's interpretation of childhood sexual abuse as mere fantasy resulted in an unfortunate legacy: many children and adults still are not believed when they disclose the trauma of abuse. Psychoanalysis, the treatment method developed from Freud's theory, is costly, lengthy, available to few, and generally not applicable to the person in crisis.

Another limitation of Freudian theory is its foundation in biology, resulting in a mechanistic model of personality. Freud's model states that the three-part system of personality—id, ego, and superego—must be kept in balance (*equilibrium*) to avoid unhealthy defense mechanisms and psychopathology. There are widespread objections to the concept of *determinism* inherent in classical psychoanalytic theory (Greenspan, 1983; Rieker & Carmen, 1984; Walsh, 1987). Determinism is based on the idea that our personalities and later life problems are determined by early childhood experiences. However, the concept of equilibrium is commonplace in the literature on crisis (for example, Aguilera, 1997). Besides appearing in the works of Freud, the concept of equilibrium can also be traced to the scientific method in the helping professions and the search for laws (as in the natural sciences) to explain human behavior.

In spite of the limitations of Freudian theory, certain psychoanalytic techniques, such as listening and *catharsis* (the expression of feelings about a traumatic event), are useful in human helping processes, including crisis intervention and brief psychotherapy (Friedman & Fanger, 1991; Littrell, 1998).

Ego Psychology

Awareness of the static nature of Freudian theory led to the development of new, less deterministic views of human beings. In the last several decades, ego psychologists such as Fromm (1941), Maslow (1970), and Erikson (1963) did much to lay the philosophical base for crisis theory. They stressed the person's ability to learn and grow throughout life, a developmental concept used throughout this book. Their views about people and human problems are based on the study of normal rather than disturbed individuals. Erikson, however, has come under critical scrutiny because his theory supports patriarchal family structures (Buss 1979, pp. 326–329; Panchuck, 1994). These traditional family structures produce increased stress for women, partly because they require women to bear disproportionately the burden of caretaking roles throughout their lives—a pattern that is changing but nevertheless dominant.

Military Psychiatry

During World War II and the Korean War, members of the military who felt distressed were treated at the front lines whenever possible rather than being sent back home to psychiatric hospitals. Studies reveal that the majority of these men were able to return to combat duty rapidly as a result of receiving immediate help, that is, crisis intervention, individually or in a group (Glass, 1957).

This approach to psychiatric practice in the military assumed that active combat was the normal place for a soldier and that the soldier would return to duty in spite of temporary problems. So even though military psychiatrists used crisis intervention primarily to expedite institutional goals, they made a useful discovery for the crisis field as a whole.

Preventive Psychiatry and Public Health

In 1942, a terrible fire raged through the Cocoanut Grove Melody Lounge in Boston, killing 492 people. Lindemann's classic study (1944) of bereavement following this disaster defined the grieving process that people went through after the sudden death of a relative. Lindemann found that the survivors of this disaster who developed serious psychopathologies had failed to go through the normal process of grieving. His findings can be applied in working with anyone suffering a serious loss. Because loss is a common theme in the crisis experience, Lindemann's work constitutes one of the most important foundations of contemporary crisis theory.

Unfortunately, decades later, many others still lack the assistance and social approval necessary for grief work following loss and instead are offered medication (see in Chapter Four the sections "Psychotropic Drugs: What Place in Crisis Intervention?" and "Loss, Change, and Grief Work"). Grief work consists of the process of mourning one's loss, experiencing the pain of such loss, and eventually accepting the reality of loss and adjusting to life without the loved person or object. Encouraging and supporting people to experience the normal process of grieving can prevent negative outcomes of crises due to loss.

Tyhurst (1957), another pioneer in preventive psychiatry, has helped us understand a person's response to community crises such as natural disasters. During the 1940s and 1950s, Tyhurst studied transition states such as migration, parenthood, and retirement. His work examined many crisis states that occur as a result of social mobility or cultural change.

Among all the pioneers in the preventive psychiatry field, perhaps none is more outstanding or more frequently quoted than Gerald Caplan. In 1964, he developed a conceptual framework for understanding crisis, including especially the process of crisis development (discussed in detail in Chapter Two). Caplan also emphasized a communitywide—that is, public health—approach to crisis intervention. Public education programs and consultation with various caretakers, such as teachers, police officers, and public health nurses, were cited as important ways to prevent destructive outcomes of crises. In his classic work *Principles of Preventive Psychiatry* (1964), Caplan's focus on prevention, mastery, and the importance of social, cultural, and material "supplies" to avoid crisis seems highly suitable to explaining the development and resolution of crisis. This public health framework resonates with a current emphasis on human rights and with the intrinsic connections between health and economic and political developments and social justice (Rodriguez-Garcia & Akhter, 2000).

Caplan's contribution to the development of crisis theory and practice is so basic that virtually all writers in the field rely on or adapt his major concepts (for example, Aguilera, 1997; Golan, 1978; Hansell, 1976). However, because of the centrality of Caplan's work in the entire crisis field, as well as the controversy surrounding his work and its disease-focused model (for instance, Brandt & Gardner, 2000; Danish, Smyer, & Nowak, 1980; Hoff, 1990; Taplin, 1971), a brief examination of his work is in order.

Caplan's conceptual framework can be questioned for its reliance on disease rather than on health concepts. This limitation is offset, however, by his emphasis on prevention rather than treatment of disease. In developing crisis theory from the foundations laid by Caplan, the useful concepts of his theory should not be rejected. Let us consider what should probably be preserved and what should be questioned. This critique lays the foundation for the next chapter, which relies heavily on Caplan in explaining the phases of crisis development, and will be supported by analysis and case examples throughout the text.

Caplan grounds his work in the mechanistic concepts set forth by Freud and in one of the most popular theories in the social and health sciences—general systems theory. The concepts of *homeostasis* and *equilibrium* are central to general systems theory. They are more suited to explaining physical disease processes than emotional crisis, yet they are pivotal in much of crisis theory. Systems authority Ludwig von Bertalanffy (1968), a biologist, cites several limitations to the systems concept of homeostasis as applied in psychology and psychiatry. For example, homeostasis does not apply to processes of growth, development, creation, and the like (p. 210). Bertalanffy also describes general systems theory as a "preeminently mathematical field" (p. vii). This mathematical base of systems theory as applied to the crisis field is illustrated by the modified square root symbol ($\checkmark$ $\curlyvee$ $\curlyvee$): the downward stroke represents the loss of functioning during crisis, and the varying positions of the horizontal line symbolize the return to higher, the same, or lower levels of equilibrium following a crisis (Jacobson, 1980, p. 8).

This interpretation of the crisis experience implies that people in crisis are unable to take charge of their lives. People who accept this view of themselves when in crisis will be less likely to participate actively in the crisis resolution process and will thereby diminish their potential for growth. General systems theory also highlights the concept of equilibrium as a static notion. This idea comes from consensus theory in the social sciences, which states that people in disequilibrium are out of kilter in respect to both their personality and the social system; they are unbalanced rather than in the ideal state of equilibrium. When a system is in equilibrium, people and behavior fit according to established norms (*consensus*). Parsons's (1951) definition of the "sick role" as a state of "deviance" is one of the most classic and controversial examples of consensus theory (Levine & Kozloff, 1978). Systems theory appeals to our desire and need for precision and a sense of order in our lives. However, the reality of our lives and the world at large suggests that dynamic, interactional theories correspond more closely to the way people actually feel, think, behave, and make sense of the crises they experience. The concept of *chaos* (Ramsay, 1997; Vicenzi, White, & Begun, 1997), also grounded in mathematics and physical science, recognizes the complexity of the human condition. Its notion of sensitive dependence on initial conditions resonates with the concept of subjectivity and the need for reassessment during the chaos of the crisis experience.

Another major criticism of the concept of equilibrium in crisis theory is that it is reductionist. It attempts to explain a complex human phenomenon in the framework of a single discipline, psychology, whereas the explanation of human behavior demands more than psychological concepts. Existential philosophy, learning, and other humanistic frameworks are ignored by this deterministic notion borrowed from mathematics, engineering, and the natural sciences (Taplin, 1971; see also McKinlay & Marceau, 1999; Weed, 1998). For example, how can the concept of equilibrium explain the different responses of people to the crises encountered in concentration camps and atomic bomb blasts or dislocation from wars of "ethnic cleansing"? Or after the death of a child, a parent's equilibrium may still waver at the thought of the tragic loss, yet the parent may have resolved this crisis within a religious framework.

Still another problem with the concept of equilibrium in crisis theory is its implications for practice, for example, in attempts to help abused women in crisis (Bograd, 1984). A systems approach here implies the importance of keeping the family intact in spite of abuse and often with heavy reliance on psychotropic drugs. Chemical restoration of homeostasis with these drugs is common. Other rationales might explain the pervasive use of medication in crisis situations, yet attention to the theory underlying this practice might reduce this prevalent but misguided approach to upset people. Chemical tranquilization practiced without humanistic crisis intervention is related to *iatrogenesis*—that is, illness induced by physicians and other health providers (McKinlay, 1990). Indeed, general systems theory supports the notion that within the complementary health delivery and economic systems, budgets can be balanced and higher profits secured if a sufficient number of drugs (in addition to other technological devices) are sold, regardless of clinical contraindications for their use. Other frameworks, such as conflict and change theory, are needed to support the awareness and social action necessary to address some of these damaging practices in agencies serving distressed people.

In summary, since human beings are more than their bodies, one might ask, Why rely so heavily on natural science models when philosophy, the humanities, and political science are also available to help explain human behavior?

Community Mental Health

Caplan's concepts about crisis emerged during the same period in which the community mental health movement was born. An important influence on crisis intervention during this era was the 1961 report of the Congressional Joint Commission on Mental Illness and Health in the United States. This book, *Action for Mental Health*, laid the foundation for the community mental health movement in the United States. It documented through five years of study the crucial fact that people were not getting the help they needed, when they needed it, and where they needed it—close to their natural social setting. The report revealed that (1) people in crisis were tired of waiting lists, (2) professionals were tired of lengthy and expensive therapy that often did not help, (3) large numbers of people (42 percent) went initially to a physician or to clergy for any problem, (4) long years of training were not necessary to learn how to help distressed people, and (5) volunteers and community caretakers (for example, police officers, teachers, and ministers) were a large untapped source for helping people in distress.

One of the many recommendations in this report was that every community should have a local emergency mental health program. In 1963 and 1965, legislation made federal funds available to provide comprehensive mental health services through community mental health centers. Hansell (1976) refined many of the findings of Caplan, Tyhurst, military psychiatry, and community mental health studies into an entire system of response to the distressed person. His work is especially important to crisis workers in community mental health agencies and primary care settings, where many people in high-risk groups go for help. However, some communities still do not have comprehensive crisis programs (Hoff & Adamowski, 1998). Even among those that do, emergency and other services are often far from ideal. Political and fiscal policies in recent decades resulted in further departures from community mental health ideals worldwide (Hoff, 1993; Marks & Scott, 1990). Reform movements in Canada, Italy, and the United States have attempted to reverse this trend (Mosher & Burti, 1994; Rachlis & Kushner, 1994; Scheper-Hughes & Lovell, 1986).

Primary Health Care

Since the Alma Ata Declaration by the World Health Organization (WHO) in 1978, international and national agencies, both public and private, have committed themselves to the concept of primary health care as fundamental to the health status of citizens (U.S. Department of Health and Human Services, 2000; Kaseje & Sempebwa, 1989). WHO's original declaration focuses on immunization, sanitation, nutrition, and maternal and child health, as well as on the economic, occupational, and educational underpinnings of health status. But health planners and policymakers are increasingly recognizing that mental health status is tied to socioeconomic and other macro factors affecting individuals in various population groups. One of the most serious implications of this interrelationship is the socioeconomic and cultural context in which violence is used as a response to individual and interpersonal stressors (Hoff, 2000). Fiscal constraints worldwide have forced even greater attention to the centrality of primary health care in various health reform efforts (Fiedler & Wight, 1990; Hoff, 1993). However, despite savings in cost and human pain, crisis intervention as part of primary care is still not fully recognized for its contribution to preventing illness and maintaining health (Paykel, 1990). In the United States, this can be traced in part to several historical themes: (1) the mind-body split in health practice (Edmands, Hoff, Kaylor, Mower, & Sorrell, 1999), (2) an individual versus population-based focus in health service delivery (Fee & Brown, 2000), and (3) a continuing bias against and disparity in health insurance coverage for those with mental or emotional illness (Ustun, 1999).

Crisis Care and Psychiatric Stabilization

Similar to the growing emphasis on primary health care is the integration of crisis approaches on behalf of those suffering from acute psychotic episodes. Typically, such persons are seen in the crisis unit of community mental health centers or in the emergency service of general hospitals, where the emphasis is on triage and rapid disposition. Psychopharmacologic agents are often used to stabilize distressed people. The strong medical orientation in such units warrants greater caution than usual by providers to ensure that crisis intervention techniques are not supplanted rather than supplemented by chemical stabilization of acutely upset persons. When these units are not tightly integrated with other services, staff burnout and rapid turnover are two of the costly results. Ideally, all mental health staff should be trained in crisis intervention. In that way, coverage of the crisis service is rotated and greater continuity of care ensured (see Hoff & Adamowski, 1998, for details).

Crisis Care and Chronic Problems

People with chronic problems (medical and psychiatric) are more vulnerable to crisis episodes in general, and their vulnerability is exacerbated by fiscal and other policies that have left thousands of seriously disturbed people without the mental health services they need after years of institutionalization (Hoff, 1993; Johnson, 1990; Perese, 1997). One result of these actions is that community-based crisis hotlines may serve by default as the routine support service to seriously disturbed people whose care is not always well coordinated among an array of agencies and providers. Another result is the expectation that primary care health providers offer the support and continued treatment needed by these individuals, whose mental status exacerbates their often precarious medical status. Routine training in crisis and psychosocial care for those serving this vulnerable population would prevent (1) a misuse of hotlines, (2) excessive prescription of psychotropic drugs by those without specialized psychiatric training, and (3) frequent readmissions to costly psychiatric services (Marks, 1985; Oakley & Potter, 1997).

Suicide Prevention and Other Specialized Crisis Services

Another influence to be noted is the suicide prevention movement. McGee (1974) has documented in detail the work of the Los Angeles Suicide Prevention Center and other groups in launching the suicide prevention and crisis intervention movement in the United States. The Los Angeles Suicide Prevention Center was born out of the efforts of Norman Farberow and Edwin Shneidman. In the late 1950s, these two psychologists led the movement by studying suicide notes. Through their many projects and those of numerous colleagues, suicide prevention and crisis centers were established throughout North America and Western Europe. The Samaritans, founded in 1953 in London by Chad Varah, is the most widespread and visible suicide prevention group, with 182 branches in the United Kingdom and 117 branches of Befrienders International now established in twenty-six countries. Another international group, Lifeline Contact Teleministry (now Contact USA), was founded in 1963 in Sydney, Australia.

The suicide prevention and crisis movement emerged in the United States during the decade when professional mental health workers had a mandate (Congressional Joint Commission on Mental Illness and Health, 1961) and massive federal funding to provide emergency services along with other mental health care. Remarkably, however, most crisis centers were staffed by volunteers and often were started by volunteer citizen groups, such as mental health or ministerial associations. Despite political and other controversy, today there is closer collaboration between volunteer and professionally staffed mental health agencies (Levine, 1981). Some crisis centers in the United States have shut down because of insufficient funds or inadequate leadership, and others have merged with community mental health programs. Still others have adapted and expanded their services or have begun new programs to meet the special needs of rape victims, abused children, runaway youths, battered women, or people with HIV-AIDS.

Currently, suicide prevention and crisis services exist in a variety of organizational frameworks. For example, many shelters for battered women that offer twenty-four-hour telephone response and physical refuge avoid traditional hierarchies in favor of a collective structure. Regardless of the models used, however, every community should have a comprehensive crisis program, including services for suicide emergencies, discharged mental patients, and victims of violence (Hoff & Adamowski, 1998).

The increasing recognition of the need for comprehensive crisis services has resulted in some relief from the dichotomy in practice between traditional psychiatric emergency care and grassroots suicide prevention, along with other specialized crisis services. The separation and territorial conflicts between these two aspects of crisis service are at best artificial and at worst a disservice to people experiencing life crises or psychiatric emergencies, the boundaries of which often overlap. For example, if an abused woman in a refuge run by volunteers becomes suicidal or psychotic, staff members without crisis intervention training usually must call on psychiatric professionals for assistance. Conversely, a health or mental health professional treating a battered woman in a hospital emergency facility may compound the problem by exhibiting victim-blaming attitudes and practices.

Greater collaboration between psychiatric and indigenous specialized crisis services is needed as survivors of abuse and increasing numbers of crisis-prone patients discharged from mental institutions seek assistance from twenty-four-hour community crisis programs.

Sociological Influences

Discussion of the evolution of crisis theory and practice thus far suggests that the momentum has come largely from psychological, psychiatric, or community sources. It is true that the strongest influences on crisis theory and practice have stressed individual rather than social aspects of crisis. Nevertheless the relative neglect of social factors in crisis theory does not reflect their unimportance but rather represents a serious omission. Caplan (1964, pp. 31–34) refers to the psychological, social, cultural, and material supplies necessary to maintain equilibrium and avoid crisis. Yet in practice, while acknowledging the place of social support in the crisis development and resolution process, most writers focus on reducing psychological tension and returning to precrisis equilibrium, without emphasizing how social factors influence these processes (see Chapter Five). Among earlier writers, psychiatrist Hansell (1976) has done the most to stress social influences on the development of crisis and its positive resolution, with particular application to the seriously and persistently mentally ill. His social-psychological approach to crisis theory and practice is explained further in Chapters Two and Three, in concert with cross-cultural influences in the field.

Cross-Cultural and Diversity Influences

Political, social, and technological developments have contributed to more permeable national boundaries and at the same time have sharpened cultural awareness, unique ethnic identities, and sensitivity to diversity issues. For instance, international relations are becoming more critical; refugees from war-torn countries are received in countries where the hosts may not know the refugees' language, and familiar supports are often minimal at best; cross-continental travel and communication are more accessible; gay, lesbian, bisexual, and transgendered activists have made visible the toll of discrimination on suicide rates among youth in this group. These observations have implications for cross-cultural and diversity issues in the experience of crisis, as well as the variance in response to distressed people. The rich data on rites of passage marking human transition states in traditional societies are another significant contribution of cultural and social anthropology to the understanding of life crises. These insights from other cultures are particularly relevant to crises around transition states, as discussed in Chapter Thirteen. In North American society, distinct contributions to crisis theory from First Nations people, from immigrant ethnic groups, and from women have illuminated the significance of crises arising out of the social structure, associated values, and various discriminatory practices (see Chapter Two).

Feminist and Victimology Influences

Women increasingly reject theories and practices that damage them outright or prevent their human growth and development (Boston Women's Health Book Collective, 1998; Mirkin, 1994). The influence of feminism on crisis theory has increased considerably, along with the growing literature on violence, as women and children are the primary objects of abuse worldwide (Hoff, 2000; Mawby & Walklate, 1994). In particular, feminist and complementary critical analysis reveals dramatically the intersection of violence, victimization, crisis, and suicide. Thus, although cross-cultural, ethnic, and feminist experiences are the newest in the historical development of contemporary crisis theory and practice, in a real sense they are also the oldest influences, as suggested earlier by the origins of crisis intervention. We thus come full circle in this historical review.

Life Crises: A Psychosociocultural Perspective

Our review of the diverse sources of crisis theory and practice suggests that understanding and helping people in crisis is a complex, interdisciplinary endeavor. Because human beings encompass physical, emotional, social, and spiritual functions, no one theory is adequate to explain the crisis experience, its origins, or the most effective approach to helping people in crisis.

Accordingly, this book draws on insights, concepts, and strategies from psychology, nursing, sociology, psychiatry, anthropology, philosophy, political science, and critical analysis to propose a dynamic theory and practice that emphasizes the following:[2]

- Individual, social, cultural, and material origins of crisis
- Development of the psychological crisis state
- Emotional, behavioral, and cognitive manifestations of crisis
- Interactive relationships between stress, crisis, and illness (physical and mental)
- Issues involved and skills needed to deal with suicidal crises, violence against others, disaster, and transition states
- Resolution of crises by use of psychological, social, material, and cultural resources
- Collaboration between the person or family in crisis and various significant others in the positive resolution of crisis
- The global social-political task of reducing the crisis vulnerability of various disadvantaged groups through social change strategies and advocacy for health in a public health and human rights framework

These elements of crisis theory and practice are illustrated relationally in the Crisis Paradigm (Figure 1.1) as a preview of Chapter Two. The Crisis Paradigm depicts (1) the *crisis process* experienced by the distressed person from origin through resolution and (2) the place of natural and formal crisis intervention in promoting growth and avoiding negative crisis outcomes. This paradigm draws on research and clinical experience with survivors of violence (Hoff, 1990), other life event literature (for example, Antonovsky, 1980; Cloward & Piven, 1979; Gerhardt, 1979), and work with survivors of man-made disasters. The inclusion of sociocultural origins of crisis extends the traditional focus of crisis intervention on situational and developmental life events, a framework found inadequate to guide practice with people intentionally injured through violence, prejudice, or neglect.

The paradigm suggests a tandem approach to crisis care—that is, attending to the immediate problem while not losing sight of the social change and public health strategies needed to address the complex sociocultural origins of certain crisis situations. This psychosociocultural perspective serves as the framework for examining life crisis situations throughout this book. Concepts in the paradigm that are shaded in other chapters depict a particular focus in the crisis care process.

Crisis Care: Intersection with Other Therapeutic Models

Approaches to crisis intervention used by helpers will vary according to their exposure to historical influences, their values, and their professional preparation in various disciplines.

---

[2] The late Sol Levine, a medical sociologist, referred to this approach as "creative integrationism," not to be confused with superficial eclecticism (personal communication, 1983).

FIGURE 1.1.   CRISIS PARADIGM.

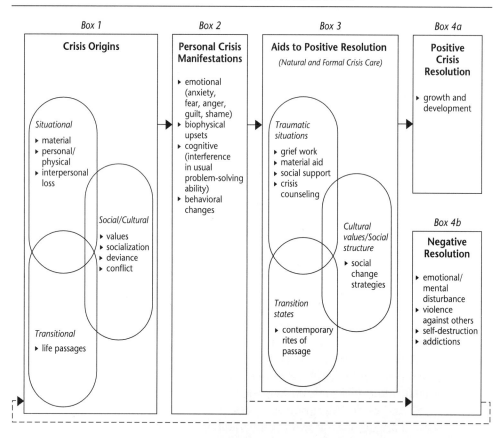

Crisis origins, manifestations, and outcomes and the respective functions of crisis care have an interactional relationship. The intertwined circles represent the distinct yet interrelated origins of crisis and aids to positive resolution, even though personal manifestations are often similar. The arrows pointing from origins to positive resolution illustrate the *opportunity for growth and development* through crisis. The broken line at bottom depicts the potential *danger of crisis* in the absence of appropriate aids. The loop between Box 4b and Box 1 denotes the *vulnerability* to future crisis episodes following negative resolution.

Differentiating Approaches to Helping People in Distress

Our approaches will vary in our effort to assist people who are acutely upset or emotionally disturbed. The following discussion illustrates the differences, overlap, and similarities among these approaches and suggests the relationship between crisis intervention and other ways of helping distressed people.

Certainly, crisis intervention should not be regarded as a panacea for all social, emotional, and mental problems. It is not synonymous with psychotherapy, even though some techniques, such as listening and catharsis, are used in both. Nor is crisis intervention intended only for poor people, reserving psychotherapy for the financially secure. The occurrence of crisis does not depend on a person's socioeconomic status, and crisis intervention can be helpful regardless of that status.

It may be just as damaging to use a crisis intervention approach when it is inapplicable as *not* to use the approach when it does apply. For example, when suicide and crisis hotlines are not linked with other mental health services, there can be negative side effects, sometimes referred to as "systems problems" (Hoff & Adamowski, 1998). Callers seeking help from crisis centers know that they must at least act as though they are in crisis in order to get attention and help. Thus, some callers may appear to be in crisis when they are not. For example, a person who is crying may or may not be in crisis. Judgment of crisis should be based on assessment of the person's total situation.

If workers are unskilled in crisis assessment, they may unwittingly encourage crisis-like behavior by discounting what distressed people say—much as the little boy crying wolf in the fable was discounted because he had cried wolf so many times when there was no wolf that no one believed him when there was. In other words, if workers assume that a person is exaggerating or pretending—crying wolf—and therefore fail to accurately assess the situation through questioning, they could miss the real and urgent message the person is trying to convey. Suicide or other-directed violence may be the unfortunate outcome.

Table 1.1 illustrates the range of services and differences among various services available to people with psychosocial problems or psychiatric illness. Crisis intervention is just one of the many services people need. Effective crisis intervention can be an important link to a person's acceptance of a referral for psychotherapy. This is because during crisis people are more likely than at other times to consider getting help for chronic problems that made them crisis prone in the first place. Crisis intervention is also a significant means of avoiding last-resort measures such as institutional care. Crisis approaches, although necessary, are usually insufficient for people with serious mental and social disabilities. Such individuals need long-term rehabilitation programs as well, including, for example, training for jobs, instruction in home management, and support in transitional facilities such as the Fountain House model (Cella, Besancon, & Zipple, 1997; Johnson, 1990; Leff, 1990).

The limitations of crisis intervention and the need to see it in a larger sociocultural and political perspective are dramatically illustrated in the following vignette. McKinlay (1990, p. 502) discusses the "manufacture of illness" and the futility of tinkering with "downstream" versus "upstream" endeavors:

> My friend, Irving Zola, relates the story of a physician trying to explain
> the dilemmas of the modern practice of medicine: "You know," he said,
> "sometimes it feels like this. There I am standing by the shore of a swiftly
> flowing river and I hear the cry of a drowning man. So, I jump into the
> river, put my arms around him, pull him to shore and apply artificial
> respiration. Just when he begins to breathe, another cry for help. So back in
> the river again, reaching, pulling, applying, breathing and then another yell.
> Again and again, without end, goes the sequence. You know, I am so busy
> jumping in, pulling them to shore, applying artificial respiration, that I have
> no time to see who the hell is upstream pushing them all in."

TABLE 1.1.   COMPARISON OF THERAPIES AND THE CRISIS INTERVENTION MODEL.

Psychotherapy	Medical-Institutional Therapy	Social-Service Rehabilitation Therapy	Crisis Intervention
Type of People Served			
Those who wish to correct neurotic personality or behavior patterns	People with serious mental or emotional breakdowns	Those who are chronically disabled	Individuals and families in crisis or precrisis states
Service Goals			
Work through unconscious conflicts	Manage, adjust, stabilize	Rehabilitation; return to normal functioning in society insofar as possible	Promote growth
Reconstruct behavior and personality patterns	Recover from acute disturbance		Promote personal and social integration
Grow personally and socially			
Service Methods			
Introspection	Medication	Work training	Social and environmental manipulation
Catharsis	Behavior modification	Resocialization	Focus on feelings and problem solving
Interpretation	Electric shock	Training in activities of daily living	Possible use of medication to promote goals
Free association	Group activities	Peer and counselor support and advocacy	Decision counseling
(Use of additional techniques depends on philosophy and training of therapist.)	(Use of additional techniques depends on philosophy of institution.)		
Activity of Workers			
Exploratory	Direct, noninvolved or indirect	Structured but less so than in crisis intervention	Active/direct (depends on functional level of client)
Nondirective			
Interpretive			

TABLE 1.1.   COMPARISON OF THERAPIES AND THE CRISIS INTERVENTION MODEL. (*continued*)

Psychotherapy	Medical-Institutional Therapy	Social-Service Rehabilitation Therapy	Crisis Intervention
Length of Service			
Usually long-term	Short or long (depends on degree of disability and approach of psychiatrist) High repeat rate	Long-term—a few months to 2–3 years	Short—usually 6 sessions or less
Beliefs About People			
Individualistic or social (depends on philosophy of therapist)	Individualistic—social aspect secondary Institutional needs and order may overshadow the needs of people	Hopeful—people can change Mental disability or a diagnosis should not spell hopelessness	Social—people are capable of growth and self-mastery
Attitudes Toward Service			
Emphasis on wisdom of therapist and 50-minute hour	Scheduled	Willingness to stick with it and observe only slow change	Flexible, any hour
Flexibility varies with individual therapist	Staff attitudes may become rigid and institutionalized	Hopefulness and expectation of goal achievement	

This story underscores the need for crisis practitioners to take the time to see their work in a broader public health perspective, not only for the sake of people in crisis but also to prevent burnout and a loss of meaning in their work. Within the array of services available to distressed people, the different helping modes obviously overlap (see Table 1.1). But charts and models are intended to clarify points in theoretical discussion rather than represent an exact picture of reality. Also, although the Crisis Paradigm presented in this book is strongly linked to public and community services, the intervention strategies outlined can be applied using telephone, face-to-face, and outreach modes in various settings: homes in different cultural milieus, primary care clinics, hospitals, and social agencies. In spite of hazy boundaries between crisis and other service models, there are fundamental differences between their purposes and assumptions about people needing help. For example, in the biomedical model, intervention consists of treatment directed toward cure or alleviation of symptoms of a person presumed ill or diseased. The focus is on the *individual*, who is generally assumed to harbor the source of difficulty within himself or herself (Barney, 1994). In contrast, the crisis model proposed in this book is embedded in the public health perspective and therefore stresses the following:

- Social, cultural, and environmental factors in addition to personal origins of crisis
- Prevention of destructive crisis outcomes such as suicide or mental breakdown (or if psychopathology was present prior to the crisis, the prevention of further breakdown and chronic pathology)
- Psychosocial growth and development as the ideal outcome of crisis—a possibility greatly enhanced through social support, environmental factors, and other crisis care strategies

Prevention strategies are usually associated conceptually with public health and primary care models. In growth and development theory, the term *enhancement* is used to describe health and development–promoting activities (Danish et al., 1980, pp. 348–359). The theoretical distinction between prevention and enhancement has not been well documented in practice. These concepts are considered together in the next section, on the assumption that crisis intervention is relevant for preventing disease (and other negative outcomes) as well as for enhancing the growth and development of individuals and, by extension, the health status of population groups.

Preventing Crisis and Promoting Emotional Growth

Viewing crisis as both an opportunity and a danger means that knowing about some upcoming events can allow us to prepare for normal life events and usually prevent the development of crises. For many people, however, these normal events do lead to hazard or danger rather than to opportunity. Although we cannot predict events such as the sudden death of a loved one, the birth of a premature child, or natural disaster, we can anticipate how people will react to them. In his study of survivors of the Cocoanut Grove fire, Lindemann (1944) demonstrated the importance of recognizing crisis responses and preventing negative outcomes of crisis. Once a population or individual is identified as being at risk of crisis, we can use a number of time-honored approaches to prevent crisis and enhance growth.

Primary Prevention and Enhancement. *Primary prevention,* in the form of education, consultation, and crisis intervention, is designed to reduce the occurrence of mental disability and promote growth, development, and crisis resistance in a community. There are several means of doing this:

1. *Eliminate or modify the hazardous situation.* The practice of immunizing children against smallpox and diphtheria, for example, is based on the fact that

failure to immunize can expose large numbers of people to the hazards of disease. Knowledge of sociopsychological hazards should inspire similar efforts to eliminate or modify these hazards. For example, we can alter hospital structures and practices to reduce the risk of crisis for hospitalized children and adults, eliminate substandard housing for crisis-prone older people and others disadvantaged by poverty, and educate people about the nature and effects of these hazards.

2. *Reduce exposure to hazardous situations.* For example, a flood warning allows people to escape disaster. In the psychosocial sphere, crisis prevention includes advising and screening people entering potentially stressful situations such as college, an unusual occupation such as working in a foreign country, or a demanding occupation such as nursing, policing, and fire fighting. With respect to the AIDS pandemic, physical and psychosocial preventive practices must be combined. The current lack of a vaccine for immunization against AIDS underscores the importance of reducing people's exposure to HIV through education and the modification of sexual behavior.

3. *Reduce vulnerability by increasing coping ability.* In the physical health sector, people with certain diseases are directed to obtain extra rest, eat certain foods, and take prescribed medicines. In the psychosocial sphere, older people, the poor, and refugees are most often exposed to the risk of urban or homeland dislocation. Extra physical resources, social services, and social action skills can counter the negative social and emotional effects of hazardous situations like ethnic conflict in a housing complex. New parents will feel less vulnerable and less prone to abuse or neglect if they are prepared for the challenge of rearing their first child or one with special needs. Marriage, retirement, or geographical relocation are other important life transitions that we can prepare for so that they become occasions for continued growth rather than deterioration.

The success of anticipatory preventive measures depends largely on a person's openness to learning, cultural values, previous problem-solving success, and general social supports. Anticipatory prevention is applicable to general target groups known to be at risk (Jacobson, Strickler, & Morley, 1968). It is similar to the developmental notion of using education to assist people at risk to better handle stressful life events.

When hazardous events or a person's vulnerability to events cannot be accurately predicted or when people are unable to respond to generic, anticipatory prevention, participatory techniques are indicated for the person or family in crisis (Caplan 1964, 1974). These involve a thorough psychosocial assessment and counseling of individuals or families by skilled crisis workers, as elaborated in later chapters. In developmental frameworks, the individual and the family participate actively in resolving the crisis. Such active participation assumes the basic human need for self-determination and the importance of providers' avoiding rescue pitfalls. For a further discussion of primary prevention in relation to crisis, see Hoff & Adamowski (1998, chap. 9).

Secondary Prevention. The term *secondary prevention* implies that some form of mental disability has already occurred because of the absence of primary activities or because a person is unable to profit from those activities. The aim of secondary prevention is to shorten the duration of disability, often by providing sustained support and easy access to crisis services. If such services are offered, emotionally and mentally disturbed people may not need psychiatric hospitalization. The disabling effects of institutional life and the increased cost are thereby avoided, as are the destructive results of removal from one's natural community. Because mentally disturbed individuals are more crisis prone than others, they need more active help during crisis than others might. When psychiatric inpatient treatment is necessary, premature discharge on financial grounds is usually counterproductive; it defeats therapeutic goals and sets in motion a vicious cycle of repeat hospital admissions. The thousands of homeless mentally ill persons illustrate this principle.

Tertiary Prevention. The goal of *tertiary prevention* is to reduce long-term disabling effects for those who are recovering from a mental disorder. Social and rehabilitation programs are an important means of helping these people return to former social and occupational roles or learn new ones (Paykel, 1990). Crisis intervention is also important for the same reasons noted in the discussion of secondary prevention. The recovery process includes learning new ways of coping with stress through positive crisis resolution. Thus, even if the precrisis state is one of mental disability, it is never too late to learn new coping devices, as implied in a growth-and-development model.

Crisis Services in a Continuum Perspective

Anticipatory and participatory techniques can be viewed as a continuum of services for people with different kinds of psychosocial problems or mental illness (see Figure 1.2). The continuum suggests that people with problems vary in their dependency on other people and agencies for help. It also illustrates the economic implications of crisis intervention in addition to its clinical and humanistic benefits. However, in the United States, health and human service workers trying to implement community-based crisis approaches in their individual practices are often frustrated by insurance reimbursement policies that underscore persistent bias against those needing mental health care (Sabin, 2000).

The five essential services illustrated in the continuum were originally mandated by the Community Mental Health Acts of 1963 and 1965 in the United States. Later federal guidelines for basic services include rehabilitation, addiction services, victim services, specialized services for the elderly and children, and evaluation programs, although policy decisions have curtailed many of these programs. Crisis intervention is now considered a key part of these mental health and social services.

Among the crisis intervention approaches and settings encompassed in this continuum, consultation and education come under the general umbrella of primary prevention and enhancement. Twenty-four-hour crisis services can also

FIGURE 1.2.   CONTINUUM OF MENTAL HEALTH SERVICES: COST AND CLIENT INDEPENDENCE.

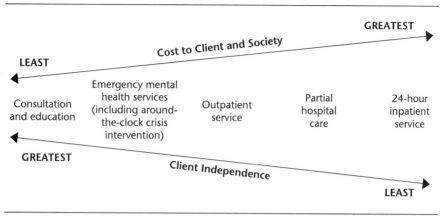

Assisting distressed people in their natural social roles (homemaker, paid worker, student) through consultation, education, and crisis services is the *least* costly means of service and allows the *greatest* client independence; institution-based care is the *most* costly means and allows the *least* client independence.

be seen as primary prevention, depending on the precrisis state of the individual in crisis. Emergency mental health is most closely related to traditional psychiatry and the management of behavioral emergencies in hospital settings (Goldman, 2000; Kravis, Warner, & Jacobs, 1993), which ideally should be linked to crisis and suicide prevention agencies. Outpatient care, partial hospital care, and twenty-four-hour inpatient care (residential) services incorporate crisis intervention while focusing on underlying emotional and mental problems (that is, secondary and tertiary prevention).

To underscore the social and cultural concepts central to the Crisis Paradigm presented here and to affirm current emphasis on community-based crisis intervention, let us consider the economy of crisis intervention in the home and its smooth linkage to other elements of comprehensive service.

For a person already in crisis, admission to a hospital for the purpose of receiving help during the crisis can itself be a hazardous event. Polak (1967) illustrated this fact in his study of 104 men admitted to a psychiatric hospital in Scotland. Polak found that these men or their families had typically requested psychiatric hospital admission following previous unresolved crises around separation, physical illness, death, and migration. However, although it offered temporary relief, admission also was frequently the occasion for another crisis because family patterns of interaction were disrupted, and the patient and the family often had disturbing and unrealistic fantasies and expectations about the purpose and meaning of hospitalization. Now, with some premature insurance-driven discharges, other crises are precipitated (Johnson, 1990).

Hansell (1976) notes how inviting a hospital environment seems to a person deprived of normal community supports. Hospitalization can also be misused by families who lack personal and social resources for relating to disturbed members. Hansell suggests that crisis can just as well lead to improved friendships as to "asylum." (See also Scott, 2000.)

Research thus not only supports the hazards of being uprooted from natural social settings but also provides a sober reminder of this social reality: agencies are indeed subcultures of the larger society in which crisis intervention by family members, friends, and neighbors is an everyday occurrence. This does not preclude the need for formal crisis intervention by persons specially trained for this task. Rather, it highlights the fact that the prospects for positive crisis resolution by individuals, families, and peer groups are enhanced and negative complications are reduced when formal crisis care occurs as close as possible to natural settings. These points are illustrated in the following account of a counselor doing crisis work in a home.

CASE EXAMPLE: RAY

Last week, another counselor and I made a home visit to a family that was very upset because the parents thought their twenty-two-year-old son Ray had "flipped out" on drugs. The parents had called with the express purpose of getting their son into psychiatric hospital care, even though he had refused to go before. I had said when they called that we would not automatically put Ray in the hospital but that we would come over to assess the situation and help the entire family through the crisis. We worked out a strategy for telling Ray directly and clearly the reasons for our visit. Ray refused to come to the phone, shouting, "They're the people who will take me to the hospital in an ambulance." When we got there, a family session revealed that Ray was the scapegoat for many other family problems. We worked out a crisis service plan, and Ray started to show some trust in us after about two hours with the whole family. He could see that we didn't just come to whisk him off to a mental hospital. In the end, even Ray's family was relieved that he didn't have to go to the hospital. Before our home visit, they had seen no other way out. They had talked with several therapists before, but no one had ever come to the house or worked with the whole family.

Although psychiatric hospitalization is necessary in some cases, its cost in both human and economic terms may not be avoided if discharge is premature and community and family supports are inadequate. Figure 1.3 illustrates these points and contrasts medical and developmental approaches in an acute situation like that of Ray and his family.

Basic Steps in Crisis Care

Because of the emotional pain of crisis, resolution will occur with or without the assistance of others. Crisis intervention can be carried out in a variety of settings, some natural, some institutional. Regardless of the context or variations in

FIGURE 1.3. NATURAL AND FORMAL CRISIS CARE.

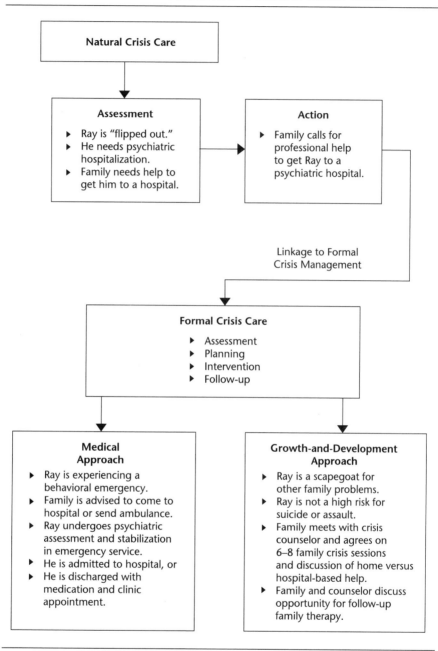

The medical approach is compared with the growth-and-development approach to formal crisis care.

personal style, the probability of positive crisis outcomes is greatly enhanced by attention to the basic steps of crisis care. These steps include the following:

1. Psychosocial assessment of the individual or family crisis, including evaluation of victimization trauma and the risk of suicide or assault on others[3]
2. Development of a plan with the person or family in crisis
3. Implementation of the plan, drawing on personal, social, and material resources
4. Follow-up and evaluation of the crisis intervention process and outcomes

The example of the Jones family illustrates these steps.

CASE EXAMPLE: THE JONES FAMILY

At 11:00 P.M., a police officer calls the twenty-four-hour telephone crisis service. A team of professional crisis workers (a psychiatric nurse with a master's degree and a volunteer with a bachelor's degree in psychology) makes an outreach visit to the home of David Jones, whom the police and the Jones family believe to be acutely suicidal, uncooperative, and in need of assessment for possible involuntary hospitalization. Mr. Jones has refused police and family recommendations for treatment. The outreach team spend one and a half hours interviewing Mr. Jones and his family in their home. Mr. Jones finally agrees to go to the emergency department of a community hospital, where he will be examined by psychiatric liaison staff for possible hospitalization. Following assessment of Mr. Jones and his family situation, he remains overnight in the emergency department holding bed. The following morning, outpatient therapy for Mr. Jones and his family takes place at the community mental health center, where the hospital has an interagency service contract for follow-up of such mental health emergency cases. The family is also given the telephone number of the twenty-four-hour telephone and outreach crisis program where the police had originally called on behalf of the family (adapted from Hoff & Wells, 1989, p. 3.).

Broadly, the steps of crisis care correspond to the problem-solving process used in medical, nursing, and social work practice, as well as in other human service protocols. The Jones case illustrates natural crisis intervention as employed by the family, as well as a formal, structured process. It underscores the fact that everyone recognizes when someone is "crazy," that is, not acting according to commonly accepted social norms. Assessment of this situation revealed the family's inability to handle the crisis alone. They managed the crisis by calling for and cooperating with professional help.

---

[3] Some health professionals may wish to include a diagnosis following this step. See Chapter Three on diagnosis and labeling theory.

A focus on early intervention and prevention of negative outcomes would include providing the average person, through public education programs, with more skills in detecting victimization and suicide or assault potential, as well as in assessing the advantages and limits of psychiatric hospitalization. Professional providers would then be less likely to simply discount what people in crisis say. After all, professional assessments must in the end rely on data presented by the traumatized, suicidal, or disturbed person, the family, police, and other laypersons.

Standards for Crisis Services

The importance of basic principles of crisis care was highlighted in 1976 by the launching of a program in the United States to certify comprehensive crisis services, including community-based agencies and programs in hospitals or community mental health centers. This program was developed and is directed by the American Association of Suicidology (AAS), a standard-setting body for suicide prevention and crisis services. Certification is intended to assure people in crisis that the services provided by a certified crisis program meet at least the minimum standards of service performance and program administration recommended by the AAS. The Ontario Association of Distress Centres has developed comparable standards. In an age when consumers are increasingly conscious of the quality of service they receive, certification is a step in the direction of ensuring such quality. For further information regarding crisis training and service standards, see Hoff & Adamowski, 1998. For information on the certification of individual crisis workers, see the Life Crisis Institute Web site at www.crisisprograms.com.

Summary

The development of crisis theory and practice has sprung from diverse sources in the health field and social sciences. Approaches to crisis intervention vary with the needs of the person in crisis and the training and experience of helpers. Preventing crises, especially the negative outcomes of crises, is central to the approach of this book. Formal crisis care consists of four steps—assessment, planning, intervention, and follow-up—carried out in a psychosociocultural framework. The development of national standards for crisis services and workers attests to the growing maturity of formal crisis intervention as a recognized field grounded in knowledge and practice.

References

Aguilera, D. C. (1997). *Crisis intervention* (8th ed.). St. Louis: Mosby-Year Book.

Antonovsky, A. (1980). *Health, stress, and coping.* San Francisco: Jossey-Bass.

Antonovsky, A. (1987). *Unraveling the mystery of health: How people manage stress and stay well.* San Francisco: Jossey-Bass.

Barney, K. (1994). Limitations of the critique of the medical model. *Journal of Mind and Behavior, 15*(1,2), 19–34.

Bertalanffy, L. von. (1968). *General systems theory* (Rev. ed.). New York: Braziller.

Bograd, M. (1984). Family systems approaches to wife battering: A feminist critique. *American Journal of Orthopsychiatry, 54*(4), 558–568.

Boston Women's Health Book Collective. (1998). *The new our bodies, ourselves for the new century.* New York: Simon & Schuster.

Brandt, A. M., & Gardner, M. (2000). Antagonism and accommodation: Interpreting the relationship between public health and medicine in the United States during the 20th century. *American Journal of Public Health, 90*(5), 707–715.

Brown, G. W. (1993). Life events and affective disorder: Replications and limitations. *Psychosomatic Medicine, 55*(3), 248–259.

Buss, A. R. (1979). Dialectics, history, and development: The historical roots of the individual-society dialectic. *Life-Span Development and Behavior, 2*, 313–333.

Caplan, G. (1964). *Principles of preventive psychiatry.* New York: Basic Books.

Caplan, G. (1974). *Support systems and community mental health.* New York: Behavioral Publications.

Caplan, G. (1981). Mastery of stress: Psycholosocial aspects. *American Journal of Psychiatry, 138*(4), 413–420.

Cella, E. P., Besancon, V., & Zipple, A. M. (1997). Expanding the role of clubhouses: Guidelines for establishing a system of integrated day services. *Psychiatric Rehabilitation Journal, 21*(1), 10–15.

Cloward, R. A., & Piven, F. F. (1979). Hidden protest: The channeling of female innovations and resistance. *Signs: Journal of Women in Culture and Society, 4*, 651–669.

Congressional Joint Commission on Mental Illness and Health. (1961). *Action for mental health.* New York: Basic Books.

Danish, S. J., Smyer, M. A., & Nowak, C. A. (1980). Developmental intervention: Enhancing life-event processes. *Life-Span Development and Behavior, 3*, 339–366.

Edmands, M. S., Hoff, L. A., Kaylor, L., Mower, L., & Sorrell, S. (1999). Bridging gaps between mind, body and spirit: Healing the whole person. *Journal of Psychosocial Nursing, 37*(10), 1–7.

Erikson, E. (1963). *Childhood and society* (2nd ed.). New York: Norton.

Farmer, P. (1999). Pathologies of power: Rethinking health and human rights. *American Journal of Public Health, 89*(10), 1486–1496.

Fee, E., & Brown, T. M. (2000). The past and future of public health practice. *American Journal of Public Health, 90*(5), 690–691.

Fiedler, J. L., & Wight, J. B. (1990). *The medical offset effect and public health policy: Mental health industry in transition.* New York: Praeger.

Friedman, S., & Fanger, M. T. (1991). *Expanding therapeutic possibilities: Getting results in brief psychotherapy.* San Francisco: New Lexington Press.

Fromm, E. (1941). *Escape from freedom.* Austin, TX: Holt, Rinehart and Winston.

Gerhardt, U. (1979). Coping and social action: Theoretical reconstruction of the life-event approach. *Sociology of Health and Illness, 1*, 195–225.

Glass, A. T. (1957). Observations upon the epidemiology of mental illness in troops during warfare. In *Symposium on prevention and social psychiatry.* Washington, DC: Walter Reed Army Institute of Research and the National Research Council.

Golan, N. (1978). *Treatment in crisis situations.* New York: Free Press.

Goldman, H. H. (2000). *Review of general psychiatry* (5th ed.). New York: Lange Medical Books and McGraw-Hill.

Greenspan, M. (1983). *A new approach to women and therapy.* New York: McGraw-Hill.

Hansell, N. (1976). *The person in distress.* New York: Human Sciences Press.

Hoff, L. A. (1990). *Battered women as survivors.* London: Routledge.

Hoff, L. A. (1993). Review essay: Health policy and the plight of the mentally ill. *Psychiatry, 56*(4), 400–419.

Hoff, L. A. (2000). Interpersonal violence. In C. E. Koop, C. E. Pearson, & M. R. Schwarz (Eds.), *Critical issues in global health* (pp. 260–271). San Francisco: Jossey-Bass.

Hoff, L. A., & Adamowski, K. (1998). *Creating excellence in crisis care: A guide to effective training and program designs.* San Francisco: Jossey-Bass.

Hoff, L. A., & Wells, J. O. (Eds.). (1989). *Certification standards manual* (4th ed.). Denver: American Association of Suicidology.

Jacobson, G. F. (1980). Crisis theory. *New directions for mental health services: Crisis intervention in the 1980s, 6,* 1–10.

Jacobson, G. F., Strickler, M., & Morley, W. (1968). Generic and individual approaches to crisis intervention. *American Journal of Public Health, 58,* 338–343.

Johnson, A. B. (1990). *Out of bedlam: The truth about deinstitutionalization.* New York: Basic Books.

Kaseje, D.C.O., & Sempebwa, E.K.N. (1989). An integrated rural health project in Saradidi, Kenya. *Social Science and Medicine, 28*(10), 1063–1071.

Kravis, T. C., Warner, C. G., & Jacobs, L. M. (Eds.). (1993). *Emergency medicine* (3rd ed.). Germantown, MD: Aspen Systems.

Leff, J. (1990). Maintenance (management) of people with long-term psychotic illness. In I. M. Marks & R. Scott (Eds.), *Mental health care delivery: Innovations, impediments and implementation* (pp. 17–40). Cambridge: Cambridge University Press.

Levine, M. (1981). *The history and politics of community mental health.* New York: Oxford University Press.

Levine, S., & Kozloff, M. A. (1978). The sick role: Assessment and overview. *Annual Review of Sociology, 4,* 317–343.

Lindemann, E. (1944). Symptomatology and management of acute grief. *American Journal of Psychiatry, 101,* 101–148. (Reprinted in H. J. Parad (Ed.), *Crisis intervention: Selected readings.* (1965). New York: Family Service Association of America.)

Littrell, J. M. (1998). *Brief counseling in action.* New York: Norton.

Marks, I. (1985). Controlled trial of psychiatric nurse therapists in primary care. *British Medical Journal, 290,* 1181–1184.

Marks, I., & Scott, R. (Eds.). (1990). *Mental health care delivery: Innovations, impediments and implementation.* Cambridge: Cambridge University Press.

Maslow, A. (1970). *Motivation and personality* (2nd ed.). New York: HarperCollins.

Mawby, R. I., & Walklate, S. (1994). *Critical victimology.* Thousand Oaks, CA: Sage.

McGee, R. K. (1974). *Crisis intervention in the community.* Baltimore: University Park Press.

McKinlay, J. B. (1990). A case for refocusing upstream: The political economy of illness. In P. Conrad & R. Kern (Eds.), *The sociology of health and illness: Critical perspectives* (3rd ed., pp. 502–516). New York: St. Martin's Press.

McKinlay, J. B., & Marceau, L. D. (1999). A tale of three tails. *American Journal of Public Health, 89*(3), 295–298.

Mirkin, M. P. (Ed.). (1994). *Women in context: Toward a feminist reconstruction of psychotherapy.* New York: Guilford Press.

Mosher, L. R., & Burti, L. (1994). *Community mental health: A practical guide.* New York: Norton.

Oakley, L. D., & Potter, L. (1997). *Psychiatric primary care.* St. Louis: Mosby-Year Book.

Panchuck, P. (1994). *The midlife experience of contemporary women: Views along the midway.* Unpublished doctoral dissertation, Lesley College, Cambridge, MA.

Parsons, T. (1951). Social structure and the dynamic process: The case of modern medical practice. In *The social system* (pp. 428–479). New York: Free Press.

Paykel, E. (1990). Innovations in mental health care in the primary care system. In I. M. Marks & R. Scott (Eds.), *Mental health care delivery: Innovations, impediments and implementation* (pp. 69–83). Cambridge: Cambridge University Press.

Perese, E. F. (1997). Unmet needs of persons with chronic mental illnesses: Relationship to their adaptation to community living. *Issues in Mental Health Nursing, 18*(1), 19–34.

Polak, P. (1967). The crisis of admission. *Social Psychiatry, 2,* 150–157.

Rachlis, M., & Kushner, C. (1994). *Strong medicine: How to save Canada's health care system.* New York: HarperCollins.

Ramsay, R. (1997). Chaos theory and crisis intervention: Toward a new meaning of equilibrium in understanding and helping people in crisis. *Child and Family, 1*(3), 23–35.

Rieker, P. P., & Carmen, E. H. (Eds.). (1984). *The gender gap in psychotherapy: Social realities and psychological processes.* New York: Plenum.

Rodriguez-Garcia, R., & Akhter, M. N. (2000). Human rights: The foundation of public health practice. *American Journal of Public Health, 90*(5), 693–694.

Sabin, J. E. (2000). Managed care and health care reform: Comedy, tragedy, and lessons. *Psychiatric Services, 51*(11), 1392–1396.

Scheper-Hughes, N., & Lovell, A. M. (1986). Breaking the circuit of social control: Lessons in public psychiatry from Italy and Franco Basaglia. *Social Science and Medicine, 23*(2), 159–178.

Scott, R. L. (2000). Evaluation of a mobile crisis program: Effectiveness, efficiency, and consumer satisfaction. *Psychiatric Services 51*(9), 1153–1156.

Taplin, J. R. (1971). Crisis theory: Critique and reformulation. *Community Mental Health Journal, 7,* 13–23.

Tyhurst, J. S. (1957). The role of transition states—including disasters—in mental illness. In *Symposium on preventive and social psychiatry.* Washington, DC: Walter Reed Army Institute of Research and the National Research Council.

U.S. Department of Health and Human Services. (2000). *Healthy people 2010: Understanding and improving health.* Washington, DC: Author.

Ustun, T. B. (1999). The global burden of mental disorders. *American Journal of Public Health, 89*(9), 1315–1321.

Vicenzi, A. E., White, K. R., & Begun, J. W. (1997). Chaos in nursing: Make it work for you. *American Journal of Nursing, 97*(10), 26–31.

Walsh, M. R. (1987). *The psychology of women: Ongoing debates.* New Haven, CT: Yale University Press.

Weed, D. L. (1998). Beyond black box epidemiology. *American Journal of Public Health, 88*(1), 12–14.

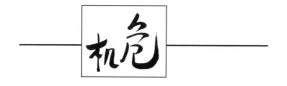

CHAPTER TWO

UNDERSTANDING PEOPLE IN CRISIS

Understanding people in crisis is the foundation for assessment, planning, intervention, and follow-up—steps intrinsic to the crisis care process. A recurring problem in the social sciences is that theories are often formulated without sufficient grounding in reality. Conversely, practitioners frequently do not study the values and theoretical assumptions implicit in research. For example, census figures reveal that mothers are awarded custody of their children in most cases. If fathers are routinely denied custody without examining the comparative parenting abilities of each parent, then a belief in biological determinism (for example, women are naturally better parents) is implied. In another example, the use of psychotropic drugs, predominantly for women in crisis, suggests theoretical assumptions about the nature of crisis and the people receiving the drugs. Also, crisis theories may rely too exclusively on the experience of ill rather than healthy individuals. As Antonovsky (1980, pp. 35–37) suggests, the crucial question may be, Why do people stay healthy? (*salutogenesis*) rather than, What makes them sick? (*pathogenesis*).

Understanding requires an examination of the central concepts of crisis theory. These concepts provide the building blocks for understanding the crisis experience and its resolution. They help answer the following questions about theory-based crisis care:

1. What are the origins of crisis?
2. How are the origins related to prediction, prevention, and resolution of crisis?
3. How is crisis related to stress and illness?
4. How does the crisis state develop, and how is it manifested?
5. How do different people resolve crises?

6. How does the interaction between natural and formal crisis intervention work to produce positive crisis outcomes?

In Chapter One, crisis was broadly linked to stress, emergencies, and emotional and mental disturbance. This chapter shows the interrelationship among human distress situations and addresses key questions about the crisis experience.

The Origins of Crisis

The importance of examining the origins of crisis is based on the assumption that insight into how a problem begins enhances our chances of dealing with it effectively. Here the term *origin* is used in the sense of the root source or beginning of a phenomenon—in this case, crisis. Considerations of origins may or may not include speculation about causes, because such an examination is associated with the so-called hard determinism found in the natural sciences. A search for cause-and-effect laws is questionable in a humanistic framework. This interpretation of origin also suggests that instead of asking what causes crisis, one would examine, for example, how some people respond to stressful events by going into crisis and others do not, or the reasons that some people resolve crisis through problem solving and growth, some by suicide, and others by chronic emotional illness (Vaillant, 1993). The following discussion clarifies the relationships among crisis origins, risk factors, manifestations, and intervention strategies, in terms of origins and development. Broadly speaking, crisis origins fall into three categories: *situational* (traditional term is *unanticipated*), *transitional state* (traditional term is *anticipated*), and *cultural and social-structural*.

Situational Origins

Crises defined as situational originate from three sources: (1) material or environmental (for example, fire or natural disaster), (2) personal or physical (for example, heart attack, diagnosis of fatal illness, loss of limb or other bodily disfigurement from accidents or disease), and (3) interpersonal or social (for example, death of a loved one or divorce (see Figure 2.1, upper circle, Box 1). Such situations are usually unanticipated. Because the traumatic event leading to possible crisis is unforeseen, one generally can do nothing to prepare for it except in an indirect sense: careful driving habits can reduce the risk of accident; changing risky lifestyle practices such as smoking can reduce the risk of heart attack or cancer; open communication may lessen the chance of divorce; a change in sexual behavior can reduce the risk of contracting HIV-AIDS. Crises arising from such situations originate, at least indirectly, from personal life choices. For example, keeping in good physical and psychological health, nurturing a social support system, and avoiding too many changes at one time prepare one indirectly to better handle unforeseen events (Turner & Avison, 1992). In the case of loss of a child

FIGURE 2.1.   CRISIS PARADIGM.

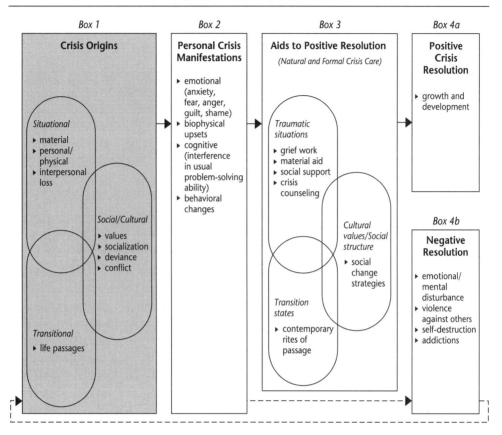

Crisis origins, manifestations, and outcomes and the respective functions of crisis care have an interactional relationship. The intertwined circles represent the distinct yet interrelated origins of crisis and aids to positive resolution, even though personal manifestations are often similar. The arrows pointing from origins to positive resolution illustrate the *opportunity for growth and development* through crisis; the broken line at bottom depicts the potential *danger of crisis* in the absence of appropriate aids. The loop between Box 4b and Box 1 denotes the *vulnerability* to future crisis episodes following negative resolution.

by *sudden infant death syndrome* (SIDS), new research (Hogberg & Bergstrom, 2000) suggests that the medically advised prone (on stomach) sleeping position is often a major factor (see Chapter Thirteen); therefore, if parents inappropriately blame themselves in the crisis response, crisis counseling and grief work will usually result in a positive outcome (unless psychopathology was present before the crisis or the death is mistakenly attributed to parental abuse). At the other end of the spectrum, crises originating from complex sociocultural or interrelated sources, the implications for intervention are also more complex. The stress and possible crisis originating from a natural event, such as being struck and injured by lightning, might be the easiest to handle, depending on the degree and type of physical injury.

Transition State Origins

The next broad category of crisis origins, transition states, consists of two types: (1) *universal*—life-cycle or normal transitions consisting of human development phases from conception to death and (2) *nonuniversal*—passages signaling a shift in social status (see Figure 2.1, lower circle, Box 1). The first type is universal in that no one escapes life passages, at least not the first and last phases. Erikson (1963) and other developmental psychologists have identified human transition states as follows:

- Prenatal to infancy
- Infancy to childhood
- Childhood to puberty and adolescence
- Adolescence to adulthood
- Maturity to middle age
- Middle age to old age
- Old age to death

During each phase, a person is subject to unique stressors. He or she faces the challenge of completing specific developmental tasks. Failure to do so stunts human growth, and one's personality does not mature according to its natural potential. Although growth toward maturity is exciting, people usually experience a higher level of anxiety during developmental transition states than at other times. The natural change in roles, body image, physical and sexual functioning, and attitudes toward oneself and the world may create internal turmoil and restlessness. Successful completion of developmental tasks requires energy as well as nurturance and social approval from others.

With appropriate support, a person is normally able to meet the challenge of growth from one stage of life to another. In this sense, developmental crises are considered normal (Panchuck, 1994) and therefore can be anticipated and prepared for. Developmental transition states need not be nightmarish; they can be rewarding times in which people enjoy a sense of self-mastery and achievement from the successful completion of developmental tasks.

Stress and turmoil can occur during periods of developmental change if the individual does not receive the normal social supports needed for the process of maturation. And each successive stage of development is affected by what took place in the previous phase. For some, the challenge of human growth is indeed a nightmare; life's turning points become crises with destructive effects rather than normal periods of change and challenge. Some people greet adolescence, middle age, and old age with suicide attempts, depression, or withdrawal to a closed, more secure, and familiar world. They approach life with a deep rejection of self and suspicion of the surrounding world.

The unique challenge in life is to move forward, not to stagnate or regress. For some, however, various situational factors make this a seemingly impossible task. Developmental challenges are particularly acute for young people today who are growing up in communities where economic security and other dreams are never borne or are quickly dashed by multiple stressors, violence, and other tragic events.

The second type of transition state, nonuniversal, includes turning points such as the change from student to worker and worker (including homemaker) to student, migration, and retirement. Crises originating from such sources differ from those arising from unanticipated hazardous events. Like the developmental transition states, nonuniversal passages are usually anticipated and can therefore be prepared for. Unlike developmental transitions, however, everyone does not experience them. And some transitions, such as relocation because of refugee status in a war-torn country, are complicated by cultural and economic factors in one's homeland (see Chapter Twelve). The transition states (universal and nonuniversal) from which some crises stem can be seen not only as markers along life's pathway but also as processes that can develop in positive or negative directions (Danish, Smyer, & Nowak, 1980, p. 342; see Chapter Thirteen).

Crises developing from situational and transitional states are the easiest to understand and to handle successfully. The personal values involved in resolving such crises generally do not clash with common interpretations of life's experiences. For example, if one loses precious possessions and is left homeless by a fire caused by arson, one's ability to handle the stress involved is generally assisted by knowledge that there are laws designed to bring the arsonist to justice, and by insurance, which may partially compensate for the material loss. To summarize, crises arising from hazardous situations and from transition states are distinct yet related. An individual in a major transition state is usually vulnerable. When the stress of an unanticipated traumatic event is added, the person is even more likely to experience a crisis because one's usual coping capacity may be strained to the limit by these combined stressors.

To illustrate, let us consider Carol and Jim, who demonstrate a capacity for growth and development around divorce.

CASE EXAMPLE: CAROL AND JIM

Carol, age thirty-eight, and Jim, age thirty-six, decide mutually to obtain a divorce. They have been married thirteen years and have two children—Dean, age twelve, and Cindy, age nine. Together they work out a custody and visiting agreement, satisfying their desires and taking the children's wishes into consideration. Carol and Jim had essentially untroubled childhoods and feel secure and confident as individuals. They can, therefore, avoid the common tactic of using their children as weapons against each other. The divorce is decidedly a source of stress to Dean and Cindy, but neither of the children (although they are not happy about the divorce) experiences it as a crisis. Both parents are mature in their marital and parental roles and do not deny their children the nurturance they continue to need from both parents. The divorce is also not the occasion of a crisis for either spouse. In fact, they both saw their marriage as stagnating their personal growth. Their decision to divorce is not a crisis; rather, as Maslow (1970) shows, it is an occasion for further self-actualization, or growth.

Many divorces, however, are more tumultuous than this couple's, or even tragic. For example, in an abusive marriage, a man may greet the news of divorce with a threat to kill first his wife and then himself (see Chapters Eight and Nine). Such cases, in their contrasting manifestations, illustrate (1) the highly subjective nature of the crisis experience, (2) the various factors that influence the development of a crisis state, and (3) the intrinsic relationship between transitional, situational, and sociocultural influences on the crisis experience.

Cultural and Social-Structural Origins

Crises arising from cultural values and the social structure include job loss stemming from discrimination on the basis of age, race, gender, disability, or sexual identity. In contrast, job loss from illness or poor personal performance can be viewed as a result of a prior crisis or illness. Job loss occurring from discriminatory treatment in the workforce is rooted in cultural values about the diversity issues noted previously—values that are embedded in the social structure. Also in this category are crises resulting from the deviant acts of others, behavior that violates accepted social norms: robbery, rape, incest, marital infidelity, and physical abuse (see Figure 2.1, right circle, Box 1). Crises from these sources are never truly expected; there is something shocking and catastrophic about them. Yet in a sense they are predictable. An older infirm woman living in a high-crime area is more vulnerable to attack than a stronger and younger person. Other examples of crises arising from sociocultural sources include violence against children and women (related to values about discipline, the role of women, and social-structural factors in the family) and residential dislocation (related to economic, class, and ethnic issues, such as *gentrification*—the displacement of the poor by the "gentry" during the "upgrading" of urban centers).

In general, crises originating from sociocultural sources are less amenable to control by individuals than are crises arising from personal action. Thus, a person of a racial minority group facing a housing crisis due to suspected discrimination and a woman in job crisis due to alleged gender discrimination must be prepared to deal with the bureaucratic justice system. To avoid the downward spiral discussed later in this chapter, *social* factors should not be misconstrued as *personal* liabilities producing crises. Consider the challenge of resolving a crisis originating from the following twist in justice: a woman is brutally beaten and threatened with her life; she and her children are left homeless, while the man who has committed the crime enjoys the comfort and security of the marital dwelling. This example of battering also illustrates the interrelationship between crisis origins. That is, an abused woman may suffer physical injury and loss of home (situational events) and be forced into a status change from married to single (transitional), but the *primary* origin of her crisis can be traced to cultural values about women, the socialization of men toward aggression, violation of basic human rights, and diversity regarding communitarian values (Tsukuda, 1999), and a widespread cultural climate approving of violence (for example, war, capital punishment, pornography) (Hoff, 2000b; Mawby & Walklate, 1994). Therefore intervention strategies focused only on the upper and lower circles (see Figure 2.1, Box 3), without attention to social change strategies and public compensation for the woman's injuries, usually will not be sufficient. Interrelated crisis origins are also apparent in the high suicide rates of gay, lesbian, bisexual, or transgendered youth and in people with AIDS, their families, and caretakers.

To illustrate further, note the difference in the element of control in two different crisis situations: (1) A heavy cigarette smoker with full knowledge of the evidence linking smoking to lung cancer receives a diagnosis of lung cancer. More than likely, insurance benefits will be available in spite of this self-chosen high-risk lifestyle. (2) A Japanese-American survivor of the nuclear bomb blast at Hiroshima receives a diagnosis of leukemia. The victim is refused insurance coverage for the required medical care by both private insurers and the U.S. government (WGBH Educational Foundation, 1982, pp. 17–18).

A more complex example of crisis from sociocultural sources involves the perpetrators of deviant acts. Here, social and personal elements are intertwined. For example, the parents of an infant whom they have abused and brought to a hospital for treatment will probably be in crisis, as will a mother who loses custody of her children because of drug abuse. Such child abuse and neglect may be rooted in cultural values about physical discipline, mothers (as opposed to mothers and fathers together) as primary child rearers, and socioeconomic status. Although such deviance may be strongly influenced by social and cultural factors, individual perpetrators of violence against others need to be carefully considered for personal liability.

These illustrations provide a preview of the relationship between origins of crisis and strategies of intervention (to be discussed in detail in later chapters). In short, whenever a crisis originates outside the individual, it is usually beyond the individual alone to control and manage successfully (Baum, Cohen, & Hall, 1993; Cloward & Piven, 1979). In such situations, the person is usually more vulnerable and has greater difficulty making sense of the traumatic event and avoiding negative coping strategies (Herman, 1992; Sales, Baum, and Shore, 1984). Public, social strategies, therefore, need to accompany any individual interventions on behalf of people whose crises originate in the sociocultural milieu.

Interrelationships Between Crisis Origins and Development

Identifying the origins of a crisis, important as it is, is only one step toward effective crisis resolution. Various situational, developmental, and sociocultural factors do not in themselves constitute a crisis state. The factors placing people at risk vary and interact to produce a crisis that is manifested in emotional, cognitive, behavioral, and biophysical responses to traumatic life events (see Figure 2.1, Box 2).

Developmentalists Danish et al. (1980, pp. 342–345) cite several factors that affect how a person responds to life events:

- *Timing.* For example, first marriage at age sixteen or fifty may be more stressful than at other times.

- *Duration.* This refers to the process aspect of life events such as pregnancy or retirement.
- *Sequencing.* For example, the birth of a child before marriage is usually more stressful than after.
- *Cohort specificity.* For example, in a reversal of traditional roles, a man becomes a househusband and a woman a corporate executive.
- *Contextual purity.* This refers to how the event relates to other events and the lives of other people.
- *Probability of occurrence.* For example, the majority of married women will become widows.

The clinical relevance of these factors can be seen in Schulberg and Sheldon's (1968, pp. 553–558) probability formulation for assessing which persons are most crisis prone:

1. *The probability that a disturbing and hazardous event will occur.* Death of close family members is highly probable, whereas natural disasters are very improbable.
2. *The probability that an individual will be exposed to the event.* Every adolescent faces the challenge of adult responsibilities, whereas fewer people face the crisis of an unwanted move from their settled dwelling.
3. *The vulnerability of the individual to the event.* The mature adult can adapt more easily to the stress of moving than can a child in the first year of school or a retired person who has lived a long time in one community.

In assessing risk, then, one should consider (1) the degree of stress stemming from a hazardous event, (2) the risk of a person being exposed to that event, and (3) the person's vulnerability (Perloff, 1983) or ability to adapt to the stress. Our awareness of these risk factors in individuals and groups enhances the success of crisis prevention and health promotion, as discussed in Chapter One.

CASE EXAMPLE: DOROTHY

Dorothy, age thirty-eight, has been treated for depression three times during the past nine years. Before her marriage and the birth of her three children, Dorothy held a job as a secretary and is now employed part-time. Dorothy's husband, a company executive, accepted a job transfer to a new location in another city. This city is known for its hostile attitudes toward African American families like Dorothy's. Dorothy dreaded the move and considered joining her husband a few months later. She thought this might allow her some time to see whether her husband's job placement might be permanent. However, she abandoned the idea because she dreaded being away from her husband for that length of time. One month after the move, Dorothy made a suicide attempt and was taken to a hospital psychiatric unit by her husband.

In this case, the initial probability of the occurrence of the hazardous event, the move, was small. The probability of Dorothy's exposure to the event was high, considering her marital status and her dependence on her husband. Her racial identity made her more vulnerable to stress from sociocultural sources such as housing discrimination. Her vulnerability in view of her past history was also very high. Taken together, these factors made Dorothy a high risk for crisis. Research on vulnerability to life events underscores the emotional cost of caretaking roles for women like Dorothy. Women are more exposed to acute life stressors because of traditional role expectations, including their response to events affecting significant others in their social network, with a consequent increased risk of depression (Conger, Lorenz, Elder, & Simons, 1993; Turner & Avison, 1992). For women like Dorothy, the risk increases if they are faced with a hazardous event such as the death of a husband.

In the Schulberg and Sheldon formulation, the probability factors that contribute to a favorable outcome of crisis include the following:

1. The person who encounters and resolves a great number and variety of difficult situations is less likely to experience a crisis in future hazardous circumstances.
2. The person who has (or thinks he or she has) the ability to resolve a problem is likely to resolve that problem successfully.
3. The person who has strong social supports is very likely to resolve life crises successfully and without destructive effects.

In another example, George Sloan, the subject of an upcoming case example, is affected by the concurrence of crisis with his son's school problem and his wife's menopause. Recalling Deborah and her family, discussed in Chapter One, if they are from a racial minority group, the chance is increased that racially related stress on the job contributed to her heart attack. Risk for future job-related crises is also increased due to her position in the social structure based on race.

The case of a family in crisis as a result of a teenager's suicide attempt also suggests the interactional aspect of crisis origins. Although the teenager's crisis may stem directly from personal feelings of failure and worthlessness and indirectly from family conflict, the family's crisis of dealing with a suicidal member is usually affected by the culturally situated stigma still attached to self-destructive behavior (see Chapter Six).

These illustrations underscore the fact that life events in themselves are not crises. Rather, the examples link the *origins* of crisis to life events, sociocultural factors, and personal values that influence the development and subjective manifestations of crisis in different individuals. This discussion highlights the need to identify specific crisis origins during assessment and to tailor intervention strategies to distinctive or interrelated origins. Appropriate strategies will increase the probability of positive crisis resolution and growth (see Figure 2.1, Box 3). Details of such assessment and intervention strategies are presented in the remainder of the book.

Stress, Crisis, and Illness

Theories and research on stress and coping occupy a prominent position in the literature of psychology, sociology, anthropology, nursing, medicine, and epidemiology (Bebbington et al., 1993; Brown, 1993; Brown & Harris, 1978; Hurwicz, Durham, Boyd-Davis, Gatz, & Bengtson, 1992; Killeen, 1990; Loustaunau & Sobo, 1997; Selye, 1956). The issue of coping with stressful life events often revolves around the relationship between stress and illness; virtually all authorities agree that stress and illness are related. The questions considered in this book are

- Do stressful life events cause illness, and if so, what is the process involved?
- Do sick people experience more stressful life events than the healthy?
- To what extent do social and psychological resources buffer the impact of stressful life events?
- What effect, if any, do "resistance resources" (Antonovsky, 1980) have on stress arising from the social structure—for example, race, class, gender, or age disparity?
- What is the relationship between stress and the concept and experience of crisis?

Imprecise definitions can create problems in answering these questions; sometimes the concepts of stress, crisis, and illness are used interchangeably (see Chapter Three on psychiatric labeling). The following definitions may clarify the discussion:

• *Stress* is described by Selye (1956, p. 15) as a specific syndrome that is non-specifically induced. Stress can also be viewed as a relationship between the person and the environment (McElroy & Townsend, 1985). For this book, stress is defined as the discomfort, pain, or troubled feeling arising from emotional, social, or physical sources and that results in the need to relax, be treated, or otherwise seek relief. Stress can be grouped into two types. *Acute stress* is brief in duration and occurs with fairly predictable manifestations and results, one of which may be crisis. *Insidious stress* is longer in duration (weeks, months, or years), with less awareness by the person experiencing it and with long-range cumulative but less clearly certain effects, which may include burnout and disease (Landy, 1977, p. 311). Stress is inherent in the process of living and may be experienced from any source: invasion of the body by organisms, trauma, internal psychological turmoil, cultural values, and social organization.

• *Burnout* is a fairly recent concept. It includes emotional exhaustion, usually stemming from work-related stressors. It is manifested in physical signs and symptoms; feelings of cynicism, anger, and resentment; and poor social performance at home and at work. Burnout is distinguished from crisis by its chronic rather than acute character. Also, people suffering from burnout often are not aware of the connection between their feelings, their behavior, and the chronic stress they are under.

- *Disease* is a pathological concept describing a condition that can be objectively verified through physical examination, observation, and various laboratory tests. The "diseased" person may or may not be aware of objective organic lesions or behavioral disturbances observable by others.
- *Illness* is related to disease but is distinguished by its subjective character. It is a cultural concept that implies the social recognition that one cannot carry out expected social roles. For instance, a person may have an early cancerous lesion but not feel ill. Once the lesion is diagnosed as cancer, though, the person is considered ill, and the social, psychological, and cultural dimensions of the disease surface: stigma, denial, fear of death. Illness may be claimed subjectively as a reason for inability to perform normally. For example, a person may say, "I don't feel well. I have a backache" (a condition not easily diagnosed), although no objective indicators of disease may be present. Illness can therefore be seen as

- *Punishment*—for example, "What did I do to deserve cancer?"
- *Deviance*—for example, Parsons's (1951) concept of the "sick role"
- *An indicator of social system performance*—for example, absenteeism due to "illness," although the real reason is job dissatisfaction
- *A social control device*—for example, attaching a psychiatric label such as *borderline personality disorder* to patients whose histories (often including childhood sexual abuse) are poorly understood (Hoff, 2000a)
- *A response to stress*—from physical, environmental, social, psychological, or cultural sources

- *Emotional breakdown* is an inability to manage one's feelings to the point of chronic interference in normal functioning; it is manifested in depression, anger, fear, and the like.
- *Mental breakdown* is a disturbance in cognitive functioning; it is manifested in the general inability to think and act normally. Biochemical imbalance and exposure to serious social stressors may be involved. It progresses to the point of interference in expression of feelings, everyday behavior, and interaction with others.
- *Crisis* is an acute emotional upset; it is manifested in an inability to cope emotionally, cognitively, or behaviorally and to solve problems by usual devices.

Research on stress, crisis, and emotional and mental breakdown reveals a lack of integration between clinical and social science insights. The imbalance between a clinical and a developmental-social analysis of coping with stressful life events needs correction (Edmands, Hoff, Kaylor, Mower, & Sorrell, 1999). Researchers trained clinically and in social science may be able to bridge some of these gaps. However, the medicalization and causal scientific models in all branches of human service practice have dominated the stress research field (McKinlay & Marceau, 1999). Conclusions from much of the research on stress point to the limitations of causal models in the analysis of stress. Increasing attention is being directed to studying the process of stress and its relationship to hazardous events, illness, coping, and social support (Caplan, 1981; Hoff, 1990; Meyer & Schwartz, 2000).

Overly simplistic psychological accounts of stress and illness are not the only problem in the crisis intervention field. Durkheim's (1897/1951) notion that people's positions in the social structure—lack of social integration and a sense of attachment to society—are causes of anomic and egoistic suicides is a prime example of sociological reductionism; it fails to account for differences in the way individuals interpret and cope with stressful life events from various sources. Although cause-and-effect laws certainly operate in regard to the physical stressors of a gunshot wound to the heart or the repeated inhalation of carcinogens—these stressors do cause death or lung cancer, respectively—a *social act*, such as suicide or violence against others, cannot be explained within the same causal framework (Hoff, 1990). What is the relevance of reductionist causal reasoning to crisis response and intervention?

Acute or chronic stress does not automatically lead to emotional imbalance or mental incompetence, abuse of alcohol and other drugs, suicide, or assault on others. If it did, humans, who by nature are rational, conscious, and responsible for their behavior, could routinely attribute their behavior to causes external to themselves and be excused from accountability. This, in fact, is the case in certain instances in which mitigating circumstances allow an excuse for some behaviors that might otherwise be punishable. In general, however, responses to stress vary. Increasingly, researchers are recognizing the importance of *context* in explaining behavior (Dobash & Dobash, 1998, pp. 9–10). Maslow's (1970) research, for example, underscores the apparent growth-promoting function of high-stress situations for achieving self-actualization, not destruction of self and others. Antonovsky's (1980) cross-cultural research on concentration camp survivors and women in menopause suggests similar conclusions. He proposes the concept of "resistance resources" (pp. 99–100), including social network support and a "sense of coherence" (SOC), as intervening variables in stressful situations. SOC includes the person's perception of events as comprehensible, manageable, and meaningful. Applied to crisis response, a person with a strong SOC will define social stressors as social rather than assuming blame for trouble that did not originate from oneself. One's resistance resources can make the difference between positive or negative responses to developmental transitions or to extreme stress (which a clinician might define as crisis), such as the catastrophic experience of concentration camp survivors. Research with battered women (Hoff, 1990) supports these views and the position taken in this book: stress, crisis, and illness (physical, emotional, and mental) are interactionally, not causally, related.

The Crisis–Psychiatric Illness Interface

Another argument about the relationship between stress, crisis, and illness concerns traditional victim blaming around crises of interpersonal violence (Ryan, 1971). The battering of women, for example, was attributed to a woman's provocative behavior, presumably arising from her own emotional or mental disturbance. This view is now widely rejected, as the global epidemic of violence against women takes center stage (Hoff, 2000b). Psychiatric and social analysis (for example, Hoff, 1990; Rieker & Carmen, 1986) reveals that the woman's emotional symptoms do not *cause* battering; rather, they occur almost invariably in the *context* of having been victimized both physically and psychologically.

Figure 2.2 illustrates this process in the downward spiral toward illness, a process that for assault victims especially usually begins with the misassignment of responsibility for the violence and abuse. Such a descent toward maladaptation can also occur in cases of oppression and discrimination based on race or sexual identity, for example. Key to this downward, possibly self-destructive or violent course is the process of *internalizing* blame or oppression originating from sociocultural sources. Once a person or group inappropriately absorbs blame for others' actions and takes on the identity of victim, helplessness or horizontal violence—venting rage or violence on people of one's own group—may prevent the proper channeling of anger toward personal healing and social change (see Figure 2.1, Box 3).

It is therefore crucial to simultaneously acknowledge the pain of victimization and oppression and keep sight of the fact that a downward spiral is not

FIGURE 2.2. ABUSE, THE DOWNWARD SPIRAL, AND ALTERNATIVE PATH.

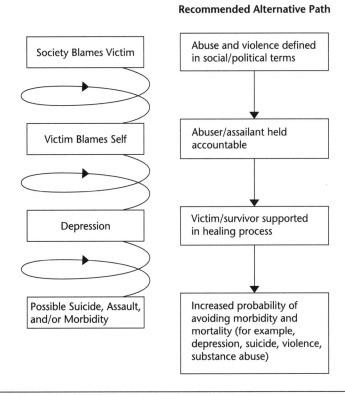

Recommended Alternative Path

Downward Spiral	Recommended Alternative Path
Society Blames Victim	Abuse and violence defined in social/political terms
Victim Blames Self	Abuser/assailant held accountable
Depression	Victim/survivor supported in healing process
Possible Suicide, Assault, and/or Morbidity	Increased probability of avoiding morbidity and mortality (for example, depression, suicide, violence, substance abuse)

Primary prevention is ideal, but intervention at *secondary* and *tertiary* levels can also prevent morbidity and save lives.

inevitable. Most important, then, for survival and growth beyond victimhood are social support and education toward a perspective that envisions the possibility of prevention and social change (Hoff, 1990; McCullough, 1995; Wendell, 1990). Note that Figure 2.2 includes these alternatives to the downward spiral.

One of the most popular notions surrounding women's crises stemming from violence is that the violent man is under high stress. To the extent that this explanation is accepted, the person's violence is excused on the basis of presumed mental incompetence. Although it is true that the extreme stress and anxiety associated with a crisis state can distort cognitive functions such as memory and decision making, mental incompetence would not be assumed if history revealed that the perpetrator's mental faculties were intact *before* the crisis (see Chapter Three). A person's decision to hit or kill his or her spouse during the high tension of a marital fight is therefore neither wise nor excusable. Social research over several decades supports the proposition that temporary insanity claims are really excuses used to evade responsibility for one's own violent behavior. This does not negate recognition that some crimes are committed by people who are diagnosed as mentally ill according to commonly accepted criteria, such as having delusions, hallucinations, or exhibiting bizarre behavior. Some recent jury acquittals of women who killed their abusive partners suggest that these women were not viewed as mentally ill; rather, the stress and danger of their circumstances after years of abuse were considered sufficient grounds for acquittal. Similarly, many men are excused from their battering, though some are convicted. One of the most striking findings of Hoff's research (1990) with abused women was their tendency to excuse their husband's violence but not their own retaliatory violence, even if the wives were under the influence of drugs or alcohol. When women are convicted of murdering their husbands, however, research suggests gross discriminatory practices (Browne, 1987).

These findings are remarkably similar to Erich Lindemann's classic study (1944): survivors of the Cocoanut Grove disaster might have been spared the negative experience of serious psychopathology if they had had assistance, such as with grief work, at the time of the crisis. Abused women without resources and assistance for constructive crisis resolution may start the downward course and become suicidal, homicidal, addicted, or emotionally disturbed, especially after repeated abuse. The reciprocal relationship between stress, crisis, and illness is observed further in the multifaceted stressors an abused woman must deal with while in crisis after a violent attack: physical injury, psychological upset, or change in her social situation—for example, disrupted marriage or residential or economic loss (see Chapter Eight, Figure 8.2, for an illustration of this relationship). Similarly, the crisis-illness relationship can be observed among the homeless. Considering how basic home and shelter are for all, the most remarkable evidence of human resilience is the survival of so many people against the greatest of odds and continuing stressors, even with the burden of serious mental disturbance (Hoff, 1993).

In a scientific sense, then, concepts of crisis, stress, and illness are imprecise and complexly associated with the political economy, a biomedical approach to people in distress, social inequality, and dominant values about people and illness in the cultural milieu—essentially an interactional, rather than causal, relationship between stress, crisis, and illness. What simplistic models miss is the influence of the distinctive individual experience of stress, crisis, and illness. Table 2.1 illustrates the distinctions and relationships between these concepts. It also links the concepts with their origins, providing a preview of the next section and remaining chapters.

Development and Individual Manifestations of Crisis

We have seen how crisis originates from physical, material, personal, social, and cultural sources, as well as how it fits into the larger picture of life's ups and downs. Let us now consider the experience of crisis at the individual, personal level.

Why People Go into Crisis

People in crisis are, by definition, emotionally upset; they are unable to solve life's problems in their usual way. A happy, healthy life implies an ability to solve problems effectively. It also implies that basic human needs are fulfilled. Our basic needs include a sense of physical and psychological well-being; a supportive network of friends, family, and associates; and a sense of identity and belonging to one's society and cultural heritage. Hansell (1976, pp. 31–49) describes our essential needs as the "seven basic attachments." All of us have a stable arrangement of transactions between ourselves and our environment. Essentially, we are attached to

1. Food, oxygen, and other physical supplies necessary to life
2. A strong sense of self-identity
3. At least one other person in a close, mutually supportive relationship
4. At least one group that accepts us as a member
5. One or more roles in which we feel self-respect and can perform with dignity
6. Financial security or a means of participating in an exchange of the goods and services we need and value
7. A comprehensive system of meaning—that is, a set of values that help us set goals and understand ourselves and the world around us

Typically, people in crisis suffer a sudden loss or threat of loss of a person or thing considered essential and important. One or several of their basic attachments are severed or are at risk of being severed. For example, the shock of the unexpected death of a loved one by car accident or heart attack can leave a person feeling incomplete and at a loss about what to do, where to turn. The individual's familiar source of support and comfort disappears without warning, with no time to adjust to the change. Similar shock occurs in response to the suicide of a friend, the threat of divorce, a diagnosis of a terminal illness such as AIDS, or an

TABLE 2.1.   DISTRESS DIFFERENTIATION.

Type of Distress or Problem	Origins	Possible Manifestations
Stress (acute)	Hazardous life events (such as heart attack, accident, death of loved one, violent attack, sudden job loss, natural disaster)	Emotional crisis General Adaptation Syndrome
	Invasion by microorganisms	General Adaptation Syndrome Disease process
	Man-made disaster	Annihilation of present civilization
Stress (chronic)	Strain in social relationships (such as marriage) Position in social structure (age, sex, race, class) Socioeconomic problems (such as unemployment) Chronic ill health Developmental transition states	Burnout Psychosomatic or stress-related illness Emotional or mental breakdown
Crisis	Traumatic situations (material, personal/physical, interpersonal) Transition states (developmental and other) Cultural values, social structure	Emotional Behavioral } Changes Cognitive Biophysical
Emotional or mental breakdown	Failure of positive response to acute stress and/or crisis Continuation of chronic stress from various sources	Neurotic and/or psychotic symptoms (such as learned helplessness or self-denigration by an abused woman)

Possible Responses		
Positive	**Negative**	**Duration**
Grief work Adaptation, emotional and social growth through healthy coping	Failure to ask for and accept help Suicide, assault, addiction, emotional/mental breakdown	Brief
Medical treatment, rest, exercise	Refusal of treatment, complications, possible premature death	
Prevention: Political action	Denial of possibility	
Lifestyle changes (such as diet, rest, exercise, leisure) Social change strategies Transition state preparation	Exacerbation of burnout All of the above, and mystification by and response to symptoms versus sources of chronic stress Inability to accomplish new role tasks	Weeks, months, years, or lifetime
Grief work Crisis coping and resolution by use of personal, social, and material resources **Prevention:** Education about sources of crisis and appropriate preventive action (such as contemporary rites of passage, action to reduce social disparities)	Same as for acute stress	Few days to 6 weeks
Reorganization or change of ineffective emotional, cognitive, and behavioral responses to stress and crisis (usually with help of therapy) Action to change social sources of chronic stress	Same as all of above, and increased vulnerability to crisis and inability to cope with acute and chronic stress	Weeks, months, years, or lifetime

operation such as a mastectomy, which seriously alters one's body. A person with AIDS, for example, not only loses health and faces the probability of a shortened life cycle but also may be abandoned by friends and family and scorned by would-be helpers.

CASE EXAMPLE: EDWARD

Edward, age forty-five, has been an outstanding assistant director of his company. When he is promoted to the vacated position of executive director, he becomes depressed and virtually nonfunctional. Edward, in spite of external signs of success, lacks basic self-confidence; he cannot face the challenge of the new job. The possibility of failure in his new position is unbearable. His anxiety about success prevents him from achieving the success he desires. Edward is one of the many people who, with the help of family and friends and perhaps a crisis counselor, can avoid possible failure and depression. He has his whole past career, including many successes, to draw on profitably in his present job. With help, he might see that failure in his present position need not mean the end of a happy and productive life.

Shock and a resulting crisis state can also occur at the time of normal role transitions. For example, Mary, age nineteen, relied very heavily on her mother for advice and support in all aspects of her life. One month after her honeymoon and the move into an apartment with her husband, she became depressed and suicidal and was unable to function at home or at work. Mary was obviously not ready for the move from adolescence to the more independent role of a young married adult.

Caplan (1964) and Tyhurst (1957) note that for some people a crisis is triggered when they face a particularly challenging psychosocial event. A crisis for such individuals represents a call to new action that they cannot face with their present resources.

CASE EXAMPLE: JOAN

Joan, age nineteen, is another person who cannot meet the challenge of increasing her personal and social resources; she cannot obtain a college credential for teaching, and she worries about coming out as a lesbian. She is paralyzed by her fear of the responsibilities involved in a teaching career. At examination time, she is unable to study and fails over half of her college courses. The conflict that Joan experiences around revealing her sexual identity is compounded by the developmental task of role transition to adulthood faced by all adolescents. Joan's challenge to increase her "supplies" in preparation for an adult teaching responsibility is more than she can face without additional resources.

How a Crisis Develops

A crisis does not occur instantaneously. There are identifiable phases of development—psychosocial in character—that lead to an active crisis state. These phases were first described by Tyhurst (1957) in his study of individual responses to community disaster. Survivors experience three overlapping phases: (1) a period of impact, (2) a period of recoil, and (3) a post-traumatic period. This breakdown of phases is applied most appropriately to crises originating from catastrophic, shocking events, such as rape and other violent attacks, war-related devastation, or sometimes the news of a terminal disease (see "Individual Responses to Disaster" in Chapter Ten for a detailed description of these phases).

Caplan (1964) describes four phases in the development of extreme anxiety and crisis. His description of phases is applicable to crises occurring in a more gradual process from less catastrophic stressors. Recognizing these phases of crisis development is useful in the important task of preventing stressful life events from spiraling into crises.

• *Phase One.* A traumatic event causes an initial rise in one's level of anxiety. The person is in a predicament and responds with familiar problem-solving mechanisms to reduce or eliminate the stress and discomfort stemming from excessive anxiety. For example, John, age thirty-four, is striving toward a career as an executive in his company when he receives a diagnosis of multiple sclerosis. His wife, Nancy, is very supportive. He adjusts to this unexpected disturbing event by continuing to work as long as he can. John also has the advantage of the most advanced medical treatment available for multiple sclerosis. In addition, John's physician is skillful in applying his knowledge of the emotional impact of John's diagnosis. At this stage, John's traumatic event does not result in a crisis for him.

• *Phase Two.* In this phase, the person's usual problem-solving ability fails, and the stimulus that caused the initial rise in tension continues. To continue with the illustration of John's case: the disease process is advancing despite excellent medical treatment. John's wife, Nancy, begins to participate less in some of her own interests, including volunteer work, so she can spend more time with her husband. The accumulating medical expenses and loss of work time strain the family's financial resources. John and Nancy receive a report from school that their son, Larry, age fourteen, is having behavioral problems. At this stage, because there is greater stress, the possibility of a crisis state for John increases, but a crisis is not inevitable. Whether it occurs or not depends on what happens next in John's life.

• *Phase Three.* In this phase, the individual's anxiety level rises further. The increased tension moves the person to use every resource available, including unusual or new means, to solve the problem and reduce the increasingly painful state of anxiety. In John's case, he fortunately has enough inner strength, confidence, and sensitivity to recognize the strain of his illness on his wife and child. He looks for new ways to cope with his increasing stress. First, he confides in his physician, who responds by taking time to listen and offer emotional support. His physician also arranges for home health services through a visiting nurse agency. This outside health assistance frees Nancy from some of her steadily increasing responsibilities. The physician also encourages John and Nancy to seek help from the school guidance counselor regarding their son, Larry, which they do.

Another way to prevent a crisis state at this phase is to redefine or change one's goals. This means of avoiding crisis is not usually possible for someone who is emotionally isolated from others and feels locked into solving a problem alone. With the help of his physician, John could accept his illness as something that changed his capacity to function in predefined, expected ways. However, he does not have to alter his fundamental ability to live a meaningful, rewarding life because of illness. As John's illness progresses, it becomes necessary to change his role as the sole financial provider in the family. John and Nancy talk openly with each other about the situation. Together they decide that Nancy will take a job to ease the financial strain. They also ask the nursing agency to increase the home health services, as Nancy is beginning to resent her confinement to the house and the increasing demands of being nurse to her husband.

• *Phase Four.* This is the state of active crisis that results when the following conditions exist.

• Internal strength and social support are lacking.
• The person's problem remains unresolved.
• Tension and anxiety rise to an unbearable degree.

An active crisis does not occur in John's case because he is able to respond constructively to his unanticipated illness. John has natural social supports and is able to use available help, so his stress does not become unbearable. The example of John illustrates how a full-blown crisis (phase four) can be avoided by various decisions and actions taken during any one of the three preceding phases.

The following example of George Sloan is in sharp contrast to that of John. George's case will be continued and discussed in subsequent chapters.

CASE EXAMPLE: GEORGE SLOAN—PHASES OF CRISIS DEVELOPMENT

George Sloan, age forty-eight, works as a machinist with a construction company. Six evenings a week, he works a second job as a taxi driver in a large metropolitan area; his beat includes high-crime sections of the city. He has just come home from the hospital after his third heart attack. The first occurred at age forty-four and the second at age forty-seven.

• *Phase One.* George is advised by his physician to cut down on his work hours. Specifically, the doctor recommends that he give up his second job and spend more time relaxing with family and friends. George's physician recognizes his patient's vulnerability to heart attacks, especially in relation to his lifestyle. George rarely slows down. He is chronically angry about things going wrong and about not being able to get ahead financially. He receives his physician's advice with mixed feelings. On the one hand, he sees the relationship between his heavy work schedule and his heart attacks; on the other hand, he resents what he acknowledges as a necessary change to reduce further risk of death by heart attack.

In any case, his health and financial problems markedly increase his usual level of anxiety. He talks superficially to his wife, Marie, about his dilemma but receives little support or understanding from her; their marital relationship is already strained. Marie suggests that in place of George's second job, she increase her part-time job to full-time. George resents this because of what it implies about his image of himself as the chief provider.

George's discouragement and anger about not getting ahead are aggravated by Marie's complaints of never having enough money for the things she wants. George also resents what he perceives as the physician's judgment that he is not strong enough to do two jobs. At this stage, George is in a precrisis state, with a high degree of stress and anxiety.

• *Phase Two.* George fails to obtain relief from his anxiety by talking with his wife. He does not feel comfortable talking with his physician about his reluctance to cut down the work stress as advised. When he attempts to do so, he senses that the physician is rushed. So he concludes that his doctor is only concerned about giving technical advice, not about how George handles the advice. The prospect of quitting his second job and bringing home less money leaves George feeling like a failure. His initial conflict and rise in tension continue. If he quits his second job, he cannot preserve his image as adequate family provider; yet he cannot reduce the risk of death by heart disease if he continues his present pace. Help from other resources seems out of his reach.

• *Phase Three.* George's increased anxiety moves him to try talking with his wife again. Ordinarily, he would have abandoned the idea based on the response he received earlier. This action therefore constitutes an unusual effort for him, but he fails again in getting the help he needs. To make matters worse, George and Marie learn that their sixteen-year-old son, Arnold, has been suspended from school for a week due to suspected drug involvement. This leaves George feeling like even more of a failure, as he is seldom home during normal family hours. In addition, Marie nags him about not spending enough time with the children. George's high level of anxiety becomes so obvious that Marie finally suggests, "Why don't you talk to the doctor about whatever's bothering you?" George knows that this is a good idea but cannot bring himself to do it, as he has always taken pride in solving his own problems. For the same reason, he cannot accept his wife's proposal to start working full-time. Personality and social factors block him from redefining or changing his goals as a means of problem resolution and crisis prevention. Financial concerns, along with the new problem of his son, further increase his anxiety level. George is in a predicament that he does not know how to resolve.

• *Phase Four.* George is at a complete loss about how to deal with all the stress in his life—the threat to his health and life if he continues his present pace, the threat to his self-image if he quits the second job, the failure to communicate with his wife, and the sense of failure and guilt in his role as a parent. His anxiety increases to the breaking point:

- He feels hopeless.
- He does not know where to turn.
- He is in a state of active crisis.

George's case illustrates situational (heart disease), maturational (adolescent changes), and sociocultural (sex-role stereotyping) factors in the development of life crises. It also highlights the subjective elements that contribute to a crisis state at different times in people's lives. George's heart disease was clearly an unanticipated, stressful—even life-threatening—event. The threat of his son's being suspended was unanticipated and a source of added stress. Yet Arnold's adolescence was anticipated as a normal phase of human development. If George's heart disease had developed at a time when his marriage was less strained, he might have received more help and support. And Arnold might have made it through adolescence without school suspension if there had been regular support from both parents. As it turned out, George and Marie had received the first report of Arnold's behavior problems in school shortly after George's first heart attack four years earlier. They were advised at that time to seek family or marital counseling; they did, but only for a single session. Finally, the socialization of George and Marie to stereotypical male and female roles was an added source of stress and a barrier to constructive crisis resolution. These contextual factors underscore the subjectivity of the crisis experience.

For another person, such as John in the previous case, or for George at another time of life, the same medical diagnosis and the same advice could have had an altogether different effect. This is also true for Arnold. A different response from his parents when he had given his first signals of distress, or a more constructive approach from school officials and counselors, might have prevented the additional stress of Arnold's school suspension. Or different cultural expectations for husbands and wives could have altered each person's interpretation of the stressful situation (to be continued in Chapter Three).

The Duration and Outcomes of Crisis

People cannot stay in crisis forever. The state of crisis and the accompanying anxiety are too painful. There is a natural time limitation to the crisis experience because the individual cannot survive indefinitely in such a state of psychological pain and turmoil. The emotional distress stemming from extreme anxiety moves the person toward action to reduce the anxiety to an endurable level as soon as possible. This aspect of the crisis experience underscores the *danger* and the *opportunity* that crisis presents.

Experience with people in crisis has led to the observation that the acute emotional upset lasts from a few days to a few weeks. The person must then move toward some sort of resolution; this is often expressed in terms such as, "I can't go on like this anymore. Something has got to give," or "Please, tell me what to do to get out of this mess. I can't stand it," or "I feel like I'm losing my mind."

What, then, happens to the person in crisis? Several outcomes are possible.

1. The person can return to the precrisis state. This happens as a result of effective problem solving, made possible by internal strength, values, and social supports. Such an outcome does not necessarily imply new psychological growth as a result of the experience; the person simply returns to his or her usual state of being.

2. The person may not only return to the precrisis state but also can grow from the crisis experience through discovery of new resources and ways of solving problems. These discoveries result from the crisis experience itself. John's case is a good example of such growth. He took advantage of resources available to him and his family, such as his physician and the school guidance counselor. He found new ways of solving problems. The result for John was a process of growth: (a) His concept of himself as a worthwhile person was reinforced in spite of the loss of physical integrity from his illness. (b) He strengthened his marriage and his ability to relate to his wife regarding a serious problem. This produced growth for both of them. (c) He developed in his role as a father by constructively handling the problem with his son in addition to his own personal stress.

3. The person responds to the problem by lapsing into neurotic, psychotic, or destructive patterns of behavior. For example, the individual may become very withdrawn, suspicious, or depressed. A person's distorted perception of events may be exaggerated to the point of blaming others inappropriately for the misfortunes experienced. Some people in crisis resolve their problems, at least temporarily, by excessive drinking or other drug abuse or by impulsive disruptive behavior. Others resort to more extreme measures by attempting or committing suicide or by abusing or killing others.

All of these negative and destructive outcomes of the crisis experience occur when the individual lacks constructive ways of solving life's problems and relieving intolerable anxiety. George, for example, came to the conclusion in his despair that he was worth more dead than alive. Consequently, he was brought to the hospital emergency department after a car crash. George crashed his car deliberately but did not die as he had planned. This was his chosen method of suicidal death, which he thought would spare his family the stigma of suicide. He felt that he had already overburdened them. George's case will be continued in Chapters Three and Four with respect to his treatment in the emergency service and his follow-up care.

Considering all of the possible outcomes of a crisis experience, the following goals become obvious.

- To help people in crisis return at least to their precrisis state
- To do all that is possible to help people grow and become stronger as a result of the crisis and effective problem solving
- To be alert to danger signals in order to prevent negative, destructive outcomes of a crisis experience

The last goal is achieved by recognizing that negative results of crisis are often not necessary but occur because of insufficient personal and family strengths or because of insensitivity and a lack of appropriate resources and crisis intervention skills in the human service sector (see Figure 2.1, Boxes 4a and 4b).

The Sociocultural Context of Personal Crisis

The contrasting cases of John (with multiple sclerosis) and George (with a heart attack) illustrate both the success and the limitations of individual approaches to life crises. Let us suppose that John and George each had identical help available from human service agencies. If George's crisis response is rooted partially in social and cultural sources—as seems to be the case—then intervention must consciously address these factors in order to be successful. Otherwise, unattended social and cultural issues can form a barrier to a strictly psychological crisis counseling approach. They also underscore McKinlay's argument (1990, p. 502) about "downstream" versus "upstream" endeavors and link individual crisis intervention efforts to complementary preventive and social change strategies.

Preventive strategies were discussed in the previous chapter. Individual and social network crisis intervention approaches are considered in detail in the remaining chapters. Social action ideas are incorporated in relevant cases throughout the book. The social change aspects of comprehensive crisis work belong to the follow-up phase of the total process. In the Crisis Paradigm (Figure 2.1), such social change strategies are illustrated in the right circle of Box 3, corresponding to sociocultural crisis origins in Box 1. However, the foundation for such action is laid in one of the cognitive aspects of healthy crisis resolution—*understanding* the traumatic event, its sources, and how it affects the way one feels during crisis. For example, a rape victim can be helped to understand that she feels guilty and dirty about being raped not because she is in fact guilty and dirty but because of the widely accepted social value that women are responsible if they are raped because they dress provocatively, hitchhike, or in a similar way allegedly provoke the attack (see Figure 2.2).

The tradition among human service workers of claiming "value neutrality" may lead some to object to including social change strategies as a formal part of service. Yet to offer only short-term crisis counseling or psychotherapy for problems stemming from cultural and social origins is value-laden in itself—that is, it suggests that the person should adjust to a disadvantaged position in society rather than develop and act on an awareness of the underlying factors contributing to depression or suicidal feelings (for example, Burstow, 1992; Cloward & Piven, 1979; McNamee & Gergen, 1992). As Johnson (1990, p. 230) points out, professionals who focus solely on purportedly neutral "clinical" material and avoid "this policy stuff" shortchange themselves and their clients whose crises are linked to various policy issues. It is therefore not a question of whether crisis workers are value-free, as such work is almost inevitably affected by our values. Rather, values should be made explicit, so that clients can make their own choices (such as accepting or acting on their disadvantaged position) from a more enlightened base.

Social Change Strategies in Comprehensive Crisis Care

As readers are perhaps less familiar with social change strategies than with other aspects of crisis care follow-up, such as psychotherapy for underlying personality problems, the following summary is offered. It highlights the principles of social change agentry as presented in the Crisis Paradigm and is adapted from the work of Chin and Benne (1969). These strategies are central to positive crisis resolution, particularly those crises originating from sociocultural sources.

Strategies Based on Reason and Research

Foremost among these strategies are research findings, new concepts, and the clarification of language to more closely represent reality as experienced by people, not as theorized by academics. These strategies rest on the assumption that people are reasonable and when presented with evidence will take appropriate action to bring about needed change. However, this strategy alone is usually not enough to move people toward change, such as enacting workplace policies that affect staff safety and injury prevention on the job.

Strategies Based on Reeducation and Attitude Change

These approaches to change are based on the assumption that people are guided by internalized values and habits and that they act according to institutionalized roles and perceptions of self. For example, some parents remain in unhappy marriages for the sake of the children. This group of strategies includes an activity central to contemporary crisis theory—fostering learning and growth in the persons who make up the system to be changed. This includes people who are in crisis because of greater vulnerability stemming from a disadvantaged position in society. This change strategy is also relevant to people whose usual coping devices leave something to be desired, such as people with learned helplessness, excessive drinking, or those who abuse others (see Figure 2.2). Prominent illustrations of this strategy include (1) the mediation and nonviolent conflict resolution programs being instituted to stem the tide of youth violence (Jenkins & Bell, 1992; Kottler, 1994) and (2) programs aimed at reclaiming values of respect for the environment and for people different from ourselves. An example of this kind of program is the Teaching Tolerance program of the Southern Poverty Law Center. Through such programs, experiencing and dealing openly with the psychic pain of the crisis experience (in contrast to resorting to violence or chronic unhealthy coping) often moves people to learn new ways of coping with life's problems.

Power-Coercive Strategies

The emphasis in these strategies is on political and economic sanctions in the exercise of power, along with such moral power moves as playing on sentiments of guilt, shame, and a sense of what is just and right. It is assumed that political action approaches will probably not succeed apart from reeducation and attitude changes. New action, such as strikes by nurses who have been traditionally socialized to a subservient role in the health care system, demands by ethnic minorities to end housing and job discrimination, or protests by gays against harassment and violence, usually requires "new knowledge, new skills, new attitudes, and new value orientations" (Chin & Benne, 1969, p. 42; Hoff, 1990; Holland, 1994).

In a similar vein, Marris (1987, pp. 156–164) proposes that new formulations of social meaning should accompany struggles to assert the ideals of society and to implement social justice policies. This presumes collective planning by people concerned with those who are distressed or in crisis because of discrimination and repressive policies—for example, feminists; racial equity groups; gay, lesbian, bisexual, and transgendered activists; and disabled persons.

The incorporation of these social change strategies into a comprehensive approach to crisis work underscores the importance of tailoring intervention strategies to correspond with the origins of stress and crisis, as illustrated in the Crisis Paradigm. For example, Cloward and Piven (1979), in their discussion of female deviance, claim that women's coping through depression, passive resistance, and lower rates of violence is related to the source of their stress. Many women have been socialized to accept the view that women's stress is determined biologically and stems from natural psychic weakness (Sayers, 1982). Women may therefore expect to simply *endure* what nature offers—not unlike survivors of natural disaster. However, social sources of stress can be *resisted*, as can the threat of man-made disaster. These ideas support the importance of raising consciousness and employing human rights and public health perspectives in crisis work. It is now common for health and mental health professionals to recommend that abused

TABLE 2.2. COMPREHENSIVE CRISIS CARE.

	Approaches to Crisis Care and Resolution		
Crisis Element	Preventive and Enhancement	Immediate or Short-Term	Long-Range (Follow-Up)
Heart attack	Lifestyle factors (such as diet, exercise, relaxation)	Life-support measures	Lifestyle factors
Marital and role strain	Marriage preparation Communication	Marriage counseling	Normative reeducative change
Midlife change and marital strain	Rites of passage (such as a support group)*	Women's support group Men's support group	Normative reeducative change strategies
Arnold's school suspension	Rites of passage (such as adolescent support group)	Family and social network crisis counseling	Family counseling or therapy
George's suicide attempt	Family support and normative reeducative change following first heart attack	Individual and family crisis counseling	Family counseling Normative reeducative change Lifestyle factors

*Contemporary substitutes for traditional rites of passage are discussed in Chapter Thirteen.

women or rape victims participate in support groups that sensitize survivors to these kinds of social and political issues.

Table 2.2 illustrates how these ideas are encompassed in a comprehensive approach with respect to the various elements of the crisis experienced by George and his family. (See Chapter Eight for an illustration of this comprehensive approach to an abused woman, Ramona.) The approaches can be grouped as preventive and enhancement, immediate or short-term, and long-range (follow-up). This diagram suggests that primary prevention and enhancement activities can abort a destructive crisis outcome like premature death. It demonstrates, too, the interactions and relationship (not necessarily an orderly sequence) between strategies, as well as the fact that various elements of comprehensive crisis care may be included in a single encounter with a person in crisis. The diagram illustrates that it is never too late to consider preventive and enhancement approaches (such as at secondary and tertiary levels), even if a suicide attempt has been made; nor is it ever too late to learn from the experience of others (Hoff & Resing, 1982).

The case of George suggests the intersection of responses relevant to crises originating from three sources: traumatic personal situations, transition states, and gender-role strain related to socialization. This case also underscores the fact that people will resolve their crises with or without the help of significant others. People rich in personal, social, and material resources are often able to resolve crises positively in a natural (as opposed to institutional) context with the help of family, friends, and neighbors. Many, however, lack such resources or for personal, cultural, and political reasons cannot mobilize them successfully during crisis. In these instances, more formal help from trained crisis workers is needed to see them through this potentially dangerous period and promote positive crisis resolution (see Figure 2.1, Box 4a). The rest of this book is devoted to the principles and strategies necessary for effective crisis intervention—assessment, planning, implementation of plan, and follow-up—the formal aspect of crisis care.

Summary

Success in crisis assessment and intervention depends on our understanding (1) the origins of crisis, (2) how crisis differs from stress and illness, and (3) the development and individual manifestations of crisis. Regardless of the origin of crisis, people in crisis have a number of characteristics in common. The probability of preventing negative outcomes for these individuals is increased by our sensitivity to the origins of crisis and the application of appropriate intervention strategies in distinct sociocultural contexts. These concepts are illustrated in the Crisis Paradigm, which provides the theoretical framework of this book.

References

Antonovsky, A. (1980). *Health, stress, and coping.* San Francisco: Jossey-Bass.

Baum, A., Cohen, L., & Hall, M. (1993). Control and intrusive memories as possible determinants of chronic stress. *Psychosomatic Medicine, 55*(3), 274–286.

Bebbington, P., Wilkins, S., Jones, P., Foerster, A., Murray, R., Toone, B., & Lewis, S. (1993). Life events and psychosis: Initial results from the Camberwell Collaborative Psychosis Study. *British Journal of Psychiatry, 162,* 72–79.

Brown, G. W. (1993). Life events and affective disorder: Replications and limitations. *Psychosomatic Medicine, 55*(3), 248–259.

Brown, G. W., & Harris, T. (1978). *The social origins of depression.* London: Tavistock.

Browne, A. (1987). *When battered women kill.* New York: Free Press.

Burstow, B. (1992). *Radical feminist therapy: Working in the context of violence.* Thousand Oaks, CA: Sage.

Caplan, G. (1964). *Principles of preventive psychiatry.* New York: Basic Books.

Caplan, G. (1981). Mastery of stress: Psychosocial aspects. *American Journal of Psychiatry, 138*(4), 413–420.

Chin, R., & Benne, K. D. (1969). General strategies for effecting change in human systems. In W. G. Bennis, K. D. Benne, & R. Chin (Eds.), *The planning of change* (2nd ed., pp. 32–57). Austin, TX: Holt, Rinehart and Winston.

Cloward, R. A., & Piven, F. F. (1979). Hidden protest: The channeling of female innovations and resistance. *Signs: Journal of Women in Culture and Society, 4,* 651–669.

Conger, R. D., Lorenz, F. O., Elder, G. H., & Simons, R. L. (1993). Husband and wife differences in response to undesirable life events. *Journal of Health and Social Behavior, 34*(1), 71–88.

Danish, S. J., Smyer, M. A., & Nowak, C. A. (1980). Developmental intervention: Enhancing life-event processes. *Life-Span Development and Behavior, 3,* 339–366.

Dobash, R. E., & Dobash, R. P. (Eds.). (1998). *Rethinking violence against women.* Thousand Oaks, CA: Sage.

Durkheim, E. (1951). *Suicide* (2nd ed.). New York: Free Press. (Original work published 1897)

Edmands, M. S., Hoff, L. A., Kaylor, L., Mower, L., & Sorrell, S. (1999). Bridging gaps between mind, body and spirit: Healing the whole person. *Journal of Psychosocial Nursing, 37*(10), 1–7.

Erikson, E. (1963). *Childhood and society* (2nd ed.). New York: Norton.

Hansell, N. (1976). *The person in distress.* New York: Human Sciences Press.

Herman, J. (1992). *Trauma and recovery: The aftermath of violence.* New York: Basic Books.

Hoff, L. A. (1990). *Battered women as survivors.* London: Routledge.

Hoff, L. A. (1993). Review essay: Health policy and the plight of the mentally ill. *Psychiatry, 56*(4), 400–419.

Hoff, L. A. (2000a). Crisis care. In B. Everett & R. Gallop (Eds.), *The link between childhood trauma and mental illness: Effective interventions for mental health professionals* (pp. 227–251). Thousand Oaks, CA: Sage.

Hoff, L. A. (2000b). Interpersonal violence. In C. E. Koop, C. E. Pearson, & M. R. Schwarz (Eds.), *Critical issues in global health* (pp. 260–271). San Francisco: Jossey-Bass.

Hoff, L. A., & Resing, M. (1982). Was this suicide preventable? *American Journal of Nursing, 82*(7), 1106–1111. (Also reprinted in B. A. Backer, P. M. Dubbert, & E.J.P. Eisenman (Eds.). (1985). *Psychiatric/mental health nursing: Contemporary readings* (pp. 169–180). Belmont, CA: Wadsworth.)

Hogberg, U., & Bergstrom, E. (2000). Suffocated prone: The iatrogenic tragedy of SIDS. *American Journal of Public Health, 90*(4). 527–531.

Holland, H. (1994). *Born in Soweto.* Harmondsworth, England: Penguin Books.

Hurwicz, M. L., Durham, C. C., Boyd-Davis, S. L., Gatz, M., & Bengtson, V. L. (1992). Salient life events in three-generation families. *Journal of Gerontology, 47*(1), 11–13.

Jenkins, E. J., & Bell, C. C. (1992). Adolescent violence: Can it be curbed? *Adolescent Medicine: State of the Art Reviews, 3*(1), 71–86.

Johnson, A. B. (1990). *Out of bedlam: The truth about deinstitutionalization.* New York:Basic Books.

Killeen, M. (1990). The influence of stress and coping on family caregivers' perceptions of health. *International Journal of Aging and Human Development, 30*(3), 197–211.

Kottler, J. A. (1994). *Beyond blame: A new way of resolving conflicts in relationships.* San Francisco: Jossey-Bass.

Landy, D. (Ed.). (1977). *Culture, disease, and healing: Studies in medical anthropology.* Old Tappan, NJ: Macmillan.

Lindemann, E. (1944). Symptomatology and management of acute grief. *American Journal of Psychiatry, 101,* 101–148. (Also reprinted in H. J. Parad (Ed.). (1965). *Crisis intervention: Selected readings.* New York: Family Service Association of America.)

Loustaunau, M. O., & Sobo, E. J. (1997). *The cultural context of health, illness, and medicine.* New York: Bergin & Garvey.

Marris, P. (1987). *Meaning and action: Community action and conceptions of change* (2nd ed.). London: Routledge.

Maslow, A. (1970). *Motivation and personality* (2nd ed.). New York: HarperCollins.

Mawby, R. I., & Walklate, S. (1994). *Critical victimology.* Thousand Oaks, CA: Sage.

McCullough, C. J. (1995). *Nobody's victim.* New York: Clarkson/Potter.

McElroy, A., & Townsend, P. K. (1985). *Medical anthropology in ecological perspective.* Boulder, CO: Westview Press.

McKinlay, J. B. (1990). A case for refocusing upstream: The political economy of illness. In P. Conrad & R. Kern (Eds.), *The sociology of health and illness: Critical perspectives* (3rd ed., pp. 502–516). New York: St. Martin's Press.

McKinlay, J. B., & Marceau, L. D. (1999). A tale of 3 tails. *American Journal of Public Health, 89*(3), 295–298.

McNamee, S., & Gergen, K. J. (Eds.). (1992). *Therapy as social construction.* Thousand Oaks, CA: Sage.

Meyer, I. H., & Schwartz, S. (2000). Social issues as public health: Promise and peril. *American Journal of Public Health, 90*(8), 1189–1191.

Panchuck, P. (1994). *The midlife experience of contemporary women: Views along the midway.* Unpublished doctoral dissertation, Lesley College, Boston.

Parsons, T. (1951). Social structure and the dynamic process: The case of modern medical practice. In *The social system* (pp. 428–479). New York: Free Press.

Perloff, L. S. (1983). Perceptions of vulnerability. *Journal of Social Issues, 39*(2), 41–61.

Rieker, P. P., & Carmen, E. H. (1986). The victim-to-patient process: The disconfirmation and transformation of abuse. *American Journal of Orthopsychiatry, 56,* 360–371.

Ryan, W. (1971). *Blaming the victim.* New York: Vintage Books.

Sales, E., Baum, M., & Shore, B. (1984). Victim readjustment following assault. *Journal of Social Issues, 40*(1), 117–136.

Sayers, J. (1982). *Biological Politics.* London: Tavistock.

Schulberg, H. C., & Sheldon, A. (1968). The probability of crisis and strategies for preventive intervention. *Archives of General Psychiatry, 18,* 553–558.

Selye, H. (1956). *The stress of life.* New York: McGraw-Hill.

Tsukuda, G. (1999). Treating Asian American clients in crisis: A collectivist approach [Commentary on the paper by Ino and Glicken]. *Smith College Studies in Social Work, 69*(3), 541–546.

Turner, R. J., & Avison, W. R. (1992). Innovations in the measurement of life stress: Crisis theory and the significance of event resolution. *Journal of Health and Social Behavior, 33*(1), 36–50.

Tyhurst, J. S. (1957). The role of transition states—including disasters—in mental illness. In *Symposium on preventive and social psychiatry.* Washington, DC: Walter Reed Army Institute of Research and the National Research Council.

Vaillant, G. E. (1993). *The wisdom of the ego: Sources of resilience in adult life.* Cambridge, MA: Harvard University Press.

Wendell, S. (1990). Oppression and victimization: Choice and responsibility. *Hypatia: A Journal of Feminist Philosophy, 4*(3), 15–46.

WGBH Educational Foundation. *Survivors* [Public television documentary]. (1982). Boston: Author.

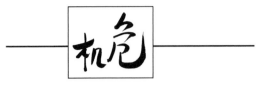

CHAPTER THREE

IDENTIFYING PEOPLE AT RISK

We know, generally, how crises originate, and we know how to predict and prevent many crises or destructive crisis outcomes in large population groups. This general knowledge, however, must be made accessible for use with individuals in actual or potential crisis. Crises from some sources are predictable and therefore more easily prepared for; preparation helps reduce the risk of crisis as well as the possibility of damaging outcomes. Common sources of predictable crises are developmental states and the role changes marking adolescence, adulthood, marriage, midlife, retirement, and old age. Typically, a person may first go to school, then get a job, find a life partner, become a parent, and reach the age of retirement. Because role changes usually are anticipated, precautions can be taken to avoid a crisis. But some people do not or cannot prepare themselves for these events; the possibility of crisis for them is increased. For example, a young person whose parents have been overindulgent and inconsistent in their responses will find it difficult to move from adolescence to adulthood. Overprotective parents stifle a child's normal development, so the move to adulthood becomes a risk and a hazard rather than an opportunity for further challenge and growth. Also, a person need not rush into marriage but can thoughtfully consider what such a major role change implies. Yet many do rush, and crises result.

Another factor affecting these predictable role changes is the element of timing (see Chapters Two and Thirteen). For example, a man or woman marrying for the first time at age forty may have planned very carefully for this life change, but altering an established pattern of living alone and being independent may lead to unanticipated stress. In addition, parental and other social supports for newlyweds are less likely to be available in later marriages. In contrast, although a planned event such as a return to school at midlife can be hazardous due to atypical timing, an older student may be less vulnerable to crisis. This is because a more mature student or life partner often has the advantage of experience, financial security, and clear-cut goals—valuable resources that younger people may possess in lesser measure.

Another aspect of a potentially hazardous role transition, even if prepared for, is its timing in connection with other life events. Many life changes are in one's control (for example, marriage or returning to school in midlife), whereas others are not (for example, menopause or death of an elderly parent). Careful planning around controllable changes can reduce a person's cumulative stress and the hazards of crisis, illness, and accidents.

Other life events are less predictable: sudden death of a loved one; serious physical illness; urban dislocation; personal and financial loss through flood, hurricane, or fire; birth of a premature infant. When these unanticipated events occur during transition states or when they originate from cultural values and one's disadvantaged social position, the probability of crisis is increased.

These examples and the interactive nature of crisis origins (discussed in Chapters One and Two) underscore the subjective nature of the crisis experience and the need to identify individuals at risk. Regardless of how predictable crisis responses might be among groups, it is important to translate *general* risk factors into an assessment of the issues and problems faced by *this* person or family at *this* particular time. Such an assessment—and assistance based on it—implies the need for precise information about individuals and families who may be at risk. For example,

1. In what developmental phase is the person or family?
2. What recent hazardous events have occurred in the life of this person or family?
3. How has this person or family interpreted these events?
4. Is there actual or potential threat to life? How urgent is the need for intervention?
5. What is the sociocultural context in which all of this is happening?

The ramifications of answers to these and related questions form the basis of this chapter on identifying and assessing people in precrisis or crisis states, the focus of Box 2 in Figure 3.1, the Crisis Paradigm.

The Importance of Crisis Assessment

The crisis worker must consider the intersections of life events, transition states, and hazardous sociocultural factors when assessing whether or not a person is in crisis. Observers may think that an emotionally upset person is obviously in a state of crisis. This is not necessarily so; thorough assessment should precede such a judgment. Still, an untrained observer may quickly dismiss the need for assessment in order to proceed to a seemingly more urgent task—to *help* the individual.

FIGURE 3.1.   CRISIS PARADIGM.

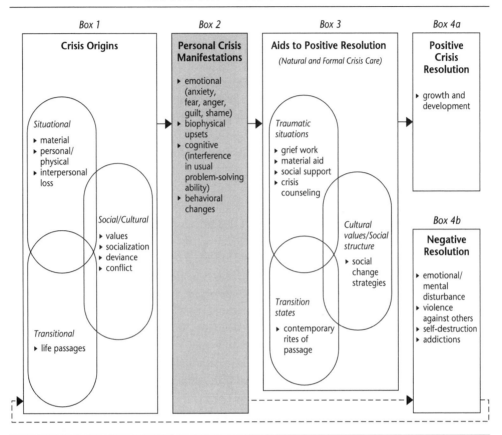

Crisis origins, manifestations, and outcomes and the respective functions of crisis care have an interactional relationship. The intertwined circles represent the distinct yet interrelated origins of crisis and aids to positive resolution, even though personal manifestations are often similar. The arrows pointing from origins to positive resolution illustrate the *opportunity for growth and development* through crisis; the broken line at bottom depicts the potential *danger of crisis* in the absence of appropriate aids. The loop between Box 4b and Box 1 denotes the *vulnerability* to future crisis episodes following negative resolution.

Such well-intentioned help sometimes has the opposite effect, however. This is most likely to happen if the urge to help springs from a helper's excessive need to be needed, thereby obscuring the distressed person's basic need for mastery and self-determination. One way to avoid misplaced helping is to be aware of and not indulge in rescue fantasies. Another is to identify people at risk through a careful assessment process.

Impediments to Adequate Assessment

Assessment can be impeded by the very nature of the crisis intervention process, a humane function that is now standard practice in health and social service settings. Helping people in crisis is immediate and often highly rewarding. However, those human service workers who are most inclined to action and who expect to obtain quick observable results often do not take time to study and evaluate their own work (Hoff & Adamowski, 1998). When the challenge of self-review is combined with the difficulty of evaluating any human helping process objectively, it is easy to see how comprehensive crisis care can flounder. This is a particularly hazardous approach in the quick-fix era of managed care, which emphasizes psychotropic drug solutions to psychosocial problems. Without a sound theoretical base and established techniques, there is little to distinguish crisis intervention from intuitive first aid.

Hazards of Inadequate Assessment and Psychiatric Labeling

The failure to assess prior to helping is often responsible for the misapplication of the crisis model. In the human service field, it is particularly unfortunate to misjudge a person in crisis due to poor observation and inadequate assessment. Ultimately, these errors result in failure to help, which can have lifelong, destructive effects. Successful crisis prediction and assessment increase the possibility of preventive intervention and make hospital admission (and its attendant risks) less likely (see "Preventing Crisis and Promoting Emotional Growth" in Chapter One). A note from the golden age of social psychiatry highlights the importance of assessment and resolution of crisis as an alternative to psychiatric hospitalization; this observation about what happens after admission is still relevant today: "The admission itself tends to promote denial of the social forces in the family and community that have produced it. The patient may then emerge as the scapegoat for these family and community problems, and psychiatric assessment [versus crisis assessment] after admission tends to focus on the patient's symptomatology [versus strengths and problem-solving ability] as the major cause of admission" (Polak, 1967, p. 153).

Institutionalization is certainly more expensive than community-based crisis intervention, but that is not the only consideration. The institutionalization of the upset person can possibly make matters worse, and certainly more complicated. After diagnosis, the person takes on the identity of a patient and falls into roles expected by the institution. The classic works of Becker (1963), Goffman (1961), and Lemert (1951) are supported by recent research (Link, Phelan, Bresnahan, Stueve, & Pescosolido, 1997) documenting the enduring negative effects of psychiatric labeling, *even* when psychiatric treatment has had positive results. Essentially, the same thing can happen to an adolescent confined to a detention home. But some families do request institutionalization for disturbed or aggressive people when they can no longer care for them at home.

Today, however, those for whom psychiatric inpatient treatment is indicated and truly necessary face triple jeopardy because of continued disparity in health insurance for the treatment of emotional and mental illness. (1) They may have to "invent" a life-threatening crisis as a ticket to hospital admission. (2) Once there, they suffer the possible negative fallout of living with the psychiatric diagnosis required for reimbursement of treatment costs. (3) Once discharged and often before recommended treatment is completed, they are at greater risk of repeat crisis episodes and readmission for hospital treatment. The human and financial costs of psychiatric recidivism from this misguided approach are enormous, tragic, and mostly preventable.

This scenario is most acute and potentially most damaging for seriously disturbed or out-of-control children and adolescents in the United States, a situation that has reached crisis proportions nationwide. Admission of these children to general pediatric wards, adult psychiatric units, or detention, combined with the administration of psychotropic drugs never tested for use with children, reveals the need for two policy actions: (1) the provision of special child and adolescent psychiatric inpatient treatment services and (2) the return to the prevention and early intervention ideals of community-based and twenty-four-hour, seven-day-a-week access to comprehensive crisis service and outpatient treatment, as recommended by the Congressional Joint Commission on Mental Health and Illness a half century ago (1961).

Older adults as well are vulnerable to the hazards of psychiatric labeling. Besides their greater risk for organically based diseases such as Parkinson's or Alzheimer's, many older people suffer from depression (Osgood, 1992). In most instances, their depression is linked to the series of losses that many have endured at this stage of the life cycle—for example, life partner, physical health or mobility, friends who have died or are unable to visit. One gerontologist advised primary care providers to apply *functional* instead of psychiatric diagnostic criteria when assessing such persons. As he aptly noted, an eighty-five-year-old man grieving the loss of his spouse and his own failing health does not need to go to his grave with a psychiatric label.

Every society has social norms—that is, expectations of how people are to interact with others. When people deviate from these norms, sanctions are applied or stigmas attached to pressure the deviant member to return to acceptable norms of behavior, suffer the consequences of their deviance, or behave in accord with their stigmatized status. Deviance can therefore be considered from three perspectives as illustrated in the following examples:

1. In Western societies, a widow may be socially ostracized if she mourns the loss of her husband beyond the generally accepted few weeks. If she does so, she deviates from the expected norm for grief and mourning in a death-denying society.
2. A person who is caught and convicted of stealing a car or molesting a child has engaged in behavior that is explicitly forbidden in most societies. Although these are clear-cut examples of deviance, the results of such violations vary. For example, an African American is more likely to be apprehended and judged harshly for the car theft than is a white person in the United States.
3. Some people are considered deviant not for particular actions but for some aspect of their being. Thus, a gay person, a woman in menopause, an old

person, or a handicapped individual carries a "mark" and can be stigmatized as a result of a physical, social, or mental attribute. The physical or social mark (difference) may become indistinguishable from the person's identity. Goffman (1963) in his classic work on stigma refers to this as "spoiled identity." Thus, a person does not *suffer* from paraplegia or schizophrenia but *is* a paraplegic or schizophrenic; the person who takes his or her own life does not just *commit* suicide but *is* a suicide; a woman with a tumultuous social history that often includes sexual abuse as a child is not just difficult to treat but *is* a "borderline" (Everett & Gallop, 2000). The person's identity becomes encompassed in a particular behavior or physical or mental characteristic.

Labeling theory, a controversial topic in social science, continues as the subject of lively debate (Gove 1975; Link et al., 1997; Scheff, 1975). Briefly, labeling theory proposes the concepts of primary and secondary deviance in an interactive relationship, as illustrated in Figure 3.2. The argument between advocates and critics of labeling theory centers on this question: Would secondary deviance occur if the person who is labeled did not experience both an altered self-concept and a change in the way others perceive him or her? An extreme view is that primary deviance could virtually be dismissed except for the detrimental effects of labeling and secondary deviance following it. In contrast, Gove (1978) suggests that the higher rates of depression among women have nothing to do with the labeling of mental illness. Rather, he says, depression among women is related to their disadvantaged position in society. This may be so, particularly if women are socialized to *endure* rather than *resist* oppression, as Cloward and Piven (1979) suggest. Each of these positions has implications for crisis assessment as well as for general mental health practice. This is because certain personal attributes or behaviors do not fall into the range of behavior and conditions commonly accepted as normal and desirable. This is primary deviance, which exists whether or not it is identified with a label. For example, some people break social rules even though they are not always caught and identified as rule breakers.

There are distinct disadvantages for those who are labeled because of gender, sexual identity, and other bias (Fausto-Sterling, 2000; Holden, 1986). People may try to "pass" or hide their identities because of the prejudices of others. For example, gay, lesbian, bisexual, and transgendered people are very careful about coming out; many women will not reveal their age, or they become avid consumers of beauty aids to keep a youthful appearance; people with a psychiatric problem may not wish to reveal the diagnosis, as they often experience prejudice in the job market. Alternatively, people may feel compelled to act as others expect. For example, misbehaving children inappropriately labeled as disabled refer to their social security disability checks as "crazy" money; convicted lawbreakers often repeat their offenses; or a person diagnosed with schizophrenia may say, "How do you expect me to succeed in this job? I'm a schizophrenic." Diagnostic labeling has also been critiqued for its inappropriate application cross-culturally (Hagey & McDonough, 1984), its ethical implications (Mitchell, 1991), and its lack of

FIGURE 3.2. RELATIONSHIP BETWEEN PRIMARY AND SECONDARY DEVIANCE.

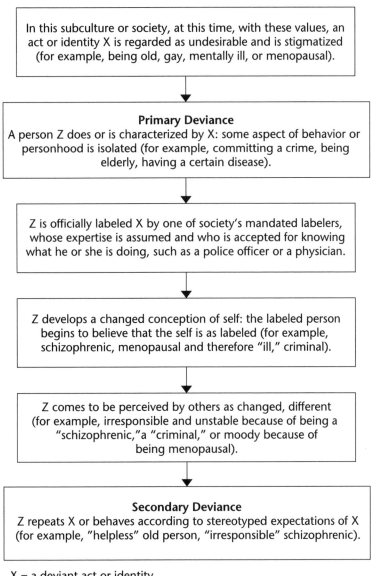

In this subculture or society, at this time, with these values, an act or identity X is regarded as undesirable and is stigmatized (for example, being old, gay, mentally ill, or menopausal).

Primary Deviance
A person Z does or is characterized by X: some aspect of behavior or personhood is isolated (for example, committing a crime, being elderly, having a certain disease).

Z is officially labeled X by one of society's mandated labelers, whose expertise is assumed and who is accepted for knowing what he or she is doing, such as a police officer or a physician.

Z develops a changed conception of self: the labeled person begins to believe that the self is as labeled (for example, schizophrenic, menopausal and therefore "ill," criminal).

Z comes to be perceived by others as changed, different (for example, irresponsible and unstable because of being a "schizophrenic," a "criminal," or moody because of being menopausal).

Secondary Deviance
Z repeats X or behaves according to stereotyped expectations of X (for example, "helpless" old person, "irresponsible" schizophrenic).

X = a deviant act or identity.
Z = a particular person labeled as deviant.

(Thanks to John McKinlay for his ideas about representing labeling theory in this format.)

scientific objectivity (Cooksey & Brown, 1998). In cases of domestic abuse, it can obscure the primary *social* issue of violence (Hoff, 2000).

Labeling theory is particularly relevant to crisis assessment practice and in the relationship of crisis to illness. If crisis is viewed as an opportunity for change and growth rather than as an illness or occasion for social or psychiatric labeling, assessment can be an important step toward growth. But crisis assessment should not be confused with traditional psychiatric diagnosis; in the view of many, psychiatry is not highly scientific, and diagnoses can often be contradictory, despite current emphasis on the biological correlates of mental illness (Cohen, 1993). The DSM, sometimes referred to as the bible of psychiatric diagnosticians, has come under particular scrutiny for its social biases and the disproportionate power it wields as a standard for the meager insurance reimbursement available under managed care for mentally disturbed people (see especially Cooksey & Brown, 1998; Caplan, 1995; and Stark, Flitcraft, & Frazier, 1979). Psychological evaluation is inherently subjective and often tinged with political considerations, as these authors attest and the conflicting opinions on the trauma and emotional health of Elián Gonzalez, the Cuban boy rescued at sea, illustrate. Another example of this is the contradictory evidence presented by psychiatrists representing the defense and the prosecution in criminal cases with insanity pleas. This does not mean that efforts to improve the objectivity of psychiatric diagnostic procedures should stop. Nor does it deny the fact that some people in crisis are also mentally disturbed and therefore diagnosable in a psychiatric framework. It simply means that a crisis experience should be assessed and approached in a crisis—not an illness—framework, so that negative outcomes such as illness are avoided. If illness was present before the crisis, the chances of its recurrence are reduced with timely crisis care. Crisis assessment and intervention should not be cast in a medical framework because this currently accessible, humane approach to helping distressed people might then become as bureaucratic and inaccessible as some aspects of the traditional health care system (Warshaw, 1989). In short, one might ask, Why attach a diagnostic label that is actually or potentially damaging, when illness may not be the central issue and when the person's subjective meaning system is central to the crisis resolution process? Anthropologist Tanya Luhrmann's (2000) extensive field study of medical residents training to be psychiatrists offers some profoundly disturbing answers to this question, many intertwined with theoretical, economic, and moral issues. See also Nehls's research (1999) regarding patients' experience of psychiatric labeling and its stigma.

The negative results of inadequate assessment and psychiatric patient identity are dramatically revealed in a study by Rosenhan (1973). The study uncovered the destructive effects of placing disturbed people in psychiatric hospitals and labeling them with a psychiatric diagnosis such as schizophrenia. Rosenhan demonstrated that the psychiatric professionals charged with the admission and diagnosis of those regarded as insane could not distinguish between pseudopatients and the truly disturbed. This was so even when the professionals were forewarned by the researcher that certain people presenting themselves for hospital admission would be pseudopatients. Once the pseudopatients were hospitalized, their subsequent behavior was interpreted within the framework of their psychiatric label, although their behavior was normal. Consequently, they had a difficult time getting released from the hospital even though they had no objective signs of mental illness. The study supports Polak's (1967) observations that psychiatric hospitalization

- Is a crisis in itself
- Is the direct result of previously undetected and unresolved crisis
- Should be avoided whenever possible
- Should be used only as a last resort when all other efforts to help have failed
- Should be substituted, whenever possible, with accurate crisis assessment and intervention in the person's natural social setting

Now that psychiatric hospitalization is less common, and thousands are discharged without housing or adequate community support, mentally disturbed people nevertheless endure similar biases and burdens in life on the streets (Hoff, 1993; Johnson, 1990).

This discussion supports the earlier recommendations about assessment and intervention in natural settings (see Chapter One). It is not that psychiatrists and other mental health professionals do not understand the difference between crisis and mental illness, but once a patient is admitted to a medical or hospital establishment, managed care policies require diagnosing them. The potentially damaging results of psychiatric labeling occur in the context of continuing cultural bias against the mentally ill, including disparity in insurance for treatment. Capponi (1992), for example, describes the challenges faced by "psychiatric survivors" of the system purportedly designed to help them.

Inadequate assessment has another negative result. When there is only the *appearance*—not the reality—of crisis, an ill-advised response might reinforce crisis-like behavior as well as the notion that the only way to get help is to convince health care providers that there is a crisis. This pattern is observed increasingly in calls to hotlines from discharged mental patients or chronically ill people who lack the longer-term treatment and support their condition requires. The complexity and danger of this situation for suicidal people is discussed further in Chapter Six. The person in crisis and the family should be advised, therefore, that there are many alternative ways of resolving life's crises (Breggin, 1992; Hoff & Adamowski, 1998; Polak, 1976).

The Distinctiveness of Crisis Assessment

The ability to discriminate, then, between a crisis and a noncrisis state requires prediction and assessment skills. Good intentions are not enough. The development of assessment skills does not take years of intensive study and training. It does require the ability to combine what is known from observing and helping distressed people with the natural tendency to assist someone in trouble. Teachers, parents, nurses, police, physicians, and clergy are on the front lines where life crises occur. In these roles, people can do a great deal to help others and prevent unnecessary casualties, especially when formal training is added to one's natural crisis intervention ability (Hoff & Adamowski, 1998).

Ivan Illich (1976) asserts that the bureaucratization of medicine has deprived ordinary people of the helping tools they could readily use on behalf of others if the system allowed their use. His point is consistent with the current emphasis on primary care and responsibility for one's own health. Bureaucracies jeopardize the human aspect of the crisis intervention approach, which has made it an accessible, inoffensive way for distressed people to receive help. Similarly, the pervasiveness of individualism and the power of biomedicine (Barney, 1994) present a temptation to medicalize the crisis assessment and intervention process. As many tools as possible should be available to people who are willing and able to help others. By sharpening the assessment and helping techniques that people have always used, frontline workers become particularly suited for prevention of acute crises. When a full-blown crisis is in progress, frontline workers such as primary care providers usually must collaborate creatively with counselors and mental health professionals, who are trained to do a more comprehensive crisis assessment. The different levels of assessment are discussed in the next section. Thus, the crisis approach can be grounded in theory and sound principles of practice without taking on the disadvantages of elitism among human service workers. The distinctiveness of crisis assessment can be summarized as follows:

1. The crisis assessment *process*, unlike traditional psychiatric diagnosis, is intricately tied to crisis *resolution*. Besides the issues already discussed, this is another compelling reason why assessment in comprehensive crisis care cannot be overstressed. For example, if a highly anxious person learns during assessment that the fear of "going crazy" is a typical crisis response, fear is relieved, and the person is already helped along the path of positive crisis resolution. Applied to a primary care office setting, this principle implies that within a single visit there must be some preliminary resolution, if only providing support and firm linkage to a mental health professional.

2. Crisis assessment occurs immediately, rather than days or weeks later as in traditional psychiatric practice.

3. The focus in crisis assessment is on immediate, identifiable problems, rather than on personality dynamics or presumed coping deficits. Once the problems are identified, assessment proceeds to ascertain the person's cognitive, emotional, and behavioral functioning in relation to them. (Primary care providers may refer to this as the Mini–Mental Status Examination, discussed under "Cognitive Response" later in this chapter.)

4. Historical material is dealt with in a special way in crisis assessment. Probing into psychodynamic issues such as unresolved childhood conflicts and repressed emotions is inappropriate. In contrast, it is not only appropriate but also necessary to obtain a person's history of solving problems, resolving crises, and

dealing with stressful life events. Such historical material is vital for assessing and mobilizing the personal and social resources needed to effect positive crisis outcomes. It can be obtained by asking, for example, "What have you done in the past that has worked for you when you're upset?"

5. Crisis assessment is not complete without an evaluation of risk to life (see Chapters Six, Eight, and Nine).

6. Crisis assessment is not something done *to* a person but is a process carried out *with* a person and in active collaboration with significant others. A service contract is therefore a logical outcome of appropriate crisis assessment.

7. Social and cultural factors and community resources are integral to a comprehensive crisis assessment because the origins and manifestations of crisis are social as often as they are individual.

The Assessment Process

Knowledge of factors that predict risk of crisis guides us in assessing particular individuals in distress. However, health and human service workers encountering a distressed person may still have many questions: What do I say? What questions should I ask? How do I find out what's really happening with someone who seems so confused and upset? How do I recognize a person in crisis? If the person in crisis is not crazy, what distinguishes him or her from someone who is mentally disturbed but not in active crisis? What roles do the family and community play on behalf of the person in crisis? In short, as in general medical care, human service workers need a structured framework for the assessment process.

Distinguishing Levels of Assessment

Two levels of assessment should be completed. Specific questions must be addressed at each level.

Level I. The following questions are key for completing a Level I assessment: Is there an obvious or potential threat to life, either the life of the individual in crisis or the lives of others? In other words, has the person been abused? And what are the risks of suicide, assault, and homicide?

Level I assessment should be done by everyone, including people in their natural roles of friend, neighbor, parent, and spouse, as well as people in various professional positions: physicians, nurses, teachers, police, clergy, welfare workers, and prison officials. *This level of assessment is critical.* It has life-and-death dimensions and forms the basis for mobilizing emergency services on behalf of the person, family, or community in crisis.

Every person in crisis should be assessed regarding victimization and danger to self and others (Hoff & Rosenbaum, 1994). (Techniques for assessment of suicidal danger are presented in detail in Chapter Six. Assessment for victimization trauma is presented in Chapter Eight. Assessing the risk of assault or homicide is discussed in Chapter Nine.) Here, a key facet of crisis work is emphasized: *no crisis assessment is complete without inquiring directly about victimization and the danger of suicide and assault or homicide.*

If a layperson, frontline health worker, or professional without special crisis training ascertains that a person is a probable risk for abuse, suicide, assault, or homicide, an experienced professional crisis worker should be consulted for Level II assessment and follow-through. Some life-threatening situations must be approached collaboratively with the police or forensic psychiatry specialists (see Chapter Nine). Most crisis and psychiatric emergency services have such collaborative relationships for handling high-risk crises (Hoff & Wells, 1989).

Level II. This more extensive assessment involves consideration of the personal and social characteristics of the distressed person and the person's family. This is usually done by a trained crisis counselor or mental health professional. Questions in Level II assessment include all Level I questions regarding victimization trauma and risk of harming self and others, plus the following: Is there evidence that the person is unable to function in his or her usual life role? Is the person in danger of being extruded from his or her natural social setting? What are the psychological, socioeconomic, and other factors related to the person's coping with life's stressors? Level II assessment is comprehensive and corresponds to the elements of the total crisis experience:

1. *Identification of crisis origins.* What hazardous events occurred? Is there turmoil associated with a stressful situation or a major transition state? What sociocultural factors are involved?
2. *Development of crisis.* Is the person in the initial or acute phase of crisis? (See "How a Crisis Develops" in Chapter Two.)
3. *Manifestations of crisis.* How does the person interpret hazardous events or situations, and what are the corresponding emotional, cognitive, behavioral, and biophysical responses to them? Are the events perceived as threat, loss, or challenge? Does the person deal with the accompanying stress effectively?
4. *Identification of resources.* These include personal, family, interpersonal, and material resources.
5. *Determination of the sociocultural milieu.* This pertains to the environment of the person or family in crisis.

All professional human service workers should acquire skill in this kind of assessment if they do not already have it. Close friends and family members are often able to make such an assessment as well. The chances for their success depend on their personal level of self-confidence, general experience, and previous success in helping others with problems. In general, however, a person unaccustomed to dealing with acutely distressed people or with no special training in crisis intervention should consult experienced professional crisis counselors. This is especially important in assessing people in complex, multiproblem, life-threatening, or catastrophic situations. The different foci and performances of Level I and Level II assessments are summarized in Table 3.1. Let us now consider the assessment process in detail.

TABLE 3.1. CRISIS ASSESSMENT LEVELS.

	Focus of Assessment	Assessment Done By
Level I	Risk to life • Victimization • Suicide (self) • Assault/homicide (child, partner, parent, mental health or community worker, police officer)	Everyone (natural and formal crisis managers) • Family, friends, neighbors • Hotline workers • Frontline workers: clergy, police officers, nurses, physicians, teachers • Crisis and mental health professionals
Level II	Comprehensive psychological and social aspects of the person's life pertaining to the hazardous event, including assessment of chronic self-destructiveness	Counselors or mental health professionals specially trained in crisis work (formal crisis managers)

Identifying Origins and Phases of Crisis Development

A basic step in crisis assessment is identification of the events or situations that led to the person's distress. Sifneos (1960, p. 177) and Golan (1969) elaborate on Caplan's concept (1964) of crisis development in phases. They differentiate between the hazardous event and the precipitating factor, which, along with the person's vulnerability, constitute the components of the crisis state. As noted in Chapter Two, stressful and shocking events can arise from personal or material sources, transition states, or sociocultural situations.

The *hazardous event* is the initial shock or situation that sets in motion a series of reactions culminating in a crisis (Golan, 1969). If the event is not already apparent, the helping person should ask directly, "What happened?" Sometimes people are so upset or overwhelmed by a series of things that they cannot clearly identify the sequence of events. In these instances, it is helpful to ask when the person began feeling so upset. Simple, direct questions should be asked about the time and circumstances of all upsetting or dangerous events. Putting events in order has a calming effect; the person experiences a certain sense of self-possession in being able to make some order out of confusion. This is particularly true for the highly anxious person who is afraid of losing control or "going crazy."

The experience of stressful, hazardous events is not in itself a crisis. It is one of several components of the crisis state. After all, just getting on with our lives implies the everyday management of stressful events. Extensive experience and research with abused women, for example, reveal them as capable survivors despite daunting odds (Hoff, 1990). The question is, How is *this* particular event unusual in terms of its timing, severity, danger, or the person's ability to handle it successfully? This component of crisis corresponds to Caplan's (1964) first phase of crisis development, which may or may not develop into a full-blown crisis, depending on personal and social circumstances (see the example of John,

Chapter Two). Early prevention and strategic intervention are pivotal in avoiding a full-blown crisis.

Because hazardous events alone are insufficient to constitute a crisis state, we need also to focus our assessment process on the *immediacy* of the person's stress—the precipitating factor. This is the proverbial straw that broke the camel's back—the final, stressful event in a series of such events or a situation that pushes the person from a state of acute vulnerability into crisis. The precipitating event is not always easy to identify, particularly when the presenting problem seems to have been hazardous for a long time.

The *precipitating factor* is often a minor incident. It can nevertheless take on crisis proportions in the context of other stressful events and the person's inability to use usual problem-solving devices. In this sense, it resembles Caplan's third phase of crisis development, following the failure of ordinary problem solving (the second phase). It corresponds to what Polak (1967) calls the final event that moves people to bring a family member to a psychiatric hospital after a series of antecedent crises. In a series of crises experienced by the same person, the precipitating factor in one crisis episode may be the hazardous event in the next. Thus, in real life—as opposed to theoretical discussion and models—hazardous events or situations and precipitating factors may be hard to distinguish. Yet, determining the mutual presence of these two components is useful in the assessment process, especially for distinguishing between *chronic stress* and an *acute crisis state*. For example, a chronic problem rather than a crisis is suggested in this interchange:

Question: What brought you here *today,* since these problems have been with you for some time now?

Response: I was watching a television program on depression and finally decided to get help for my problems.

Careful assessment can prevent the mistake of referring to a person experiencing repeated crisis episodes as one in *chronic crisis*—a contradiction in terms. A review of histories revealing repeated crisis experiences suggests that (1) comprehensive crisis care was not implemented, or (2) providers mistakenly assumed that crisis intervention alone would address serious problems demanding longer-term treatment. Such examples underscore a key concept in this book: *crisis care is necessary but not always sufficient*—the limitations of managed care policies notwithstanding.

Assessing Individual Crisis Manifestations

In crisis assessment, the identification of hazardous events or situations and the precipitating factor must be placed in meaningful context. This is done by ascertaining the subjective reaction of the person to stressful events. Sifneos (1960) and Golan (1969) refer to this component of crisis assessment as the "vulnerable state." It corresponds to Caplan's second and fourth phases of crisis development. Its focus is on the emotional, biophysical, cognitive, and behavioral responses that the person makes to recent stressful events. A person's subjective response can be elicited by questions such as those illustrated in Table 3.2. The answers to questions like these are important for several reasons:

- They provide essential information to determine whether or not a person is in crisis.
- They suggest whether the person's problem-solving ability and usual coping devices are, for example, healthy or unhealthy, and how these ways of coping are related to what Caplan calls the personal, material, and sociocultural supplies needed to avoid crisis.
- They provide information about the meaning of stressful life events to various people and about the individual's particular definition of the situation, which is essential to a personally tailored intervention plan.
- They link the assessment process to intervention strategies by providing baseline data for action and for learning new ways of coping.

TABLE 3.2. ASSESSING PERSONAL RESPONSES.

Sample Assessment Questions	Possible Verbal Responses	Interpretation in Terms of Personal Crisis Manifestations (Emotional, Cognitive, Behavioral)
How do you feel about what happened? (for example, divorce or rape)	*Divorce:* I don't want to live without her. If I kill myself, she'll be sorry.	Feelings of desperation, acute loss, revenge (emotional)
(Or if the feelings have already been expressed spontaneously), I can see you're really upset.	*Rape:* I shouldn't have accepted his invitation to have a drink. I suppose it's my fault for being so stupid.	Guilt, self-blame (emotional, cognitive)
What did you do when she told you about wanting a divorce?	I figured, good riddance. I only stayed for the kids' sake. But now that she's gone, I'm really lonely, and I hate the singles' bar scene.	Relief, ambivalence (emotional, cognitive)
	Or: I went down to the bar and got drunk and have been drinking a lot ever since.	Unable to cope effectively, desire to escape loneliness (emotional, behavioral)
How do you usually handle problems that are upsetting to you?	I generally talk to my closest friend or just get away by myself for a while to think things through.	Generally effective coping ability (behavioral, cognitive)
Why didn't this work for you this time?	My closest friend moved away, and I just haven't found anyone else to talk to that I really trust.	Realization of need for substitute support (cognitive, behavioral)

The relationship between hazardous events or situations, people's responses to them (their vulnerability), and the precipitating factor is illustrated in Figure 3.3.

The answers to our assessment questions provide a broad picture of what Hansell (1976) calls "crisis plumage," the distinguishing characteristics of a person in crisis compared with one who is not. This plumage consists of distress signals that people send to others when they experience a loss or a threat of loss, are abused or in danger, or are challenged to increase their supplies—their basic needs or life attachments. Signals of distress include the following:

1. Difficulty in managing one's feelings
2. Suicidal or homicidal tendencies
3. Alcohol or other drug abuse
4. Trouble with the law
5. Inability to effectively use available help

FIGURE 3.3.   COMPONENTS OF THE CRISIS STATE.

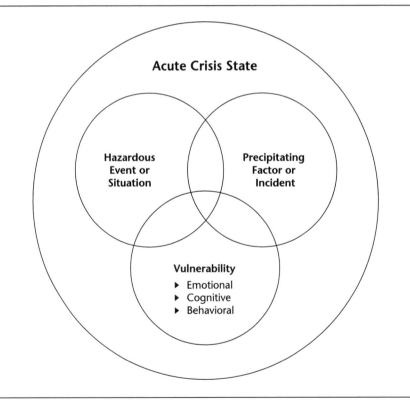

The components in the intertwining circles represent the interactional process that characterizes the crisis experience.

These signals usually indicate that a person is coping ineffectively with a crisis and needs assistance to forestall negative crisis outcomes. In short, people proceed through life with material, personal, and sociocultural resources, as well as problem-solving devices for dealing with various stressors. When these resources are intact, people generally avoid the possible negative outcomes of stressful life events. For example, in assessing the vulnerability of an assault victim, careful attention must be paid to the circumstances of victimization (Sales, Baum, & Shore, 1984). In contrast, if the attack is linked to the victim's character traits, we are very close to victim blaming, which hampers the person's recovery and may contribute to the downward spiral depicted in Figure 2.2, Chapter Two. When psychosocial resources are lacking, the person in crisis usually seeks help from others to compensate for a temporary inability to deal constructively with life's stressors. The help received is crisis intervention. If the help obtained is from human service institutions or professionals, it is known as *formal crisis care,* as distinguished from *natural crisis care.* However, in order to be part of the crisis solution rather than the problem, crisis workers must assess in greater detail the parameters of the individual's vulnerability. To do so requires understanding the emotional, biophysical, cognitive, and behavioral responses to hazardous events. Let us consider, then, the specific characteristics of crisis plumage—how people in crisis feel, think, and act (see Figure 3.1, Box 2).

Feelings and Biophysical Response. People in crisis experience a high degree of anxiety and tension—in short, severe emotional pain. Another common theme is a sense of loss or emptiness. This feeling springs directly from an actual or threat-ened loss in self-esteem, physical well-being, material goods, social relationships, or a failure to reach a life goal, such as promotion or retirement. Other feelings frequently experienced are fear, shock, anger, guilt, embarrassment, or shame. Fear is often expressed in terms of losing control or not understanding why one is responding in a certain way. Anger is often directed inward for not being able to manage one's life or at a significant other for leaving, dying, or inflicting physical or sexual abuse. Guilt and embarrassment often follow anger that does not seem justified. How can one be angry at a dead person when considering one's luck in being alive from an accident or disaster? People who are abused by someone they love often feel ashamed—an outcome of the victim-blaming legacy.

Of all feelings common to the crisis experience, anxiety is probably the most familiar. A certain degree of tension is a normal part of life; it serves to move us to make plans for productive action. Without it, we become nonpro-ductive. For example, Terri, a student, has no anxiety about passing or failing a course. She therefore does not exert the effort required to study and achieve a passing grade. When a person is excessively anxious, however, negative results usually occur. Acute anxiety is one of the most painful experiences a human being can have. However, this does not necessarily imply the presence of a psychiatric disorder.

Anxiety is manifested in a number of ways. Some characteristics will be peculiar to the person concerned. Commonly experienced signs of anxiety are

- Sense of dread
- Fear of losing control
- Inability to focus on one thing
- Physical symptoms—sweating, frequent urination, diarrhea, nausea and vomiting, tachycardia (rapid heartbeat), headache, chest or abdominal pain, rash, menstrual irregularity, and sexual disinterest

---

CASE EXAMPLE: DELAINE

Delaine, age forty-five, feels bereft after the recent death of her husband. Her friends have been supportive since his death from chronic heart disease. She chides herself and feels guilty about not being able to take the loss any better. She knew her husband's condition was precarious; nevertheless, she had depended on him as a readily available source of reassurance. Because she is basically a cheerful person, always on hand to support others in distress, she is embarrassed by what she perceives as weakness following her husband's death.

Because she cries more than usual, Delaine is afraid she may be losing control. At times, she even wonders whether she is going crazy. It should be noted that Delaine is in a major developmental transition to middle age. Also, the oldest of her three children was recently married, leaving her with a sense of loss in her usual mothering role. An additional, but anticipated, loss is the recent news that one of her close friends will soon be leaving town. This threatens to further erode Delaine's base of support. Delaine feels angry about all the losses in her life, asking, "Why does all this have to happen to me all at once?" But she also feels guilty about her anger; after all, her friend deserves the opportunity that the move will afford her and her husband, and Delaine knows her daughter has every right to get married and live her own life.

Complicating Delaine's emotional upheaval, she has developed gastrointestinal symptoms, including bouts of lower abdominal pain and diarrhea. She has avoided her friend's advice to seek counseling but did see her primary care provider around her physical symptoms and requested something to ease her "embarrassing" crying bouts (to be continued in Chapter Four).

What Delaine does not realize are these facts:

- She has a right to her feelings about these disturbing events.
- She has a right and a need to express those feelings.
- Her feelings of loss and anger do not cancel the good feelings and support she can continue to have from her daughter and friend, though in an altered form.
- Her physical symptoms are probably related to the psychosocial facets of her life.

Were it not for these developmental and situational factors, Delaine might not have experienced her husband's death as a crisis. The stability of Delaine's life was disrupted on several counts:

- Her role as wife was changed to that of widow.
- Her role as mother of her oldest daughter was altered by her daughter's marriage.
- Her affectional attachment to her husband was completely severed.
- Her affectional attachment to her friend will be altered in terms of physical distance and immediacy of support.
- Her notion of a full life includes marriage, so she must adjust, at least temporarily, to a change in that perception.
- Her unanticipated physical symptoms need medical attention.

Delaine's case underscores the importance of (1) incorporating crisis assessment strategies—at a minimum, Level I—into primary health care and (2) sorting out through physical examination and laboratory tests the separate and interacting relationship between physical and emotional symptoms (Edmands, Hoff, Kaylor, Mower, & Sorrell, 1999). Primary care providers should not assign a psychiatric diagnosis of *anxiety disorder* without a Level II crisis assessment, which typically includes mental health specialty skills. Implications for treatment based on assessment are discussed in the continuation of Delaine's case in Chapter Four.

Overall the Mental Status Examination (MSE) incorporates cognitive, emotional (for example, mood, anxiety symptoms), and behavioral functioning and is intended for use by trained mental health professionals. Rote decontextualized use of the Mini–Mental Status Examination (MMSE) in primary care can be a barrier, therefore, to truly understanding a distressed person. As Lyness (1997, p. 144) notes, the patient loses MMSE points for wrong answers no matter how close or far off the response is, but clinically, it matters greatly whether a person is off by a day or a century (see also Luhrmann, 2000).

Primary care health providers are cautioned in the use of the MMSE, a thirty-point scale designed for screening cognitive deficits in certain populations, for example, an older person with beginning symptoms of Alzheimer's disease.

In the United States, the constraints of managed care, the disparity in insurance reimbursement for mental health treatment, and the policy requirements of a medical-psychiatric (that is, the *Diagnostic and Statistical Manual of Mental Disorders*, known as DSM-IV) diagnosis are a grim reality facing health professionals. Primary care providers who must practice within these constraints as a prelude to policy changes that might address these issues are urged to assign a diagnosis from Axis V of the DSM-IV—that is, *global assessment of functioning* (GAF). This diagnostic category encompasses many of the items of the Comprehensive Mental Health Assessment form presented in this chapter and has the fewest hazards of a psychiatric label. Health providers should also note that the DSM was developed with the original intent of use by psychiatric–mental health specialists.

In short, mental health providers' assessment skills include the necessary *general* knowledge about medical phenomena to make an appropriate initial response followed by referral to medical specialists; primary care (nonpsychiatric) providers' assessment skills include the necessary *general* knowledge of psychosocial and psychiatric phenomena to make an empathic response, apply crisis intervention strategies such as ensuring safety of self and others, and implement referral to crisis or mental health specialists for comprehensive assessment and care. Instead of concluding that a person suffering the emotional and physiological consequences of stressful events and insufficient supports has an anxiety disorder, a crisis-trained provider would realize that emotional pain is the predictable and normal response to life's normal upheavals and upsetting events and is experienced by most people over the life span. These responses do not require a DSM-IV diagnosis to warrant a health provider's appropriate response, and they *should not* require such a psychiatric label for prepaid insurance coverage (see Luhrmann, 2000, chap. 6, "The Crisis of Managed Care").

Cognitive Response: Thoughts, Perceptions, and Interpretations of Events.

Feelings—especially of high anxiety—have great impact on perceptions and thinking processes. In crisis, one's attention is focused on the acute shock and anguish being experienced and a few items concerning the crisis event. As a consequence, the person's usual memory and way of perceiving may be altered. The person may have difficulty sorting things out. The relationship between events may not seem clear. Acutely anxious people feel caught in a maze of events they cannot fit together. They often have trouble defining who they are and what their skills are. The state of anguish and resulting confusion can alter a person's ability to make decisions and solve problems, the very skills needed during acute anxiety states. This disturbance in perceptual processes and problem-solving ability increases the individual's already heightened state of anxiety. Sometimes the person fears losing control.

The distorted perceptual process observed in crisis states should not be confused with mental illness, in which a person's *usual* pattern of thinking is disturbed, or with acute confusional states (*delirium*), in which altered perceptions are also apparent. In a crisis state, the disturbance arises from and is part of the crisis experience. There is a rapid return to normal perception once the crisis is resolved.

CASE EXAMPLE: JOAN

Joan, age thirty-four, called a mental health center stating that her husband had just left the house with his rifle and that she did not know where he was going. She was afraid for her life, as they had had an argument the night before during which she had complained about his drinking and he had threatened her. On further questioning, it turned out that Joan's husband had left the house at his usual time for work in a neighboring town. He had left with the rifle the previous evening after the argument, although on occasion he also took his gun along to work in case he had a chance to go hunting. After three hours, he had returned, apparently calmed down, and put away the gun. The gun was still in the house in a safe place when Joan called. There was nothing in the interaction to lead an outside observer to conclude that Joan's husband would not be home as usual after a day at work.

Noteworthy in this example is Joan's disturbed perceptual process. On questioning, she cannot recall certain details without help and cannot put all the facts into logical order. Joan is obviously very anxious about her safety, a factor requiring serious attention, especially given the presence of a gun. Complicating this feeling of anxiety is her sense of guilt about her role in precipitating the argument with her husband by mentioning his drinking. Her anxiety is consistent with her perception—not necessarily the reality—of a threat to her safety. The determining factor is how she *perceives* the event. Nevertheless marital discord and the presence of a gun underscore the importance of assessing thoroughly for a history of abuse and safety resources for a woman like Joan. One of the most common complaints from abused women and their advocates is that people do not believe them or take their stories seriously.

The feelings of people in crisis are usually consistent with their perception of the situation (Dressler, 1973). Recognition of this fact should decrease the possibility of casting people with similar problems into a common mold. The perception of the event is one of the factors that makes an event a crisis for one person but not for another.

Joan's case illustrates how excessive anxiety interferes with effective problem solving. If Joan were not so anxious, she would probably have arrived at an obvious way to ensure her immediate safety—that is, removing the gun or leaving the house herself and seeking help. Joan probably knows that the use of weapons is intrinsically connected with their availability, but her anxiety prevents her from using that knowledge.

Other aspects of cognitive functioning spring from different socialization processes and value systems that influence how particular events are interpreted. Illness, for example, has a different meaning and crisis potential for various ethnic and religious groups (see Chapter Eleven). A state legislator who was jailed for a minor offense killed himself hours after being imprisoned. For this elected figure, the transgression meant loss of reputation, whereas a person arrested for repeated drunken driving may interpret the event differently because of having less to lose. People socialized to feel incomplete without marriage will probably experience the loss of a spouse as an occasion of crisis, whereas others grow from the challenges of greater independence. These examples illustrate the importance of being culturally sensitive and not imposing our own values and behavior norms on others. No situation or disturbance affects two people in the same way, and the same person may respond differently to similar events at different times in life. Thus, interpersonal *process*—not rote mental status examination—should be central as we assess varying subjective interpretations of life events.

Behavior. Behavior usually follows from what people think and feel and from their interpretations of life events. A person who feels anxious and has a distorted perception of events is likely to behave in unusual ways. However, what may seem unusual, distorted, or crazy to an outsider may be considered normal behavior within certain cultural groups. In order to determine whether a person's behavior is normal or deviant, we need to start with *that* person's cultural definition of what is usual, not our own. This is particularly important if the crisis worker and the person in distress are from different cultures, classes, or ethnic groups. If the distressed person is too upset to provide this kind of information, it should be elicited from family or friends whenever possible. Failing that, a consultation with someone of the person's ethnic or cultural group would be useful.

A significant behavioral sign of crisis is the individual's inability to perform normal vocational functions in the usual manner—for example, when a person cannot do necessary household chores, concentrate on studies, or work at an outside job. Another sign is a change in social behavior, such as withdrawing from friends, making unusual efforts to avoid being alone, or becoming clingy or demanding (Hansell, 1976). As social connections break down, the person may also feel detached or distant from others. Some people in crisis act on impulse. They may drive a car recklessly, make a suicide attempt, or attack others as a desperate means of solving a problem (see Chapters Six and Nine).

Some people will go out of their way to reject the assistance offered by friends. Often this response arises out of the person's sense of helplessness and embarrassment at not being able to cope in the usual manner. The person fears that acceptance of help may be misinterpreted as a confirmation of perceived weakness. To allay such fears, it is paramount that crisis workers examine the attitudes and any biases they may bring to the assessment milieu. People in crisis are also observed to behave in ways that are inconsistent with their thoughts and feelings. For example, a young woman witnessed a shooting accident that caused the death of her boyfriend. Initially, she was visibly upset by the event. She was brought by her family to a mental health emergency clinic. During the interview with a counselor, she laughed inappropriately when talking about the shooting and death she had witnessed, a behavior suggesting very high anxiety. Another behavioral signal of crisis is atypical behavior, such as driving while intoxicated by an individual with no previous record of such behavior.

In summary, when assessing vulnerability, it is important to find out how *this* person is reacting *here and now* to whatever happened. The simplest way to assess a person's vulnerability is to ask, "How do you feel about what happened? What do you usually do when you're upset?" and similar questions suggested in Table 3.2.

Family and Community Assessment

Our discussion of the assessment process thus far has focused primarily on techniques to determine the hazardous events or situations precipitating the crisis and the individual's vulnerability as revealed in personal responses to these events—emotional, cognitive, behavioral, and biophysical. Crisis assessment, however, is incomplete without evaluating the person's social resources and cultural milieu. This includes inquiring whether the person perceives family and other social contacts as real or potential assets or as liabilities. Asking whether network members are part of the problem or part of the solution is often the full extent of social assessment in much of crisis practice, in spite of historical emphasis on sociocultural factors (Caplan, 1964). In this book, social assessment means that the person's social network members are deliberately—not just incidentally—included in the assessment process. This is not difficult to do, but it does require the worker's knowledge of its importance and the willingness to make the effort. Often workers cite a lack of time or inaccessibility of the family as reasons for limiting the assessment to the upset individual. But this probably obscures their own lack of conviction or skills in the use of social approaches. In view of what is known about the social aspects of crisis responses, these issues should be examined in order to refine crisis assessment and intervention strategies.

Including a social approach in crisis assessment reduces misidentifying who is in crisis. That is, sometimes the person who appears or is brought in for help may be upset but not in crisis. A complete assessment could reveal that an entire family is in crisis, as could happen, for example, when a teenager tries to commit suicide.

Evaluation of the sociocultural context and community resources is related to family assessment; the context may figure in the origin and resolution of crises, as illustrated in the Crisis Paradigm. Evaluation should include questions about whether the person has received necessary help from community resources, as well as inquiries about cultural and socioeconomic factors that may contribute to the person's vulnerability and ability to resolve crises constructively. For example, negative factors, such as racial unrest, or positive ones, such as opportunities for welfare mothers to become economically self-sufficient, should be considered. These aspects of comprehensive crisis assessment and their implications for intervention are discussed further in Chapter Five.

The individual and sociocultural aspects of crisis assessment are summarized and illustrated with examples in Table 3.3. This diagram elaborates on the concept of healthy and unhealthy coping. It outlines the relationship between crisis origins and personal manifestations of crisis (see Figure 3.1, Boxes 1 and 2). It also links the crisis assessment process to various intervention techniques. For example, if assessment reveals that a person is coping well in general terms—emotional, biophysical, cognitive, and behavioral—the information received can be used to help the person cope more effectively. Careful assessment can also show when not to intervene—in areas where the person's coping is adequate or the person chooses to do without our services. Even a person who is acutely upset can be helped to realize that he or she is coping adequately in *some* aspects of life (for example, at work but not at home or vice versa). In short, a skilled crisis worker avoids doing either too little or too much. An old adage applies here: "if it's not broken, don't fix it."

TABLE 3.3.   DIFFERENTIATION: EFFECTIVE AND INEFFECTIVE CRISIS COPING ACCORDING TO CRISIS EPISODE.

Crisis Episode			Crisis Coping	
Hazardous Event	**Origin**	**Personal Manifestations**	**Ineffective**	**Effective**
Loss of child by death	*Situational:* Unexplained physical malfunctioning of child, for example, SIDS	Emotional	Depression	Grief work
		Biophysical	Stomach or other ailments	
		Cognitive	Conviction of having done something wrong to cause death of the child	Recognizing and accepting that one used all available knowledge to prevent the death
		Behavioral	Inability to care for other children appropriately (for example, overprotectiveness)	Attending peer support group
Physical battering by partner	*Sociocultural:* Values and other factors affecting relationships	Emotional	Crying, depression, feelings of worthlessness, self-blame, and helplessness	Anger, shock (How could he do this to me?), outrage at the fact that it happened
		Cognitive	Assumption that the beating was justified: inability to decide what to do	Conviction of inappropriateness of violence between men and women, decision to leave and/or otherwise reorder one's life free of violence
		Behavioral	Alcohol abuse, abuse of children, excusing of partner's violence	Seeking refuge in nonviolent shelter, initiating steps toward economic independence, participating in peer group support and social change activities

The next section describes a structured approach to carrying out the assessment process, using the concepts discussed so far.

An Assessment Interview

An interview (see Table 3.4) with George Sloan, age forty-eight, is conducted by an emergency department nurse. George is brought to the hospital by police following an attempt to commit suicide by crashing his car. (This case illustration is continued from Chapter Two.)

Besides the technical aspects of asking clear, direct questions, this interview excerpt illustrates another important point. The nurse reveals an understanding of George's problem and empathizes with the despair he must be feeling when she says,

- "So your car accident was really an attempt to kill yourself?"
- "Sounds like you've been having a rough time, George."
- "I can see that your illness and all the other troubles have left you feeling pretty bad."
- "George, I can see that you're feeling desperate about your situation."
- "I'm glad your suicide attempt didn't work."

The nurse clearly comes through as a human being with feelings and concern about a patient who is in despair. Concern is conveyed by a gentle tone of voice and unstylized manner. Furthermore the nurse is able to express feelings without sounding sentimental and shocked and apparently is not afraid to be with a person in the acute emotional pain of crisis. As shown by this interview, effective assessment techniques are not highly complicated or veiled in mystery. The techniques require the following:

- A straightforward approach with simple direct questions
- The ability to empathize or appreciate the other person's perspective
- An ability to grasp the depth of another's despair and share the feelings this evokes
- The courage not to run away from frightening experiences like suicide attempts

The interview also shows that ascertaining suicide risk (Level I assessment) is an integral part of thorough crisis assessment. Parents, teachers, friends, and police can augment their natural tendencies to help by learning these assessment techniques. Failure to use the techniques can mean the difference between life and death for someone like George Sloan. It is not uncommon for people in his condition to be treated medically or surgically without anyone finding out about his intention to commit suicide. If he receives only medical or surgical treatment and nothing else changes in his life, George Sloan is at risk of committing suicide within six to twelve months. He is already in a high-risk category (see Chapter Six).

TABLE 3.4.   ASSESSMENT INTERVIEW EXAMPLE.

Assessment Techniques	Interview Between George Sloan and Emergency Department Nurse
Signals of Distress and Crisis to Be Identified	*Nurse:* Hello, Mr. Sloan. Would you like to be called Mr. Sloan or George? *George:* George is fine. *Nurse:* Will you tell me what happened, George? *George:* I had a car accident. Can't you see that without asking? (slightly hostile and seemingly reluctant to talk) *Nurse:* Yes, I know, George. But the police said you were going the wrong way on the expressway. How did that happen?
Active Crisis State: Extreme anxiety to the breaking point	*George:* Yes, that's right. (hesitates) Well, I just couldn't take it anymore, but I guess it didn't work. *Nurse:* Sounds like you've been having a rough time, George. Can you tell me what it is you can't take anymore?
Hazardous Event/ Situation: Physical illness	*George:* Well, I've got heart trouble . . .
Vulnerable State: Loss of external social supports or inability to use them	It's gotten to be too much for my wife. I can't expect her to do much more.
Loss of personal coping ability	We're having trouble with our 16-year-old son, Arnold.
Inability to communicate stress to significant others	I just couldn't take it anymore. I figured I'd do everybody a favor and get rid of myself.
High-lethal suicide attempt	*Nurse:* So your car accident was really an attempt to kill yourself? *George:* That's right. That way, at least my wife wouldn't lose the insurance along with everything else she's had to put up with. *Nurse:* I can see that your heart trouble and all your other troubles have left you feeling pretty bad.
Depression	*George:* That's about it, too bad I came out alive. I really feel I'm worth more dead than alive. *Nurse:* I can see that you're feeling desperate about your situation. How long have you felt this way? *George:* I've had heart trouble for about four years. After my last heart attack, the doctor told me I had to slow down or it would probably kill me. Well, there's no way I can change things that I can see.
Precipitating Factor: Inability to perform in expected role as father	*Nurse:* What happened this past week that made you decide to end it all? *George:* Well, our kid Arnold got suspended from school—that did it! I figured if a father can't do any better with his son than that, what's the use? *Nurse:* I gather from what you say and feel that you just couldn't see any other way out.

TABLE 3.4. ASSESSMENT INTERVIEW EXAMPLE. (*continued*)

Assessment Techniques	Interview Between George Sloan and Emergency Department Nurse	
State of Active Crisis: Vulnerability: Fixation on role expectations, inability to use outside helping resources	*George:*	That's right. Money is really getting tight; my wife was talking about getting a full-time job, and that really bothers me to think that I can't support my family anymore. And if she starts working more, things might get even worse with Arnold. There was no one to talk to. Suicide's the only thing left.
	Nurse:	With all these problems, George, have you ever thought about suicide before?
History of poor coping ability	*George:*	Yes, once, after my doctor told me to really watch it after my last heart attack. I felt pretty hopeless and thought of crashing my car then. But things weren't so bad then between me and my wife, and she talked me out of it and seemed willing to stick with me.
	Nurse:	I see, but this time you felt there was nowhere else to turn. Anyway, George, I'm glad your suicide attempt didn't work. I'd really like to help you consider some other ways to deal with all these problems.
	George:	I don't know what they could be. I really feel hopeless, but I guess I could see what you've got to offer.
	Nurse:	There are several things we can discuss.

(To be continued in Chapter Four, "Helping People in Crisis").

Another objective of the initial interview is to provide the person in crisis with concrete help. If George had not felt the nurse's acceptance and concern, he would not have dropped his initial resistance to sharing his dilemma. The nurse opened the discussion of alternatives to suicide.

Once an individual is identified as being in a state of crisis, the helping person proceeds to give or obtain whatever assistance is indicated. In complex situations or in circumstances involving life and death, the helper should engage the services of professional crisis workers (Hoff & Adamowski, 1998).

Once the state of crisis is ascertained, the professional crisis worker engages the person in a comprehensive evaluation (Level II assessment) of his or her problems. Such assessment techniques are currently practiced in many crisis and counseling clinics and community mental health programs. A framework and a sample tool from an assessment protocol is discussed next.

Comprehensive Crisis Assessment

A well-organized worker uses tools that aid in the assessment process. If a crisis worker lacks direction and a sense of order, this adds to the confusion felt by acutely anxious people. Tools emphasize a structured approach to the assessment process, but no record system or mechanical tool, such as computer analysis, can substitute for the empathy, knowledge, and experience of a skilled clinician.

Records are to complement, not displace, clinical judgment and expertise in the psychosocial interview process. Nor should record-keeping procedures be allowed to depersonalize interaction with a distressed person.

Philosophy and Context of Record System

The framework and sample tool recommended to guide and record the crisis care process as conceived in this book was selected because it illustrates the principles that should guide any crisis-sensitive record system. The example presented here

- Is based on the understanding of crisis in the psychosociocultural perspective emphasized in this text
- Is client centered in that it includes the person's self-evaluation as an integral aspect of the assessment process
- Assumes that the client is a member of a social network—not simply an individual in psychological disequilibrium—and that disruption or threat of disruption from essential social attachments is often the occasion of crisis and therefore provides significant members of the person's social network an opportunity to participate actively in the assessment process
- Provides a structured, standardized framework for gathering data while including subjective, narrative-style information from the client
- Focuses on a view of the person in crisis as a human being functioning at varying degrees of adequacy or inadequacy, not merely as a diagnostic entity
- Assists in fostering continuity between the various steps of the crisis intervention process (assessment, planning, implementation, follow-up) by providing relevant, organized information so that the client's level of functioning, goals, and methods for attaining these goals can be sharply defined and used as a guide in the course of service
- Provides supervisory staff with information necessary to monitor service and ensure quality care to clients on an ongoing basis
- Provides administrative staff the database needed for monitoring and evaluating service program outcomes in relation to stated objectives

Genesis of Record System

The record system of which this sample tool is a part was developed by a special task force in the Erie County Mental Health System in Buffalo, New York. It is unique in that it incorporates crisis care principles into the assessment and record-keeping requirements of a state and county mental health department, while retaining its client-centered focus. Clients at risk for crisis who were served in this mental health system included (1) people experiencing various unanticipated hazardous life events, who were therefore at risk of extrusion from their natural social setting, and (2) people vulnerable to crisis in relation to chronic mental or emotional disturbance, chemical dependence, or disadvantaged social circumstances. Some of the case examples cited in this book are drawn from people who requested service in this crisis-sensitive mental health system.

The original record system was tested in the 1970s with crisis and mental health workers in the community mental health agencies that adopted the system. Included were the majority of publicly funded programs serving urban, suburban, and rural communities in a metropolitan area with a population of 1.25 million. Participants in testing the system also included people receiving service. A client was considered an active partner in developing the record and had full access to it. Examples of client feedback include the following:

- "I'm not so bad off as I thought."
- "This takes some of the mystery out of mental health."
- "Getting help with a problem isn't so magical after all."
- "Now I have a diary of how I worked out my problems and got better."

The revised version presented here was evaluated for validity and interrater reliability in six comparable agencies in Massachusetts and in Ontario and British Columbia, Canada.

This record system's philosophical underpinning is in the civil rights movement (including the rights of psychiatric patients) and the nationwide program of deinstitutionalizing the mentally ill and providing community-based, easily accessible services; the goal was to restore and maintain people in noninstitutional settings and thereby prevent readmission to psychiatric facilities whenever possible. Today most public mental hospitals have shut down, and many former patients of these facilities roam the streets homeless and without adequate treatment and social support (Perese, 1997). Fortunately, however, some ideal community-based services are being developed—for example, the Club House transition service modeled on the empowerment value of the civil rights movement (Cella, Besancon, & Zipple, 1997; Farrell & Deeds, 1997). For these and other mental health services built on the WHO People 2010 goals, which emphasize health promotion, risk prevention, clients' active involvement in their own health, and moving beyond quick-fix drug approaches to complex mental health problems, this record system holds promise. Managed care policies around treatment goals and evidence indicating progress toward achieving them underscore the need for tools that aid in service delivery without compromising the importance of provider-client team efforts. The tool also captures key features of emotional and mental disturbance or disability without the disadvantage of a psychiatric label.

Staff members using the forms receive formal training in crisis intervention and in using the record system according to written specifications. Although the category "violence experienced" was added in 1982 and published in Hoff & Rosenbaum (1994) and three earlier editions of this text, research (Ross, Hoff, & Coutu-Wakulczyk, 1998; Tilden et al., 1994; Woodtli & Breslin, in press) documents that education and clinical application on this topic, although increasing, are still far from routine, despite growing public concern about violence and health professionals' roles in prevention and the treatment of survivors (Hoff, 2000). See Chapters Six, Eight, and Nine for a more detailed discussion of this topic, a suggested triage tool for use at all entry points to the health and social service system, and an illustration of the tool's use with abused women.

Service Forms

The following description for using the forms is excerpted from the complete specifications.[1] Because of the life-and-death implications of certain items, specifications and rating scales are included for three of the twenty-one items: item 13, violence/abuse experienced; item 14, injury to self; and item 15, danger to others. This is essentially a Level I assessment. They are included in Chapters Eight, Six, and Nine, respectively. The forms included here illustrate assessment information in reference to the case example of George Sloan, continued from Chapter Two. The twenty-one items in the Assessment Worksheet illustrate the "basic life attachments" (items 1–12) and the "signals of distress" (items 13–21) discussed in this and the previous chapter. Items 19, 20, and 21 are used when the rating for item 13, violence/abuse experienced, is 2 or higher. The same twenty-one items are used for client assessment and program evaluation purposes at (1) completion of the service contract (discharge) and (2) periods designated for formal follow-up, especially of high-risk clients, for example, six or twelve months postdischarge.

Initial Contact Sheet

This form (see Exhibit 3.1) is intended to provide basic demographic and problem information at the time the client requests service or is presented for service by another person or agency. This information should provide the worker with sufficient data to make several key decisions early in the crisis care process:

- How urgent is the situation?
- Who is to be assigned responsibility for proceeding with the next step?
- What type of response is indicated as the next step?

This form is used chiefly by the worker designated to handle all incoming calls and on-site requests for service during a specified period of time, sometimes called a triage worker. The "Crisis Rating" section of the form should be completed according to the following guidelines:

---

[1]For complete forms and specifications for their use and for information about reliability and validity studies, the reader is referred to the author, who can be contacted through the publisher. See also Hoff, Hanrahan, & Gallop, 2000.

EXHIBIT 3.1.   INITIAL CONTACT SHEET.

Today's Date:_____*2-15-01*_____   I.D.:_____*101*_____

Name:_____*George O. Sloan*_____

Age:__*48*__   Relationship Status: Married ___*X*___   Single_____   Other_____

Address: ___*33 Random Avenue, Middletown 01234, Central County*_____

_____

Telephone:_____*(444) 123-0987*_____

Have you talked with anyone about this? No_____*X*_____   Yes_____

If yes, to whom?_____   Date of last contact:_____

Significant other (name and phone):_*wife, Marie Sloan (444) 123-0987*_____

Are you taking any medication now? No_____   Yes_____*X*_____

If yes, what?_____*nitroglycerine*_____

Crisis rating: 1   2   3   4   ⑤
                 Not urgent   Very urgent

Probability of engaging in counseling/treatment contract:

          1   2   ③   4   5
       Very high   Very low

Summary of presenting problem or situation and help-seeking goal: *George Sloan, 48, was brought to E.R. by police following a suicide attempt by car crash. His intention was to die, as he saw no way out of his personal and family problems. Has had heart trouble for 4 years. Was urged to quit second job and take office job in Police Dept. His 16-yr. old son's suspension from school adds to his sense of failure. Feels he has no one to talk to. Had considered suicide after last heart attack, but support from his wife prevented him then from crashing his car. While initially reluctant, Mr. Sloan now seems open to counseling assistance.*

Disposition and Recommendation: *Referred tp Psychiatric Liaison Service. Recommend Mr. Sloan receive full assessment and crisis counseling while being treated for injuries from suicidal car accident, plus follow-up with entire family.*

Signature (intake/triage person): *Jane Doe, R. N.*_____Date:_*2-15-01*___

Crisis Rating: How Urgent Is Your Need for Help?

> *Very Urgent.* Request requires an immediate response (within minutes)—for example, crisis outreach; medical emergency requiring an ambulance, such as overdoses, severe drug reaction; or police needed if situation involves extreme danger or weapons.
>
> *Urgent.* Response should be rapid but not necessarily immediate (within a few hours)—for example, low to moderate risk of suicide or mild drug reaction.
>
> *Somewhat Urgent.* Response should be made within a day (twenty-four hours)—for example, planning conference in which key persons are not available until the following evening.
>
> *Slightly Urgent.* Response is required within a few days—for example, client whose funding runs out within a week needs public assistance.
>
> *Not Urgent.* Situation has existed for a long time and does not warrant immediate intervention (a week or two is unlikely to cause any significant difference)—for example, child with a learning disability; couple that needs marital counseling.

Assessment Worksheet

The Assessment Worksheet (see Exhibit 3.2) can be used in two ways: (1) it can serve as an interview guide in a face-to-face session with the client, or (2) the client (if not acutely upset) can be given the form to complete *on-site,* after which the items are discussed in a face-to-face interview. Such use of this form assumes that *the record belongs to the client.* This principle needs shoring up because psychiatric groups have used legal channels to keep mental health clients from gaining access to their records. A client-centered record also reflects the view that they are in charge of their lives and that the helping process should not be mysterious to them. The worksheet is *never* to be used without a personal interview, nor should it simply be given to the client to complete at home. An abuse victim or a potentially suicidal person could perceive such action as a dismissal of one's immediate concerns. The Child Screening Checklist (see Exhibit 3.3) can be used in a similar fashion. (The complete record system includes the Significant Other Worksheet, which is designed for similar use).

A cautionary note is in order here: forms can never substitute for rapport, time, and sensitivity to the unique needs of each distressed person. Clinicians bombarded with management information systems must be careful to avoid recording more and more about doing less and less. A client-centered record system like this that clearly documents progress in treatment goals based on systematic assessment may even advance the cause of parity in insurance coverage for mental health services rendered.

EXHIBIT 3.2.   ASSESSMENT WORKSHEET: GEORGE SLOAN.

1. <u>Physical Health</u>: How do you judge your physical health in general?

1	2	(3)	4	5
Excellent	Good	Fair	Poor	Very poor

Comments: *No problems except for heart. Feel OK except for chest pain, which is getting more frequent.*

2. <u>Self-Acceptance/Self-Esteem</u>: How do you feel about yourself as a person?

1	2	3	(4)	5
Very good	Good	Fair	Poor	Very poor

Comments: *Not very good—especially when I think about my son's trouble—that it's probably my fault. Seems like I'm no good at anything lately.*

3. <u>Vocational/Occupational</u> (includes student, homemaker, volunteer): How would you judge your work/school situation?

1	2	(3)	4	5
Very good	Good	Fair	Poor	Very poor

Comments: *I can still do patrol work, but the doctor says I should slow down.*

4. <u>Immediate Family</u>: How would you describe your relationship with your family?

1	2	3	(4)	5
Very good	Good	Fair	Poor	Very poor

Comments: *Ever since my first heart attack, we seem to be going from bad to worse, especially with our son Arnold.*

5. <u>Intimacy/Significant Other Relationship(s)</u>: Is there anyone you feel really close to and can rely on if you're very upset or in a life-threatening situation?

1	2	3	(4)	5
Always	Usually	Sometimes	Rarely	Never

Comments: *Not really. Things used to be better between my wife and me, but we seem to be drifting apart.*

6. <u>Residential/Housing</u>: How do you judge your housing situation?

(1)	2	3	4	5
Very good	Good	Fair	Poor	Very poor

Comments: _____

EXHIBIT 3.2. ASSESSMENT WORKSHEET: GEORGE SLOAN. (*continued*)

7. <u>Financial Security</u>: How would you describe your financial situation?

1	②	3	4	5
Very good	Good	Fair	Poor	Very poor

Comments: *As long as I have my second job, it's O.K., but I don't like the idea of my wife working full time.*

8. <u>Decision-Making Ability</u>: How satisfied are you with your ability to make life decisions?

1	2	③	4	5
Always very satisfied		Somewhat dissatisfied		Always very dissatisfied

Comments: *Mostly around the problems we have with Arnold.*

9. <u>Problem-Solving Ability</u>: How would you judge your ability to solve everyday problems?

1	2	③	4	5
Very good	Good	Fair	Poor	Very poor

Comments: *I thought I was doing pretty well before this heart trouble got in the way of my second job.*

10. <u>Life Goals/Spiritual Values</u>: How satisfied are you with how your life goals (and things you value most) are working for you?

1	2	③	4	5
Always very satisfied		Somewhat dissatisfied		Always very dissatisfied

Comments: *I almost always felt satisfied before the heart trouble started 4 years ago.*

11. <u>Leisure Time/Community Involvement</u>: How satisfied are you with the availability of leisure time and ability to relax and take part in activities beyond everyday duties?

1	2	③	4	5
Always very satisfied		Somewhat dissatisfied		Always very dissatisfied

Comments: *I don't have much free time, but I really like my work. I suppose our whole family could use more time together.*

12. <u>Feelings</u>: How comfortable are you with your feelings? (For example, do you often feel anxious or fearful?)

1	2	③	4	5
Always comfortable		Sometimes uncomfortable		Always uncomfortable

Comments: *Just during the last few months I really started feeling depressed. My wife says I bottle everything up.*

EXHIBIT 3.2. ASSESSMENT WORKSHEET: GEORGE SLOAN. (*continued*)

13. Violence/Abuse Experienced: To what extent have you been injured or troubled by physical, sexual, or emotional abuse?

    ①   2   3   4   5
Never   Several times recently   Routinely (every day or so)

Comments/Describe:_____
_____
_____

Note: If rating of item 13 is 2 or above, answer items 19, 20, and 21 below.

14. Injury to Self: Do you have any thoughts of suicide or a plan to hurt yourself in any way?

    1   2   3   4   ⑤
No risk whatsoever   Moderate risk   Very serious risk

Comments/Describe: *I still can't see any way out except suicide, but right now I feel a little better from talking with you.*
_____

15. Danger to Other(s): Do you have any thoughts about violence or a plan to physically harm someone?

    ①   2   3   4   5
No risk whatsoever   Moderate risk   Very serious risk

Comments/Describe:_____
_____
_____

16. Substance Use/Abuse (alcohol and/or other drugs): Does the use of alcohol or other drugs concern you or interfere with your life in any way (work, family)?

    ①   2   3   4   5
Never   Rarely   Sometimes   Frequently   Constantly

Comments/Describe:_____
_____
_____

17. Legal: What is your tendency to get in trouble with the law?

    ①   2   3   4   5
No   Slight   Moderate   Great   Very great

Comments/Describe:_____
_____
_____
_____
_____

EXHIBIT 3.2. ASSESSMENT WORKSHEET: GEORGE SLOAN. (*continued*)

18. <u>Agency Use</u>: How satisfied are you with getting the help you need from doctors or other health providers?

1	2	3	4	5
Always very satisfied		Somewhat dissatisfied		Always very dissatisfied

Comments: *I don't like going to doctors and avoid it if at all possible. My heart doctor told me to slow down, but that's easier said than done.*

<u>Note</u>: If item 13, Violence/Abuse Experienced, is rated 2 or higher, answer items 19, 20, and 21.

19. <u>Relationship with Abuser</u>: How would you describe your relationship with the person who has abused you?

1	2	3	4	5
No contact or conflict now		Occasional conflict		Great conflict and turmoil

Comments/Describe: _____

20. <u>Safety—Self</u>: How safe do you feel now?

1	2	3	4	5
Very safe		Sometimes unsafe		Very unsafe

Comments/Describe: _____

21. (if there are children) <u>Safety—Children</u>: How safe do you think your children are?

1	2	3	4	5
Very safe		Sometimes unsafe		Very unsafe

Comments: _____

<u>Additional Items</u>: Do you have any other issues, concerns, or problems that you wish to discuss with a counselor?
No, not really.

<u>Urgency/Importance</u>: Among the items noted, which do you consider the most urgent or in need of immediate attention?
Well, I wish I could do right by my family, but I just can't get through to my wife.

Name: *George Sloan*
Address: *33 Random Avenue*
Middletown 01234 Central County
Telephone: *(444) 123-0987*
Date: *2-15-01*

EXHIBIT 3.3.   CHILD SCREENING CHECKLIST.

Child's Full Name_____ Gender_____ Date of Birth_____

Family Relationship Concerns:

Does not get along with mother____ father____ brother(s)____ sister(s)____ refuses to participate in family activities____ refuses to accept and perform family responsibilities____ frequently absent parent____ marital problems/domestic violence____ rotating "parents" (parents' girlfriends or boyfriends)____ inadequate child care arrangements____ family health problems____ financial insecurity/homelessness____ family transitions (move, divorce, remarriage, incarceration, death)____ rejection of child____ other____

School Concerns:

Poor grades/underachievement____ lack of motivation/disinterest/failure to do home-work____ frequent absences or tardiness____ warnings, detentions, suspensions____ does not get along with students____ does not get along with teachers____ other____

Peer Relationship Concerns:

Inability to get along with peers____ lack of friends____ prefers to be alone____ prefers to be with adults____ does not associate with peers____ not accepted by peers____ bullied/harassed by peers____ reluctant to leave parent/home____ other____

Dyssocial Behavioral Concerns:

Excessive lying____ stealing____ vandalism____ fire setting____ aggression/fighting/violence____ runaway____ early sexual behavior____ inappropriate sexual behavior____ substance abuse____ court involvement____ homicidal____ suicidal____ other____

Personal Adjustment Concerns:

Temper tantrums____ easily upset____ clinging/dependent____ sleep disturbances ____ nervous mannerisms____ thumb sucking ____ speech problems____ eating problems____ wetting, soiling, retention____ lacks self-confidence/self-esteem____ other____

Emotional Concerns:

Loneliness____ boredom____ being different____ frustration____ anger/hostility____ anxiousness____ fearfulness____ negativism____ depression____ other____

Medical and Developmental Concerns:

Acute illness____ chronic illness____ disabilities____ allergies____ accident prone____ seizures____ physical complaints____ lengthy or frequent clinic/hospital visits____ medication____ surgery____ mental retardation____ other____

Strengths and assets:

_____

_____

_____

Comments:

_____

_____

_____

Screened by_____

_____

Summary

Some people are at greater risk of crisis than others. Identifying groups of people who are most likely to experience a crisis is helpful in recognizing individuals in crisis. People in crisis have typical patterns of thinking, feeling, and acting. There is no substitute for a thorough assessment of whether a person is or is not in crisis. The assessment is the basis of the helping plan. It can save lives and avoid many later problems, including unnecessary placement of people in institutions, and can address issues of managed care as it affects people in serious need of mental health services.

References

Barney, K. (1994). Limitations of the critique of the medical model. *Journal of Mind and Behavior, 15*(1,2), 19–34.

Becker, H. S. (1963). *Outsiders: Studies in the sociology of deviance.* New York: Free Press.

Breggin, P. (1992). *Beyond conflict: From self-help and psychotherapy to peacemaking.* New York: St. Martin's Press.

Caplan, G. (1964). *Principles of preventive psychiatry.* New York: Basic Books.

Caplan, P. (1995). *They say you're crazy: How the world's most powerful psychiatrists decide who's normal.* Reading, MA: Addison-Wesley.

Capponi, P. (1992). *Upstairs in the crazy house.* Toronto: Penguin Books.

Cella, E. P., Besancon, V., & Zipple, A. M. (1997). Expanding the role of clubhouses: Guidelines for establishing a system of integrated day services. *Psychiatric Rehabilitation Journal, 21*(1), 10–15.

Cloward, R. A., & Piven, F. F. (1979). Hidden protest: The channeling of female innovations and resistance. *Signs: Journal of Women in Culture and Society, 4,* 651–669.

Cohen, C. I. (1993). The biomedicalization of psychiatry: A critical overview. *Community Mental Health Journal, 29,* 509–521.

Congressional Joint Commission on Mental Health and Illness. (1961). *Action for mental health.* New York: Basic Books.

Cooksey, E. C., & Brown, P. (1998). Spinning on its axes: DSM and the social construction of psychiatric diagnosis. *International Journal of Health Sciences, 28*(3), 525–554.

Dressler, D. M. (1973). The management of emotional crises by medical practitioners. *Journal of American Medical Women's Association, 28*(12), 654–659.

Edmands, M. S., Hoff, L. A., Kaylor, L., Mower, L., & Sorrell, S. (1999). Bridging gaps between mind, body and spirit: Healing the whole person. *Journal of Psychosocial Nursing, 37*(10), 1–7.

Everett, B., & Gallop, R. (2000). *The link between childhood trauma and mental illness: Effective interventions for mental health professionals.* Thousand Oaks: CA: Sage.

Farrell, S. P., & Deeds, E. S. (1997). The clubhouse model as exemplar. *Journal of Psychosocial Nursing, 35*(1), 27–34.

Fausto-Sterling, A. (2000). *Sexing the body.* New York: Basic Books.

Goffman, E. (1961). *Asylums.* New York: Doubleday.

Goffman, E. (1963). *Stigma.* Englewood Cliffs, NJ: Prentice Hall.

Golan, N. (1969). When is a client in crisis? *Social Casework, 50,* 389–394.

Gove, W. (Ed.). (1975). *The labeling of deviance.* New York: Wiley.

Gove, W. (1978). Sex differences in mental illness among adult men and women: An examination of four questions raised regarding whether or not women actually have higher rates. *Social Science and Medicine, 12,* 187–198.

Hagey, R., & McDonough, P. (1984). The problem of professional labeling. *Nursing Outlook, 32*(3), 151–157.

Hansell, N. (1976). *The person in distress.* New York: Human Sciences Press.

Hoff, L. A. (1990). *Battered women as survivors.* London: Routledge.

Hoff, L. A. (1993). Review essay: Health policy and the plight of the mentally ill. *Psychiatry, 56*(4), 400–419.

Hoff, L. A. (2000). Interpersonal violence. In C. E. Koop, C. E. Pearson, & M. R. Schwarz (Eds.), *Critical issues in global health* (pp. 260–271). San Francisco: Jossey-Bass.

Hoff, L. A., & Adamowski, K. (1998). *Creating excellence in crisis care: A guide to effective training and program designs.* San Francisco: Jossey-Bass.

Hoff, L. A., Hanrahan, P., & Gallop, R. (2000). *Comprehensive mental health assessment: A functional approach.* Unpublished manuscript.

Hoff, L. A., & Rosenbaum, L. (1994). A victimization assessment tool: Instrument development and clinical implications. *Journal of Advanced Nursing, 20*(4), 627–634.

Hoff, L. A., & Wells, J. O. (Eds.). (1989). *Certification standards manual* (4th ed.). Denver: American Association of Suicidology.

Holden, C. (1986). Proposed new psychiatric diagnoses raise charges of gender bias. *Science, 231,* 327–328.

Illich, I. (1976). *Limits to medicine.* Harmondsworth, England: Penguin Books.

Johnson, A. B. (1990). *Out of bedlam: The truth about deinstitutionalization.* New York: Basic Books.

Lemert, W. M. (1951). *Social pathology.* New York: McGraw-Hill.

Link, B. G., Phelan, J. C., Bresnahan, M., Stueve, A., & Pescosolido, B. A. (1997). Public conceptions of mental illness: Labels, causes, dangerousness, and social distance. *American Journal of Public Health, 89*(9), 128–133.

Luhrmann, T. M. (2000). *Of two minds: The growing disorder in American psychiatry.* New York: Knopf.

Lyness, J. M. (1997). *Psychiatric pearls.* Philadelphia: F. A. Davis.

Mitchell, G. (1991). Nursing diagnosis: An ethical analysis. *Image: Journal of Nursing Scholarship, 23*(2), 99–103.

Nehls, N. (1999). Borderline personality disorder: The voice of patients. *Research in Nursing and Health, 22*(4), 285–293.

Osgood, N. (1992). *Suicide in later life: Recognizing the warning signs.* San Francisco: New Lexington Press.

Perese, E. F. (1997). Unmet needs of persons with chronic mental illness: Relationship to their adaptation to community living. *Issues in Mental Health Nursing, 18*(1), 19–34.

Polak, P. (1967). The crisis of admission. *Social Psychiatry, 2,* 150–157.

Polak, P. (1976). A model to replace psychiatric hospitalization. *Journal of Nervous and Mental Disease, 162,* 13–22.

Rosenhan, D. L. (1973). On being sane in insane places. *Science, 179,* 250–258. (Also reprinted in H. D. Schwartz & C. S. Kart. (1976). *Dominant issues in medical sociology.* Reading, MA: Addison-Wesley; and in P. J. Brink (Ed.). (1976). *Transcultural nursing.* Englewood Cliffs, NJ: Prentice Hall.)

Ross, M., Hoff, L. A., & Coutu-Wakulczyk, G. (1998). Nursing curricula and violence issues: A study of Canadian schools of nursing. *Journal of Nursing Education, 37*(2), 53–60.

Sales, E., Baum, M., & Shore, B. (1984). Victim readjustment following assault. *Journal of Social Issues, 40*(1), 117–136.

Scheff, T. J. (Ed.). (1975). *Labeling madness.* Englewood Cliffs, NJ: Prentice Hall.

Sifneos, P. E. (1960). A concept of "emotional crisis." *Mental Hygiene, 44,* 169–179.

Stark, E., Flitcraft, A., & Frazier, W. (1979). Medicine and patriarchal violence: The social construction of a "private" event. *International Journal of Health Services, 9,* 461–493.

Tilden, V. P., Schmidt, T. A., Limandri, B. J., Chiodo, G. T., Garland, M. J., & Loveless, P. A. (1994). Factors that influence clinicians' assessment and management of family violence. *American Journal of Public Health, 84*(4), 628–633.

Warshaw, C. (1989). Limitations of the medical model in the care of battered women. *Gender and Society, 3*(4), 506–517.

Woodtli, A., & Breslin, E. (in press). Violence-related content in the nursing curriculum: A follow-up national survey. *Journal of Nursing Education.*

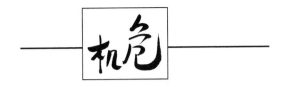

CHAPTER FOUR

HELPING PEOPLE IN CRISIS

Understanding the crisis model lays the foundation for assessing people at risk. The focus in this chapter is on the interpersonal context of crisis care and on specific strategies for assisting people who are acutely upset. Specifically, communication and rapport, planning, contracting, and working through the crisis toward a positive outcome will be discussed. The principles and techniques suggested can be applied in a wide variety of crisis intervention settings: primary care agencies, homes, hospitals, clinics, hotlines, and alternative crisis services. These principles and techniques can be varied and adapted according to professional training, personal preference, and setting, but the fundamental ideas remain the same.

Communication and Rapport: The Immediate Context of Crisis Work

Crisis intervention strategies are not likely to work if a crisis worker has failed to establish rapport with the person in crisis. Just as assessment is part of the helping process, rapport and effective communication are integrated throughout all stages of crisis care: assessment, planning, intervention, and follow-up.

The Nature and Purpose of Communication

Human beings are distinguished from the nonhuman animal kingdom by our ability to produce and use symbols and to create meaning out of the events and circumstances of our lives. Through language and nonverbal communication, we let our fellow humans know what we think and feel about life and about one another. For example, a man might say, "Life is not worth living without her." He may be contemplating suicide after divorce because he sees life without his cherished companion as meaningless. A rape victim or terminally ill woman might say, "What did I do to deserve this?" thus accounting for the situation by blaming herself. Communication is the medium through which we

- Struggle to survive (for example, by giving away prized possessions or saying, "I don't care anymore" as a cry for help after a serious loss)
- Develop meaningful human communion and maintain it (for example, by giving and receiving support during stress and crisis)
- Bring stability and organization into our lives (for example, by sorting out the chaotic elements of a traumatic event with a caring person)
- Negotiate social and political struggles at national and international levels

When communication fails, a person may feel alone, abandoned, worthless, and unloved, or conflict and tension may be created in interpersonal relations. The most tragic result of failed communication is violence toward self and others; at the societal level, this translates into war. Such destructive outcomes of failed communication are more probable in acute crisis situations. Given the importance of communication in the development and resolution of crisis, let us consider some of the factors that influence our interactions with people in crisis.

Factors Influencing Communication

Many sources provide theoretical knowledge about human communication: psychology, sociology, cultural anthropology, ecology, and sociolinguistics (for example, Dahnke & Clatterbuck, 1990; Loustaunau & Sobo, 1997; Storti, 1994). These sources provide important insights into communication as it applies to crisis work.

Psychology. As noted in Chapter Three, cognitive functions are significant in crisis response and coping. The way a person perceives stressful events influences how that person feels about these events and communicates feelings about them. When an event and a person's perception of the meaning of the event are incongruous and thus lead to a culturally inappropriate expression of feelings, this may indicate mental impairment and greater vulnerability to stress. For example, a person who feels depressed and unworthy of help will usually have difficulty expressing feelings such as anger, which might be appropriate after a traumatic event such as a violent attack. A human services provider who feels insecure with the crisis model of helping can have difficulty communicating effectively; the worker may talk too much or may fail to be appropriately active when the situation calls for worker initiative.

Sociology. Sociological factors affecting communication in crisis situations spring from society at large as well as from the subcultures of various crisis service delivery systems. These include status, role, and gender factors and political and economic factors (Campbell-Heider & Pollock, 1987). For example, a nurse may not communicate concern to a person in the hospital who is suspected of being suicidal, assuming that assessment for suicide risk is someone else's responsibility. Or the policies and economics of insurance and hospital care may obscure the fact that community-based help is often more appropriate than hospital care. Similarly, the predominance of individualistic approaches may obscure the highly effective group medium of helping people in crisis.

Cultural Anthropology. Insights from cultural anthropology are pivotal in communication with people in crisis. Our sensitivity to another person's values and beliefs is crucial to understanding what life events mean to different people. Members of particular cultural groups are almost invariably characterized by a degree of *ethnocentrism*—the conviction that one's own value and belief system is superior. At its best, ethnocentrism is a necessary ingredient of cultural identity and a person's sense of belonging to a social group. At its worst, ethnocentrism can become exaggerated and destructive, for example, in resolving community problems among different ethnic groups. Members of a cultural group may impose their values on others, assume an attitude of superiority about their own customs, or be disdainful toward people unlike themselves. Ethnocentric attitudes can interfere with effective communication.

It is important to remember in crisis work that for many people certain values are worth dying for. Needless to say, if an *imposed*—rather than a negotiated—crisis management plan contradicts dearly held values and threatens a person's sense of self-mastery, the chances of success are minimal. Examples of values that may be critical include a person's (1) idea of the meaning of death, illness, and health, (2) feelings about whether to seek and accept help, and (3) opinion about how help should be offered. For example, a person contemplating suicide but seeking one last chance to get help may interpret a prescription for sleeping pills as "an invitation to die" (Jourard, 1970). Crisis workers should also be aware that many human service professionals in the United States and other Western societies hold values of the white, middle-class majority.

Ecology. Environmental factors are intricately tied to cultural values regarding privacy. Examples from the previous chapters suggest that the environment in which crisis service is offered influences the outcome of the crisis. If a person lacks privacy, such as in a busy hospital emergency department, the likelihood of successful communication during crisis is reduced. A serious commitment to crisis service delivery in emergency settings, therefore, would provide for separate rooms to facilitate the kind of communication necessary for acutely upset people. A worker's skills are useless if staffing and material factors prevent the effective application of those skills (Hoff & Adamowski, 1998).

Similarly, in crisis work done by police officers and outreach staff, such as mediating a marital fight, spatial factors can be critical in saving lives. The expression "A man's home is his castle" symbolizes a personalized and defended territory. Inattention to these unstated but culturally shared experiences can result in violent behavioral—that is, nonverbal—communication about this hidden dimension of public and private life. Police officers often refer to the "sixth sense" they develop through street experience and sensitivity to environmental factors related to crisis. Potential victims in high-crime areas and stressful work environments should also sensitize themselves to elements in their milieu that may signal a crisis of violence, so they can protect themselves. Police or neighborhood associations are good sources of this kind of information.

Sociolinguistics. Sociolinguistics is the study of social theories of language. Scholars examine how social factors such as race, gender, class, region, and religion influence language and how language can both influence health status (Pennebaker, 1993) and condition thought and social action. Language is the common medium for verbal communication between particular linguistic communities and the most observable way to ascertain the ideas, beliefs, and attitudes of various cultural groups. Insensitivity to an individual's linguistic interpretation can reflect a lack of appreciation of cultural values. Effective crisis workers should have something in common linguistically with various ethnic groups if they are to serve people in the groups within the framework of their value systems.

Language, then, serves as an important link between individual and social approaches to crisis. For example, in *individual* crisis work with a victim of rape or racially motivated violence, a worker helps the person talk about the event, work through feelings, and develop a plan of action, such as reporting to the police. The *sociocultural* element in this kind of crisis situation is the message to women and ethnic minority groups that they are responsible for their own victimization (Ryan, 1971). Such cultural messages are revealed in conversation: "Women and blacks are their own worst enemies," or "Why does she [a battered woman] stay?" Such messages influence how women and members of racial minorities respond emotionally, cognitively, and behaviorally to violent events.

The written word similarly conveys the beliefs and values of a cultural community. For example, you may have observed many pages ago that the language in this book is nonmedical and nonsexist. This usage is based on the recognition that language is a powerful conveyor of social and cultural norms governing social status and behavior. Relationships between women and men and the contrast between medical and developmental approaches to crisis intervention can be revealed through language (Vetterling-Braggin, Elliston, & English, 1977, pp. 105–170).

Crisis workers will discover other examples in which sensitivity in communication affects interactions with people in crisis. Communication is not only necessary for carrying out the crisis intervention process, but it is also an integral aspect of the helping process itself.

Relationships, Communication, and Rapport

The most technically flawless communication skills are useless in the absence of rapport with the person in crisis. Conversely, if our values, attitudes, and feelings about a person are respectful, unprejudiced, and based on true concern, those values will almost always be conveyed to the person, regardless of any technical errors in communication. This point cannot be overemphasized. For example, it is commonplace to hear, "I thought he was suicidal, but I didn't say anything because I was afraid I'd say the wrong thing." This argument represents a gross misconception of the nature of language. If we truly are concerned about whether a person lives or dies, this concern will almost invariably be conveyed in what we say unless we

- Deliberately say the opposite of what we mean
- Are mentally disturbed, with an accompanying distortion and contradiction between thought and language
- Lack knowledge about suicidal people or feel anxious about how the person will respond to our sincere message and therefore fail to deliver it (see Chapter Six)

Crisis workers therefore must learn the technical aspects of skillful communication with people who are upset (Haney, 1991; Thompson, 1988). They must avoid asking why and refrain from asking questions that lead to yes or no answers; they must not make judgments or offer unrealistic reassurance. But it is equally important to establish rapport and foster the relationship necessary for a distressed individual to accept help. Although theoretical and technical knowledge is important in facilitating positive outcomes with people in crisis, the quality of the relationship we establish is far more important. In particular, this includes the worker's ability to convey empathy, caring, and sincerity. Truax and Carkhuff (1967) found that nonprofessional persons are highly capable of creating such relationships and that mental health professionals' demonstrations of empathy *decrease* as the length of time after their original training *increases*—findings still relevant today.

In our efforts to establish rapport, two objectives are central:

1. We should aim to make the distressed person feel understood. We can convey understanding by using reflective statements, such as, "You seem to be very hurt and upset by what has happened," and "Sounds like you're very angry." If our perception of what the person is feeling is incorrect, the words *seem to be* and *sounds like* provide an opening for the person to explain his or her perception of the upsetting or traumatic event. The expression "I understand" should generally be avoided, as it may be perceived as presumptuous; there is always the possibility that we do not truly understand. Parents who suffer the loss of a child say that no one but a similarly grieving parent can truly understand.

2. If we are unclear about the nature or extent of what the person feels or is troubled by, we should convey our wish to understand by asking, for example, "Could you tell me more about that?" or "How do you feel about what has happened?" or "I'm not sure I understand. Could you tell me what you mean by that?"

Besides these techniques for establishing rapport, there are several other means of removing barriers to effective communication (Pluckhan, 1978, pp. 116–128; Arnold & Boggs, 1999):

- Become aware of the internal and external noises that may inhibit our ability to communicate sincerely.
- Avoid double messages. For example, we may convey concern at a verbal level but contradict our message by posture, facial gestures, or failure to give undivided attention. Traditionally, this is known as the "double bind" in communication (Bateson, 1958).
- Avoid unwarranted assumptions about other people's lives, feelings, and values (Kottler, 1994).
- Keep communication clear of unnecessary professional and technical jargon; when technical terminology is unavoidable, translate it.
- Be aware of the trust-risk factor in communication. We must periodically examine whether we are trustworthy and what kind of social, cultural, and personal situations warrant the trust needed to accept help from another (Pluckhan, 1978, pp. 88–89; Northouse & Northouse, 1998). Also keep in mind that some people are distrustful not because of us but because they have been betrayed by others they trusted.
- Take advantage of opportunities to improve self-awareness, self-confidence, and sensitivity to factors affecting communication (human relations courses, biofeedback training, assertiveness workshops).

These suggestions represent a small part of the communication field as it pertains to crisis work. Because communication is inseparable from culture and human life, its importance in helping people in crisis can hardly be overestimated (Haley, 1987). Keeping in mind these contextual aspects of crisis work, let us proceed to specific strategies of planning, intervention, and follow-up in the crisis care process. In the Crisis Paradigm, these steps are illustrated in the intertwined circles in Box 3 (see Figure 4.1).

Planning with a Person or Family in Crisis

There is no substitute for a good plan for crisis resolution. Without careful planning and direction, a helper can only add to the confusion already experienced by the person in crisis. Some may argue that in certain crisis situations there is no time to plan, as life-and-death issues may be at stake. Rather than excusing the need for planning, this only underscores its urgency. A good plan can be formulated in a few minutes by someone who knows the signs of crisis, is confident in his or her own ability to help, and is able to enlist additional, immediate assistance in cases of impasse or life-and-death emergency.

FIGURE 4.1.   CRISIS PARADIGM.

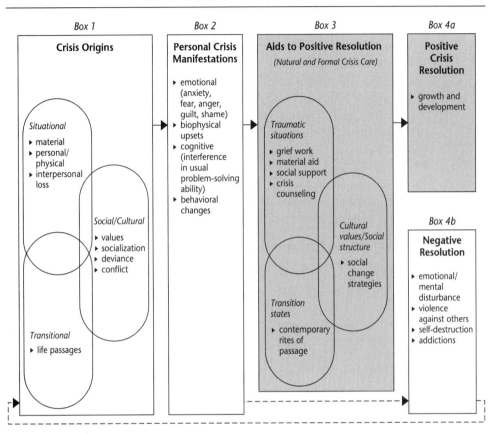

Crisis origins, manifestations, and outcomes and the respective functions of crisis care have an interactional relationship. The intertwined circles represent the distinct yet interrelated origins of crisis and aids to positive resolution, even though personal manifestations are often similar. The arrows pointing from origins to positive resolution illustrate the *opportunity for growth and development* through crisis; the broken line at bottom depicts the potential *danger of crisis* in the absence of appropriate aids. The loop between Box 4b and Box 1 denotes the *vulnerability* to future crisis episodes following negative resolution.

CASE EXAMPLE: ROBERT

A police officer was called to the home of Robert, who had recently been discharged from a hospital. He had angrily barricaded himself in the bathroom and was making threatening comments to his family. On arrival, the officer learned that a psychiatrist–social worker team was already at the home. They were frightened by Robert's threats and were unable to persuade him to unlock the door. The officer identified himself and asked Robert to open the door. He refused. The officer then forced the door open. There was no formal discussion between the officer and the mental health team. Robert became frightened and stabbed the officer in the shoulder with a kitchen knife.

This case illustrates several points:

1. Action occurred *before* planning. As a result, the resources of the professional mental health and police systems were not used to their fullest capacity.
2. When police officers and others are injured by mentally disturbed persons, the injury is often related to the worker's inadequate training in crisis intervention (see Chapter Nine). Because most police officer training now includes crisis intervention, police deaths and injuries on the job have declined.
3. The time spent *planning*—even if it is only a few minutes—can prevent injuries and save lives.

Research on similar work-related injuries documents that many of these injuries might have been prevented (Chappell & Di Martino, 1998).

Assessment and Planning Linkage

A useful plan consists of more than vague or haphazardly formulated intentions. Planning with a person for crisis resolution follows assessment that the person is in a crisis or precrisis state. The information needed for the plan is obtained from careful assessment. The following key questions, in the context of a skilled interview, represent a more general summary of the twenty-one items included in the assessment forms presented in Chapter Three:

- To what extent has the crisis disrupted the person's normal life pattern?
- Is the person able to go to school or hold a job?
- Can the person handle the responsibilities of daily life, for example, eating and personal hygiene?
- Has the crisis situation disrupted the lives of others?
- Has the person been victimized by crime?
- Is the person suicidal, homicidal, or both?
- Is the person coping through substance abuse?
- Does the person seem to be close to despair?
- Has the high anxiety level distorted the person's perception of reality?
- Is the person's usual support system present, absent, or exhausted?
- What are the resources of the individual helper or agency in relation to the person's assessed needs?

The answers to such questions provide the worker with essential data for constructing the intervention plan. This involves, first, thinking through the relationships between events and the way the person is thinking, feeling, and acting and then formulating some possible solutions with the person and the family.

To ensure that the plan is specific to the person's crisis response and corresponding needs, a worker may set priorities by checking the assessment form for ratings of 3, 4, or 5 (the levels designating ineffective or impaired functioning). The worker should then ask the person which problem or issue seems the most urgent—for example, "It seems there are a lot of things upsetting you right now. Which of these is the most important for you to get help with immediately?"

Decision Counseling

Skill in decision counseling (Hansell, 1970) is intrinsic to the crisis assessment, planning, and intervention process. Decision counseling is cognitively oriented and allows the upset person to put distorted thoughts, chaotic feelings, and disturbed behavior into some kind of order. The person is encouraged to

- Search for the boundaries of the problem. ("How long has this been troubling you?" or "In what kind of situation do you find yourself getting most upset?")
- Appraise the meaning of the problems and how they can be mastered. ("How has your life changed since your wife's illness?")
- Make a decision about various solutions to the problem. ("What do you think you can do about this?" or "What have you done so far about this problem?")
- Test the solutions in a clear-cut action plan that is documented in a service contract.

In decision counseling, the crisis worker facilitates crisis resolution by helping the person decide

- What problem is to be solved? ("Of the things you are troubled by, what is it you want help with now?")
- How can it be solved? ("What do you think would be most helpful?")
- When should it be solved? ("How about coming in after school today with your husband and your son?")
- Where should it be solved? ("Yes, we do make home visits. Tell me more about your situation, so we can decide if a home or office visit is best.")
- Who should be involved in solving it? ("Who else have you talked to about this problem who could be helpful?")

Decision counseling also includes setting goals for the future and forming an alternative action plan to be used if the current plan fails or goals are not achieved.

In decision counseling, the counselor must have thorough knowledge of the person's functional level and network of social attachments. Used effectively, this technique makes maximum use of the turmoil of crisis to (1) assess current coping ability, (2) develop new problem-solving skills, (3) establish more stable emotional attachments, (4) improve the person's social skills, and (5) increase the person's competence and satisfaction with life patterns.

Developing a Service Contract

Once an action plan is agreed on by the person in crisis and the worker, it is important to confirm the plan in a service contract (see Exhibit 4.1). The nature of the contract is implied in the fact that the plan for crisis intervention is *mutually arrived at by the helper and the distressed person*. If the person comes to the attention of professional crisis counselors or mental health professionals with training in crisis intervention, the service contract should be formalized in writing. The following conditions are implicit in the contract:

- The person is essentially in charge of his or her own life.
- The person is able to make decisions.
- The crisis counseling relationship is one between partners.
- Both parties to the contract, the person in crisis and the crisis counselor, have rights and responsibilities, as spelled out in the contract.
- The relationship between the helper and the person in crisis is complementary rather than hierarchical, as between a supervisor and a subordinate.

Institutional psychiatry and traditional mental health professions in North America have come under serious attack for violating civil rights (Kelly & Weston, 1974; Rodriguez-Garcia & Akhter, 2000). Individuals have been locked up, medicated, and given electric shock against their will in mental institutions. Protests and demands for appropriate treatment by human rights and consumer groups have led to certain reforms, although this is still contested terrain (Capponi, 1992; Cohen, 1993; Hoff, 1993). Currently, groups like the National Alliance for the Mentally Ill and the Ontario Psychiatric Survivors Association do advocacy work around these issues. The fiftieth anniversary of the Universal Declaration of Human Rights, adopted by the United Nations in 1948, has brought renewed attention to the issue, which makes drawing up contracts as safeguards against abuse of those rights more important than ever.

People have the right to either use or refuse services; the formal service contract protects that right. In addition, the contract establishes the following:

- What the client can expect from the counselor
- What the counselor can expect from the client
- How the two parties will achieve the goals on which they have agreed
- The target dates for achieving the goals defined in the contract

Nothing goes into a contract that is not mutually developed by client and counselor through decision counseling. Both parties sign the contract and retain copies. Receiving help on a contractual basis has these effects: (1) reducing the possibility that the helping relationship will degenerate into a superior-subject or rescuer-victim stance, (2) enhancing the self-mastery and social skills of the client, (3) facilitating growth through a crisis experience, (4) reducing the incidence of

EXHIBIT 4.1. SERVICE CONTRACT.

Date: _____

Code: _____

1. Physical health
2. Self-acceptance/self-esteem
3. Vocational/occupational
4. Immediate family
5. Intimate relationship(s)
6. Residential/housing
7. Financial security

8. Decision-making ability
9. Problem-solving ability
10. Life goals/spiritual values
11. Leisure time/community involvement
12. Feelings
13. Violence/abuse experienced
14. Injury to self

15. Danger to other(s)
16. Substance use/abuse
17. Legal
18. Agency use
19. Relationship with abuser
20. Safety—self
21. Safety—children

Stress Rating Code: 1 = low stress/very high functioning   5 = high stress/very low functioning

Item/Stress Rating	Problem/Issue Specification	Strategies/Techniques (planned actions of client and health provider)

Signatures: Client _____   Crisis Worker _____

failure in helping a person in crisis, and (5) documenting for insurance purposes the goals and outcomes of crisis care and mental health treatment. The example of a service contract is adapted from the record system described in Chapter Three.

Evaluating the Crisis Intervention Plan

A plan can be used in several ways: (1) as a self-evaluation tool, (2) as a checklist for evaluating what might be missing or determining why progress seems elusive, (3) as a means by which supervisors can monitor client service, (4) as data for consultants who are brainstorming with workers about complex or difficult crisis situations. A good plan should have the following characteristics:

1. *Developed with the person in crisis.* A good intervention plan is developed in active collaboration with the person in crisis and the significant people in the person's life. The underlying philosophy is that people can help themselves with varying degrees of help from others. Doing things to, rather than with, a distressed person can lead to failure in crisis intervention. If the goals for crisis intervention and problem solving are formulated by the helper alone, those goals are practically worthless—no matter how appropriate they appear. Inattention to this important element of the planning process is probably responsible for more failures in healthy crisis resolution than any other single factor. Making decisions *for* rather than *with* the person in crisis violates the growth-and-development concept that is basic to effective crisis intervention. If a worker takes over, this implies that the person cannot participate in matters of vital concern. The person in crisis may feel devalued. Also, when a counselor assumes control, other important characteristics of the plan may be overlooked, for example, attention to the person's cultural pattern and values.

2. *Problem oriented.* The plan focuses on immediate, concrete problems that directly contribute to the crisis—that is, the hazardous event or situation and the precipitating factor. For example, a teenage daughter has run away, a woman gets a diagnosis of breast cancer, or a man learns he has AIDS. The plan should avoid probing into personality patterns or underlying psychological or marital problems contributing to the risk of crisis. These are properly the aim of psychotherapy or ongoing counseling, which the individual may choose after the immediate crisis is resolved. Exploration of previous successes and failures in problem solving is appropriate in the crisis model.

3. *Appropriate to a person's functional level and dependency needs.* The helper assesses how the person is thinking, feeling, and acting. If the individual is too anxious to think straight and make decisions (as assessed through decision counseling), the helper takes a more active role than might otherwise be indicated. In general, a crisis worker should never make a decision for another unless thorough assessment reveals that the person is unable to make decisions independently.

If the person is feeling pent up with emotion, the plan should include adequate time to express those feelings. It is legitimate to give directions for action if the person's behavior and thinking are chaotic. Success in this kind of action plan is based on a belief in a person's ability to reassume independence once the acute crisis phase is over. A firm, confident approach, based on accurate assessment and respect for the person, inspires confidence and restores a sense of order and independence to the individual in crisis.

Success in this aspect of planning implies an understanding of human interdependence. Healthy *inter*dependence is keeping a good balance between dependence and independence needs. Some individuals are too dependent most of the time; others are too independent most of the time. The excessively independent person will probably have a hard time accepting the need for more dependence on others during a crisis. Asking for help is viewed as a loss of self-esteem. In contrast, the very dependent person will tend to behave more dependently during a crisis than the situation warrants.

These considerations underscore the need for thorough assessment of a person's strengths, resources, and usual coping abilities. A good rule of thumb is never to do something *for* a person until it is clear that the person cannot do it alone. We all resent extreme dependence on others, as it keeps us from growing to our full potential. It is equally important that helpers not fail to do for a person in crisis what assessment reveals the person cannot do alone. The crisis intervention model calls for active participation by the worker. However, the crisis counselor needs to know when to let go, so the person can once again take charge of his or her life. This is more easily done by workers who are self-aware and self-confident.

4. *Consistent with a person's culture and lifestyle.* Inattention to a person's lifestyle, values, and cultural patterns can result in the failure of a seemingly perfect plan. We must be sensitive to the person's total situation and careful not to impose our own value system on a person whose lifestyle and values are different. Various cultural, ethnic, and religious groups have distinct patterns of response to events such as death, physical illness, divorce, and pregnancy out of wedlock. A sincere interest in people different from ourselves conveys respect, elicits information relevant to health, and curbs ethnocentric tendencies.

5. *Inclusive of the person's significant other(s) and social network.* If acutely upset people are viewed as social beings, a plan that excludes their social network is incomplete. Because crises occur when there is a serious disruption in normal social transactions or a person's self-perception in interpersonal situations, planning must attend to these important social factors. This is true even when the closest social contacts are hostile and are contributing significantly to the crisis.

It is tempting to avoid dealing with family members who appear to want a troubled person out of their lives. Still, significant others should be brought into the planning, at least to clarify whether or not they are a future source of help. In the event that the person is no longer wanted (for example, by a divorcing spouse or parents who abandon their children), the plan will include a means of helping the individual accept this reality and identify new social contacts. A child not helped to face such harsh realities may spend years fantasizing about reuniting a broken family. Put another way, our plan should include information about whether the family (or other significant person) is part of the problem or part of the solution (see Chapter Five).

6. *Realistic, time limited, and concrete.* A good crisis intervention plan is realistic about needs and resources. For example, a person who is too sick or who has no transportation or money should not be expected to come to an office for help. The plan should also contain a clear time frame. The person or family in crisis needs to know that actions A, B, and C are planned to occur at points X, Y, and Z. This kind of structure is reassuring to someone in crisis. It provides concrete evidence that

- Something definite will happen to change the present state of discomfort.
- The seemingly endless confusion and chaos of the crisis experience can be handled in terms familiar to the person.
- The entire plan has a clearly anticipated ending point.

For the person who fears going crazy, is threatened with violence, or finds it difficult to depend on others, it is reassuring to look forward to having events under control again within a specified time.

An effective plan is also concrete in terms of place and circumstances—for example, "Family crisis counseling sessions will be held at the crisis clinic at 7 P.M. twice a week; one session will be held at daughter Nancy's school and will include her guidance counselor, the school nurse, and the principal." Or "Police will provide transportation for a victim of violence."

7. *Dynamic and renegotiable.* A dynamic plan is not carved in marble; it is alive, meaningful, and flexible. It is specific to a particular person with unique problems and allows for ongoing changes in the person's life. It should also include a mechanism for dealing with changes if the original plan no longer fits the person's needs, so that expected outcomes will not be perceived as failures.

A person who doubts whether anything can be done to help should be assured, "If this doesn't work, we'll examine why and try something else." This feature of a plan is particularly important for people who distrust service agencies or who have experienced repeated disappointment in their efforts to obtain help.

8. *Inclusive of follow-up.* Finally, a good plan includes an agreement for follow-up contact after the apparent resolution of the crisis. This feature is too often neglected by crisis and mental health workers. If it is not initially placed in the plan and the service contract, it probably will not be done. In life-threatening crisis situations, a follow-up plan literally can mean the difference between life and death.

Careful attention to these planning criteria reduces the probability of negative crisis outcomes (Figure 4.1, Box 4b). These unhealthy outcomes increase one's vulnerability to future crisis episodes.

CASE EXAMPLE: MARY

Mary calls a crisis hotline at 11 P.M. She is very upset over the news of her husband's threat of divorce. After forty-five minutes, she and the telephone counselor agree that she will call a local counseling center the next day for an appointment. She is given the name and phone number to help her make the contact. The plan includes an agreement that Mary will call back the hotline for renegotiation if for any reason she is unable to keep the appointment.

Working Through a Crisis: Intervention Strategies

Effective crisis care fosters growth and avoids negative, destructive outcomes of traumatic events. Helping a person through healthy crisis resolution means carrying out the plan that was developed after assessment. The worker's crisis intervention techniques should follow from the way the person in crisis is thinking, feeling, and acting and should be tailored to the distinct origins of the crisis (see Figure 4.1, Boxes 1 and 3).

The manifestations of ineffective crisis coping in the case of George Sloan are spelled out on the assessment form illustrated in Chapter Three. The items designating life areas and signals of distress represent a detailed picture of biophysical, emotional, cognitive, and behavioral functioning. Ineffective coping in any of these realms can be thought of as a red flag signaling possible negative crisis outcomes. The signals indicate that help is needed and that natural and formal crisis intervention strategies should be mobilized. Using any psychosocial techniques of intervention requires assessing the need for emergency medical services and establishing access to them if necessary. Common instances of such intervention are in the event of self-inflicted injury, victimization by crime, or injury by accident, as discussed in Chapters Seven, Eight, and Eleven. Having assessed the person's coping ability in each of the functional areas, the crisis worker helps the person avoid negative outcomes and move toward growth and development while resolving the crisis. The following crisis intervention strategies are suggested as ways to achieve this goal.

Loss, Change, and Grief Work

No matter what the origin of distress, a common theme observed in people in crisis is that of loss, including loss of

- Spouse, child, or other loved one
- Health, property, and physical security
- Job, home, and country
- A familiar social role
- Freedom, safety, and bodily integrity
- The opportunity to live beyond youth

From this it follows that a pivotal aspect of successful crisis resolution is grief work. Bereavement is the response to any acute loss. Our rational, social nature implies attachment to other human beings and a view of ourselves in relationship to the rest of the world: our family, friends, pets, and home. Death and the changes following any loss are as inevitable as the ocean tide, but because loss is so painful emotionally, our natural tendency is to avoid coming to terms with it immediately and directly.

Grief work, therefore, takes time. Grief is not a set of symptoms to be treated; rather, it is a process of suffering that a bereaved person goes through on the way to a new life without the lost person, status, or object of love. It includes numbness and somatic distress (tightness in the throat, need to sigh, shortness of breath, lack of muscular power), pining and searching, anger and depression, and finally a turning toward recovery (Lindemann, 1944; Parkes, 1975). Care of the bereaved is a communal responsibility. Traditional societies, however, have assisted the bereaved much more effectively than have industrialized ones. Material prosperity and the high value placed on individual strength and accomplishment tend to dull awareness of personal mortality and the need for social support. This issue will be discussed more fully in Chapter Thirteen. Because reconciliation with loss is so important in avoiding destructive outcomes of crises, the main features of bereavement reactions are included here.

- A process of realization eventually replaces denial and the avoidance of memory of the lost person, status, or object.
- An alarm reaction sets in, including restlessness, anxiety, and various somatic reactions that leave a person unable to initiate and maintain normal patterns of activity.
- The bereaved has an urge to search for and find the lost person or object in some form. Painful pining, preoccupation with thoughts of the lost person or role and events leading to the loss, and general inattentiveness are common.
- Anger may develop toward the one who has died, or oneself, or others: "Oh John, why did you leave me?" or "Why didn't I insist that he go to the hospital?" are typical reactions.
- Guilt about perceived neglect is typical—neglect by self or others—as is guilt about having said something harsh to the person now dead or guilt about one's own survival—Lifton and Olson's (1976) "death guilt." There may also be outbursts against the people who press the bereaved person to accept the loss before he or she is psychologically ready.
- Feelings of internal loss or mutilation are revealed in such remarks as, "He was a part of me," or "Something of me went when they tore down our homes and neighborhood." The "urban villagers" (Gans, 1962) in Boston's West End are still mourning the loss of their community to an urban renewal project several decades later.
- By adopting the traits and mannerisms of the lost person or by trying to build another home of the same kind, the bereaved person re-creates a world that

has been lost. This task of grief work is monumental for refugees who have lost family members and everything but the clothes on their backs.

- A pathological variant of normal grief may emerge—that is, the reactions just described may be excessive, prolonged, inhibited, or inclined to take a distorted form. This is most apt to happen in the absence of social support. Variants of normal grief also happen in the case of *ambiguous loss,* situations in which it is not clear whether the lost person is dead or a prisoner of war, for example, or cases in which there is delay or uncertainty of ritual closure, such as waiting for recovery of remains after an airliner crash or other catastrophe (see Boss, 1999).

These reactions have been observed in widows, disaster survivors, persons who have lost a body part or who have lost their homes in urban relocation, and among people who have lost a loved one, especially if the death is an untimely one, as in the case of SIDS or AIDS (Ericsson, 1993; Lindemann, 1944; Marris, 1974; Moffatt, 1986; Parkes, 1975; Silverman, 1969).

Both normal and pathological reactions are influenced by factors existing before, during, and after a loss. These are similar to the personal, material, demographic, cultural, and social influences affecting the outcome of any other crisis. Examples of factors affecting the response to loss include an inflexible approach to problem solving, poverty, the dependency of youth or old age, cultural inhibition of emotional expression, and the unavailability of social support. Assisting the bereaved in avoiding pathological outcomes of grief is an essential feature of a preventive and developmental approach to crisis work. Grief work, then, can be viewed as integral to any crisis resolution process in which loss figures as a major theme.

Normal grief work (Harvey, 1998; Johnson-Soderberg, 1981; Lindemann, 1944; Parkes, 1975) consists of the following:

1. *Acceptance of the pain of loss.* This means dealing with memories of the deceased.
2. *Open expression of pain, sorrow, hostility, and guilt.* The person must feel free to mourn the loss openly, usually by weeping, and to express feelings of guilt and hostility.
3. *Understanding of the intense feelings associated with loss.* For example, the fear of going crazy is a normal part of the grieving process. When these feelings of sorrow, fear, guilt, and hostility are worked through in the presence of a caring person, they gradually subside. The ritual expression of grief, as in funerals, greatly aids in this process.
4. *Resumption of normal activities and social relationships without the person lost.* Having worked through the memories and feelings associated with a loss, a person acquires new patterns of social interaction apart from the deceased.

Many bereaved persons find support groups particularly helpful. Being with others who have suffered a similar loss provides understanding as well as some relief of the social isolation that may follow an acute loss. When people do not do grief work following any profound loss, serious emotional, mental, and social problems can occur. All of us can help people grieve without shame over their losses. This is possible if we are sensitized to the importance of expressing feelings openly and to the various factors affecting the bereavement process.

Those whose needs around grief work extend beyond the few crisis counseling sessions should have the benefit of individual or group psychotherapy. This may include persons who have suffered several serious losses in a short time or those with pathological grief reactions accompanied by serious depression. Children are of special concern around loss and grief because they may be overlooked as adults focus on their own grief. Linda Goldman (1994, 1996) has produced informative guides for laypersons and professionals, focusing on the particular needs of grieving children (see also Perschy, 1997, for helping grieving adolescents).

Other Intervention and Counseling Strategies

Some additional crisis care strategies include the following:

1. *Listen actively and with concern.* When a person is ashamed of his or her ability to cope with a problem or feels that the problem is too minor to be so upset about, a good listener can dispel some of these feelings. Being listened to helps a person feel important and deserving of help no matter how trivial the problem may appear. Effective listening demands attention to possible listening barriers, such as internal and external noise and the other factors influencing communication discussed earlier. Comments such as, "Hmm," "I see," and "Go on" are useful in acknowledging what a person says; they also encourage more talking and build rapport and trust. The failure to listen forms a barrier to all other intervention strategies.

2. *Encourage the open expression of feelings.* Listening is a natural forerunner of this important crisis intervention technique. One reason that some people are crisis prone is that they habitually bottle up feelings such as anger, grief, frustration, helplessness, and hopelessness. Negative associations with expressing feelings during childhood seem to put a damper on such expression when traumatic events occur later in life. The crisis worker's acceptance of a distressed person's feelings often helps the person feel better immediately. It also can be the beginning of a healthier coping style in the future. This is one of the rewarding growth possibilities for people in crisis who are fortunate enough to get the help they need.

A useful technique for fostering emotional expression is role playing or role modeling. For example, the worker could say, "If that happened to me, I think I'd be very angry," thus giving the distressed person permission to express feelings that one may hesitate to share, perhaps out of misdirected shame.

For extreme anxiety and accompanying changes in biophysical function, relaxation techniques and exercise can be encouraged. The increase in energy that follows a crisis experience can be channeled into constructive activity and socially approved outlets, such as assigning tasks to disaster victims or providing athletic facilities in hospitals. The current popular emphasis on self-help techniques, such as physical exercise and leisure for stress reduction, should be encouraged as a wholesome substitute for chemical tranquilizers during crisis.

As important as listening and emotional and physical expression are, they do not constitute crisis intervention in themselves. Without additional strategies, these techniques may not result in positive crisis resolution. Used together, grief work, listening, and facilitating the expression of feelings address the emotional responses to crisis, but the cognitive and behavioral elements of the crisis are also important. The next several strategies focus on these facets of the crisis resolution process.

3. *Help the person gain an understanding of the crisis.* The individual may ask, "Why did this awful thing have to happen to me?" This perception of a traumatic event implies that the event occurred because the person in crisis was bad and deserving of punishment. The crisis worker can help the person see the many factors that contribute to a crisis situation and thereby curtail self-blaming. The individual is encouraged to examine the total problem, including his or her own behavior or physical symptoms, as they may be related to the crisis. Thoughtful reflection on oneself and one's behavior can lead to growth and change rather than self-deprecation and self-pity.

4. *Help the person gradually accept reality.* Respond to a person's tendency to adopt a victim role or to blame problems on others. An individual in crisis who adopts the victim role can be helped to escape that role (McCullough, 1995). It may be tempting to agree with the person who is blaming others, especially when the person's story, as well as the reality, reveal especially cruel attacks, rejections, or other unfair treatment. Those whose crises stem primarily from social sources do not just *feel* victimized, they *are* in fact victimized. Such abused people, though, are also survivors (Hoff, 1990); their survival skills can be tapped for constructive crisis resolution by encouraging them to channel their anger into action to change oppressive social arrangements and policies (see Figure 4.1, right circle, Box 3).

The tendency to blame and scapegoat is especially strong in family and marital crises. The crisis counselor should help such people understand that victim-persecutor relationships are not one-sided. This can be done effectively when the counselor has established an appropriate relationship with the person. If the counselor has genuine concern and is not engaging in rescue fantasies, the distressed person is more likely to accept the counselor's interpretation of his or her own role in the crisis event. The victim-rescuer-persecutor syndrome occurs frequently in human relationships of all kinds and is common in many helping relationships. People viewed as victims are not rescued easily, so counselors who try it are usually frustrated when their efforts fail. Their disappointment may move them to "persecute" their "victim" for failure to respond. At this point, the victim turns persecutor and punishes the counselor for a well-intentioned but inappropriate effort to help (Haley, 1969b; James & Jongeward, 1971; McKinlay, 1990). Figure 4.2 illustrates the pitfalls of engaging in rescue or power struggles in crisis work or other human relationships.

FIGURE 4.2. VICTIM-RESCUER-PERSECUTOR TRIANGLE.

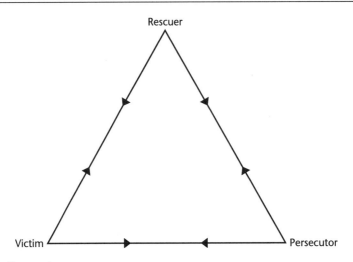

Key Concepts

Rescuer Role:

- Cannot be enacted without a complementary "victim"
- May suggest provider's excessive "need to be needed"
- Impedes growth and empowerment of client

Victim Role:

- Threatens basic need for self-mastery and self-determination
- Even if overt message is demand for rescue, more help covertly leads to resentment and role switch to "persecutor"

Practice Implications:

- Emphasize self-awareness and focus on empathy versus sympathy
- Conduct data-based assessment of client's actual needs
- Provide neither more nor less than needed
- Promote interdependence (versus excessive dependence or independence)
- Be clear about necessary limits and rationale for same
- Avoid power and control tactics

Adapted from transactional analysis.

In such "meta-complementary" relationships (Haley, 1969a), the egalitarian aspects of the service contract are sabotaged—that is, one person allows or pressures another to define a relationship in a certain way. For example, if person A acts helpless and provokes person B to take care of him or her, A is actually in control while being manifestly dependent. Translated to the helping relationship, a counselor may not wish to be controlled any more than a client would, hence the initiation of the troublesome victim-rescuer-persecutor cycle that is so difficult to disrupt once started. (See "Social Network Strategies" in Chapter Five for an effective means of interrupting the cycle and Chapter Six for rescue implications with self-destructive persons.)

5. *Help the person explore new ways of coping with problems.* Instead of responding to loss and crises as helpless victims or with suicide and homicide attempts, people can learn new responses. Sometimes people have given up on problem-solving devices that used to work for them.

CASE EXAMPLE: JANE

Jane, age thirty-eight, was able to weather a lot of storms until her best friend died. After her friend's death, she somehow could not find the energy necessary to establish new friendships. Exploration revealed that Jane had never worked through the grief she had experienced over the death of her friend. The lack of healthy resolution of this crisis left Jane more vulnerable than she might otherwise have been when her daughter, age eighteen, left home and married. Jane had temporarily given up and stopped using her effective problem-solving devices.

In Jane's case, a crisis worker might ask about previous successful coping devices and find out whether Jane thinks any of these might work for her now. Jane could also be assisted with delayed grief work and with exploring avenues for developing new friendships (see also Littrell, 1998; Walter & Peller, 2000).

6. *Link the person to a social network.* The technique of exploring new coping devices leads naturally to this important facet of crisis care. Just as disruption of social ties is an important precursor of crisis, the restoration of those ties (or if they have been permanently lost, the formation of new ones) is one of the most powerful means of resolving a crisis in a healthy way. The crisis counselor takes an active role in reestablishing a person with his or her social network. This aspect of crisis care is also known as social network intervention—the ecological approach—and is discussed in detail in the next chapter.

Another way to enhance social network linkage is through "contemporary rites of passage" (see Figure 4.1, lower circle, Box 3). Such ritual support mechanisms are especially important in dealing with the common theme of loss during crisis, whether through unanticipated events or role changes. Chapter Thirteen discusses this strategy in detail.

7. *Reinforce the newly learned coping devices, and follow up after crisis resolution.* The person is given time to try the proposed solutions to the problem. Successful problem-solving mechanisms are reinforced; unsuccessful solutions are discarded, and new ones are sought. In any case, the person is not cut off abruptly.

A follow-up contact is carried out as agreed to in the initial plan. Some workers argue that follow-up contact maintains people in an unnecessary state of dependency. Others think that contacting a person later constitutes an invasion of privacy and an imposition of therapy on an unwilling client. Rarely does this argument hold when the person being helped has initiated the helping process, and follow-up is included in a mutually negotiated service contract. Unquestionably, premature or pressured referrals for psychotherapy or other services on people who do not want them would be unethical. Yet we need to consider whether the "invasion of privacy" and similar arguments may be covering a dearth of sensitively designed and integrated follow-up programs (Hoff & Adamowski, 1998). As already noted, in the managed care milieu, the practice of collabora- tively developed "contracting"—whether in counseling or primary health care settings—enhances the prospect of client responsibility for self-care and follow- through, while serving as a structured framework for continued service, evaluation of same, and avoidance of recidivism and systems problems (see "Service Forms" in Chapter Three).

Follow-up is more likely to be successful and less likely to be interpreted as an unwanted intrusion if

- It is incorporated into the total service plan rather than added as an afterthought or an unexpected telephone call.
- It is based on the principle of self-determination (even if a person is in crisis) and on the avoidance of "savior" tactics as well as any denigration of others' values and abilities by counselors.

When carefully designed, then, follow-up work can often be the occasion for reaching people who are unable to initiate help for themselves *before* a crisis occurs. This is especially true for those people who are suicidal and very depressed, those threatened with violence, those whose medical and emotional problems are com- plexly intertwined, and those especially vulnerable because of severe psychiatric illness. In such life-threatening situations, a person often feels worthless and is un- able to reach out for help (see Chapters Six, Seven, Eight, and Eleven).

These crisis intervention techniques can be mastered by any helping person who chooses to learn them. Human service workers and community caretak- ers, volunteer counselors, social workers, nurses, physicians, police officers, teach- ers, and clergy increasingly incorporate crisis intervention as a part of their professional training in caring for distressed people. Whether in offices, institutions, homes, or mobile outreach programs, effective helping techniques save time and effort spent on problems that can develop from ineffectively resolved crises (Haley, 1987; Hoff & Adamowski, 1998; Zealberg, Santos, & Fisher, 1993). Primary prevention is much less costly in both human and economic terms. These basic strategies can be applied in a variety of settings and circumstances to be discussed in the remaining chapters. In highly charged and potentially violent crisis situations (both individual and group), additional techniques are indicated (see Part Two).

Psychotropic Drugs: What Place in Crisis Intervention?

Advertisements bombard us constantly with the idea that drugs are a solution for many problems. We hear, Do you feel down or upset? Can't sleep? Can't control your kids? Take pills. The inclusion of a question in this section's title mirrors the controversy and questions that abound in any discussion of drugs among professionals and laypersons alike. These controversies, prominent across media sources, are situated in historical, cultural, and economic realities commonly discussed by patients, their families, health and mental health providers, policymakers and others. The purpose for this book is *not* a comprehensive review or critique of the issues or individual drugs and their indications. Health providers with prescriptive authority (physicians and some advanced practice nurses) are obliged to keep current on drugs and their use. The focus here is to consider how psychotropic drugs can be used responsibly or misused in crisis work. Some common historical facts, related questions, and results of research and practice with psychotropic agents are therefore presented as context for criteria that should guide drug use for some clients in crisis situations.

1. People have been using mind-altering substances over many centuries. It is therefore unlikely that a particular "war on drugs" will significantly alter this pattern. What, then, is the significance today of having legalized one of these substances, alcohol (at one time legally prohibited in the United States), but not others?

2. How did so many people, both professionals and the general public, come to believe that chemical tranquilization is a preferred way to deal with life's stresses and crises? For example, some parents and teachers insist on drugs for "attention deficit hyperactivity disordered" children. When confronted with a client's demand for drugs, it is not uncommon to hear practitioners say, "But they want the pills. They don't want to talk about or deal with what's troubling them or what's going on in the family. What am I supposed to do?" Of note here is the fact that the advertising industry and professional practice have enormous influence on what the public comes to accept as a norm. Also of note is the national crisis in the United States resulting from inadequate counseling and psychiatric services for disturbed children, services that would alleviate excessive reliance on drugs for children. Of further policy significance is the requirement of some insurance companies to have a child evaluated for medication very early in the course of treatment as a condition for covering other psychotherapeutic services.

3. The media are increasingly addressing the problem of prescription drugs, their overuse, and their escalating costs; many Americans go to Canada to purchase an identical drug at a fraction of the cost. What does the profit motive have to do with the overuse of some drugs and the prices U.S. citizens are expected to pay in comparison with others? Given this pattern of dependency on and overuse of prescription drugs, why does the political war on drugs continue to focus on foreign production of illegal drugs rather than on prevention and treatment among users at home? And why—in the United States—are the main victims of this war mostly poor inner-city black youth rather than those profiting from the illegal drug traffic?

4. At least a half century of research-based knowledge and experience regarding psychotropic drugs establishes that their greatest efficacy is when used in

combination with other therapeutic modalities, such as psychotherapy and support in rehabilitation programs. These outcomes have been demonstrated even in the treatment of bipolar illness and schizophrenia, the mental disorders with strong biological correlates. Yet the disparity in insurance coverage for treatment and rehabilitation of the mentally ill beyond psychotropic medications continues.

Clearly, the benefits of psychotropic drugs when used responsibly are accepted by professionals and laypersons alike. It is their misuse and overdependence that are in dispute. With this overview of the problem, let us consider the criteria for use of psychotropic drugs (usually, antianxiety agents and antidepressants) for distressed people.

Tranquilizers taken during crisis temporarily relieve anxiety but do nothing about the problem's root cause. At best, they are a crutch. At worst, they can be addictive and can displace effective problem solving at the psychosocial level. For the person in crisis, psychotropic drugs should *never* be used as a substitute for crisis counseling and problem solving. However, there are times when a tranquilizer can be used in addition to the crisis intervention techniques outlined previously. These instances are (1) when a person is experiencing extreme anxiety, has frequent crying spells, or fears losing control, (2) when a person is so distraught that it is impossible to engage him or her in the problem-solving process, and (3) when a person's extreme anxiety prevents sleep for a significant period of time. Sleeping pills should always be avoided. Exercise and nonchemical means of relaxation should be encouraged (see Chapter Seven, "Drug Treatment for Depression"). The increasingly popular alternative or complementary medical techniques should also be encouraged—for example, biofeedback, acupuncture, herbal remedies, and so forth, for certain bodily responses to stress.

Apart from these special circumstances, psychotropic drugs should be avoided whenever possible while dealing with a critical life event. By relieving anxiety on a temporary basis, tranquilizers can have the effect of reducing the person's motivation to effectively resolve a crisis. With chemical tranquilization, the person loses the advantages of increased energy during a crisis state. The *opportunity* for psychosocial growth is often lost due to the temporary tranquility of a drugged psyche, while the *danger* is increased—including possible overdose or unpleasant and even dangerous side effects from interactions among drugs that are not carefully monitored. Some drugs can complicate rather than alleviate the original symptoms for which they were sought.

Caution is also suggested to crisis workers who have physician or psychiatrist consultants available to them. Sometimes crisis workers ask for psychiatric consultation simply because of their own lack of clinical experience, not because the distinct service of a psychiatrist is needed. As long as the psychiatrist shares the worker's values regarding crisis care and has additional crisis intervention skills, there is no problem. However, this is not true of all psychiatrists;

some have little or no training or experience in crisis intervention but have the legal right to prescribe drugs. A similar dynamic may apply to other health providers with prescriptive authority. Of note is the fact that the majority of psychotropic drug prescriptions are written by providers who lack specialty training in psychopathology and its treatment (Lessig, 1996), underscoring the importance of consultation with a psychiatrist or advanced practice psychiatric nurse (see Edmands, Hoff, Kaylor, Mower, & Sorrell, 1999).

Although the traditional psychiatric management of behavioral emergencies has some features in common with crisis intervention, it should not be equated with the crisis model if a strictly biomedical approach (relying heavily on chemical stabilization) is used (see Cohen, 1993, and Luhrmann, 2000, Chapter Four). The nonmedical crisis worker should remember that a consultation request may result in a distressed person's receiving a drug prescription when actually what is needed is the experience of highly skilled crisis specialists. Such specialists include—but are not limited to—psychiatrists. Conversely, a comprehensive plan for certain individuals in crisis may include measures available only through the professions of medicine and psychiatry. Psychiatrists have a medical degree and the skills and legal powers unique to their training and position in the field of medicine. Unlike nonmedical counselors or psychiatric practitioners—social workers, for example—psychiatrists can prescribe medications, admit people to hospitals, and make distinctions between psychological, psychiatric, and neurological disturbances. Psychiatrists also diagnose and treat the symptoms of drug overdose. In the United States, advanced practice nurses and psychologists can also prescribe medication in some jurisdictions. Ideally, psychiatric stabilization programs, such as those in emergency departments with holding beds, should include the services of skilled crisis counselors.

In short, all steps taken by the crisis intervention movement to reduce the large-scale dependence on drugs for problem solving during crisis and at other times will be steps forward (see also Barney, 1994; Breggin & Breggin, 1994; Doweiko, 1995; Hamilton, Jensvold, Rothblum, & Cole, 1995; Luhrmann, 2000; Ray & Ksir, 1993; Zito et al., 2000).

Crisis Intervention Illustrations

Two cases, continued from Chapters Two and Three, illustrate the use of the techniques discussed in this chapter.

Crisis Care in an Emergency Setting

An interview with George Sloan (continued from Chapters Two and Three) illustrates crisis planning and intervention in an emergency department following a high-lethal suicide attempt (see Table 4.1).

TABLE 4.1. CRISIS CARE IN AN EMERGENCY SETTING.

Intervention Techniques	Interview Between George Sloan and Emergency Department Nurse
Exploring resources	*Nurse:* You said you really can't talk to your wife about your problems. Is there anyone else you've ever thought about talking with?
	George: Well, I tried talking to my doctor once, but he didn't really have time. Then a few months ago, my minister could see I was pretty down and he stopped by a couple of times, but that didn't help.
Facilitating client decision making	*Nurse:* Is there anyone else you think you could talk to?
	George: No, not really—nobody, anyway, that would understand.
Suggesting new resources	Nurse: What about seeing a regular counselor, George? We have connections here in the emergency room with the psychiatric department of our hospital, where a program could be set up to help you work out some of your problems.
	George: What do you mean? You think I'm crazy or something? (defensively) I don't need to see a shrink.
Listening, accepting client's feelings	*Nurse:* No, George, of course I don't think you're crazy. But when you're down and out enough to see no other way to turn but suicide—well, I know things look pretty bleak now, but talking to a counselor usually leads to some other ways of dealing with problems if you're willing to give it a chance.
	George: Well, I could consider it. What would it cost? I sure can't afford any more medical bills.
Involving client in the plan Facilitating client decision making Making the plan concrete and specific Involving significant other	Nurse: Here at our hospital clinic, if you can't pay the regular fee, you can apply for medical assistance. How would you like to arrange it? I could call someone now to come over and talk with you and set up a program, or you can call them yourself tomorrow and make the arrangements.
	George: Well, I feel better now, so I think I'd just as soon wait until tomorrow and call them—besides, I guess I should really tell my wife; I don't know how she'd feel about me seeing a counselor. But then I guess suicide is kind of a coward's way out.
Reinforcing coping mechanism Actively encouraging	*Nurse:* George, you sound hesitant, and I can understand what you must be feeling. Talking again with your wife sounds like a good idea. Or you and your wife might want to see the counselor together sometime. But I hope you do follow through on this, as I really believe you and your family could benefit from some help like this. After all, you've had a lot of things hit you at one time.
Expressing empathy	*George:* Well, it's hard for me to imagine what anyone could do, but maybe at least my wife and I could get along better and keep our kid out of trouble. I just wish she'd quit insisting on things I can't afford.

TABLE 4.1.   CRISIS CARE IN AN EMERGENCY SETTING. (*continued*)

Intervention Techniques	Interview Between George Sloan and Emergency Department Nurse	
Conveying realistic hope that things might get better	*Nurse:*	That's certainly a possibility, and that alone might improve things. How about this, George: I'll call you tomorrow afternoon to see how you are and whether you're having any trouble getting through to the counseling service?
Initiating follow-up plan	*George:*	That sounds fine. I guess I really should give it another chance. Thanks for everything.
	Nurse:	I'm glad we were able to talk, George. I'll be in touch tomorrow.

Crisis and Psychosocial Care in a Primary Care Setting

Applying crisis care to Delaine's case (continued from Chapter Three, p. 80), the primary care provider, either a physician or an advanced practice nurse, would have made a mental connection between her request for something to ease her crying bouts, her gastrointestinal symptoms, and the series of losses she has suffered. Without discounting or minimizing any of Delaine's presenting symptoms, the provider would listen attentively and make an empathic response affirming the realistic basis for her distress—for example, "You've certainly been through a lot in a very short time. It's not surprising that you feel sad and a bit overwhelmed with many losses and big changes from what you're used to."

The provider would also use the office visit to teach about the essential normality of physical symptoms like Delaine's in response to coping with major life stressors. Such teaching would serve as a context for explaining to Delaine the limitations of psychotropic medication if not accompanied by social support and counseling around her many losses.

Delaine's history of coping suggests her positive response to this approach. Ideally, the physician or advanced practice nurse develops the following plan with Delaine.

1. Laboratory tests to aid diagnosis and follow-up treatment of gastrointestinal symptoms
2. A referral to the on-site mental health service (usually staffed by a social worker or advanced practice psychiatric–mental health nurse) for crisis counseling around loss and guilt
3. A one-week prescription of an antianxiety medication to be monitored in concert with follow-up counseling by the mental health specialist
4. A recommendation to consider joining a support group for widows (resource information is given, with the suggestion to discuss this further in follow-up counseling)
5. A follow-up appointment for review of laboratory results and general progress

Exhibit 4.2 sets out the basics for assessment and crisis work in primary care.

EXHIBIT 4.2. BASICS OF PSYCHOSOCIAL ASSESSMENT AND CRISIS WORK IN PRIMARY CARE.

1. Detection (implies routine inquiry in health assessment protocols)
2. Assessment of risk (includes emotional trauma from victimization and danger of injury to self and others)
3. Empathic, supportive response (constitutes public recognition of trauma from abuse)
4. Safety planning for self (and for mothers and their children as well)
5. Linkage, effective referral, and follow-up (implies collaboration with crisis, mental health, or trauma specialist)

Summary

Without communication and rapport—the immediate context for crisis work—success will probably elude us. Resolution of crisis should occur in a person's or a family's natural setting whenever possible. Planning well and using good crisis intervention skills are the best ways to avoid extreme measures such as hospitalization and lengthy rehabilitation programs. The active involvement of a distressed person in a plan for crisis resolution is essential if crisis intervention is to succeed as a way of helping people. The service contract symbolizes this active involvement. The use of tranquilizers decreases such involvement and can sabotage the growth potential of the crisis experience.

References

Arnold, E., & Boggs, K. U. (1999). *Interpersonal relationships: Professional communication skills for nurses* (3rd ed.). Philadelphia: Saunders.

Barney, K. (1994). Limitations of the critique of the medical model. *Journal of Mind and Behavior, 15*(1,2), 19–34.

Bateson, G. (1958). *Naven* (2nd ed.). Palo Alto, CA: Stanford University Press.

Boss, P. (1999). *Ambiguous loss*. Cambridge, MA: Harvard University Press.

Breggin, P., & Breggin, G. R. (1994). *Talking back to Prozac: What doctors won't tell you about today's most controversial drug*. New York: St. Martin's Press.

Campbell-Heider, N., & Pollock, D. (1987). Barriers to physician-nurse collegiality: An anthropological perspective. *Social Science and Medicine, 25*(5), 421–425.

Capponi, P. (1992). *Upstairs in the crazy house*. Toronto: Penguin Books.

Chappell, D., & Di Martino, V. (1998). *Violence at work*. Geneva: International Labour Organisation.

Cohen, C. I. (1993). The biomedicalization of psychiatry: A critical overview. *Community Mental Health Journal, 29*, 509–521.

Dahnke, G. L., & Clatterbuck, G. W. (1990). *Human communication: Theory and research*. Belmont, CA: Wadsworth.

Doweiko, H. E. (1995). *Concepts of chemical dependency* (3rd ed.). Pacific Grove, CA: Brooks/Cole.

Edmands, M. S., Hoff, L. A., Kaylor, L., Mower, L., & Sorrell, S. (1999). Bridging gaps between mind, body and spirit: Healing the whole person. *Journal of Psychosocial Nursing, 37*(10), 1–7.

Ericsson, S. (1993). *Companion through the darkness: Inner dialogues on grief.* New York: Harper-Collins.

Gans, H. (1962). *The urban villagers.* New York: Free Press.

Goldman, L. (1994). *Life and loss: A guide to help grieving children.* Philadelphia: Taylor & Francis.

Goldman, L. (1996). *Breaking the silence: A guide to help children with complicated grief: Suicide, homicide, AIDS, violence and abuse.* Philadelphia: Taylor & Francis.

Haley, J. (1969a). *Strategies of psychotherapy.* Philadelphia: Grune & Stratton.

Haley, J. (1969b). The art of being a failure as a therapist. *American Journal of Orthopsychiatry, 39*(4), 691–695.

Haley, J. (1987). *Problem-solving therapy.* San Francisco: Jossey-Bass.

Hamilton, J. A., Jensvold, M. F., Rothblum, E. D., & Cole, E. (Eds.). (1995). *Psychopharmacology from a feminist perspective.* New York: Harrington Park Press.

Haney, W. (1991). *Communication and interpersonal relations: Text and cases* (6th ed.). Burr Ridge, IL: Irwin.

Hansell, N. (1970). Decision counseling. *Archives of General Psychiatry, 22,* 462–467.

Harvey, J. H. (Ed.). (1998). *Perspectives on loss: A source book.* Philadelphia: Taylor & Francis.

Hoff, L. A. (1990). *Battered women as survivors.* London: Routledge.

Hoff, L. A. (1993). Review essay: Health policy and the plight of the mentally ill. *Psychiatry, 56*(4), 400–419.

Hoff, L. A., & Adamowski, K. (1998). *Creating excellence in crisis care: A guide to effective training and program designs.* San Francisco: Jossey-Bass.

James, M., & Jongeward, D. (1971). *Born to win.* Reading, MA: Addison-Wesley.

Johnson-Soderberg, S. (1981). Grief themes. *Advances in Nursing Science, 3*(4), 15–26.

Jourard, S. M. (1970). Suicide: An invitation to die. *American Journal of Nursing, 70*(2), 269, 273–275.

Kelly, V. R., & Weston, H. B. (1974). Civil liberties in mental health facilities. *Social Work, 19,* 48–54.

Kottler, J. A. (1994). *Beyond blame: A new way of resolving conflicts in relationships.* San Francisco: Jossey-Bass.

Lessig, D. Z. (1996). Primary care diagnosis and pharmacologic treatment of depression in adults. *Nurse Practitioner, 21*(10), 74–87.

Lifton, R. J., & Olson, E. (1976). The human meaning of total disaster: The Buffalo Creek experience. *Psychiatry, 39,* 1–18.

Lindemann, E. (1944). Symptomatology and management of acute grief. *American Journal of Psychiatry, 101,* 101–148. (Also reprinted in H. J. Parad (Ed.). (1965). *Crisis intervention: Selected readings.* New York: Family Service Association of America.)

Littrell, J. M. (1998). *Brief counseling in action.* New York: Norton.

Loustaunau, M. O., & Sobo, E. J. (1997). *The cultural context of health, illness, and medicine.* New York: Bergin & Garvey.

Luhrmann, T. M. (2000). *Of two minds: The growing disorder in American psychiatry.* New York: Knopf.

Marks, I. M., & Scott, R. (Eds.). (1990). *Mental health care delivery: Innovations, impediments, and implementation.* Cambridge: Cambridge University Press.

Marris, P. (1974). *Loss and change.* London: Routledge.

McCullough, C. J. (1995). *Nobody's victim.* New York: Clarkson/Potter.

McKinlay, J. B. (1990). A case for refocusing upstream: The political economy of illness. In P. Conrad & R. Kern (Eds.), *The sociology of health and illness: Critical perspectives* (3rd ed., pp. 502–516). New York: St. Martin's Press.

Moffat, B. (1986). *When someone you love has AIDS: A book of hope for family and friends.* Santa Monica, CA: IBS Press, in association with Love Heals.

Northouse, L. L., & Northouse, P. G. (1998). *Health communication: Strategies for health professionals* (3rd ed.). East Norwalk, CT: Appleton & Lang.

Parkes, C. M. (1975). *Bereavement: Studies of grief in adult life.* Harmondsworth, England: Penguin Books.

Pennebaker, J. W. (1993). Putting stress into words: Health, linguistic, and therapeutic implications. *Behavior Research & Therapy, 31*(6), 539–548.

Perschy, M. K. (1997). *Helping teens work through grief.* Philadelphia: Taylor & Francis.

Pluckhan, M. L. (1978). *Human communication.* New York: McGraw-Hill.

Ray, O. S., & Ksir, C. (1993). *Drugs, society, & human behavior.* St. Louis: Mosby-Year Book.

Rodriguez-Garcia, R., & Akhter, M. N. (2000). Human rights: The foundation of public health practice. *American Journal of Public Health, 90*(5), 693–694.

Ryan, W. (1971). *Blaming the victim.* New York: Vintage Books.

Silverman, P. (1969). The widow-to-widow program: An experiment in preventive intervention. *Mental Hygiene, 53,* 333–337.

Storti, C. (1994). *Cross-cultural dialogues: Seventy-four Brief encounters with cultural difference.* Yarmouth, ME: Intercultural Press.

Thompson, T. L. (1988). *Communication for health professionals.* Lanham, MD: University Press of America.

Truax, C. B., & Carkhuff, R. R. (1967). *Toward effective counseling and psychotherapy.* Hawthorne, NY: Aldine de Gruyter.

Vetterling-Braggin, M., Elliston, F. A., & English, J. (Eds.). (1977). *Feminism and philosophy, Part 3: Sexism in ordinary language* (pp. 105–170). Totowa, NJ: Littlefield, Adams.

Walter, J. L., & Peller, J. E. (2000). *Recreating brief therapy.* New York: Norton.

Zealberg, J. J., Santos, A. B., & Fisher, R. K. (1993). Benefits of mobile crisis programs. *Hospital and Community Psychiatry, 44*(1), 16–17.

Zito, J. M., Safer, D. J., dosReis, S., Gardner, J. F., Boles, M., & Lynch, F. (2000). Trends in the prescribing of psychotropic medications to preschoolers. *Journal of the American Medical Association, 283*(8), 1025–1030.

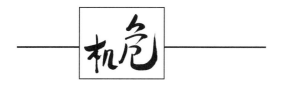

CHAPTER FIVE

FAMILY AND SOCIAL NETWORK STRATEGIES DURING CRISIS

We are conceived and born in a social context. We grow and develop among other people. We experience crises around events in our social milieu. People near us—friends, family, community—help or hinder us through crises. And finally, death, even for those who die alone and abandoned, demands some response from the society left behind.

Social Aspects of Human Growth

Multidisciplinary research increasingly has supported a shifting emphasis from individual to social approaches to helping distressed people (for example, Antonovsky, 1980, 1987; Boissevain, 1979; Hoff, 1990; Mitchell, 1969). Despite the prevalence of individual intervention techniques, overwhelming evidence now shows that social networks and support are primary factors in a person's susceptibility to disease, the process of becoming ill and seeking help, the treatment process, and the outcome of illness, whether that is rehabilitation and recovery or death (for example, Berkman & Syme, 1979; Loustaunau & Sobo, 1997; Robinson, 1971; Sarason & Sarason, 1985). The work of clinicians during the golden age of social psychiatry supports the prolific social science literature on social approaches to distressed people (see Garrison, 1974; Langsley & Kaplan, 1968; Polak, 1971). After using family and social network approaches, clinicians seldom return to predominantly individual practice (for example, Yalom, 1995; Satir, Stackowiak, & Taschman, 1975; Speck & Attneave, 1973). Hansell (1976) casts his entire description of persons in crisis in a social framework.

Caplan (1964) laid the foundation for much of this work. The Crisis Paradigm (see Figure 5.1) in this book similarly stresses the pivotal role of sociocultural factors in the development, manifestation, and resolution of crises. This chapter presents an overview of social approaches to crisis intervention and suggests strategies for family, social network, and group practice.

An interrelated assumption underlies this discussion: people often avoid social approaches because they have not been trained to use them, or their usefulness is still questioned. In addition, individual approaches often are not evaluated for either their effectiveness or their underlying assumptions. The treatment bias favoring individualistic measures is compounded by heavy reliance on psychoactive

FIGURE 5.1. CRISIS PARADIGM.

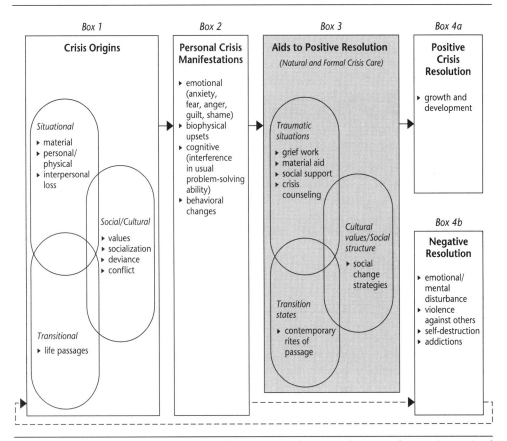

Crisis origins, manifestations, and outcomes and the respective functions of crisis care have an interactional relationship. The intertwined circles represent the distinct yet interrelated origins of crisis and aids to positive resolution, even though personal manifestations are often similar. The arrows pointing from origins to positive resolution illustrate the *opportunity for growth and development* through crisis; the broken line at bottom depicts the potential *danger of crisis* in the absence of appropriate aids. The loop between Box 4b and Box 1 denotes the *vulnerability* to future crisis episodes following negative resolution.

drugs, whereas evidence of sociocultural variables affecting health and illness often takes second place (McKinlay & Marceau, 1999; Meyer & Schwartz, 2000). Social strategies contrast strongly with approaches in which upsets are seen primarily as the result of personality dynamics and internal conflicts. Advocates of the latter view do not entirely disregard social factors, nor do advocates of social-interactional approaches ignore individual factors. Rather, their differences are in emphasis and in their conviction of what constitutes an appropriate helping process.

A social network may consist of a person's family, friends, neighbors, relatives, bartender, employer, hairdresser, teacher, welfare worker, physician, lawyer—anyone with whom a person has regular social intercourse. Different individuals have different networks. The following interview with a cocktail waitress illustrates the diversity of social network support and how the *natural* crisis care process works.

CASE EXAMPLE: THE COCKTAIL WAITRESS

This is the dumpiest bar I've ever worked in, but I really enjoy it. I like the people. When I quit my last job and came here, a lot of old men followed me. There are all kinds of bars, but if it weren't for bars like this, a lot of old people and "down and outers" wouldn't have any place to go. Our regulars don't have anything or anyone, and they admit it. I feel like a counselor a lot of times. One of my customers, a pretty young woman, has had several children taken away. When her caseworker called me to ask if I thought she was ready to have her child back, I said no—and I told the woman so.

I think the people I feel closest to are the old men who are lonesome or widowed. One guy who shouldn't drink at all stayed on the wagon for quite a while, then went on a three-week binge. His girlfriend told him that she didn't want him anymore if he didn't stop drinking. So he came in here and got sick after two drinks. He fell on the floor and hurt himself. I called the police and asked them to take him to the hospital. I called the girlfriend, and she and I both convinced him to finally get some help to control his drinking. When he got out, he came in and thanked me. This is really rewarding.

I work hard at helping people get on the right track, and I'm really tough on people who don't do anything with their lives, like these old guys. I know just how much they can drink. Take Ben, he can drink only three and I tell him, "OK, you can have them either all at once, or you can stick around for a while." I was brought up to respect my elders, and I don't want to see these guys go out and fall on their faces. I have a good friend who's a priest. We argued for years about my work in the bar. Finally, he agreed that it wasn't a bad thing to do. Someone has to do it.

The next case example highlights the individual, as opposed to the social, approach to *formal* crisis care.

CASE EXAMPLE: ELLEN

Ellen, age sixteen, ran away from home. Shortly after police returned her, she attempted suicide with approximately ten aspirin and five of her mother's tranquilizers. Ellen had exhibited many signs of depression. She was seen for individual counseling at a mental health clinic for twelve sessions. Ellen's parents were seen initially for one session as part of the assessment process. The counselor learned that Ellen was always somewhat depressed and withdrawn at home and that she was getting poor grades in school.

Counseling focused on Ellen's feelings of guilt, worthlessness, and anger, cen-tered on her relationship with her parents. She complained that her father was aloof and seldom available when there was a problem. She felt closer to her mother but said her mother was un-reasonably strict about her friends and hours out. At the conclusion of the indi-vidual counseling sessions, Ellen was less depressed and felt less worthless, al-though things were essentially the same at home and school. Two months after termination of counseling, Ellen made another suicide attempt, this time with double the amount of aspirin and tranquilizers.

This case reveals that the involvement of Ellen's family and the school counselor—primary people in her social network—was not an integral part of the helping process. In contrast, a social approach to Ellen's problem would have attended to her feelings of depression and worthlessness, but these feelings would have been viewed in the context of her interactions with those closest to her, not as the result of her withdrawn personality. In other words, in crisis intervention, people and their problems are seen in a psychosocial rather than a psychoanalytic context.

Within the psychosocial framework, Ellen's counselor would have included at least her family and the school counselor in the original assessment and counsel-ing plan. This initial move might have revealed still other people who were im-portant to Ellen and would be able to help. For example, when Ellen ran away, she went to her Aunt Dorothy's house; she felt closer to Dorothy than to her parents.

Social support is central to the process of human growth, development, and crisis intervention. Ellen is in a normal transition stage of development. The way she handles the natural stress of adolescence depends on the people in her social network: her parents, brothers and sisters, friends, teachers, and relatives. Her relationship with these people sets the tone for the successful completion of developmental tasks. A counselor with a social view of the situation would say that necessary social supports were lacking at a time in Ellen's life when stress was already high. So instead of normal growth, Ellen experienced a degree of stress that resulted in a destructive outcome—a suicide attempt. This was a clear message that support from members of her social network was weak.

Even when stress becomes so great that suicide seems the only alternative, it is not too late to mobilize a shaky social network on behalf of a person in crisis. Failure to do so can result in the kind of outcome that occurred for Ellen—that is, another crisis within two months. Individual crisis counseling was not necessarily bad for Ellen; it simply was not enough.

Before considering the specifics of how a person's social network is engaged or developed in crisis resolution, let us examine two important facets of the social network—the family and the community in crisis.

Families in Crisis

Although social relations are important for an individual in crisis, often the members of a person's social network are themselves in crisis. The family unit can experience crises just as individuals can. Researchers consider family troubles in terms of sources, effect on family structure, and type of event affecting the family (Hill, 1965; Parad & Caplan, 1965). If the source of trouble is within the family, an event is usually more distressing than if the source is external, such as a flood or racial prejudice. Often an individual in crisis may precipitate a family crisis. For example, if family members make suicide attempts or abuse alcohol, the family usually lacks basic harmony and internal adequacy, as suggested in the case of Ellen, discussed in the previous section.

Family troubles must be assessed according to their effect on the family configuration. Families experience stress from *dismemberment* (loss of family member), *accession* (an unexpected addition of a member), *demoralization* (loss of morale and family unity), or a combination of all three (Hill, 1965). This classification of stressor events casts in a family context the numerous traumatic life events associated with crises. Death and hospitalization, which are crisis-precipitating events for individuals, are examples of dismemberment for families. Unwanted pregnancy, a source of crisis for the girl or woman, is also an example of accession to the family and therefore a possible precipitant of family crisis as well. A person in crisis because of trouble with the law for delinquency or drug addiction may trigger family demoralization and crisis (Bishop & McNally, 1993; Seelig, Goldman-Hall, & Jerrell, 1992). Divorce and acquisition by children of stepparents and stepfamilies (Stanton, 1986) also constitute dismemberment and accession. The Stepfamily Association of America estimates from remarriage rates that 35 percent of children born today will live in a stepfamily (sometimes called blended or combined families) before their eighteenth birthday. Role and relationship loss are sources of significant stress. Divorce, suicide, homicide, illegitimacy, imprisonment, or institutionalization for mental illness are examples of demoralization and dismemberment or accession.

The nuclear family (father, mother, and children) is the norm in most Western societies, whereas the extended family (including relatives) is the norm in most non-Western societies. Among immigrant Mexican women in the United States, relatives of the family of origin are more important sources of emotional support than friends (Vega, Kolody, Valle, & Weir, 1991). According to U.S. census figures, only 36 percent of American families consist of a married couple and their young children, and only half of children live with two parents. It is now widely recognized and accepted that the traditional form of the nuclear family is being replaced by a variety of family forms. For example, the American Association of Retired Persons (AARP) notes that of 60 million American grandparents, about 3 percent are raising their grandchildren, and another 8 percent assist in the process.

Communal or "New Age" families may provide more avenues of support for some people than do traditional nuclear families. A current variation on these themes is the Cohousing approach, which is designed to address some of the family issues faced by all. Cohousing was initiated by a Danish divorced mother seeking greater support for rearing her children. Developed from the utopian ideal put forth by Thomas More (1516/1965) in the sixteenth century, the concept encompasses several features intended to

- Provide privacy through separate, self-contained units for individuals and families
- Relieve isolation and alienation and promote community by an arrangement of clustered homes, a shared common house, a shared garden, play and work space, community dinners, and perhaps a computer center
- Encourage diversity by welcoming a broad range of residents and lifestyles
- Promote a sense of ownership and empowerment by participatory planning and design from the start

Pioneered primarily in Denmark during the 1970s and 1980s, the Cohousing movement "reestablishes many of the advantages of traditional villages within the context of late twentieth-century life" (McCamant & Durrett, 1988, p. 7). Hundreds of Cohousing communities exist in Western Europe and North America or are in start-up stages.

Increasingly, people call on friends and peers for essential material and social support that traditionally came from one's extended family. However, these new family forms can also be the source of unanticipated conflict when lines of authority are unclear, when opinions differ about privacy and intimacy, and when the group cannot reach consensus about how to get necessary domestic work done.

Whether or not stressful events lead to crisis depends on a family's resources for handling such events. Hill (1965, p. 33) gives a vivid description of the nuclear family and its burden as a social unit:

> Compared with other associations in society, the family is badly handicapped organizationally. Its age composition is heavily weighted with dependents, and it cannot freely reject its weak members and recruit more competent teammates. Its members receive an unearned acceptance; there is no price for belonging. Because of its unusual age composition and its uncertain gender composition, it is intrinsically a puny work group and an awkward decision-making group. This group is not ideally manned to withstand stress, yet society

has assigned to it the heaviest of responsibilities: the socialization and orientation of the young, and the meeting of the major emotional needs of all citizens, young and old.

The family holds a unique position in society. It is the most natural source of support and understanding, which many of us rely on when in trouble, but it is also the arena in which we may experience our most acute distress or even abuse and violence. All families have problems, and all families have ways of dealing with them. Some are very successful in problem solving; others are less so. Much depends on the resources available in the normal course of family life. Despite the burdens many face that can be traced to family stress, discord, or abuse, crisis workers can enhance individuals' prospects of moving beyond their family troubles. The labeling of so many families as "dysfunctional" can be just as damaging as the psychiatric labeling of individuals (Hillman & Ventura, 1992; Wolin, 1993).

In addition to the ordinary stressors affecting families in recent years, U.S. families have faced extraordinary stress stemming from a laissez-faire approach to public policy affecting families. Note the following:

- Approximately 40 million Americans have no health insurance coverage, and many lack money for the most basic health care.
- Because affordable, high-quality child care is unavailable for many, millions of children are left alone. Although available on-site child care for employees is increasing, their access to it is by no means the norm.
- Caretakers in the day-care centers that exist earn poverty-level wages or less, and 90 percent of women caring for children in their homes earn at that level (Trotter, 1987, p. 38).
- Millions of families cannot afford to buy a home, and millions of others are homeless, due primarily to cuts in federal housing programs since 1981 (see Chapter Thirteen).
- The majority of mothers are in the labor force, and most are there not only for personal fulfillment but also because they need the money; yet North American women earn only about 75 percent of what similarly qualified men earn, in spite of civil rights legislation decades ago.

Traditional caretaking patterns in the home are additional sources of stress for families, particularly for women (Reverby, 1987; Sommers & Shields, 1987). James Levine, director of the Fatherhood Project at the Family and Work Institute in New York, urges fathers to assume more active roles in parenting. Research by Peisner-Feinberg et al. (in press) affirms the dominant importance of family—not day care—in shaping children, despite the guilt many wage-earning mothers often feel for not being home full-time for parenting. The disproportionate burden of caretaking placed on women is even more stark in less industrialized societies. This source of stress on families will only increase with the AIDS crisis and the increasing numbers of old people needing care, unless the prevailing attitude and practice regarding the caretaking role shifts radically (see Chapters Eleven and Thirteen).

A family's vulnerability to crisis is also determined by how it defines a traumatic event. For some families, a divorce or a pregnancy without marriage is regarded as nearly catastrophic; for others, these are simply new situations to cope with. Much depends on religious and other values. Similarly, financial loss for an upper-middle-class family may not be a source of crisis if there are other reserves to draw on. In contrast, financial loss for a family with very limited material resources can be the last straw; such families are generally more vulnerable. If the loss includes a loss of status, however, the middle-class family that values external respectability will be more vulnerable to crisis than the family with little to lose in prestige.

As important as a family perspective is, one also needs to look beyond the family for influences on family disharmony and crisis. A well-known example of the failure to look further is Senator Daniel Patrick Moynihan's report, *The Negro Family, the Case for National Action* (1965). Moynihan concluded that causal relationships existed between juvenile delinquency and black households headed by women and between black women wage earners and "emasculated" black men. When these factors were examined in relation to poverty, however, there was no significant difference between black and white female-headed households. This study is now largely discredited for its race, class, and gender bias, but it still represents a sophisticated example of blaming the victim and using scientific "evidence" that masks economic injustice.

Current welfare reform policies in most states require mothers with inadequate job skills to work for poverty-level wages, which compounds the issue of affordable child care. If such mothers are also denied education and training opportunities to improve their economic status, children already at risk face even greater odds in healthy development. Overall, draconian policies often fail to recognize the interrelatedness of poverty, race, and gender bias and widespread urban decay—the roots of problems instead of obvious symptoms (Allen & Baber, 1994; Medoff & Sklar, 1994; Wilson, 1987). These policy failures and the continuing pattern in numbers of children born to single mothers is particularly revealing in light of the correlation between falling birthrates and the improvement in women's educational and economic status, regardless of race or ethnicity. This correlation has been established over five generations of women. It is easier, of course, to blame women for their dependency than to address the socioeconomic and cultural origins of welfare dependency.

Such blaming of families that are in crisis due to deeply rooted social problems becomes more significant when considering that the United States is the only industrialized country without a national family policy to deal with issues such as maternity and paternity leaves, child care, and flexible work schedules, even though the two-income family is the norm rather than the exception (see Chapter Thirteen). Although the U.S. Congress passed a bill permitting unpaid family leave in medium to large companies without threat of job loss, few wage-earning parents can afford the loss of a regular paycheck. In contrast, most Western European parents can take such leave *with* pay.

Despite debates about whether day care is harmful or helpful for infants and toddlers, as well as passionate arguments about abortion, the impending collapse of the family (according to some people), and traditional as opposed to alternative family structures, everyone agrees that human beings need other human beings for development and survival. In short, support from social network members—or the lack of it—influences the outcome of everyday stress, crisis, and illness whether the resolution of crisis is human growth or death. The probability, then, of people receiving support during crisis *includes* family issues but is not limited to them. Community stability and resources as well as public policies that affect individuals and families must also be considered (see Chapter Thirteen).

Communities in Crisis

Just as individuals in crisis are entwined with their families, so are families bound up with their community. An entire neighborhood may feel the impact of an individual in crisis. In one small community, a man shot himself in his front yard. The entire community, to say nothing of his wife and small children, was affected by this man's crisis. Of course, the murder or abduction of a child in a small community invariably incites communitywide fear on behalf of other children. A crisis response to the entire community, including special sessions for school children, is indicated in these situations (National Organization for Victim Assistance, 1987). Incidents of violence targeted to schools and their children and teachers call for planning similar to disaster preparedness, as discussed in Chapter Ten. Watson and colleagues (Watson, Poda, Miller, Rice, & West, 1990) offer detailed suggestions for preventing and containing crises in schools.

Clearly then, communities ranging from small villages to sprawling metropolitan areas experience crisis. In small communal or religious groups, the deprivation of individual needs or rebellion against group norms can mushroom into a crisis for the entire membership. Social and economic inequities among racial and ethnic groups or police brutality can trigger a large-scale community crisis (Holland, 1994; West, 1993). The risk of crisis for these groups is influenced by

- Social and economic stability of individual family units within a neighborhood
- Level at which individual and family needs are met within the group or neighborhood
- Adequacy of neighborhood resources to meet social, housing, economic, and recreational needs of individuals and families
- Personality characteristics and personal strengths of the group's members

Psychosocial needs must be met if individuals are to survive and grow. In the context of Maslow's (1970) hierarchy of needs, as a person meets the basic survival needs of hunger, thirst, and protection from the elements, other needs emerge, such as the need for social interaction and pleasant surroundings. We cannot actualize our potential for growth if we are barely surviving and using all our energy just to keep alive. To the extent that people's basic needs are unmet, they are increasingly crisis prone.

This is true, for example, of millions of people worldwide who suffer from hunger, war, and other disasters and of those living in large, inner-city housing projects. Poverty is rampant. Slum landlords take advantage of people who are already disadvantaged; there is a constant threat of essential utilities being cut off for persons with inadequate resources to meet skyrocketing rates, leaving them vulnerable to death by exposure. An elderly couple in an eastern state, unable to pay their bills, died of exposure after a utility company cut off their heat. Emergency medical and social services are often inadequate or inaccessible through the bureaucratic structure.

The social and economic problems of the urban poor have been complicated further by the recent trend toward gentrification—the upgrading of inner-city property so that it is only affordable by the well-to-do. In a partial reversal of an earlier "white flight" from inner-city neighborhoods, middle-class and upper-middle-class professionals (mostly white) are returning to the city. Housing crises or homelessness are the unfortunate outcome for many who are displaced (see Chapter Twelve).

Similar deprivations exist on North American Indian reservations, among migrant farm groups, and in sprawling cities with shantytowns (especially in the Southern Hemisphere), where millions of the world's poorest people eke out a way to survive. As a result of the personal, social, and economic deprivations in these communities, crime becomes widespread, adding another threat to basic survival. Another crisis-prone setting is the subculture of the average jail or prison. Physical survival is threatened by poor health service, and there is danger of suicide. Prisoners fear rape and physical attack by fellow prisoners. Social needs of prisoners go unmet to the extent that the term *rehabilitation* does not apply to what happens in prisons. This situation, combined with community attitudes, unemployment, and poverty, makes ex-offenders highly crisis prone after release from prison (see Chapter Nine).

Natural disasters such as floods, hurricanes, and severe snowstorms and real or threatened acts of terrorism are other sources of community crisis (see Chapter Ten). This is true not only in internationally publicized cases but also in small communities. In one small town, families and children were threatened and virtually immobilized by an eighteen-year-old youth suspected of being a child molester. Another small community feared for everyone's safety when three teenagers threatened to bomb the local schools and police station in response to their own crises: the teenagers had been expelled from school and were unemployed.

Communities in crisis have several characteristics in common with those observed in individuals in crisis. First, within the group, an atmosphere of tension and fear is widespread. Second, rumor runs rampant during a community crisis.

Individuals in large groups color and distort facts out of fear and lack of knowledge. Third, as with individuals in crisis, normal functioning is inhibited or at a standstill. Schools and businesses are often closed; health and emergency resources may be in short supply.

However, as is the case with families, traumatic events can also mobilize and strengthen a group or nation (Holland, 1994; Medoff & Sklar, 1994). Examples include class-based prejudice, bombing by an enemy country, Nazi persecution of the Jews in Europe, and survivors of South Africa's apartheid policies.

Individual, Family, and Community Interaction

Individuals, families, and communities in crisis must be considered in relation to one another. Basic human needs and the prevention of destructive outcomes of crises form an interdependent network.

Privacy, Intimacy, Community

Human needs in regard to the self and the social network are threefold:

1. The need for privacy
2. The need for intimacy
3. The need for community

To lead a reasonably happy life free of excessive strain, people should have a balanced fulfillment of needs in each of these three areas. Many people support the Cohousing concept because it addresses the problem of meeting those needs. With a suitable measure of privacy, intimate attachments, and a sense of belonging to a community, people can avoid the potentially destructive effects of the life crises they encounter. Figure 5.2 illustrates these needs concentrically.

In the center of the interactional circle is the individual, with his or her personality, attributes and liabilities, view of self, view of the world, and goals, ambitions, and values. The centered person who is self-accepting has a need and a capacity for privacy. Well-adjusted people can retreat to their private world as a means of rejuvenating themselves and coming to terms with self and with the external world.

We all have differing needs and capacities for privacy. However, equally vital needs for intimacy and community affiliation should not be sacrificed to an excess of privacy. The need for privacy can be violated either by a consistent deprivation of normal privacy or by retreat into an excess of privacy, that is, isolation. Privacy deprivation can occur, for example, when families are crowded into inadequate housing or when marriage partners are extremely clingy.

The excessively dependent and clinging person is too insecure to ever be alone in his or her private world. Such an individual usually assumes that there can be

FIGURE 5.2. PRIVACY, INTIMACY, COMMUNITY INTERACTION.

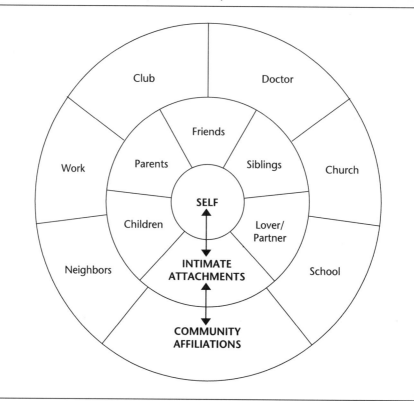

no happiness alone; the person's full psychosocial development has been stunted and the capacity for privacy is therefore unawakened. The person does not see how unfulfilling an overly dependent relationship can be. For example, a man involved in this kind of relationship is a prime candidate for a suicide attempt when his wife threatens to divorce him; the wife is also deprived of essential privacy and feels exhausted by the demand to relate continually to another person.

The problem of too much privacy leads to a consideration of the needs for intimacy and community. A person can seldom have too much privacy if social needs are being met. An example of social-need deprivation is the isolated person who eventually commits suicide because of extreme loneliness and feelings of rejection by others. The concentric circle of needs illustrates the continuous interaction between privacy, intimacy, and community.

The Individual's Extension Beyond Self

Individuals who feel in charge of themselves and capable of living in their private world are at a great advantage as they reach out and establish intimate attachments. They may have a mature marital relationship or a small circle of intimate friends to rely on (see Figure 5.2). Need fulfillment in this second circle enables the individual to establish and enjoy additional relationships in the work world and the larger community. The development of this interactional system can be halted in many situations: (1) if a person feels too insecure to establish intimate or communal attachments, (2) if a person is handicapped by mental illness, has been institutionalized for a long time, or has a history of rejection by family and others, (3) if a couple establishes an intimate attachment that is essentially closed and turned inward, thus limiting need fulfillment from the larger community (Dowrick, 1994), (4) if a small communal group (for example, a religious cult) turns in on itself and fails to relate to society outside of its confines. In all of these situations, healthy interaction is halted; an extreme example of this is the mass suicides of some cult groups.

Social Network Influences on the Individual

The capacity of individuals to live comfortably with themselves and to move with ease in the world is influenced by families and communities. A child born into a chaotic, socially unstable family may find it difficult to settle into a hostile world. Such a child is more crisis prone at developmental turning points, such as entering school or beginning puberty. The child's family, in turn, is affected by the surrounding community. Both the child and the family are influenced by factors such as economic and employment opportunities; racial, ethnic, or other types of prejudice; the quality of available schools; family and social services; and recreational opportunities for youth. When a sufficient number of individuals and families are adversely affected by these factors, the whole community is more prone to crisis.

This concept of individuals, families, and communities interacting underscores the importance of assessing and managing human crises in a social framework. Certainly, a person in crisis needs individual help. But this should always be offered in the context of the person's affectional and community needs. The psychiatrist Halleck (1971) urged a social approach to human problems and crises that is still relevant today (see Luhrmann, 2000). Halleck suggests that it may be unethical for a therapist to spend professional time focusing on a single individual in prison who has made a suicide attempt. Rather than tending only to the individual in crisis, the therapist would be taking a more responsible approach by using professional skills to influence the prison system that contributes to suicidal crises. As violence escalates and the subcultures of U.S. prisons explode with overcrowding and more violence, the crises in these communities will only increase as long as the socioeconomic and cultural roots of aggression are ignored (see Chapter Nine).

Gil (1987), discussing the social roots of violence, extends this argument. He suggests that emergency treatment of abused children and others must be combined with attention to social institutions such as schools and beliefs about parenting that perpetuate violent behavior. Work with survivors of abuse and sexual assault supports similar conclusions: these individuals' crises originate from society's values about women, marriage, the family, and violence (see Figure 5.1, the Crisis Paradigm).

Social Network and Group Process in Crisis Intervention

The foundations have been in for a crisis paradigm that stresses the dynamic relationship between individual, family, and sociocultural factors. The task now is to consider the application of this perspective in actual work with distressed people.

A Social Network Framework

Social approaches to crisis intervention never lose sight of the interactional network between individuals, families, and other social elements. Helping people resolve crises constructively involves helping them reestablish themselves in harmony with intimate associates and with the larger community. In practice, this might mean, for example,

- Relieving the extreme isolation that led to a suicide attempt
- Developing a satisfying relationship to replace the loss of one's partner or a close friend
- Reestablishing ties in the work world and resolving job conflicts
- Returning to normal school tasks after expulsion for truancy, drug abuse, or violence
- Establishing stability and a means of family support after desertion by an alcoholic parent
- Allaying community anxiety concerning bomb threats or child safety
- Identifying why a client complains that "no one is helping me" when, in fact, five agencies (or more) are officially involved

In each of these instances, an individual, psychotherapeutic approach is often used. However, a social strategy, for all of these examples, is so appropriate and evidence supporting it seems so extensive that one wonders why so many practitioners rely primarily on individual approaches—including psychotropic drugs—to crisis resolution. The reasons are complex, of course, and related to issues such as the medicalization of life problems and to the political and economic factors influencing illness and its treatment (see Chapters One and Four).

Increasing numbers of practitioners, however, are choosing social strategies for helping distressed people. In an era before biological psychiatry became dominant (Cohen, 1993), the experience of social psychiatrists (for example, Halleck, 1971; Hansell, 1976; Polak, 1971) and nonmedical practitioners (for example, Garrison, 1974) suggested that social network techniques are among the most practical and effective available to crisis workers. Hansell (1976) refers to such network strategies as the *screening-linking-planning conference method*. This method was developed and used extensively in community mental health systems in Chicago and

Buffalo on behalf of high-risk former mental patients and others. Polak (1971) called this method *social systems intervention* in his community mental health work in Colorado. The use of network strategies in resolving highly complex crisis situations is unparalleled in mental health practice. Their effectiveness is based on recognition and acceptance of the person's basic social nature. Social network techniques, therefore, are essential crisis worker skills. They should not be neglected in favor of excessive reliance on medications, a pattern traceable in part to cost containment measures and disparity in health insurance for those needing mental health care. As noted in Chapter Four, psychoactive drugs are often highly effective but rarely are sufficient without other forms of therapy.

An effective crisis worker has faith in members of a person's social network and in the techniques for mobilizing these people on behalf of a distressed person. A worker's lack of conviction translates into a negative self-fulfilling prophecy—that is, the response of social network members is highly dependent on what the worker expects will happen. A counselor skilled in social network techniques approaches people with a positive attitude and conveys an expectation that the person will respond positively and will have something valuable or essential to offer the distressed individual. Such an attitude eliminates the need to be excessively demanding, which could alienate the prospective social resource. Workers confident in themselves and in the use of social network techniques can successfully use an assertive approach that yields voluntary participation by those whose help is needed.

Social Network Strategies

Besides confidence in the usefulness of social approaches, the crisis worker also needs practice skills. Social network strategies can be used at any time during the course of service: at the beginning of intervention, when an impasse has been reached and evaluation suggests the need for a new strategy, or at the termination of service (Hansell, 1976; Garrison, 1974; Polak, 1971). The social network approach is particularly effective when chronic problems and crisis episodes intersect (see Figure 5.3). Its relevance is underscored by the worldwide trend toward community-based primary care, as discussed in Chapter One.

Putting social network strategies into operation involves several steps:

1. *Clarify with the client and others the purpose of a network strategy and their active participation in it.* A person who seeks help usually expects an individual approach and may be surprised at the social emphasis. Tradition, after all, dies hard. Educating clients, based on our own convictions, is therefore an essential aspect of success with social network strategies. Similarly, clients may be surprised to learn that they not only have an *opportunity* but are *expected* to participate actively in the crisis resolution process. This is especially true for people who may have developed unhealthy dependencies on agencies: the "agency shopper," the "revolving door

FIGURE 5.3. COMPARISON OF CHRONIC PROBLEMS AND CRISES AND INTERVENTION STRATEGIES.

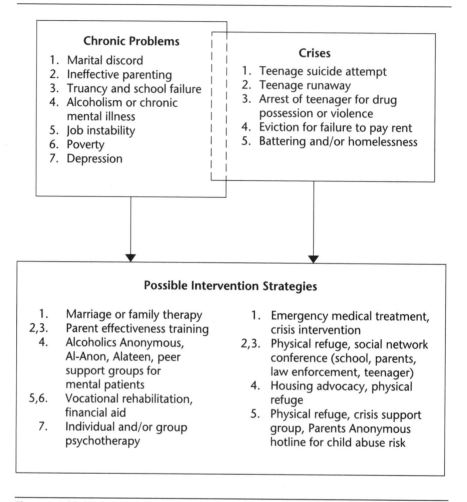

Chronic Problems

1. Marital discord
2. Ineffective parenting
3. Truancy and school failure
4. Alcoholism or chronic mental illness
5. Job instability
6. Poverty
7. Depression

Crises

1. Teenage suicide attempt
2. Teenage runaway
3. Arrest of teenager for drug possession or violence
4. Eviction for failure to pay rent
5. Battering and/or homelessness

Possible Intervention Strategies

1. Marriage or family therapy	1. Emergency medical treatment, crisis intervention
2,3. Parent effectiveness training	2,3. Physical refuge, social network conference (school, parents, law enforcement, teenager)
4. Alcoholics Anonymous, Al-Anon, Alateen, peer support groups for mental patients	4. Housing advocacy, physical refuge
5,6. Vocational rehabilitation, financial aid	5. Physical refuge, crisis support group, Parents Anonymous hotline for child abuse risk
7. Individual and/or group psychotherapy	

The permeable boundaries between the two types of distress suggest the mutual influence these situations have on each other.

client," the multiproblem family (Lynch & Tiedje, 1991), the repeat caller, or the person with "chronic stress" (Worthington, 1992).

The purpose of a network conference can be clarified with a statement such as this: "John, you've been coming here for some months now, each time with a new crisis around an old problem, it seems. We don't seem to be helping you with what you need. And you say other agencies aren't helping you either. I think we should all get together and try to figure out what's going wrong. Whatever it is we're doing now doesn't seem to be working." A positive presentation like this usually elicits a positive response.

2. *Identify all members of the social network.* This "laundry list" should include everyone involved with the person either before or because of the individual's crisis. The comprehensive assessment suggested in Chapter Three is very useful in accomplishing this step.

Identification includes brainstorming and creative thinking with the client about possible substitutes for missing elements of a support network. This includes social resources that are currently unused but that could lead to successful crisis resolution, for example, transitional housing or support for job training. People who lack a *natural* support network (such as discharged mental patients who have been institutionalized for many years and have little or no family support) may rely extensively on institutional network support. When such support is suddenly withdrawn, they are particularly vulnerable to recurring crises and need substitute sources of support (Farrell & Deeds, 1997; Hoff, 1993; Johnson, 1990). This problem has been particularly acute in U.S. communities where adequate community-based services were not developed in concert with the virtual emptying of state mental institutions (see "Homelessness and Vulnerability to Violence" in Chapter Twelve). The excerpt from a networking session with Alice illustrates these points. Rather than pressuring Alice to go back home, Mr. Higgins is engaged as a new network member. A network conference about such problems may also yield the necessary evidence for community political action to alleviate these problems.

CASE EXAMPLE: ALICE—EXCERPT FROM NETWORKING SESSION

Mr. Rothman (by telephone): Mrs. Barrett, this is Mr. Rothman at the crisis clinic. Your daughter Alice is here and refuses to go home. Alice and I would like to have you join us in a planning conference.

Mrs. Barrett: So that's where she is. I've done everything I know of to help that girl. There's nothing more I can do.

Mr. Rothman: I know you must feel very frustrated, Mrs. Barrett, but it's important that you join us even if it's agreed that Alice doesn't go back home.

After a few more minutes, Mrs. Barrett agrees to come to the clinic with her husband. (Alice is age thirty-four, has been in and out of mental hospitals, and cannot hold a job. She and her mother had a verbal battle about household chores.

Mrs. Barrett threatened to call the police when Alice started throwing things. Alice left and went to the crisis clinic.) During the session at the clinic, the conference leader addresses questions to those attending and facilitates discussion:

To Alice: Alice, will you review for everyone here how you see your problem?

To Mr. Higgins, the counselor from the emergency hostel: Will you explain your emergency housing service, eligibility requirements, and other arrangements to Alice and her parents?

To Alice: How does this housing arrangement sound to you, Alice?

To Alice's parents: What do you think about this proposal?

3. *Identify the "symptom bearer" for a family or social network.* This is the person whose crisis state is most obvious. Sometimes this individual is called "crazy." Mental health workers often refer to this person as the *identified client*—recognizing that the entire family or community is, in fact, the client, but their role in the individual's crisis is unclear. The symptom bearer is also commonly called the scapegoat for a disturbed social system.

4. *Establish contact with the resource people identified and explain to them the purpose of the conference.* Elicit the cooperation of these people in helping the person who is stalled in the therapy process and therefore is increasingly vulnerable to repeat crisis episodes. Explain how you perceive the troubling situation and how you think someone can be of help to the distressed person. Finally, arrange the conference at a mutually satisfactory time and place.

If our approach is positive, others involved with a multiagency client will usually express relief that someone is taking the initiative to coordinate services. The families of people with repeated crisis episodes often respond similarly. Problems at this stage may occur because the crisis worker is not convinced that there is a need for the conference, or people from other agencies may raise the issue of confidentiality. This is actually not an issue, because the client has been actively involved in the process of planning the conference: "Why, of course John consents. He's right here with me now." Consent forms should not be a problem if the client participates actively. A straightforward approach is the most successful when using this method.

People may be concerned that conference participants will work together against the client. This is another nonissue, as the purpose of the conference is problem solving for the client's benefit, not punishment. If intentions are sincere, if the purposes of the conference are adhered to, and if the leader is competent, the group process should yield constructive, not destructive, results. People tend to surpass their own expectations in situations like this—even the worker who is frustrated by dependent self-destructive persons. Often the conference represents hope of success. This hope in turn is conveyed to the client. Another recommended strategy for defusing fears about a client being harmed is to appoint a client advocate, someone who will ensure that the client's interests are not sacrificed in any way during the conference. Staff should therefore work in teams of two in conducting these conferences.

5. *Convene the client and network members.* The network conference should be held in a place that is conducive to achieving the conference objectives. This might be the home, office, or hospital emergency department.

6. *Conduct the network conference with the distressed person and with his or her social network.* During this time, starting with the client's view, the problem is explored as it pertains to everyone involved. The complaints of all parties are aired, and possible solutions are proposed and considered in relation to available resources.

7. *Conclude the conference with an action plan for resolving the crisis or other problem.* For example, link the troubled person to a social resource such as welfare, emergency or transitional housing, emergency hospitalization, or job training.

The details of the action plan are clearly defined: everyone knows *who* is to do *what* within a designated time frame. A contingency plan specifies what is to be done if the plan fails (see "Planning with a Person or Family in Crisis" in Chapter Four). This facet of the formal network strategy is what distinguishes it most from a haphazard or unsystematic involvement of a client's family or other network members.

8. *Establish a follow-up plan.* This involves determining the time, place, circumstances, membership, and purpose of the next meeting. Experience reveals that many seemingly intractable problems can be traced to a failure to examine why an established action plan did not turn out as anticipated.

9. *Record the results of the conference and distribute copies to all participants.* This step is based on the principles of contracting discussed in Chapter Four. It also provides the basis for evaluating progress or for finding out what went wrong if the plan fails. This step is particularly important in cases in which both the client and staff feel hopeless about further progress.

Workers who have tried social network techniques are very confident in them; the strategy usually yields highly positive results. Its success can be traced to two key factors: (1) the power and effective implementation of *group process* techniques and (2) *active client involvement* in every step of the process. The client's empowerment and responsibility for self-care that are thereby implied are powerful antidotes to hopelessness and a failure to follow through on recommended treatment. For example, a client can scarcely continue to protest that no one is helping when confronted with six to eight people whose explicit purpose is to brainstorm together about ways to help more effectively. Nor can agency representatives continue to blame the victim for repeated suicide attempts or lack of cooperation when confronted with evidence that part of the problem may be

- Lack of interagency coordination
- Cracks and deficits in the system that leave the client's needs unmet
- Lack of financial resources to pay rent and utility bills
- Previous failure to confront the client (individuals and family) in a united, constructive manner

As increasing numbers of discharged mental patients call crisis hotlines for routine support, the social networking technique suggested here is more relevant than ever. Social network strategies are also effective in avoiding unnecessary hospitalization. Certainly, individual help and sometimes hospital treatment are indicated for a person in crisis. But once the person enters the subculture of a hospital, the functions of the natural family unit are disrupted. In the busy, bureaucratic atmosphere of institutions, it is all too easy to forget the family and community from which the individual came, although some hospital staffs do excellent work with families. Even when social network members (natural and institutional) contribute to the problem rather than offer support, they should be included in crisis resolution to help the person in crisis clarify the positive and negative aspects of social life. Steps of the social network intervention process are illustrated in Figure 5.4.

A final observation is offered for readers who are new to this approach or feel intimidated by it. Social network principles—if not all the steps outlined here—can be applied in varying degrees. In noninstitutional crisis settings, for example, some

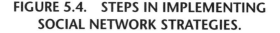

FIGURE 5.4. STEPS IN IMPLEMENTING SOCIAL NETWORK STRATEGIES.

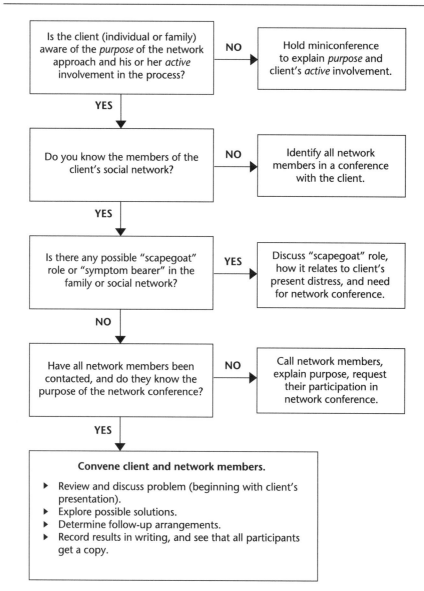

of the steps may be unnecessary. The example of Ramona illustrates a very simple version of network intervention in a highly charged situation. Years of special training are not required for success in network techniques. Yet professionals and others trained in group process should be comfortable in applying this method even in complex situations.

CASE EXAMPLE: RAMONA

Ramona was one of a group of eight abused women in a shelter with no overnight staffing. This shelter, like most, screens its residents for acute suicidal tendencies, addictions, and mental disturbance. Ramona became suicidal nevertheless, and one night she locked herself in the parlor to protect herself from acting on her suicidal tendencies with kitchen knives. When she slept, she did so on the office sofa so she would not have to be alone. Ramona had not told her fellow house members why she did these things, although the other women did know that she was suicidal. Tension among the residents grew because they did not understand Ramona's behavior. They were afraid that if they asked about it, she would become more suicidal (see Chapter Six regarding this popular myth). One of the residents said she would leave the house if the staff did not get rid of Ramona.

Assessing the total situation, Diane, a volunteer staffer who was also a registered nurse trained in crisis intervention, called a meeting to discuss the problem. She explained to Ramona that other residents were worried about her and asked, "Are you willing to meet with them and explain what's happening with you?" Ramona replied, "Sure," and eagerly jumped off the sofa. The volunteer added that she had experience with suicidal people and was not afraid to discuss suicide. This brought a sigh of relief and a "Thank God!" from Ramona. (Ramona was on the waiting list for admission to a local hospital psychiatric unit for treatment of other problems.)

In the group meeting, Ramona explained her behavior as self-protection, not hostility, as her fellow residents had perceived, and shared with the group that she felt most protected and least suicidal when another resident had gone for a walk with her. Ramona also reassured everyone that in the event she hurt herself or died, it was her responsibility, not theirs. All residents expressed relief at having the problem openly discussed and agreed to keep open future communication with Ramona instead of trying to second-guess her.

Crisis Groups

The idea of helping people in groups developed during and after World War II. Because so many people needed help and resources were limited, it was impossible to serve everyone individually; group therapies were instituted. This experience, along with the success of the method, established the group mode of helping as often the method of choice rather than expediency. Whether or not workers use group modes in crisis intervention is influenced by their training and experience. Attitudes have been strongly influenced by psychiatric practice models that emphasize individual rather than social factors.

The traditional emphasis on individual rather than group approaches has contributed to the relative lack of study of group methods in crisis intervention (Walsh & Phelau, 1974). As is true of social network techniques, success in working with groups depends on workers' conviction that the method is appropriate in the crisis intervention process. Group work is indicated in several instances:

1. *As a means of assessing a person's coping mechanisms.* This can be uniquely revealed through interaction with a group. Direct observation of a person in a group setting can uncover behaviors that may have contributed to the crisis situation. The individual is helped to grasp the reality and impact of his or her behavior in relation to others, which can lead to the discovery of more constructive coping mechanisms. The group is an ideal medium for such a process.

2. *As a means of crisis resolution.* This can be accomplished through the helping process inherent in a well-defined and appropriately led group. For the group members in crisis, the number of helpers is extended from one counselor to the whole group. The process of helping others resolve crises restores a person's confidence and can relieve a member's fear of going crazy or losing control.

3. *As a means of relieving the extreme isolation of some individuals in crisis.* For persons almost completely lacking in social resources or the ability to relate to others, the crisis group can be a first step in reestablishing a vital social network.

4. *As a means of immediate screening and assessment.* This is especially useful in settings where large numbers of people come for help and the number of counselors is limited. This is the case in some metropolitan areas where the population is more crisis prone due to housing, financial conditions, employment, violence, and physical health problems.

Crisis Assessment in Groups

A crisis assessment group should be used only when counseling resources are so limited that the people asking for help would otherwise not be seen at all or would be placed on a waiting list. The chief value of a crisis assessment group is to screen out and assist people in most serious need of help before helping those in less critical need. This kind of screening is often necessary in busy emergency mental health clinics. Not all the people who come to such clinics are in crisis. The crisis assessment group is a means of quickly identifying those persons in need of immediate help. This method of assessment should not be used as a substitute for a comprehensive evaluation of individuals, including active involvement of the person's social network members. In essence, it should be considered a group approach to triage—that is, quickly identifying those whose needs are most urgent.

Suggested Procedure for Group Crisis Assessment

Ideally, crisis assessment group work proceeds as in the following example:

1. Several people appear for service in an emergency mental health clinic within one hour: Joe, age twenty-eight, Jenny, age thirty-six, Charles, age thirty-nine, and Louise, age nineteen. Only two counselors are available for assessment, one of whom is involved in an assessment interview.

2. Each person is asked whether he or she is willing to be seen for initial assessment with a group of people who also desire crisis counseling. During this initial presentation, each person is also told that (a) the reason for the group assessment is to give some immediate assistance and prevent a long period of waiting due to staff shortages and (b) the group assessment is not a substitute for individual assessment and counseling needs that are revealed in the group. Those who refuse are reassured of being seen individually as soon as a counselor is available.

3. The crisis counselor explores with each group member the nature of the problem. Each is asked to share the reason for coming to the emergency mental health service. Members are specifically asked why they came *today* rather than on another day. This line of questioning usually reveals the precipitating event as well as the person's current coping ability. Some responses might be as follows:

Joe: I had another argument with my wife last night, and I felt like killing her. I couldn't control myself and got scared. Today I couldn't face going to work, so I thought I'd come in.

Jenny: I've been feeling so depressed lately. The only reason I happened to come in today is that I was talking with my best friend, and she convinced me I should get some help.

Charles: I've been so nervous at work. I just can't concentrate. Today I finally walked off and didn't tell anyone. I'm afraid to face my wife when I get home because we really need the money, so I decided to come here instead.

Louise: I took an overdose of pills last night, and they told me at the hospital emergency room to come in here today for some counseling.

4. Coping ability and resources are explored in detail. The counselor ascertains in each case the degree of danger to self or others. Group members are asked how they have resolved problems in the past. They are invited to share and compare problem areas and ways of solving them:

Joe: Usually, I go out drinking or something just to keep away from my wife. Maybe if I'd have done that last night, too, I wouldn't have felt like killing her. No, I've never hit her, but I came pretty close to it last night.

Jenny: Usually, it helps a lot to talk to my friend. We both think I should get a less stressful job, but my husband thinks it's too risky to quit right now. No, I've never planned anything in particular to kill myself.

Charles: I find, too, that it helps to talk to someone. My wife has been really great since I've had this trouble on the job. She convinced me to talk with the company doctor. Maybe I could do that tomorrow and get medical leave or something for a while.

Louise: My mother said I had to come in here. They think I'm crazy for taking those pills last night. I feel like you, Joe. I can't stand going back home, but I don't know where else to go. Maybe if someone else could just talk to my folks.

5. Action plans are developed with the members. Again, members are invited to share ideas:

Joe's plan: An individual assessment is scheduled for later in the afternoon. A call to Joe's wife, asking her to participate in the assessment, is also planned. Joe is extremely tense and uses alcohol to calm his nerves. This, in turn, upsets his wife, so a referral to Alcoholics Anonymous (AA) will be considered after the full assessment.

Jenny's plan: An individual assessment interview is planned for Jenny three days later, as Jenny is depressed but not in crisis or in immediate danger of harming herself. She is also given the agency's emergency number should she become upset between now and her scheduled appointment (see "Assessment of the Suicidal Person" in Chapter Six). Jenny is also given the names and telephone numbers of private psychotherapists accepting referrals.

Charles's plan: He agrees to talk with the company doctor the next day and request medical leave. He will call in the results and return for a detailed assessment and exploration of his problem soon thereafter.

Louise's plan: A telephone call is planned to Louise's parents to solicit their participation in working with the counselor on Louise's behalf. If they refuse to come in, a home visit will be planned within twenty-four hours.

This example illustrates the function of the crisis assessment group as a useful way to focus helping resources intensely on people whose problems are most urgent without neglecting others. The crisis assessment group rapidly reveals the degree of stress that people are feeling and their ability to cope with problems. It is apparent, for example, that Jenny has a problem with which she needs help, although she is not in crisis.

Mental health agencies with limited counseling resources need to develop techniques to ensure that those in crisis or in life-and-death emergencies receive immediate attention (Hoff & Adamowski, 1998). The assessment worker who uses social resources and network techniques also facilitates the use of resources outside the agency and the individual. Charles, for example, is supported in his self-preservation plan to see the company doctor for medical leave; he intends to resolve his problem through counseling.

As is true with crisis groups generally, crisis assessment groups develop rapid cohesion. Members receive immediate help in a busy agency. Sharing their problems voluntarily with others and assisting fellow group members with similar or more difficult problems give people a sense of self-mastery. It also strengthens their sense of community. An appropriately conducted crisis assessment group can lay the foundation for (1) network techniques in each individual's own social milieu, (2) later participation in a crisis counseling group that may be recommended as part of the total plan for crisis resolution, (3) participation in self-help groups such as AA, widows' clubs, and Parents-in-Crisis.

Crisis Counseling in Groups

An important facet of crisis intervention is determining when group work is indicated. Counselors should guard against unnecessarily protecting people in crisis from groups. This attitude is often revealed in workers' statements, such as, "I'll see her individually just for a few sessions," or "She's not ready for a group yet." These statements can be interpreted in several ways:

1. A person actually needs individual crisis counseling.
2. A person is so terrified of the prospect of a group experience that he or she is, in fact, not ready.
3. The counselor believes that counseling people individually is always better and that a group approach is indicated only when there is not enough time for individual work.

Consider the following responses to these interpretations:

1. The need for individual crisis counseling does not negate the need for group crisis counseling. If both are indicated, both should be offered simultaneously.
2. If a person is indeed terrified of a group experience, this may suggest an even greater need for it. In the individual sessions preparatory to the group experience, the counselor should convey the expectation that group work will be a helpful process. An overprotective attitude will confirm the person's fear that groups are basically destructive, and this can limit the person's learning of new coping skills.
3. If the counselor believes in group work only as an expedient measure to be taken in certain instances rather than as the intervention of choice, the counselor will not use this effective method of crisis counseling even when its use is indicated.

Group Structure

Other facets of crisis counseling in groups are the structure, content, and conduct of the group itself. Some crisis workers recommend structuring the group to a strict limit of six sessions. A more flexible approach takes into consideration the different coping abilities and external resources available to individuals. In general, group members should be asked to attend sessions once or twice a week (average session length of one and one-half to two hours) for a minimum of six sessions, but they might be permitted a maximum of ten sessions if a particular crisis situation warrants it. Group crisis counseling that extends beyond ten sessions indicates that (1) the counselor does not recognize the difference between crisis counseling and longer-term therapy, (2) the person in crisis has an underlying, chronic mental health problem that should be dealt with in a traditional group therapy setting, or (3) the person in crisis may be substituting the group meetings for other, more regular social contacts, and the counselor is inadvertently fostering such restricted social engagement by not limiting the number of group sessions.

The content and conduct of the crisis counseling group are determined by its purpose—resolution of crisis by means of a group process. The sessions therefore focus on the crises identified by group members. Individual histories and feelings not associated with the crisis are restricted from group discussion. There is a continued focus on resolving the crisis that brought the person to the group. All techniques employed in crisis care for individuals should be used: encouraging expression of feelings appropriate to the traumatic event, gaining an understanding of the crisis situation, exploring resources and possible solutions to the problem, and examining social change strategies that might reduce crisis risk in the future (see Chapter Four).

A major difference between group and individual work is that in group work the counselor facilitates the process of group members' helping one another in the resolution of crises. Another difference is that individuals in crisis feel less isolated socially as a result of the bonds created in the group problem-solving process. The relief people feel at no longer being isolated, along with an accompanying sense of group solidarity, can be an important forerunner of other social action they can take to prevent future crises. For example, peer support groups are strongly recommended for people with cancer, parents who have lost a child, battered women, or widowed people.

We also need to consider whether a crisis group should be open or closed. The size of the agency and the potential number of clients can partially determine this. In an agency where many in crisis are seen daily, closed groups are indicated— that is, six or eight people are assigned to a crisis counseling group with the understanding of the contracted six- to ten-session limit, and no new members are admitted to the group once it is formed.

In an agency with fewer clients, where it is difficult to form an initial group of even five people, the group might be structured in an open fashion. This means that new members can be admitted up to a maximum of eight or ten. To avoid constantly dealing with the initiation of new members, admissions are best limited to every second or third session. Even though the group is open to new members, each individual is expected to abide by the six- to ten-session contract. The nature and structure of the group are explained to prospective members in orientation sessions conducted by the group crisis counselor.

Admission to and termination of the group can serve as a medium for discussion about the events that are often an integral part of life crises: loss, admission of a new family member by birth of a baby, revelation of minority sexual orientation, divorce, unwanted pregnancy, rape, death, or absence of a family member through illness. As individuals come and go in the group, members are provided an opportunity to work through possible feelings associated with familiar personal losses. Crisis groups can also be viewed as contemporary substitutes for traditional rites of passage, an idea explored more fully in Chapter Thirteen.

Group counseling is a valuable means of facilitating individual and social growth from a crisis experience. More counselors are now availing themselves of this method of helping people in crisis.

Counseling Families in Crisis

Group crisis work resembles family crisis work, but scapegoating and established family patterns and roles make helping families in crisis more complex. Determining who the scapegoat (or identified symptom bearer) is, along with that person's social network, will reveal the purpose of a person's symptoms in maintaining a family's function—unhealthy and maladjusted as the family may appear at times. For example, Julie, age fifteen, is identified by the school as a "behavior problem." She violates all the family rules at home. John, age seventeen, is seen as a "good boy." Through this convenient labeling process, the mother and father can overlook the chronic discord in their marital relationship and child-rearing practices. Julie's mother and father always seem to be fighting about disciplining Julie. It is therefore easy for them to conclude that they would not be fighting if it were not for Julie's behavior problems. Julie becomes very withdrawn, threatens to kill herself, and finally runs away from home to her friend's house. A naive counselor could simply focus on Julie as the chief source of difficulty in the family. If, however, the counselor were attuned to the principles of human growth, development, and life crises in a social context, the analysis would be different. Julie would be viewed as the symptom bearer for a disturbed family. The entire family would be identified as the client.

Crisis intervention for a family such as Julie's includes the following elements:

1. Julie's mother brings her to the crisis or mental health clinic as recommended by the school guidance counselor.
2. Julie and her mother are seen in individual assessment interviews.
3. A brief joint interview is held in which the counselor points out the importance and necessity of a family approach if Julie is to get any real help with

her problem. The mother is directed to talk with her husband and son about this recommendation, with the understanding that the counselor will assist in this process as necessary.

4. Individual assessment interviews are arranged with the husband and son.

5. The entire family is seen together, and a six- to eight-session family counseling contract is arranged.

6. Crisis counseling sessions are conducted with all family members participating. Julie does indeed have a problem, but the family is part of it. For example, Julie's mother and father give conflicting messages regarding their expectations: John is an "ideal boy," and Julie "never does anything right." Julie feels that her father ignores her. The guidance counselor had asked Julie's parents to come to the school for a conference, but they "never had time."

   The sessions will focus on helping Julie and her parents reach compromise solutions regarding discipline and expected task performance. The parents are helped to recognize and change their inconsistent patterns of discipline. All family members are helped to discover ways to give and receive affection in needed doses. John and his parents are helped to see how John's favored position in the family has isolated Julie and contributed to her withdrawing and running away.

7. A conference is held after the second or third session with the entire family, the school guidance counselor, and Julie's friend. This conference will ensure proper linkage to and involvement of the important people in Julie's social network.

8. During the course of the family sessions, basic marital discord between Julie's mother and father becomes apparent. They are referred to a marital counselor from a family service agency.

9. Family sessions are terminated with satisfactory resolution of the crisis, as manifested by the family symptom bearer, Julie.

10. A follow-up contact is agreed on by the family and the counselor.

In some families, the underlying disturbance is so deep that the symptom bearer is forced to remain in the scapegoat position. For example, if Julie's father and mother refused to seek help for their marital problems, Julie would continue her role in the basic family disturbance. Unfortunately, these situations often get worse before they improve. For example, if in her desperation Julie becomes pregnant or carries out her suicide threat, the family might be jolted into doing something about the underlying problems that can lead to such extreme behavior.

For children and adolescents in crisis, family crisis counseling is the preferred helping mode in nearly all instances. Bypassing this intervention method for young people does a grave disservice and ignores the concepts of human growth and development as well as the key role of family in this process. Decades ago, Langsley and Kaplan (1968) demonstrated the effectiveness of family crisis intervention in other situations as well (see McKenry & Price, 2000; Minuchin, 1993). The current widespread practice of prescribing antidepressants and other psychoactive drugs for children is a disturbing example of such disservice. Fortunately, family and pediatric specialty groups, the Federal Drug Administration, and the media are revealing the damaging results of this reductionist approach to complex social and behavioral problems (Waters, 2000; Zito et al., 2000).

When dealing with suicidal persons, family approaches may be lifesaving (see Chapter Seven; Hoff & Resing, 1982). Figure 5.3 highlights the relationship between crises and chronic problems. It also illustrates

- The interface between crisis and longer-term help for families such as Julie's and Ellen's
- The greater crisis vulnerability of people with chronic problems
- The inherent limitations of applying only a crisis approach to chronic problems
- The possible threat to life when crisis assistance is unavailable to people with chronic problems
- The consequent need to use a tandem approach to situations that contain elements of both a chronic and a crisis nature

Self-Help Groups

Whereas social network and family groups are typically led by trained mental health professionals, self-help groups emphasize the strengths of the group members themselves. With roots in the consumer movement, self-help groups play an important part in all phases of crisis care: in the acute phases, in prevention, and in follow-up support. Key factors in the success of such groups are the climate of empowerment that is created and the bonding among members that so often occurs. Among self-help groups, AA and Al-Anon are the most familiar. Many self-help groups have adopted the AA twelve-step model and should be considered valuable sources of support by professionals working with distressed people.

Grieving people who share with others an acute loss, such as the death of a child from SIDS or the stress of having a child with AIDS, may feel less isolated. The group is also a source of affirmation and information and a potential protection against suicide. Survivors of abuse, for example, can encourage one another to externalize their misfortunes rather than blaming themselves. Self-help groups exist in most communities for practically every kind of problem or health issue (for example, parents of murdered children, incest survivors, families of people with AIDS, mastectomy patients). Although professionals do not usually lead or facilitate such groups, they can help as catalysts and as resources for getting self-help groups started. They can also be a source of referrals. As a resource for people in crisis and with chronic problems, self-help groups have assumed growing importance in an era of increased consumer awareness of responsibility for one's own health. However, such groups should never become a substitute—at least not because of fiscal constraints—for the comprehensive professional health services to which every community member is entitled.

Summary

Individuals, families, and communities interact with one another in inseparable ways. Crises arise out of this interaction network and are resolved by restoring people to their natural place. Attention to these principles can be the key to success in crisis intervention; inattention to the social network is often a source of destructive resolution of crises. In spite of the heavy influence of individualistic philosophies in all helping professions, a social network approach is being used effectively by increasing numbers of human service workers.

References

Allen, K. R., & Baber, K. M. (1994). Issues of gender: A feminist perspective. In P. C. McKenry & S. J. Price (Eds.), *Families and change: Coping with stressful events* (pp. 21–39). Thousand Oaks, CA: Sage.

Antonovsky, A. (1980). *Health, stress, and coping.* San Francisco: Jossey-Bass.

Antonovsky, A. (1987). *Unraveling the mystery of health: How people manage stress and stay well.* San Francisco: Jossey-Bass.

Berkman, L. F., & Syme, S. L. (1979). Social networks, host resistance, and mortality: A nine-year follow-up study of Alameda County residents. *American Journal of Epidemiology, 109,* 186–204.

Bishop, E. E., & McNally, G. (1993). An in-home crisis intervention program for children and their families. *Hospital and Community Psychiatry, 44*(2), 182–184.

Boissevain, J. (1979). Network analysis: A reappraisal. *Current Anthropology, 20*(2), 392–394.

Caplan, G. (1964). *Principles of preventive psychiatry.* New York: Basic Books.

Cohen, C. I. (1993). The biomedicalization of psychiatry: A critical overview. *Community Mental Health Journal, 29,* 509–521.

Dowrick, S. (1994). *Intimacy and solitude.* New York: Norton.

Farrell, S. P., & Deeds, E. S. (1997). The clubhouse model as exemplar. *Journal of Psychosocial Nursing, 35*(1), 27–34.

Fausto-Sterling, A. (2000). *Sexing the body.* New York: Basic Books.

Garrison, J. (1974). Network techniques: Case studies in the screening-linking-planning conference method. *Family Process, 13,* 337–353.

Gil, D. (1987). Sociocultural aspects of domestic violence. In M. Lystad (Ed.), *Violence in the home: Interdisciplinary perspectives* (pp. 124–149). New York: Brunner/Mazel.

Halleck, S. (1971). *The politics of therapy.* New York: Science House.

Hansell, N. (1976). *The person in distress.* New York: Human Sciences Press.

Hill, R. (1965). Generic features of families under stress. In H. J. Parad (Ed.), *Crisis intervention: Selected readings* (pp. 32–52). New York: Family Service Association of America.

Hillman, J., & Ventura, M. (1992, May/June). Is therapy turning us into children? *New Age,* 60–65, 136–141.

Hoff, L. A. (1990). *Battered women as survivors.* London: Routledge.

Hoff, L. A. (1993). Review essay: Health policy and the plight of the mentally ill. *Psychiatry, 56*(4), 400–419.

Hoff, L. A., & Adamowski, K. (1998). *Creating excellence in crisis care: A guide to effective training and program designs.* San Francisco: Jossey-Bass.

Hoff, L. A., & Resing, M. (1982). Was this suicide preventable? *American Journal of Nursing, 82*(7), 1106–1111. (Also reprinted in B. A. Backer, P. M. Dubbert, & E.J.P. Eisenman (Eds.). (1985). *Psychiatric/mental health nursing: Contemporary readings* (pp. 169–180). Belmont, CA: Wadsworth.)

Holland, H. (1994). *Born in Soweto.* Harmondsworth, England: Penguin Books.

Johnson, A. B. (1990). *Out of bedlam: The truth about deinstitutionalization.* New York: Basic Books.

Langsley, D., & Kaplan, D. (1968). *The treatment of families in crisis.* Philadelphia: Grune & Stratton.

Loustaunau, M. O., & Sobo, E. J. (1997). *The cultural context of health, illness, and medicine.* New York: Bergin & Garvey.

Luhrmann, T. M. (2000). *Of two minds: The growing disorder in American psychiatry.* New York: Knopf.

Lynch, I., & Tiedje, L. B. (1991). Working with multiproblem families: An intervention model for community health nurses. *Public Health Nursing, 8*(3), 147–153.

Maslow, A. (1970). *Motivation and personality* (2nd ed.). New York: HarperCollins.

McCamant, K., & Durrett, C. (1988). *Cohousing: A contemporary approach to housing ourselves.* Berkeley, CA: Ten Speed Press.

McKenry, P. C., & Price, S. J. (Eds.). (2000). *Families and change: Coping with stressful events and transitions.* (2nd ed.). Thousand Oaks, CA: Sage.

McKinlay, J. B., & Marceau, L. D. (1999). A tale of three tails. *American Journal of Public Health, 89*(3), 295–298.

Medoff, P., & Sklar, H. (1994). *Streets of hope: The fall and rise of an urban neighborhood.* Boston: South End Press.

Meyer, I. H., & Schwartz, S. (2000). Social issues as public health: Promise and peril. *American Journal of Public Health, 90*(8), 1189–1191.

Minuchin, S. (1993). *Family healing: Strategies for hope and understanding.* New York: Simon & Schuster.

Mitchell, S. C. (Ed.). (1969). *Social networks in urban situations.* Manchester, England: Manchester University Press.

More, T. (1965). *Utopia.* London: Penguin Classics. (Original work published 1516)

Moynihan, D. P. (1965). The Negro family, the case for national action. In L. Rainwater & W. Yancy (Eds.), *The Moynihan Report and the politics of controversy.* Cambridge, MA: MIT Press.

National Organization for Victim Assistance. (1987). *Crisis response.* Washington, DC: Author.

Parad, H. J., & Caplan, G. (1965). A framework for studying families in crisis. In H. J. Parad (Ed.), *Crisis intervention: Selected readings* (pp. 53–74), New York: Family Service Association of America.

Peisner-Feinberg, E., Burchinal, M., Clifford, R., Culkin, M., Howes, C., Kagan, S., & Yazejian, N. (in press). The relation of pre-school quality to children's cognitive and social developmental trajectories through second grade. *Child Development.*

Polak, P. (1971). Social systems intervention. *Archives of General Psychiatry, 25,* 110–117.

Reverby, S. (1987). *Ordered to care.* Cambridge: Cambridge University Press.

Robinson, D. (1971). *The process of becoming ill.* London: Routledge.

Sarason, A. G., & Sarason, B. R. (Eds.). (1985). *Social support: Theory, research and application.* The Hague: Martinus Nijhoff.

Satir, V., Stackowiak, J., & Taschman, H. A. (1975). *Helping people to change.* Northvale, NJ: Aronson.

Seelig, W. R., Goldman-Hall, B. J., & Jerrell, J. M. (1992). In-home treatment of families with seriously disturbed adolescents in crisis. *Family Process, 31*(2), 135–149.

Sommers, T., & Shields, L. (1987). *Women take care: The consequences of caregiving in today's society.* Gainesville, FL: Triad.

Speck, R., & Attneave, C. (1973). *Family networks.* New York: Pantheon Books.

Stanton, G. (1986, May/June). Preventive intervention with stepfamilies. *Social Work,* 201–206.

Trotter, R. J. (1987). Project daycare. *Psychology Today, 21*(12), 32–38.

Vega, W. A., Kolody, B., Valle, R., & Weir, J. (1991). Social networks, social support, and their relationship to depression among immigrant Mexican women. *Human Organization, 5*(2), 154–162.

Walsh, J. A., & Phelau, T. W. (1974). People in crisis: An experimental group. *Community Mental Health Journal, 10,* 3–8.

Waters, R. (2000, March/April). Generation RX: The risk of raising our kids on pharmaceuticals. *Networker,* 34–43.

Watson, R. S., Poda, J. H., Miller, C. T., Rice, E. S., & West, G. (1990). *Containing crisis: A guide to managing school emergencies.* Bloomington, IN: National Educational Service.

West, C. (1993). *Race matters.* New York: Beacon Press.

Wilson, W. J. (1987). *The truly disadvantaged: The inner city, the underclass, and public policy.* Chicago: University of Chicago Press.

Wolin, S. (1993). *The resilient self: How survivors of troubled families rise above adversity.* New York: Random House.

Worthington, J. G. (1992). Managing a crisis in a rehabilitation facility. *Rehabilitation Nursing, 17*(4), 187–196.

Yalom, I. D. (1995). *The theory and practice of group psychotherapy* (4th ed.). New York: Basic Books.

Zito J. M., Safer, D. J., dosReis, S., Gardner, J. F., Boles, M., & Lynch, F. (2000). Trends in the prescribing of psychotropic medications to preschoolers. *Journal of the American Medical Association, 283*(8), 1025–1030.

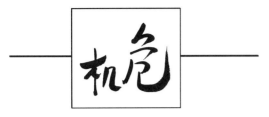

PART TWO

VIOLENCE AS ORIGIN OF AND RESPONSE TO CRISIS

The Crisis Paradigm presented in Part One links the origins of crisis with their possible outcomes. In Part Two, violence is discussed, both as an origin of and a response to crisis (see Crisis Paradigm). Violence toward oneself and others is a major, life-threatening factor for individuals, families, and whole communities in many crisis situations. Chapters Six and Seven focus on assessing and helping people who respond to crisis by suicide or other forms of self-destructiveness. Chapters Eight and Nine deal with violence toward others, including the crises of both victims and perpetrators of violence. In Chapter Ten, violence affecting entire communities—disaster—is traced to natural and human sources. Because the effects of violence are destructive and often irreversible, the theme of prevention is reemphasized in discussing crisis and violence.

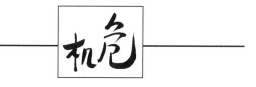

CHAPTER SIX

SUICIDE AND OTHER SELF-DESTRUCTIVE BEHAVIOR: UNDERSTANDING AND ASSESSMENT

Some people respond to life crises by suicide or other self-destructive acts. George Sloan, whose case was noted in previous chapters, tried to kill himself in a car crash when he saw no other way out of his crisis (see Figure 6.1, Box 4b).

A Framework for Understanding Self-Destructive Behavior

Suicide is viewed as a major public health problem in many countries. In the United States, it is the ninth leading cause of death (Moscicki, 1999, p. 41). Suicide among adolescents and young adults continues as a serious problem. Among young people ages fifteen to nineteen, it is the third-ranking cause of death after accidents and homicide (Goldman & Beardslee, 1999) and the fifth leading cause of death among children under age fifteen. The highest rates of suicide in the United States are among older white males, although suicide is not the leading cause of death in older people, male or female (Moscicki, p. 41). Adolescent suicides constitute about 20 percent of all suicides nationwide. Among black men, American Indian, and Alaska Natives, however, the highest rates occur between ages twenty and twenty-nine (Moscicki, p. 41). This suggests racial minority groups' continuing struggle with devastating social and individual circumstances. There is a strong association between suicide risk and bisexuality in males that is only recently commanding research attention (Remafedi, French, Story, Resnick, & Blum, 1998). Homosexuals are estimated to account for 30 percent of adolescent suicides, despite constituting only 5 to 10 percent of the general population (Remafedi, Farrow, & Deisher, 1991). In contrast, Rich, Fowler, Young, and

FIGURE 6.1. CRISIS PARADIGM.

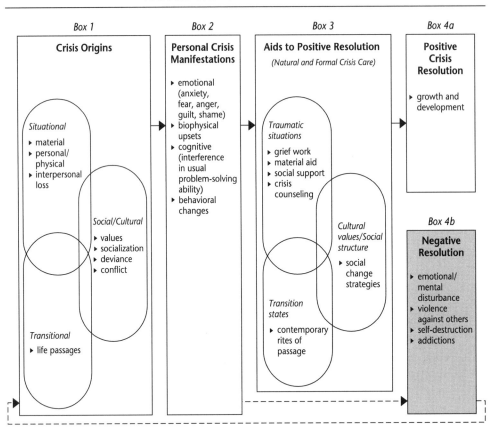

Crisis origins, manifestations, and outcomes and the respective functions of crisis care have an interactional relationship. The intertwined circles represent the distinct yet interrelated origins of crisis and aids to positive resolution, even though personal manifestations are often similar. The arrows pointing from origins to positive resolution illustrate the *opportunity for growth and development* through crisis; the broken line at bottom depicts the potential *danger of crisis* in the absence of appropriate aids. The loop between Box 4b and Box 1 denotes the *vulnerability* to future crisis episodes following negative resolution.

Blenkush (1986) found little difference in suicide rates between adult homosexual and heterosexual men. The rate of suicide for all ages and groups in the United States is about 12 per 100,000 (approximately 30,000 annually) and has remained relatively constant over several decades (National Center for Health Statistics, 1995).

In the United States, firearms are the suicide method of choice for both men and women, whereas the second most common method used by men is hanging and by women is poisoning (Maris, 1991, p. 9). White women's rates peak at around age fifty, whereas rates for nonwhite women remain low and fairly constant through old age (Canetto, 1992).

Suicide attempts occur at least ten times more frequently than suicides, with a total of approximately 300,000 annually. Among adolescents, particularly females, the attempt rate may be twenty to fifty times higher. Many of these adolescents have been physically or sexually abused. Stephens's research (1985, 1987) on suicidal women suggests strong links to conflict and abuse in intimate relationships. She suggests that women with histories of exaggerated passivity may be at greater risk of suicide than those who are rebellious. Women have higher rates of depression than men, which is commonly attributed to socioeconomic disparities (Badger, McNiece, & Gagan, 2000). However, research remains to be done on why greater numbers of women who are abused or otherwise disadvantaged do not kill themselves.

Internationally, the wide range of suicide rates reveals further the complexity of the suicide problem. In Canada, the age-adjusted suicide rate is 13.6. In England, France, Italy, Denmark, and Japan, the rates for men are consistently higher than for women. England has the lowest rate for old people, Hungary the highest rates in the world, and Italy the lowest rate for the young. In most European countries, the rates are lowest among those of Catholic tradition (Kerkhof & Clark, 1993; United Nations, 1996). In Japan, the rate for women between fifteen and twenty-four is half that for men (McGinnis, 1987, p. 25), whereas in India, for every hundred suicides, seventy are women (R. Menon, personal communication, June 26, 1988). Because reporting systems differ widely, there are probably more suicides than are reported. Cultural taboos, insurance policies, and other factors strongly influence the reporting of suicide. Some coroners, for example, will not certify a death as suicide unless there is a suicide note. However, everyone who commits suicide does not leave a suicide note. Research supports the claim that the compilation of suicide statistics, like suicide itself, is a social—not strictly scientific—process affected by cultural, social, and economic considerations (Atkinson, 1978). Because of all these factors, we lack accurate and comprehensive data. Statistics about suicide, therefore, should be used primarily as an indicator of trends, not as a substitute for sensitive interpersonal work with suicidal people. For example, because suicide rates among adolescents and ethnic minority groups have increased the most dramatically in recent years, greater public attention is warranted than earlier, lower rates seemed to indicate.

Suicide as a response to crisis is used by all classes and kinds of people with social, mental, emotional, and physical problems—possibly including our relatives and neighbors. In short, people of every age, sex, religion, race, sexual identity, and social or economic class commit suicide. Perhaps most important of all, in the ethic of most world religions, suicide is generally considered the most stigmatizing sort of death.

In this and the following chapter, suicide and self-destructive behavior are discussed in the contexts of the Judeo-Christian value system and the development of social science, crisis theory, and public health. The discussion assumes the psychosociocultural perspective presented in earlier chapters, with particular emphasis on themes of growth and empowerment despite the specter of death as a response to psychic pain during crisis. Inasmuch as suicide has occurred since the beginning of recorded history—the similar age-old response of distressed and despairing people—the holistic, preventive model of this book contrasts with the current widespread tendency to treat suicide as a psychiatric disorder (United Nations, 1996; see also Figure 6.1). This is not to disclaim what contemporary psychiatry offers; rather, the intent is to avoid "pathologizing" a phenomenon that is much more complex than is implied by a diagnosis such as subclinical depression or major depressive disorder (MDD).

Suicide universally conveys the value that "death is preferred over life," making this discussion relevant in cross-cultural terms as well. However, particular belief systems will influence how and why suicide occurs and is interpreted in various non-Western societies. For a fuller cross-cultural discussion of suicide, see Counts (1987), Farberow (1975), and the journal *Crisis*.

Perspectives, Myths, and Feelings About Self-Destructive People

Nearly everyone has had contact with self-destructive people. Some of us have relatives and friends who have committed suicide or made suicide attempts. We know others who slowly destroy themselves by excessive drinking or abuse of other drugs. Among the readers of this book, a certain percentage will have responded to a life crisis by some kind of self-destructive act. For example, the suicide rates among physicians and dentists are some of the highest among occupational groups. Also, narcotic addiction, as a way of coping with stress, is prevalent among physicians and nurses. It is a tragedy that those whose main work is service to others often find it difficult to ask for help for themselves when in crisis. All too often, physicians and nurses, particularly those who are in direct contact with people who have cut their wrists, attempted to kill themselves in a car crash, or overdosed on pills, will attempt to drown their own troubles in alcohol. These are only a few of the many consequences of self-destructive incidents commonly addressed by emergency service personnel.

Volunteers and other workers in suicide and crisis centers are another group that has frequent contact with self-destructive people. About 20 percent of callers to these centers are in suicidal crisis. Counselors and psychotherapists also work with self-destructive people.

These workers, as well as other people, have varying degrees of knowledge about suicide and self-destructive people. Unfortunately, myths and misleading beliefs about suicidal people are widespread. The following are some of the most common myths and facts about suicide (Motto, 1999; Shneidman, 1981, pp. 213–214):

Myth: People who commit suicide have a psychiatric illness, are "crazy."
Fact: Diagnosable mental illness is not the dominant factor in most suicides, although people who commit suicide are usually in emotional turmoil. (See this chapter's "Assessment of the Suicidal Person" section for the suicide-depression link.)

Myth: Good circumstances—a comfortable home or a good job—prevent suicide. This view is revealed in the surprised expression following the suicide of a talented student: "He had everything going for him." *Fact:* Suicide cuts across class, race, age, and sex differences, although its frequency varies among different groups in society.

Myth: When gay, lesbian, bisexual, and transgendered people recognize the "sinfulness" of their lives, most of them kill themselves. *Fact:* Although a significant number of this group commit suicide or make suicide attempts, they do so most often because of the prejudice, hatred, and sometimes violence they have endured from mainstream society.

Myth: People who talk about suicide are not a serious risk for suicide. *Fact:* People who die by suicide almost invariably talk about suicide or give clues and warnings about their intention through their behavior, even though the clues may not be recognized at the time.

Myth: People who threaten suicide, superficially cut their wrists, or do not succeed with other attempts are not at risk for suicide. *Fact:* The majority of people who succeed in killing themselves have a history of previous suicide attempts. All threats and self-injury should be taken seriously. Not to do so may precipitate another attempt.

Myth: Talking about suicide to people who are upset will put the idea in their heads. This myth prevails as a misguided protection for those who do not know how to help and therefore are uncomfortable bringing up the subject. *Fact:* Suicide is much too complex a process to occur as a result of a caring person asking a question about suicidal intent.

Myth: People who are deeply depressed do not have enough energy to commit suicide. *Fact:* The energy level of another person is subjective and difficult to assess. People may kill themselves when depressed or following improvement; frequent and repeated assessment is therefore indicated, regardless of the level of depression.

Some of these myths can probably be recognized among ourselves, family, friends, and associates. Even among health professionals, these ideas are more common than one would expect.

Professional *suicidologists* (those trained in the study of suicide and suicide prevention) believe that suicide prevention is everybody's business—a difficult order considering how many unfounded beliefs about suicide still persist. But often, even nurses and physicians may resist dealing with self-destructive people by telling themselves, "That's somebody else's job." To be fair, people can hardly deal with something they know little about, and there are a number of difficulties in trying to learn more about self-destructive people:

- Cultural taboos against suicide
- Strong feelings about suicide and other self-destructive acts

- Limitations of doing research on human beings
- The intrinsic difficulty of examining the self-destructive process in those who commit suicide, because study is limited to determining the probable reasons for suicide from survivors closely associated with the person

In spite of these limitations, research and direct work with self-destructive persons have yielded promising results. *Suicidology,* the study of suicide and suicide prevention, is still by no means an exact science. Yet the scientific practices developed in the past few decades are a considerable advancement over responses based on myths and taboos. Knowledge alone, however, does not guarantee the use of that knowledge. Many misguided perceptions about self-destructive people and responses to them persist because of intense feelings about suicide, death, and dying. What are some of the most common feelings people have about a self-destructive person? And why are these feelings particularly intense in the helper-client interaction?

As we interact with or observe self-destructive people, we may feel sadness, pity, helplessness, desire to rescue, anger, or frustration. Some of these feelings are mirrored in the following comments:

> *Curious bystander:* "Oh, the poor thing."
>
> *Friendly neighbor:* "What can I possibly do?"
>
> *Family:* "Why did she have to disgrace us this way?"
>
> *Health provider:* "I can't stand wasting my time on these people who are just looking for attention."

After a suicide, several feelings are common among survivors: *anxiety* that something we did or did not do caused the suicide; *relief,* which is not uncommon among family members or therapists who have exhausted themselves trying to help the suicidal person; or *guilt,* which often follows feelings of disgust or relief that the desperate person has died.

Understanding these feelings and their sources is crucial if we are to keep them from becoming impediments to helping distressed people find alternatives to suicide. Our feelings about suicide and responses to self-destructive persons can be clarified from three perspectives: social, psychological, and cultural.

Social Perspective

Physicians, nurses, and other providers are often frustrated in working with self-destructive people. This can be traced, in part, to the socialization these professionals receive in their role of helping the sick person return to health. Success in this role depends partly on whether patients behave according to expectations of people in the "sick role." Parsons (1951, pp. 436–437) identified the following exemptions and responsibilities associated with the sick role:

1. Depending on the nature and severity of the illness, the person is exempt from normal social responsibility. This implies that the illness has been legitimized

by a "mandated labeler," usually a physician (Becker, 1963; see also Chapter Three). Such legitimation gives moral approval to being sick and prevents people from using sickness inappropriately for secondary gains (Ehrenreich & Ehrenreich, 1978; Zola, 1978).

2. The sick person is expected to accept help and depend as necessary on the caregiver; it is understood that the person cannot improve merely by an act of will.

3. The person is obligated to want to get well as expeditiously as possible.

4. The person must seek technically competent help and cooperate with the helper.

This concept of the sick role is unproblematic if applied to acute illness such as appendicitis or extreme pain caused by kidney stones. In fact, the study of persons with precisely such acute physical conditions resulted in Parsons's sick role formulation. However, the concept is inadequate if applied to chronic illnesses or to any condition with significant social, psychological, or cultural components—in short, any condition in which lifestyle or a willful act, such as smoking, drinking, or sexual contact by the individual, is directly related to the malady (Levine & Kozloff, 1978).

If so-called social illnesses do not fit the traditional sick role–helper model, think of the model's limitations when applied to a person who is self-destructive. Not only do suicidal people defeat the medical role of fostering and maintaining life, but self-injury appears to flout deliberately the natural instinct to live. The self-destructive person is requesting, directly or indirectly, a departure from the usual roles of patient and health service provider. If such providers deal with suicidal people according to rigid role expectations, the helper-patient relationship can lead to conflict. And if helping is limited to a medical approach when the problem is as philosophical, religious, and social as it is medical, the trouble that health professionals have when working with suicidal persons becomes more understandable. Attention to these social and sick role concepts is particularly relevant in today's managed care system that provides limited insurance coverage for "talk" therapies.

Psychological Perspective

Role conflicts are complicated further if helpers have an unrecognized or excessive need to be needed or to rescue the self-destructive person. Not only is the helper denied the fulfillment of traditional role expectations, but the suicidal person says, in effect, "I don't need you. How can you save me when I don't even want to save myself?" This is a very good question, considering what we know about the failure of therapy without the client's voluntary collaboration.

The most complex manifestation of the social-psychological roots of conflict with suicidal people is in the victim-rescuer-persecutor triangle discussed in Chapter Four. Of all the phases of crisis work, it is most important here that we are sensitive to a person's need for self-mastery, as well as to our own need to control any rescue fantasies we might have. Not to do so could result in a vicious cycle of results that are exactly the opposite of our intentions:

- Our misguided rescue attempts are rejected.
- We feel frustrated in our helper role.
- We persecute the suicidal person for failing to cooperate.
- The suicidal person feels rejected.
- The suicidal person repeats the self-injury.
- The helper feels like a victim.

Preventing and interrupting the victim-rescuer-persecutor cycle is one of the most challenging tasks facing the crisis worker, especially in dealing with self-destructive people. The social network strategies discussed in Chapter Five are particularly helpful in this task.

Cultural Perspective

Self-destructive behavior takes on added meaning when placed in cultural-historical perspective. Suicide and self-destructive behavior have been part of the human condition from the beginning of time. Views about it—whether it is honorable or shameful—have always varied. In the Judeo-Christian tradition, neither the Hebrew Bible nor the New Testament prohibits suicide. Jews (defenders of Masada) and Christians (martyrs) alike justified suicide in the face of military defeat or personal attack by pagans. Later, however, suicide took on the character of a sinful act.

Over the centuries, we have seen suicide considered first from a religious standpoint and more recently from a legal and medical perspective as well. Today these three major social institutions overlap in their interpretations of suicide. In spite of professionals' and civil libertarians' sophistication about the topic, suicide is still largely taboo. Now suicide is seen less as a moral offense than as a socially disgraceful act, a response to crisis, or a manifestation of psychiatric illness.

When suicide is viewed in social, psychological, and cultural perspective, our beliefs and feelings about it are not surprising. We are, after all, members of a cultural community with distinct values about life, ourselves, and other people, as well as views about how people should behave. These cultural facts of life are even more complex when considering the multiethnicity of North American societies and the current emphasis on preserving one's unique cultural heritage. It is impossible for us to know in detail the beliefs and customs of cultures to which we have had little direct exposure. What we can do, however, is educate ourselves about ethnocentrism (see "Factors Influencing Communications" in Chapter Four) and refrain from imposing our values on others. For example, in some belief systems the idea of an afterlife is meaningless, whereas for others suicide might be precisely the avenue toward a better life after reincarnation.

It is easier to accept and deal with our feelings if we remember that they have historical roots and are complicated by contemporary socialization to professional roles. Failing to recognize this can prevent us from being helpful to self-destructive people, which places an especially heavy burden on emergency and rescue personnel. Human service workers need an opportunity to express and work through their feelings about self-destructive behavior. Dealing with feelings and their origins, then, is a basic step in a worker's acquiring the knowledge and skills necessary to help people in suicidal crisis. Team relationships, peer support groups, and readily accessible consultation are some of the avenues that should be available to people working with suicidal persons.

Ethical Issues Regarding Suicide

Closely related to coping with feelings about self-destructive behavior are our positions on the right to die and the degree of our responsibility for the lives of others. In professional circles of suicidology, philosophy, and psychiatry, and among the general public, the following are hotly debated topics (Battin & Mayo, 1980; Humphrey, 1992; Richman, 1992):

- The right to die by suicide
- The right and the responsibility to prevent suicide
- The right to euthanasia and abortion (related topics)

Several ethical and legal questions have implications for the crisis worker.

- How do we respond to a person's declaration: "I have the right to commit suicide, and you don't have the right to stop me"?
- If our own belief system forbids suicide, how might this belief influence our response to such a person?
- If a person commits suicide, whose responsibility is it?
- If we happen to believe the suicidal person alone is responsible, why do we often feel guilty?
- What is the ethical basis for depriving a person of normal, individual rights by commitment to a mental health facility to prevent suicide?
- What do we do if someone close to us requests our assistance in committing suicide?

The intent of these questions is not to persuade the reader to give up cherished beliefs or to impose a libertarian view about suicide. Rather, it is to provide an ethical and clinical basis for dealing with the issues without either abandoning our own beliefs or imposing them on others.

Some workers may confuse suicide prevention efforts with a distorted sense of obligation to prevent any and all suicides whenever physically possible and by whatever means possible. The term *distorted* is used to emphasize these facts:

1. It is physically impossible to prevent suicide in some instances unless we place a person in a padded cell and strip him or her of all clothing. This does not

mean that suicide is inevitable; it means that if psychological aid and social support are lacking, physical protection alone is inadequate.

2. Forced physical protection attacks a person's basic need for mastery and self-determination and may result in the opposite of what is intended in the long run, even though suicide may be prevented in the short run. Such suicide prevention efforts may (a) impose on others the belief that people do not have the right to commit suicide or (b) result in the worker's unresolved "savior complex."

These beliefs and unconscious conflicts often accompany a lack of scientific knowledge about self-destructive behavior and the inability to assess suicidal risk. The results may promote rather than prevent suicide through such practices as these:

1. *Placing a hospitalized suicidal person in isolation.* This is done to allow closer observation, but it increases the person's sense of abandonment, which, for someone suicidal, is already acute.
2. *Committing a suicidal person involuntarily to a psychiatric facility.* This practice assumes the belief that others know what is best for a suicidal person. This can be an attack on the person's sense of dignity and self-worth, yet mental health laws in many states and provinces may encourage the practice among those working in public agencies or mental health professions. There is often little awareness that restricting individual freedom is a counterproductive power play that can give the suicidal person one more reason to choose death over life.
3. *Engaging in punitive practices or discounting the seriousness of self-injury.* When this occurs, the self-destructive person feels attacked and more worthless than ever.

The hidden function of these practices is probably the expression of anger against the self-destructive person for violating the suicide taboo and for frustrating the worker's helping role. The suicidal person has little or no ability to understand such messages. He or she already has an overdose of emotional pain or self-hatred. Rejection by helpers as they carry out their service responsibilities can only increase a person's self-destructiveness.

Opinions differ regarding the issue of responsibility to save others, the right to determine one's own death, and differentiating between adults and children in regard to rights and responsibilities. The *ethical* and *legal* aspects of certain issues must be distinguished. For example, many people believe that suicide is ethically acceptable in certain circumstances, but regardless of personal beliefs, it is illegal in the United States and in most other countries to assist another in the act of suicide. The passage in Oregon of a ballot measure regarding physician-assisted suicide is an exception to this rule. Other states are considering similar legislation. In contrast, although abortion is legal in the United States, people differ about whether it is ethically or morally acceptable. Crisis workers must consider the relevance of theoretical debates to their everyday interaction with suicidal people. The following case analyses illustrate some of the ethical questions.

CASE EXAMPLE: RACHEL'S "RIGHT" TO COMMIT SUICIDE

Rachel, age sixty-nine, lived with her daughter and son-in-law and was dying of cancer. The community health nurse learned that she was considering suicide. In fact, Rachel spoke openly of her right to kill herself, although she had no immediate plan. Basically, Rachel felt she was a burden to her daughter. Although the daughter voluntarily had invited Rachel to live in her home, she acknowledged the extra stress of caring for her mother. After the nurse worked with the daughter and explored her feelings regarding her dying mother, the relationship between the daughter and mother improved. The daughter was put in touch with a respite service for families of cancer patients. Rachel was no longer suicidal and decided not to exercise her right.

This case demonstrates the philosophical dilemma posed by rational versus "manipulated" suicide (Battin, 1980). Among the rank and file of health and social service workers, the idea of manipulation is commonplace, especially with respect to suicidal people. But several things are noteworthy about this usage. When someone is unsuccessful in a suicide attempt, the assumption is that the person is inappropriately trying to *manipulate* the staff, a family member, or others. The term therefore has a moral connotation. Yet human service workers often do not acknowledge that manipulation is common in all social life. For example, the average person manipulates to get a larger salary, a different work shift, or better housing. When considering the right to commit suicide, we need to examine whether we, as members of a suicidal person's social world, have manipulated a person into "choosing" suicide. A person like Rachel can be manipulated into suicide through material and social circumstances and through ideology (see Bernardi, 1995).

Rachel's case illustrates (1) her social circumstances, highlighted by her relationship with her daughter and changed through home health care given to the daughter, and (2) her ideology—that is, her belief about her value as an older person dying of cancer. As her view of herself changed, from feeling nonproductive and worthless to feeling valuable in the eyes of her daughter and herself, she stopped arguing about her right to commit suicide. The argument about the right to die, then, becomes moot if the reasons for choosing suicide are the failure to (1) relieve intolerable pain, (2) provide relief to family caretakers, and (3) examine critically a value system that holds no place for the "nonproductive" old, ill, or disabled.[1] Despite continuing trends to pathologize suicide, it is useful to recall Jourard's (1970) definition of suicide as "an invitation [from social network members] to die." Rachel's case suggests that the right-to-commit-suicide argument can cloak hidden social processes and values at work. Paradoxically, acknowledging

[1]Current debates on voters' ballots about physician-assisted suicide and action intersect with people's concerns about the adequacy of health and social services during terminal illness and their dread of the prospect of "high-technology" death in institutions, which is discussed at length in Chapter Thirteen.

a person's right to commit suicide can have a curious suicide prevention effect. Even if our own belief system disallows such a right, it is empowering (and therefore life promoting) to respect and acknowledge others' beliefs.

CASE EXAMPLE: DIANE—YOUNG ADULT SUICIDE

Diane, a college student, age twenty-two, resisted all alternatives to suicide as proposed by a crisis counselor. She learned she was pregnant, was rejected by her lover, and could not share her distress with her parents or friends. Abortion was not an acceptable alternative to her. She feared that continuing the pregnancy would mean failure to graduate. The counselor agreed with Diane's assertion of her basic right to commit suicide but expressed regret if Diane were to follow through on that decision during the peak of her crisis. This acknowledgment seemed to give Diane a sense of dignity and control over her life and a new will to live, even though the only resource she perceived at the moment was the counselor.

This and other examples of distressed youth invite us to consider the alarming increase in adolescent suicides. We could profitably ask ourselves the following questions:

- What are our children telling us about the life and the world we have created for them if they choose death over life at a time when life has just begun?
- Have we "manipulated" our children into suicide by creating a material and social world and value system that they feel are not worth staying alive for?
- If we acknowledge the "right" of a young person to commit suicide, do we ignore a larger question about reasons for hope or despair among young people?

CASE EXAMPLE: JOHN—MENTAL HEALTH COMMITMENT

John, age forty-eight, was placed in a mental health facility against his will when he became highly suicidal after his wife had divorced him. He also had a serious drinking problem. John had two very close friends and a small business of his own. The main reason for hospitalizing John was to prevent him from committing suicide. John found the hospital worse than anything he had experienced. He had no contact with his friends while in the hospital. After two weeks, John begged to be discharged. He was no longer highly suicidal but was still depressed. John was discharged with antidepressant medicine and instructed to return for a follow-up appointment in one week. He killed himself with sleeping pills (obtained from a private physician) and alcohol two days after discharge. The staff of the mental hospital did not understand how they had failed John.

John's case represents the complexity of the debate between a commitment to protect against suicide and infringement on the right to self-determination. Mental health laws in North America include provisions for involuntary commitment for observation, evaluation, and treatment of persons considered a serious danger to themselves, either by overt suicidal behavior or by neglect of necessary self-care. But as the paralyzed hero of a movie by the same title put it, "Whose life is it, anyway?" He was speaking of his resistance to the treatment that kept him alive. Even though suicide can be seen as rational in certain circumstances, John's decision could also be seen as "not in his own best interest." Cases like John's reveal the ethical basis for depriving a person of personal freedom in the name of suicide prevention and treatment. In this case, John had friends and by objective standards something to live for, even though he could not see that when he killed himself. It could be argued, therefore, that extreme rescue action by helpers is justified (see Bongar et al., 1998).

John's eventual suicide, though, illustrates the care that must be taken in implementing mental health laws on behalf of suicidal people. First of all, the decision to commit a person must be based on a thorough assessment. Second, even if John had been found to be a serious risk for suicide, involuntary hospitalization seemed to contribute to rather than prevent John's suicide. Hospitalization is indicated for suicidal people only when natural social network resources (such as John's friends) are not present. This case is analyzed further in "Team Analysis Following a Suicide" in the next chapter.

Some people choose suicide even after considering the alternatives with caring people. Public and controversial examples include the planned suicide of artist Jo Roman in the United States and the case of Sue Rodriguez in Canada. Roman's suicide plans and discussion with her family and friends were aired on national public television, followed by an interdisciplinary panel discussion of the issues by authorities on the topic.

CASE EXAMPLE: PAUL—RATIONAL SUICIDE?

Paul, age sixty-four, had chronic heart disease. He had been depressed since his wife's death three months earlier. When he was laid off from his job, he became suicidal and talked with his doctor. Paul's doctor referred him to a community mental health center for therapy. He received individual and group psychotherapy and antidepressant drugs. After three months, Paul's depression lifted somewhat, but he was still unconvinced that there was anything left to live for. He had been very dependent on his wife and seemed unable to develop other satisfying relationships, even through the support group for widowed people that he had joined. Paul killed himself by carbon monoxide poisoning after terminating therapy at the mental health center.

Paul's situation does not imply that suicide is inevitable. Instead it suggests the rationality of Paul's decision to commit suicide rather than live in circumstances to which he apparently could not adjust. However, Paul's case also shows us what can be done to help lonely older people find alternatives to suicide, even though these alternatives may be rejected. The people who tried to help Paul can take comfort in the fact that they acted humanely on his behalf, although they may still feel regret. But we must recognize our limitations in influencing the lives of other people (see "Support and Crisis Invention for Survivors" in the next chapter).

Rational suicide as well as assisted suicide continue as points of discussion in professional and lay circles—including the periodic efforts to test these issues in the voting booth, as states consider laws similar to the one passed in Oregon.

CASE EXAMPLE: DENNIS—RATIONAL SUICIDE?

Dennis, age thirty-three, held a good job as a university professor when he was diagnosed with AIDS. Initially, Dennis was overwhelmed with shock, rage, and despair. He had been successful in his career, enjoyed a supportive circle of friends, and was comfortable with his gay identity. He had decided to kill himself, but after surviving an antigay physical attack and helping two of his friends cope with a similar episode of violence, he became involved in a local activist group and no longer felt suicidal. Dennis reserves for himself, though, the possibility of suicide at a future time if AIDS progresses to the point of dementia for him.

Dennis's case illustrates the importance of control and self-determination for anyone in crisis. Although we need to respect the decisions of people like Dennis, we must be particularly careful in reference to AIDS not to proffer rational suicide as a substitute for our humane response to this worldwide crisis (see Chapter Eleven).

The following is offered as a practical guideline to helpers with respect to rights and responsibilities regarding suicide: each person has the final responsibility for his or her own life. This includes the right to live as one chooses or to end life. We have a communal responsibility to do what we reasonably can to help others live as happily as possible. This includes preventing suicide when it appears to be against a person's own best interests—for example, when suffering from major depression without the benefit of treatment. It also involves examining values and social practices that inadvertently lead people to choose suicide only because they are socially disadvantaged and see no other way out. This same principle applies to the issue of euthanasia and assisted suicide: for many, the ethical concern is the "slippery slope" that is too close to the Nazi experience of exterminating people on grounds of ethnicity, religion, sexual identity, or perceived "uselessness" in a society that is bigoted or lacks policies guaranteeing equal access to health and social services (see Fuller, 1997; U.S. Public Health Service, 1999). And if ethical arguments do not support legalized physician-assisted suicide, neither does an economic argument. Emanuel and Battin (1998) found that in the wealthy United States, total end-of-life health care expenditures would be reduced by only 0.07 percent if physician-assisted suicide were legalized. The choice of assisted suicide in these instances is not truly free. Our social responsibility does not require that we prevent a suicide at all costs. We need to recognize that misguided savior tactics can result in suicide if overbearing help is interpreted as control. However, workers in human service professions such as nursing, medicine, mental health, and law enforcement have an additional responsibility: they should learn as much as they can about self-destructive people and advocate strongly to help despairing people find alternatives to suicide.

Characteristics of Self-Destructive People

To be understood is basic to the feeling that someone cares, that life is worth living. When someone responds to stress with a deliberate suicide attempt, those around the person are usually dismayed and ask *why*. The wide range of self-destructive acts adds to the observer's confusion; there are many overlapping features of self-destructive behavior. For example, Mary, age fifty, has been destroying herself through alcohol abuse for fifteen years, but she also takes an overdose of sleeping pills during an acute crisis.

Volumes have been written about suicide—by philosophers, the clergy, psychiatrists and psychologists, nurses, and crisis specialists. Academics and researchers have profound discussions and varied opinions regarding the process, meanings, morality, and reasons involved in the act of self-destruction. While these debates continue, the focus in this book is on the *meaning* of self-destructive behavior and the importance of understanding and reaching out to those in emotional pain (see O'Carroll, 1993; Shneidman, 1993). Suicidology founder Edwin Shneidman calls this emotional pain *psychache*, the "hurt, anguish, or ache that takes hold of the mind. It is intrinsically psychological; it is the . . . pain of negative emotions, such as guilt, shame, anguish, fear, panic, anger, loneliness, helplessness. . . . Suicide occurs when the psychache is deemed to be unbearable and when death is actively sought in order to stop the unceasing flow of intolerable consciousness" (1999, pp. 86–87). Precise definitions and a clear understanding of such behavior are complex and difficult to achieve. However, in spite of academic differences, most people agree that self-destructive behavior signals that a person is in turmoil or "perturbation" (Shneidman, 1976, p. 53). We can enhance our effectiveness in working with suicidal people by becoming familiar with several aspects of self-destructive behavior and with intervention practices widely accepted by experts:

- The range and complexity of self-destructive behavior
- Communication and the meaning of self-destructive behavior
- Ambivalence and its relevance to suicide prevention
- The importance of assessing for suicidal risk
- Sensitivity to ethical issues as an aid to understanding, assessment, and appropriate intervention

Self-Destructiveness: What Does It Include?

Self-destructive behavior includes any action by which a person emotionally, socially, and physically damages or ends his or her life. Broadly, the spectrum of self-destructiveness includes biting nails, pulling hair, scratching, cutting one's wrist, swallowing toxic substances or harmful objects, smoking cigarettes, banging one's head, abusing alcohol and other drugs, driving recklessly, neglecting life-preserving measures such as taking insulin, attempting suicide, and committing suicide (Farberow, 1980; Menninger, 1938).

At one end of the spectrum of self-destructiveness is Jane, who smokes but is in essentially good emotional and physical health. She knows the long-range effects of smoking and chooses to live her life in such a way that may in fact shorten it. However, Jane would hardly be regarded as suicidal on a lethality assessment scale. Smoking by Arthur, who has severe emphysema, is another matter. His behavior could be considered a slow form of deliberate self-destruction. At the other end of the spectrum is James, who plans to hang himself. Unless saved accidentally, James will most certainly die by his own hand.

There are four broad groups of self-destructive people:

1. *Those who commit suicide.* Suicide is defined as a fatal act that is self-inflicted, consciously intended, and carried out with the knowledge that death is irreversible. This definition of suicide generally excludes young children because a child's conception of death as final develops around age ten (Pfeffer, 1986). Self-destructive deaths in young children are usually explained in terms of learning theory; the child learns—often by observing parents—that physical and emotional pain can be relieved by ingesting pills or banging one's head.

Classically defined, suicide is one of four modes of death; the others are natural, accidental, and homicidal. Shneidman (1973, p. 384) emphasizes the role of intention in an individual's death and proposes a reclassification of death as (a) intentioned, (b) subintentioned, (c) unintentioned. If full information is not available about the person's intentions, it is difficult to determine whether the act is suicidal or accidental. Suicide is not an illness or an inherited disease, as popular opinion and some professional practice seem to imply.

2. *Those who threaten suicide.* This group includes those who talk about suicide and whose suicidal plans may be either very vague or highly specific. Some in this group have made suicide attempts in the past; others have not. Note that only suicidal people threaten suicide; all suicide threats should be taken seriously and considered in relation to the person's intention and social circumstances.

3. *Those who make suicide attempts.* A suicide attempt is any nonfatal act of self-inflicted damage with self-destructive intention, however vague and ambiguous. Sometimes the individual's intention must be inferred from behavior. Technically, the term *suicide attempt* should be reserved for those actions in which a person attempts to carry out the intention to die but for unanticipated reasons, such as failure of the method or an unplanned rescue, the attempt fails. Other self-destructive behavior can more accurately be defined as *self-injury.* The neutral term self-injury should be substituted for the term *suicide gesture,* as the latter suggests that the behavior need not be taken seriously or that the person is "just seeking attention."

Some suicidal persons are in a state of acute crisis—in contrast to some who are chronically self-destructive—and therefore experience a high degree of emotional turmoil. As noted in Chapter Three, people in crisis may experience a temporary upset in cognitive functioning. This upset can make it difficult for a person to clarify his or her intentions, or it may interfere with making wise decisions. This feature of the crisis state is the basis for the general wisdom of delaying serious decisions such as getting married, selling one's house, or moving to a foreign country while in crisis. Certainly, then, it is similarly unwise to make an irrevocable decision such as suicide when in a state of emotional turmoil and crisis.

The ambiguity arising out of the crisis state should not be confused with a psychotic process, which may or may not be present. Nor should one subscribe to the prevalent myth that "only a crazy person could seriously consider, attempt, or commit suicide." Loss of impulse control influences some suicide attempts and completed suicides. In the large majority of instances, however, self-destructive behavior is something that people consciously and deliberately plan and execute.

4. *Those who are chronically self-destructive.* People in this group may habitually abuse alcohol or other drugs and are often diagnosed with personality disorders. For many First Nations people, self-destructive behaviors are embedded in the abject poverty, unemployment, and other results of colonialism and the near destruction of Native cultures (Philp, 1993). The complex relationship between multiple self-harm episodes and suicide risk is discussed further in "Assessment of the Suicidal Person" later in this chapter. Other people may destroy themselves by the deliberate refusal to follow life-sustaining medical programs for such conditions as heart disease or diabetes. Still others engage in high-risk lifestyles or activities that bring them constantly into the face of potential death. Such individuals seem to need the stimulation of their risky lifestyles to make life seem worth living. These behaviors are not, of course, explicitly suicidal. However, individuals who engage in them may become overtly suicidal. This complicates whatever problems already exist.

When considering chronic self-destructiveness, Maris's concept of *suicidal careers* (1981, pp. 62–69) is relevant. In this framework, suicide can be seen as "one product of a gradual loss of hope and the will and resources to live, a kind of running down and out of life energies, a bankruptcy of psychic defenses against death and decay" (p. 69). Or as Shneidman (1987) puts it, "People reach 'the point of no return' in response to unendurable psychological pain."

It is important to distinguish here between self-destructive persons and those who engage in self-mutilating activity (for example, cutting, scraping, and bruising) that generally has no dire medical consequences, although some may end up killing themselves. Unlike suicidal behavior, self-mutilation is not characterized by an intent to die. Rather, it is a way of coping and is usually employed by women. Many of these women are survivors of extreme childhood sexual abuse who have internalized their oppression (see Burstow, 1992, pp. 187–220; Everett & Gallop, 2000; Hoff, 2000).

The Path to Suicide

Suicidal behavior can be viewed on a continuum or as a *highway leading to suicide*. The highway begins with the first suicide threat or attempt and ends in suicide. As in the case of any trip destined for a certain end point, one can always change one's mind, take a different road to another destination, or turn around and come back. The highway to suicide can be conceived either as a short trip—acute crisis—or as a long trip—chronic self-destructiveness extending for years or over a lifetime. But in either case, it suggests that suicide is a process involving

- One's perception of the meaning of life and death
- Availability of psychological and social resources
- Material and physical circumstances making self-destruction possible (for example, when a gun or pills are available or when a bedridden, helpless person is capable of self-destruction only through starvation)

The continuum concept is also useful in understanding suicides that appear to result from impulsive action, as sometimes happens with adolescents. Even with adolescent suicides, though, examination and hindsight usually reveal a process including, for example, alienation, an acute loss, developmental issues, family conflict, abuse, depression, self-doubt, and cynicism about life.

A destiny of suicide is not inevitable. Whether one continues down the highway to suicide depends on a variety of circumstances. People traveling this highway usually give clues to their distress, so the suicide continuum can be interrupted at any point: after a first attempt, a fifth attempt, or as soon as clues are recognized. Much depends on the help available and the ability of the suicidal person to accept and use help. It is never too late to help a despairing person or to change one's mind about suicide.

Lacking help, some suicidal persons try to relieve their pain by repeated self-injury; each time, their gamble with death becomes more dangerous. As they move along the suicide highway repeating their cries for help, they are often labeled and written off as manipulators or attention seekers. This usually means that professional helpers and others regard them as devious and insincere in their demands for attention. Some conclude that a person who was really serious about suicide would try something that "really did the job." Such a judgment implies a gross misunderstanding of the meaning of a suicidal person's behavior and ignores the person's real needs.

Individuals who are thus labeled and ignored will probably continue to injure themselves. The suicidal episodes typically become progressively more serious in the medical sense, signaling increasing desperation for someone to hear and understand their cries for help. They may also engage in the "no-lose game" as they plan the next suicide attempt (Baechler, 1979). The no-lose game goes something like this: "If they (spouse, friend, family) find me, they care enough and therefore life is worth living. (I win by living.) If they don't find me, life isn't worth living. (I win by dying.)"

The suicide method chosen is usually lethal but includes the possibility of rescue, such as swallowing pills. No-lose reasoning is ineffective in instances when one cannot reasonably expect rescue (for example, a family member rarely checks a person at 2 A.M.). It nevertheless indicates the person's extreme distress and illustrates the logic of the no-lose game.

The Messages of Self-Destructive People

Despite differing explanations for suicide, most people agree that self-destructive acts are a powerful means of communicating; suicidal people are trying to tell us something by their behavior. Interrupting the suicide continuum depends on understanding and responding appropriately to messages of psychic pain, distress, or despair.

Most individuals get what they need or want by simply asking for it. Or friends and family are sensitive and caring enough to pick up the clues to distress before the person becomes desperate. Some people, however, spend a lifetime trying to obtain, without success, what they need for basic survival and happiness. This may be because they cannot express their needs directly, either because their needs are insatiable and therefore unobtainable or because others do not listen and try to meet their needs. Finally, these people give up and attempt suicide as a last effort to let someone know that they are hurting and desperate.

Typically, then, suicidal people have a history of unsuccessful communication. Their problems with communication follow two general patterns:

1. In the first pattern of communication problems, people habitually refrain from expressing feelings and sharing their concerns with significant others. People in this group use the "stiff upper lip" approach to life's problems. Men socialized to be cool and rational in the face of adversity and women socialized to be the social and emotional experts for everyone but themselves contribute to the withholding of feelings. This kind of failure in communication is typified by the following:
    a. A successful businessman, who obtains a promotion, is threatened by his fear of not being able to handle his new responsibilities and kills himself.
    b. A mother of five children, who works devotedly and without complaint for her children and husband and is considered an ideal mother, one day kills two of her children and then herself.
    c. A boy, age seventeen, who is an honor student, plans to go to law school, and is the pride of his parents and the school, is found dead of carbon monoxide poisoning in the family car.

In each of these cases, the response is great shock and consternation: "He seemed to have everything. I wonder why. There doesn't seem to be any reason." Yet hindsight usually reveals that there were clues. Subtle changes in behavior, along with a tendency to repress feelings, should be regarded as quiet cries for help. The messages of these suicidal people are less explicit, and there often is no history of suicidal behavior. Caring others, therefore, need great sensitivity; they need to encourage the suicidal person to share life's joys, troubles, and suicidal fantasies without feeling like an "unmanly" man, a "failure" as a wife and mother, or a "sissy" as an adolescent. Lacking invitations to share and live instead of die, these people's despair may be forever unexpressed in the eternity of death.

2. The second pattern of communication problems is less subtle than the first. People in this group typically include those who threaten suicide or have actually injured themselves. Their suicidal messages are quite direct and are often preceded by other cries for help (Farberow & Shneidman, 1961). Consider, for example, an adolescent girl's signals that something is wrong:
   Age 11: sullenness and truancy from school
   Age 12: experimentation with drugs
   Age 13: running away from home
   Age 14: pregnancy and abortion
   Age 15: first suicide attempt

After a person's first suicide attempt, family members and other significant people in the individual's life are usually shocked. They often are more disturbed by a suicide attempt than by anything else the person might have done. Typically, a parent, spouse, or friend will say, "I knew she was upset and not exactly happy, but I didn't know she was that unhappy." In other words, the first suicide attempt is the most powerful of a series of behavioral messages or clues given over a period of time.

We should all be familiar with suicidal clues or cries for help, such as

- "You won't be seeing me around much anymore."
- "I've about had it with this job. I can't take it anymore."
- "I'm angry at my mother. She'll really be sorry when I'm dead."
- "I can't take any more problems without some relief."
- "I can't live without my boyfriend. I don't really want to die; I just want him back or somebody in his place."
- "I can't take the pain and humiliation [from AIDS, for example] anymore."
- "There's nothing else left since my wife left me. I really want to die."

Behavioral clues may include making out a will, taking out a large life insurance policy, giving away precious belongings, being despondent after a financial setback, or engaging in unusual behavior.

Studies reveal that a majority of persons who commit suicide have made previous attempts. In the absence of attempts, 80 percent have given other significant clues of their suicidal intent (Brown & Sheran, 1972; Shneidman and Farberow, 1957). These behavioral, verbal, and affective clues can be interpreted in two general ways: (1) "I want to die," or (2) "I don't want to die, but I want something to change in order to go on living," or "If things don't change, life isn't worth living. Help me find something to live for."

It is up to the interested helping person to determine the *meaning* of suicidal behavior and to identify clues in the distressed person's words and attitudes. This is done not by inferring the person's meaning but by *asking,* for example,

- "What do you mean when you say you can't take your problems anymore? Are you thinking of suicide?"
- "What did you hope would happen when you took the pills (or cut your wrists)? Did you intend to die?"

There is no substitute for *simple, direct communication* by a person who cares. Besides providing the information we need in order to help, it is helpful to the suicidal person. It tells the person we are interested and concerned about her or his motives for the contemplated suicide. Often self-destructive people have lacked the advantages of communicating directly about their feelings all of their lives.

Unfortunately, many people lack the knowledge or resources to respond helpfully to a suicidal person. The self-destructive person is often surrounded by others who potentially could help but whose own troubles prevent them from providing what the self-destructive person needs. Some families are so needy that the most they can do is obtain medical treatment for the suicidal person. This situation is not helped by the fact that twenty-four-hour crisis services are not accessible in some communities.

Some would-be helpers fail to communicate directly about suicide in the false belief that talking to the person about suicide intentions may trigger such ideas if the person does not already have them. The process of deciding to commit suicide is much more complicated than such reasoning implies. A person who is not suicidal will not become so as a result of a question from someone intending to help. In fact, experience reveals that suicidal people are relieved when someone is sensitive enough to respond to their despair and help protect them from themselves.

For three reasons, then, communication is crucial in our work with people who respond to crisis by self-destructive behavior.

1. It is a key element in discerning the *process* of self-destruction (understanding).
2. It is the most effective means of ascertaining the person's intention regarding death (assessment of risk).
3. It is an essential avenue for helping the person feel reconnected to other human beings and find a reason to live (crisis intervention).

Ambivalence: Weighing Life and Death

Suicidal people usually struggle with two irreconcilable wishes—the desire to live and the desire to die. They simultaneously consider the advantages of life and death, a state of mind known as *ambivalence.* As long as the person has ambivalent feelings about life and death, it is possible to help the individual consider choices on the side of life. Suicide is not inevitable. People can change their minds if they find realistic alternatives to suicide. The concept of ambivalence is basic to the purpose of suicide prevention and crisis work; those who are no longer ambivalent do not usually come to an emergency service, see their physician, or call crisis hotlines.

CASE EXAMPLE: SALLY

Sally, age sixteen, made a suicide attempt by swallowing six sleeping pills. In medical terms, this was not a serious attempt. Although she contemplated death, she also wanted to live. She hoped that the suicide attempt would bring about some change in her miserable family life, so that she could avoid the last resort of suicide itself. Before her suicide attempt, Sally was having trouble in school, ran away from home once, experimented with drugs, and engaged in behavior that often brought disapproval from her parents.

All of these behaviors were Sally's way of saying, "Listen to me! Can't you see that I'm miserable, that I can't control myself, that I can't go on like this anymore?" Sally had been upset for several years by her parents' constant fighting and playing favorites with the children. Her father drank heavily and frequently was away from home. When Sally's school counselor recommended family counseling, the family refused out of shame. Sally's acting out was really a cry for help. After her suicide attempt, her parents accepted counseling. Sally's behavior improved generally, and she made no further suicide attempts.

If Sally had not obtained the help she needed, it is probable that she would have continued down the highway to suicide. The usual pattern in such a case is that the attempts become medically more serious, the person becomes more desperate, and finally he or she commits suicide. Helping the ambivalent person move in the direction of life is done by understanding and responding to the meaning of the person's behavior.

Assessment of the Suicidal Person

Communication leads to understanding, which is the foundation for decision and action. Helping suicidal people without understanding what their behavior means and without ascertaining the degree of suicide risk is difficult. *Suicide risk assessment* is the process of determining the likelihood of suicide for a particular person. *Lethality assessment* refers to the degree of physical injury incurred by a particular self-destructive act. Sometimes these terms are used interchangeably. *Suicide prediction*, in terms of current research, is "not very precise or useful" (Maris, 1991, p. 2) and according to Motto (1991, p. 75) should probably be eliminated from scientific terminology. The main focus here is to provide clinicians with guidelines about the risk of suicide that are based on clinical experience and on empirical and epidemiological findings. Clinical assessment tries to answer this question: What is the risk of death by suicide for *this individual* at *this time*, considering the person's life as a whole?

Some workers use lethality assessment scales, which are primarily research tools, to assess suicidal risk. Most of these scales are not very effective (Brown & Sheran, 1972). Motto (1985, p. 139) states, "The use of a scale has never been intended to predict suicide, but simply to supplement clinical judgment at the time an evaluation is done." Nor can a rating scale ever substitute for a clinician's sensitive inquiry (Motto, 1991)—for example, "Can you tell me what's happening to cause you so much pain?" The problem with most scales is that they do not exclude the nonsuicidal population. For example, let us consider depression as a predictive sign. A large number of people who commit suicide (approximately 60 percent) have been diagnosed as depressed; however, the majority of depressed people do not commit suicide. Of the twenty million or so persons with a depressive disorder, only 0.1 percent commit suicide; Jacobs (2000, p. 32) notes the striking fact that 99.9 percent of persons diagnosed annually with depression do not commit suicide. Similarly, the majority of people who commit suicide have made previous suicide attempts, yet eight out of ten people who attempt suicide never go on to commit suicide. These statistics do not invite complacency; they simply indicate the complexity of suicide risk assessment, the limits of psychiatric diagnostic criteria, and the fact that something changed for a particular person at risk—for example, a cry for help was heard.

The Importance of Assessing Suicide Risk

The importance of suicide risk assessment can be compared with the importance of diagnosing a cough before beginning treatment. Effective assessment of suicide risk should accomplish the following:

- Cut down on guesswork in working with self-destructive people
- Reduce the confusion and disagreement that often occur among those trying to help suicidal people
- Provide a scientific base for service plans for self-destructive people
- Ensure that hospitalization of suicidal persons is used appropriately
- Decrease a worker's level of anxiety in working with suicidal persons

Failure to assess the degree of suicide risk results in unnecessary problems, such as failure to institute follow-up counseling following emergency medical treatment for self-injury. Another problem arising out of guesswork about suicide risk is unnecessary hospitalization. It is inappropriate to hospitalize a suicidal person when the degree of suicide risk is very low and other sources of protection are available. A person who hopes, by a suicide attempt, to relieve isolation from family may feel even more isolated in a psychiatric hospital. This is especially true when community and family intervention are indicated instead.

Sometimes community and hospital workers hospitalize suicidal people because of their own anxiety about suicide. Unresolved feelings of guilt and responsibility about suicide usually precipitate such action. Conversely, hospitals can be places in which isolation can be relieved and suicide prevented when social supports in the community are lacking. As with personal factors, assumptions about the presence or absence of social supports should not be made without a systematic social assessment (see Chapters Three and Five).

Signs That Help Assess Suicide Risk

Risk assessment techniques are based on knowledge obtained from the study of completed suicides. Such research is among the most difficult of scientific studies (Maris, 1991; Smith & Maris, 1986), but the study of completed suicides has explained much about the problem of risk assessment. Maris (1992), Brown and Sheran (1972), and others have identified signs that help us assess the degree of risk for suicide. The most reliable indicators help us distinguish people who commit suicide from the population at large and also from those who only attempt suicide. These signs, however, have their limitations. For instance, there is not enough research on suicide to warrant general conclusions about suicide for different population groups (Smith & Maris, 1986). One should never be overconfident in applying signs to a suicidal person. It is impossible to predict suicide in any absolute sense; the focus for clinicians should be on assessing immediate and long-term risk. However, attention to the known signs of suicide risk is a considerable improvement over an approach based on myth, taboo, and unresearched guesswork. The chaos of a crisis situation and anxiety about suicide can be reduced by thoughtful attention to general principles based on research.

The following material regarding signs that help us assess suicide risk is summarized from the works of Alvarez (1971), Brown and Sheran (1972), Brown and Harris (1978), Durkheim (1897/1951), Farberow (1975), Furst and Huffine (1991), Hatton, Valente, and Rink (1984), Hendin (1982), Litman (1987), Maris (1981, 1992), and Shneidman (1985). These principles for assessing suicide risk apply to *any* person in *any* setting contacted through *any* helping situation: telephone, office, hospital, home, work site, jail, nursing home, school, or pastoral care. *Functional* assessment (emotional, cognitive, behavioral) is the focus, although psychiatric *pathology* may be present in some instances. The discussion is based on research in Western societies; suicide signs and methods vary in other cultural settings (see United Nations, 1996). Sensitivity to these differences, however, is important in helping various immigrant and ethnic groups in distress in North America.

Suicide Plan. Studies reveal that the majority of persons who die by suicide deliberately planned to do so. Without a high-lethal plan with available means, suicide cannot occur. In respect to the plan, people suspected of being suicidal should be asked several direct questions concerning the following subjects:

1. *Suicidal ideas.* "Are you so upset that you're thinking of suicide?" or "Are you thinking about hurting yourself?"
2. *Lethality of method.* "What are you thinking of doing?"

High-Lethal Methods

Gun

Hanging

Barbiturate and prescribed sleeping pills

Jumping

Drowning

Carbon monoxide poisoning

Aspirin (high dose) and acetaminophen (Tylenol)

Car crash

Exposure to extreme cold

Antidepressants

Low-Lethal Methods

Wrist cutting

Nonprescription drugs (excluding aspirin and acetaminophen [Tylenol])

Tranquilizers (antianxiety agents)

The helper should also determine the person's knowledge about the lethality of the chosen method. For example, a person who takes ten tranquilizers with the mistaken belief that the dose is fatal is alive more by accident than by intent.

3. *Availability of means.* "Do you have a gun? Do you know how to use it? Do you have ammunition? Do you have pills?" Lives have often been saved by removing very lethal methods such as guns and sleeping pills. A highly suicidal person who calls a crisis center is often making a final effort to get help, even while sitting next to a loaded gun or a bottle of pills. Such an individual will welcome a direct, protective gesture from a telephone counselor, such as, "Why don't you put the gun away?" or "Why don't you throw the pills out, and then let's talk about what's troubling you." When friends and family are involved, they too should be directed to get rid of the weapon or pills. In disposing of lethal weapons, it is important to engage the suicidal person actively in the process, keeping in mind that power ploys can trigger rather than prevent suicide. If trust and rapport have been established, engaging the suicidal person is generally not difficult to do.

4. *Specificity of plan.* "Do you have a plan worked out for killing yourself?" "How do you plan to get the pills?" "How do you plan to get the gun?" A person who has a plan that is well thought out—including time, place, and circumstances—with an available high-lethal method is an immediate and very high risk for suicide. We should also determine whether any rescue possibilities are included in the plan—for example, "What time of day do you plan to do this?" or "Is there anyone else around at that time?" We should also inquire about the person's intent. Some people really do intend to die; others intend to bring about some change that will help them avoid death and make life more livable.

We can seldom discover a person's suicide plan except through direct questioning. Someone who believes in the myth that talking about suicide may suggest the idea will hesitate to ask direct questions. The suicide plan is a less important sign of risk in the case of people with a history of impulsive behavior. This is true for some adults and for adolescents in general, who are inclined to be impulsive as a characteristic of their stage of development.

History of Suicide Attempts. In the North American adult population, suicide attempts occur eight to ten times more often than actual suicide. Among adolescents, there are about fifty attempts to every completed suicide. Most people who attempt suicide do not go on to commit suicide. Usually, some change occurs in their psychosocial world that makes life more desirable than death. But it is also true that the majority of people who kill themselves have made previous suicide attempts. A history of suicide attempts (65 percent of those who have completed suicide) is especially prominent among suicidal people who find that self-destructive behavior is the most powerful means they have of communicating their distress to others. Those who have made previous high-lethal attempts are at greater risk for suicide than those who have made low-lethal attempts. Another historical indicator is a change in method of suicide attempt. A person who makes a high-lethal attempt after several less lethal attempts that elicited increasingly indifferent responses from significant others is a higher risk for suicide than a person with a consistent pattern of low-lethal attempts. This is particularly true in the case of suicidal adolescents. Suicide attempts as a risk factor should also be considered in relation to depression. Among the 929 severely depressed patients in the Collaborative Depression Study, suicide attempt was not a predictor of suicide within one year but was a predictor of suicide within two to ten years (Fawcett, 2000, p. 38). This finding underscores a pivotal point in suicide prevention work—the need to *reassess* for suicide risk.

We should also determine the outcome of previous suicide attempts—for example, "What happened after your last attempt? Did you plan any possibility of rescue, or were you rescued accidentally?" A person living alone who overdoses with sleeping pills and then has unexpected company and is rescued is alive more by accident than by intent. This person falls into a high-risk category for future suicide if there are other high-risk indicators as well. Suicide risk is also increased if the person has a negative perception of a psychiatric hospital or counseling experience. This finding underscores the importance of extreme caution in employing mental health laws to hospitalize suicidal people against their will for self-protection.

Resources and Communication with Significant Others. Internal resources consist of strengths, problem-solving ability, and personality factors that help one cope with stress. External resources include a network of persons on whom one can rely routinely as well as during a crisis. Communication as a suicide sign includes (1) the statement to others of intent to commit suicide and (2) the disruption of bonds between the suicidal person and significant others. A large number of people who finally commit suicide feel ignored or cut off from significant people around them, some to the point of feeling there are no significant people in their lives. This is extremely important in the case of adolescents, especially regarding their attempts to communicate with their parents. Research suggests that most adolescents who kill themselves are at odds with their families and feel very misunderstood or have experienced various external stressors (Berman & Jobes, 1991; Brent et al., 1993).

Institutionalized racism and the unequal distribution of material resources in the United States appear to contribute to the rapidly increasing rate of suicide among minority groups. This is especially true among young (under thirty) people who realize early in life that many doors are closed to them. Their rage and frustration eventually lead to despair, suicide, and other violent behavior. An example of violence that is closely linked to suicide is *victim-precipitated homicide*. In this form of homicide, the person killed is suicidal, but instead of committing suicide, the victim incites someone else to kill, thus precipitating the homicide (see Parent, 1998, for a discussion on when such deaths involve police).

Others may have apparent resources, such as a supportive, caring spouse, but the conviction of their worthlessness prevents them from accepting and using such support. This is especially true for suicidal people who are also extremely depressed. Adequate personality resources include the ability to be flexible and to accept mistakes and imperfections in oneself. Some people who kill themselves seem to have happy families, good jobs, and good health. Observers therefore assume that these people have no reason to kill themselves. Research by Breed (1972) reveals that this kind of person perceives himself or herself in very rigid roles imposed by culture, sexual identity, or socioeconomic status. A typical example is the middle-aged male executive who rigidly commits himself to success by climbing up the career ladder in his company. A threatened or actual failure in this self-imposed and rigid role performance can precipitate suicide for such a person.

Such perceived failure is usually sex specific—work failure for men (Morrell, Taylor, Quine, & Kerr, 1993) and family or mate failure for women (Stephens, 1985). Other research, however, suggests that a woman might commit suicide in response to "superwoman" demands that she be both the perfect, unpaid domestic worker and the perfect paid public worker (Hoff, 1985). Investigation of completed suicides reveals that a person with rigid role perceptions commits suicide after receiving, for example, a long-anticipated promotion, an event that leads the person to doubt his or her ability to fulfill higher expectations (Perrah & Wichman, 1987). Such rigidity in personality type is also revealed in the person's approach to problem solving. The individual sees narrowly, perceiving only one course of action or one solution to a problem—suicide. This has sometimes been described as telescopic or *tunnel vision* (Hatton et al., 1984, p. 29; Shneidman, 1987, p. 57). Such people typically are candidates for psychotherapy to help them develop more flexible approaches to problem solving. We should recognize this rigidity as a possible barrier in our efforts to help suicidal people consider alternatives. A person of this type whose personal and social resources are exhausted and whose only remaining communication link is to a counselor or helping agency is a high risk for suicide.

Research and clinical experience suggest that workers should look not only at such signs of risk but also at the complex *patterning* of signs (Brown & Sheran, 1972; Farberow, 1975), in concert with clinical judgment (Motto, 1991). Let us apply this evidence to the pattern of the signs considered previously. If the person (1) has a history of high-lethal attempts, (2) has a specific, high-lethal plan for suicide with available means, and (3) lacks both personality and social resources, and cannot communicate with available resources, the immediate and long-range risk for suicide is very high, regardless of other factors. The risk increases, however, if factors such as those discussed next are also present.

Sex, Age, Race, Marital Status, and Sexual Identity. The suicide ratio among North American men and women is approximately three males to one female, although female suicides are increasing at a faster rate than male suicides. Among children between the ages of ten and fourteen, the suicide rate averages 0.8 per 100,000. Because suicide implies an understanding of death as irreversible, in the case of children below the age of ten, designating suicide as a cause of death should be done cautiously. Surely there is psychic pain, but learned self-destructive behavior may be more accurate. Suicide risk increases with age only for white males. Among blacks, Chicanos, and First Nations people, the suicide rate reaches its peak under the age of thirty (for additional statistics, see United Nations, 1996).

The overall suicide rate among white persons is three times that among black persons. However, among young, urban, African American men between twenty and thirty-five years of age, the rate is twice that of white men the same age. In Native North American communities, the suicide rate varies from group to group. In general, suicide rates are increasing among adolescents and racial minority groups and among youth experiencing sexual-identity crisis.

If a person is separated from a spouse, widowed, or divorced, the risk of suicide increases. Those who are married or who have never been married are at less risk (Smith, Mercy, & Conn, 1988). This seems related to the loss factor among suicidal people but does not seem to apply to two specific groups—older, married, white men who are simply tired of living and married black people who have lost a love relationship. See Motto (1991) regarding limitations of statistical data to predict suicide in particular individuals.

Recent Loss. Loss or the threat of loss of a spouse, parent, status, money, or job increases a person's suicide risk. Loss is a very significant suicide indicator among adolescents. Loss should also be kept in mind as a common theme in most people's experience of crisis (see "Loss, Change, and Grief Work" in Chapter Four).

Physical Illness. Studies reveal that many people who kill themselves are physically ill. Three out of four suicide victims have been under medical care or have visited their physician within four to six months of their death. The visit to a physician does not necessarily imply that the person is physically ill. However, it highlights the fact that a large number of people with any problem seek out either physicians or the clergy. In the case of suicidal people, the visit may be their last attempt to find relief from distress.

These facts suggest the influential role primary care providers can have in preventing suicide if they are attentive to clues. The provider's failure to ascertain the suicide plan or to examine the depression disguised by a complaint with no physical basis often leads to the common practice of prescribing a psychotropic drug without listening to the person and making a referral for counseling. Such a response by a physician or advanced practice nurse can be interpreted by the individual as an invitation to commit suicide (see Chapter Eleven).

The possibility of suicide is even greater if a person receives a diagnosis that affects his or her self-image and value system or demands a major switch in lifestyle—for example, AIDS, degenerative neurological conditions, heart disease, breast cancer, amputation of a limb, or cancer of the sex organs (see Rodin, 2000).

Drinking and Other Drug Abuse. Drinking increases impulsive behavior and loss of control and therefore increases suicide risk, especially if the person has a high-lethal means available. Alcohol also reduces the number of sleeping pills needed for a lethal overdose. Among those diagnosed with alcoholism, a significant number die by suicide (Motto, 1980). Often adolescents who die by suicide were involved in drug or alcohol abuse before their death. People with liver damage from alcohol abuse may die from a low-lethal method like wrist cutting because of interference with the normal clotting time.

Physical Isolation. If a person is isolated both emotionally and physically, risk of suicide is greater than if he or she lives with close significant others. According to Durkheim (1897/1951), *egoistic suicide* occurs among people who feel they do not belong to society; *anomic suicide* occurs among people who cannot adjust to change and social demands. One of the basic human needs is approval by others of our performance in expected roles. The lack of such approval leads to social isolation.

Negative reactions from significant people are incorporated into the hurt and painful sense of self. Rejection from significant others can lead to a conviction of worthlessness. When this happens, people believe that others also see them as worthless. People who suffer from discrimination are at risk for egoistic suicide. However, studies indicate that once minority groups and women achieve equality and better conditions, their risk for anomic suicide will increase. If white society or male dominance can no longer be blamed, the person may internalize failure. This process can lead to suicide. As one black person put it, "Being on the ground floor left no room to jump." Thus upward mobility may increase suicide risk.

A person who is physically alone and socially isolated is often a candidate for hospitalization or other extraordinary means to relieve isolation. In such cases, hospitalization can be a lifesaving measure.

Unexplained Change in Behavior. Changes in behavior, such as reckless driving and drinking by a previously careful and sober driver, can be an indicator of suicide risk. It is particularly important to observe behavior changes in adolescents, as these changes are often clues to inner turmoil. Again, direct communication about observed behavior changes can be a lifesaving measure, signaling that someone cares and is sensitive to another's distress, even though talking about it initially may seem impossible.

Depression. Depressed people may experience sleeplessness, early wakening, slowed-down functioning, weight loss, menstrual irregularity, loss of appetite, inability to work normally, disinterest in sex, crying, and restlessness. Feelings of hopelessness are an even more important indicator of suicidal danger than depression (Beck, Steer, Beck, & Newman, 1993). Those with bipolar illness, especially early in the illness, are also at risk (Solomon, Keitner, Miller, Shea, & Keller, 1995). Depressed adolescents are often overactive (agitated depression); they may fail in school or withdraw from usual social contacts. Although not all people who kill themselves show signs of depression, enough suicide victims are depressed to make this an important indicator of risk. This is particularly true for the depressed person who feels worthless and is unable to reach out to others for help. Because most depressed people do not kill themselves (Fawcett, 2000, p. 38) and because a useful predictor must distinguish between the general population and those who make suicide attempts, we should refrain from declaring depression as a significant predictor of suicide. That said, *depression is a significant avenue for opening direct discussion of possible suicide plans:* "You seem really down. Are you so depressed that perhaps you've considered suicide?"

Social Factors. Social problems such as family disorganization, a broken home, and a record of delinquency, truancy, and violence against others increase a person's risk of suicide. Many adolescents who kill themselves had prior physical fights with their families. A person with a chaotic social background is also likely to follow the suicide attempt pattern of significant others. Suicide risk also increases for people who are unemployed or forced to retire or move, especially when these upsets occur during a developmental transition stage. Among women who attempt suicide, many have a history of sexual or other abuse (Egmond, Garnefski, Jonker, & Kerkhof, 1993; Hoff, 2000; Stephens, 1985).

Psychosis. Some people falsely believe that only a mentally ill person could commit suicide. If an individual with a thought disorder hears voices directing him or her to commit suicide, the risk of suicide is obviously increased. However, the number of individuals who fall into this category is extremely small. Risk may also increase following remission if the person interprets effective treatment as freedom from illness and then discontinues antipsychotic medication only to have the perception of being "cured" dashed by another psychotic episode (Motto, 1999, pp. 227–228). People who are diagnosed as psychotic should routinely be assessed for suicide risk according to the criteria outlined in this section.

Table 6.1 illustrates how signs of suicide risk help distinguish people who kill themselves from those who injure themselves nonlethally and from the general population. In the next section, the pattern of these signs is described in a typology of suicide risk.

Typology of Suicidal Behavior: Assessing Immediate and Long-Range Risk

People tend to classify the seriousness of self-destructive behavior according to whether there is immediate danger of death. A person might engage in several kinds of self-destructive behavior at the same time. For example, an individual who chronically abuses alcohol may threaten, attempt, or commit suicide—all in one day. We should view these behaviors on the continuum noted earlier; all are serious and important in terms of life and death. The difference is that for some the danger of death is immediate, whereas for others it is long-range. Still others are at risk because of a high-risk lifestyle, chronic substance abuse, and neglect of medical care.

Distinguishing between immediate and long-range risk for suicide is not only a potential lifesaving measure, it is also important for preventing or interrupting a vicious cycle of repeated self-injury. If immediate risk is high, and we do not uncover it in assessment, a suicide can result (see Hoff & Resing, 1982). Conversely, if immediate risk is low, as in medically nonserious cases of wrist slashing or swallowing a few sleeping pills, but we respond medically as though life were at stake while failing to address the *meaning* of this physical act, we run the risk of *reinforcing* self-destructive behavior. The person, in effect, is told by our behavior, "Do something more serious (medically), and I'll pay attention to you." In reality, medically nonserious self-injury is a life-and-death issue—that is, if the person's cries for help are repeatedly ignored, there is high probability that eventually the person will accept the invitation to do something more serious and actually commit suicide. The Collaborative Depression Study (Fawcett, 2000) affirms this decades-long clinical observation.

The following schema assists in assessing suicide risk by means of a structured guide, as presented in Chapter Three (see Table 6.2). Examples illustrate the application of risk criteria to people at low risk, moderate risk, and high risk. This assessment guide highlights the importance of the patterns of signs and the use of clinical judgment, along with a database—not simply a mechanical rating—in evaluating suicidal risk (Motto, 1991).

Low-Risk Suicidal Behavior. This includes verbal threats of suicide with no specific plan or means of carrying out a plan. This category also includes self-injury by a person who knows that the effects of the method do not involve physical danger or clearly provides for rescue. Ambivalence in low-risk behavior tends more in the direction of life than death.

The immediate risk of suicide is low, but the risk of an attempt, a repeat attempt, and eventual suicide is high, depending on what happens after the threat or attempt. The risk is increased if the person abuses alcohol and other drugs. Social and personal resources are present but problematic for people in this behavior group.

TABLE 6.1.   SIGNS COMPARING PEOPLE WHO COMPLETE OR ATTEMPT
SUICIDE WITH THE GENERAL POPULATION.

Signs	Suicide	Suicide Attempt	General Population
Suicide plan*	Specific, with available, high-lethal method; does not include rescue	Less lethal method, including plan for rescue; risk increases if lethality of method increases	None, or vague ideas only
History of suicide attempts*	65 percent have history of high-lethal attempts; if rescued, it was probably accidental	Previous attempts are usually low lethal; rescue plan included; risk increases if there is a change from many low-lethal attempts to a high-lethal one	None, or low lethal with definite rescue plan
Resources* Psychological Social	Very limited or nonexistent; or person *perceives* self with no resources	Moderate, or in psychological and/or social turmoil	Either intact or able to restore them through nonsuicidal means
Communication*	Feels cut off from resources and unable to communicate effectively	Ambiguously attached to resources; may use self-injury as a method of communicating with significant others when other methods fail	Able to communicate directly and nondestructively for need fulfillment
Recent loss	Increases risk	May increase risk	Is widespread but is resolved nonsuicidally through grief work, and so forth
Physical illness	Increases risk	May increase risk	Is common but responded to through effective crisis management (natural and/or formal)
Drinking and other drug abuse	Increases risk	May increase risk	Is widespread but does not in itself lead to suicide
Physical isolation	Increases risk	May increase risk	Many well-adjusted people live alone; they handle physical isolation through satisfactory social contacts
Unexplained change in behavior	A possible clue to suicidal intent, especially in teenagers	A cry for help and possible clue to suicidal ideas	Does not apply in absence of other predictive signs
Depression	60 percent have a history of depression	A large percentage are depressed	A large percentage are depressed

TABLE 6.1.   SIGNS COMPARING PEOPLE WHO COMPLETE OR ATTEMPT SUICIDE WITH THE GENERAL POPULATION. (*continued*)

Signs	Suicide	Suicide Attempt	General Population
Social factors or problems	May be present	Often are present	Widespread but do not in themselves lead to suicide
Psychosis	May be present	May be present	May be present
Age, sex, race, marital status, sexual identity	Statistical predictors that are most useful for identifying whether an individual belongs to a high-lethal risk group, not for clinical assessment of individuals	May be present	May be present

*If all four of these signs exist in a particular person, the risk for suicide is very high regardless of all other factors. If other signs also apply, the risk is increased further.

TABLE 6.2. LETHALITY ASSESSMENT SCALE: SELF.

Key to Scale	Danger to Self	Typical Indicators
1	No predictable risk of suicide now	Has no suicidal ideation or history of attempt, has satisfactory social support system, and is in close contact with significant others
2	Low risk of suicide now	Has suicidal ideation with low-lethal methods, no history of attempts or recent serious loss, has satisfactory support network, no alcohol problems, basically wants to live
3	Moderate risk of suicide now	Has suicidal ideation with high-lethal method but no specific plan or threats. Or has plan with low-lethal method, history of low-lethal attempts; for example, employed female, age 35, divorced, with tumultuous family history and reliance on psychotropic drugs for stress relief, is weighing the odds between life and death
4	High risk of suicide now	Has current high-lethal plan, obtainable means, history of previous attempts, is unable to communicate with a significant other; for example, female, age 50, living alone, with drinking history; or black male, age 29, unemployed and has lost his lover, depressed and wants to die
5	Very high risk of suicide now	Has current high-lethal plan with available means, history of suicide attempts, is cut off from resources; for example, white male, over 40, physically ill and depressed, wife threatening divorce, is unemployed, or has received promotion and fears failure

Adapted from specifications for use of forms discussed in Chapter Three.

CASE EXAMPLE: SARAH

Sarah, age forty-two, took five sleeping pills at 5:00 P.M. with full knowledge that the drug would not kill her and obtained the temporary relief she wanted in sleep. When her husband found her sleeping at 6:00 P.M., he had at least some message of her distress. Sarah is troubled by her marriage and has a limited social circle (her husband never liked any of her friends). She is employed part-time as a secretary. She really wants a divorce but is afraid she cannot easily make it on her own. Sarah also takes an antidepressant drug every day. She has not made any other suicide attempts.

Suicide risk for Sarah: Sarah's immediate risk of suicide is low (rating scale: 2). The risk of repeat suicide attempts is moderate to high, depending on what Sarah is able to do about her problem.

Moderate-Risk Suicidal Behavior. This includes verbal threats with a plan and available means more specific and potentially more lethal than those involved in low-risk behavior. Also included are attempts in which the possibility of rescue is more precarious. The chosen method, although it may result in temporary physical disability, is not fatal, regardless of whether or not there is rescue. Ambivalence is strong; life and death are seen more and more in an equally favorable light. The immediate risk for suicide is moderate. The risk for a repeat suicide attempt and eventual suicide is higher than for low-risk behavior if emotional pain is not relieved and no important life changes occur after the attempt or revelation of the suicide plan. The risk is significantly increased in the presence of chronic alcohol or other drug abuse.

CASE EXAMPLE: SUSAN

Susan, age nineteen, came alone in a taxi to a local hospital emergency department. She had taken an overdose of her antidepressant prescription (three times the usual dose) a half hour earlier. Susan and her three-year-old child, Debbie, live with her parents. She has never gotten along well with her parents, especially her mother. Before the birth of her child, Susan had a couple of short-lived jobs as a waitress. She dropped out of high school at age sixteen and has experimented off and on with drugs. Since the age of fifteen, Susan had made four suicide attempts. She took overdoses of nonprescription drugs three times and cut her wrists once. These attempts were assessed as being of low lethality.

At the emergency department, Susan had her stomach pumped and was kept for observation for a couple of hours. She and the nurses knew one another from emergency service visits after her other suicide attempts. She was discharged with a recommendation that she seriously consider previous referrals for follow-up counseling. This emergency department did not have on-site crisis or psychiatric consultants. While there, Susan could sense the impatience and disgust of the staff. A man with a heart attack had come in around the same time. Susan felt that no one had the time or interest to talk with her. Twice before, Susan had refused referrals for counseling, so the nurses assumed that she was hopeless and did not really want help.

Suicide risk for Susan: Susan is not in immediate danger of suicide (rating scale: 3). She does not have a high-lethal plan and has no history of high-lethal attempts, although overdosing on a prescription antidepressant signifies a change toward increased risk. As already noted, most antidepressants are considered high-lethal methods, depending on the particular drug and the age and weight of the patient. In general, a lethal dose is ten times the prescribed dose. Susan's overdose of three times the prescribed dose therefore falls in the moderate-risk category. Best practice includes calling local poison control centers when there is any question about dosage and lethality. Susan's personal coping ability is poor. She used drugs and failed in school, but she is not cut off from her family, despite their disturbed relationship. She has not suffered a serious personal loss. However, because there is no follow-up counseling or evidence of any changes in her troubled social situation, she is at risk of making more suicide attempts in the future. If such attempts increase in their medical seriousness, Susan's risk of eventual suicide also increases significantly. On the ambivalence scale, life and death may begin to look the same for Susan if her circumstances do not change.

High-Risk Suicidal Behavior. This includes a threat or a suicide attempt that would probably be fatal without accidental rescue and sophisticated medical or surgical intervention. Such behavior also includes instances when a suicide attempt fails to end in death as expected, such as in a deliberate car crash. Another example is a threat that will be carried out unless a potential rescuer, such as a friend, family member, or crisis worker, can convince the person that there are good reasons to go on living. Ambivalence in high-risk behavior tends more in the direction of death than life.

The present and long-range risk of suicide is very high unless immediate help is available and accepted. Chronic self-destructive behavior increases the risk even further.

CASE EXAMPLE: EDWARD

Edward, age forty-one, had just learned that his wife, Jane, had decided to get a divorce. He threatened to kill himself with a gun or carbon monoxide on the day she filed for the divorce. Jane's divorce lawyer proposed that their country home and the twenty adjoining acres be turned over completely to Jane. Edward told his wife, neighbors, and a crisis counselor that his family and home were all he had to live for. Indeed, all Edward could afford after the divorce was the rental of a single shabby room. He and Jane have four children. Edward also has several concerned friends but does not feel he can turn to them, as he always kept his family matters private. Jane's decision to divorce Edward has left him feeling like a complete failure. He has several guns and is a skilled hunter. A major factor in Jane's decision to divorce Edward was his chronic drinking problem. He had threatened to shoot himself eight months earlier after a violent argument with Jane when he was drinking, and Jane kept urging him to get help from AA.

Several strong signs of high risk can be identified in Edward's case.

1. He has a specific plan with an available high-lethal means—the gun.
2. He threatened suicide with a high-lethal method eight months previously and is currently communicating his suicide plan.
3. He is threatened with a serious interpersonal loss and feels cut off from what he regards as his most important social resources, his family and home.
4. He has a rigid expectation of himself in his role as husband and provider for his family. He sees himself as a failure in that role and has a deep sense of shame about his perceived failure.
5. His coping ability is apparently poor, as he resorts to the use of alcohol and is reluctant to use his friends for support during a crisis.
6. He is also a high risk in terms of his age, sex, race, marital status, and history of alcohol abuse.

Suicide risk for Edward: Edward is in immediate danger of committing suicide (rating scale: 5). Even if he makes it through his present crisis, he is also a long-range risk for suicide because of his chronic self-destructive behavior—abuse of alcohol and threats of suicide by a readily available, high-lethal means.

CASE EXAMPLE: BARBARA

Barbara, age seventy-seven, is noted in the nursing care facility for her disagreeable personality and suspiciousness of staff and other residents. She has diabetes, heart disease, and asthma, the symptoms of which are exacerbated when she has an unpleasant encounter with others. Barbara has been moved to several different wings of the institution because staff "can take only so much of her." After her last move, Barbara refused to eat or receive visits from other residents, resisted taking her medication, and said she just wanted to die. Barbara has a daughter and son-in-law who see her every few months. She also attends religious services routinely, the only activity she has continued.

Suicide risk for Barbara: Barbara is a high risk for suicide both immediately and in the future (rating scale: 4). The outcome of her self-destructive behavior will depend on how staff and her family understand and respond to her distress. On the ambivalence scale, unless her circumstances change, Barbara will probably continue to see death as more desirable than life (see Moore, 1997).

CASE EXAMPLE: SHIRLEY

A woman went to visit her mother, Shirley, at a psychiatric facility, though she was advised on arrival not to see her mother at that time; Shirley was hearing voices telling her to kill herself and had therefore been placed in a special room with restraints. Her treatment consisted of psychotropic drugs and periodic checks by staff members. After the staff convinced the daughter that a visit would not benefit Shirley, the daughter asked to be allowed to see her mother through the peek hole, unobserved by her mother. The daughter had had a dream about her mother dying and told the psychiatrist she would not be able to forgive herself if her mother did die and she had not seen her. The psychiatrist refused, claiming then to be protecting the daughter.

Suicide risk for Shirley: Shirley is an immediate and long-range risk for suicide (rating scale: 5). Shirley's physical restraint decreased her immediate risk; however, it is now known that social isolation only promotes suicidal tendencies. Hallucinations directing her to kill herself also increase risk. The long-range probability of suicide by Shirley is further increased by the coercive measures used and by the psychiatrist's refusal to allow a caring daughter to visit. The immediate and long-range risks of these suicidal behaviors are summarized in Table 6.3.

Understanding and Assessing Risk in Special Populations

This chapter describes the wide range of people who are self-destructive and need help. The general principles of assessment apply to all people who are actually or potentially suicidal—the old, the young, different ethnic and sexual-identity groups, institutionalized people, the unemployed, the educated, patients in medical and surgical wards, and psychotic and nonpsychotic persons in psychiatric settings. Still, trends and issues in the suicidology field suggest the need to highlight the special needs of adolescents, distinct ethnic groups, and suicidal people in hospitals and other institutions.

TABLE 6.3.   SUICIDE RISK DIFFERENTIATION.

Suicidal Behavior		Ambivalence Scale	Rescue Plan	Immediate Risk	Long-Range Risk	
Low risk	Life	Desires life more than death	Present	Low	High	Depending on immediate response, treatment, and follow-up
Moderate risk		Life and death seem equally desirable	Ambiguous	Moderate	High	
High risk	Death	Desires death more than life	Absent, or rescue after past attempts was accidental	Very high	High	

Young People

As we have seen, suicidal behavior is a cry for help, a way to stop the pain when nothing else works. Unnecessary death by suicide is a tragedy regardless of age, gender, class, race, or sexual identity and regardless of variations in suicide rates among these different groups. But suicidal death by those who have barely begun life's journey is particularly poignant—for the victims themselves, their families, and all of society. The tragedy of youth suicide must not be missed in statistical comparisons with other at-risk groups. Young people who kill themselves not only prefer death over life, but they are telling us in powerful behavioral language that they do not even want to try out the society we have created for them. The question is *why*. What can we do to prevent these premature deaths? And how is youth suicide related to other problems, such as substance abuse, violence against others, and entrenched social problems?

Increased public attention to these questions has resulted in a recent surge in literature on the topic (for example, Berman & Jobes, 1991; Deykin & Buka, 1994; Holinger, Offer, Barter, & Bell, 1994; Leenaars & Wenckstern, 1991; Pfeffer, 1986; Recklitis, Noam, & Borst, 1992; Workman & Prior, 1997). The general criteria for assessing risk of suicide, as already discussed, are similar for adolescents and adults, except for adolescents' greater tendency toward imitation and impulsivity as seen in cluster suicides (Coleman, 1987; Velting & Gould, 1997). However, the issues are complex, and the answers are not always clear. Recognition of the individual developmental, familial, and societal factors that interact in self-destructive youth will enhance the understanding and empathic communication necessary for risk assessment and suicide prevention among young people. Providers face a challenging ethical issue involving confidentiality and parental rights when a young person divulges suicidal intentions but does not want the listener or school authority to inform his or her parents. (See Chapter Seven, "Young People," for suggestions regarding this ethical delimma.)

Teens in North America and other industrial societies today feel great pressure to avoid failure in a social milieu that is very achievement oriented, while facing employment uncertainties affected by global economic shifts and turmoil. As a distinct and increasingly prolonged phase in the life cycle, adolescence exaggerates the challenge of finding one's place in the world, while cultural messages emphasize that anything can be had in modern society if one only works hard and takes advantage of opportunities. This means, among other things, that traumatic life events, such as failing an exam or the breakup of a relationship, are perceived as disasters by at-risk teens. Furthermore the brutal reality for many is that individual efforts are not enough to overcome obstacles such as race and class divisions, which are deeply embedded in the social structure and cultural values. This is particularly true for black and Hispanic urban males in the United States, who face disproportionately high unemployment rates, and for Native youth on reservations, whose futures are even more bleak. Development of the Tribal Colleges system portends some relief for Native Americans.

Complicating teenagers' lives today are the flux and change occurring throughout many societies, particularly in traditional roles for women and men. All adolescents face normal role confusion and sexual-identity issues, but family instability and the frequency of divorce create additional stresses for children. Thousands of teens also encounter problems with alcoholism, violence, and incest. (Chapter Eight discusses in greater detail the relationship between victimization and self-destructiveness. See also Figure 2.2 in Chapter Two.) Many suicidal runaway teens are victims of these family problems. Considered together, these factors make a teenager's hopelessness and disillusionment with planning a career and entering adult life understandable.

This is not to suggest that living in an era of global change and unrest causes teen suicide. Rather, an attitude of cultural pessimism, financial uncertainties, and a widening gap between rich and poor combine with individual stressors, family, and other social factors to create a climate from which many teens today will want to escape (see Chapters One and Two on crisis origins). These issues are elaborated further in Chapters Eight, Nine, and Thirteen.

Distinct Ethnic and Sexual Orientation Groups

The tragedy of suicide among ethnic minority and Native groups in U.S. society is often hidden behind the predominant presence of the white majority. Similarly, research about suicide among gay, lesbian, bisexual, and transgendered people has been neglected in favor of the heterosexual majority. Social and cultural factors have been cited as the origin of many crises, especially among those disadvantaged by the economic, political, and related factors stemming from personal and institutionalized racism and homophobia (Berlin, 1987; Hendin, 1987; Nisbet, 1996; Remafedi, 1994; Remafedi et al., 1991; Rofes, 1983; also see Chapter Thirteen). Understanding and assessing individual pain and suicide risk in these instances is incomplete without attention to the cultural context of this pain. It is incongruous to speak of the right of disadvantaged people to commit suicide when the basic rights of life are not enjoyed on an equal basis. Our common humanity demands a renewed effort to combine understanding of individuals in crisis with keen sensitivity to the social and political origins and ramifications of these crises (see Figure 6.1, the right circle in Boxes 1 and 3).

People in Hospitals and Other Institutions

Finally, a number of people are in institutions because they are suicidal or for other reasons: illness, infirmity, crime, or behavioral problems. Admission to an institution is often a crisis in itself. Not infrequently, the culture shock experienced in this process is so extreme that suicide seems the only way out. Osgood's (1992) research supports the relationship between adverse environmental factors (for example, frequent staff turnover) and suicidal behavior and death in long-term care facilities, as in the case example of Barbara. Such factors also contribute to the greater frequency of suicide in temporary holding centers than in prisons. Often a person already suicidal feels so disempowered by the experience of institutionalization that suicide is the single action that says, "I am in charge of my life (and death)."

Preventing suicide, self-injury, and indirect self-destruction in institutions demands that

- We do not use hospitals as a "catchall" to prevent suicide.
- We abandon the notion that when a patient is under a physician's care, responsibility for intelligent assessment and intervention by others ceases.
- We recognize that the general principles of suicidology and risk assessment apply equally to institutionalized and other people. If physical and social isolation and powerlessness increase suicidal risk, people in hospitals and other institutions who are isolated and powerless are at increased suicide risk (Farberow, 1981; Haycock, 1993).

Despite decades of knowledge about therapeutic milieu, public placards declaring patients' rights, and experience with the fact that authoritarian attitudes and power tactics in institutional settings are always counterproductive, it is shocking to read and hear about abusive approaches to distressed people in institutions, some of which result in violent retaliation against staff (see Chapter Nine).

This discussion of special population groups and the previous case examples is continued in the next chapter.

Two final points about the assessment of suicide risk must be noted.

1. *Suicide risk assessment is an ongoing process.* A person at risk should be reassessed continually. If important social and attitudinal changes occur as a result of a suicide attempt, the person who is suicidal today may not be suicidal tomorrow or ever again. The opposite is also true: a crucial life event or other circumstance can drastically affect a person's view of life and death. Someone who has never been suicidal may become so.

2. *Suicide risk assessment is an integral aspect of the crisis assessment process.* No assessment of a person who is upset or in crisis can be considered complete if evaluation of suicide risk is not included. See Chapter Three for interview examples of how to incorporate these suicide risk assessment principles and techniques into routine crisis and mental health practice in emergency settings and elsewhere.

Summary

Suicide and self-destructive behavior are extreme ways in which some people respond to crisis. The pain and turmoil felt by a self-destructive person can be compared with the confusion and mixed feelings of those trying to help. People destroy themselves for complex reasons. Understanding what a self-destructive person is trying to communicate is basic to helping that person find alternatives to suicide. Assessment of suicide risk is a difficult task, but it is made possible by recognition of signs that portend the likelihood of suicide for particular individuals. Assessment of suicide risk is an important basis for appropriate response to self-destructive people.

References

Alvarez, A. (1971). *The savage god.* London: Weidenfield and Nicolson.

Atkinson, J. M. (1978). *Discovering suicide: Studies in the social organization of death.* Pittsburgh: University of Pittsburgh Press.

Badger, T. A., McNiece, C., & Gagan, M. J. (2000). Depression, service need, and use in vulnerable populations. *Archives of Psychiatric Nursing, 14*(4), 173–182.

Baechler, J. (1979). *Suicide.* New York: Basic Books.

Battin, M. P. (1980). Manipulated suicide. In M. P. Battin and D. J. Mayo (Eds.), *Suicide: The philosophical issues* (pp. 169–182). New York: St. Martin's Press.

Battin, M. P., & Mayo, D. J. (Eds.). (1980). *Suicide: The philosophical issues.* New York: St. Martin's Press.

Beck, A. T., Steer, R. A., Beck, J. S., & Newman, C. F. (1993). Hopelessness, depression, suicidal ideation, and clinical diagnosis of depression. *Suicide & Life-Threatening Behavior, 23*(2), 120–129.

Becker, H. (1963). *Outsiders: Studies in the sociology of deviance.* New York: Free Press.

Berlin, I. N. (1987). Suicide among American Indian adolescents: An overview. *Suicide & Life-Threatening Behavior, 17*(3), 218–232.

Berman, A. L., & Jobes, D. A. (1991). *Adolescent suicide: Assessment and intervention.* Washington, DC: American Psychological Association.

Bernardi, P. J. (1995, May 6). The hidden engines of the suicide rights movement. *America,* 14–17.

Bongar, B., Berman, A. L., Maris, R. W., Silverman, M. M., Harris, E. A., & Packman, W. L. (1998). *Risk management of suicidal patients.* New York: Guilford Press.

Breed, W. (1972). Five components of a basic suicide syndrome. *Suicide & Life-Threatening Behavior, 2,* 3–18.

Brent, D. A., Perper, J. A., Moritz, G., Baugher, M., Roth, C., Balach, L., & Schweers, J. (1993). Stressful life events, psychopathology, and adolescent suicide: A case control study. *Suicide & Life-Threatening Behavior, 23*(3), 179–187.

Brown, G. W., & Harris, T. (1978). *The social origins of depression.* London: Tavistock.

Brown, T. R., & Sheran, T. J. (1972). Suicide prediction: A review. *Suicide & Life-Threatening Behavior, 2,* 67–97.

Burstow, B. (1992) *Radical feminist therapy: Working in the context of violence.* Thousand Oaks, CA: Sage.

Canetto, S. (1992). Gender and suicide in the elderly. *Suicide & Life-Threatening Behavior, 22*(1), 80–97.

Coleman, L. (1987). *Cluster suicides.* London: Faber & Faber.

Counts, D. A. (1987). Female suicide and wife abuse: A cross-cultural perspective. *Suicide & Life-Threatening Behavior, 17*(3), 194–204.

Deykin, E. Y., & Buka, S. L. (1994). Suicidal ideation and attempts among chemically dependent adolescents. *American Journal of Public Health, 84*(4), 634–639.

Durkheim, E. (1951). *Suicide* (2nd ed.). New York: Free Press. (Original work published 1897)

Egmond, M. V., Garnefski, N., Jonker, D., & Kerkhof, A.J.F.M. (1993). The relationship between sexual abuse and female suicidal behavior. *Crisis, 14*(3), 129–139.

Ehrenreich, B., & Ehrenreich, J. (1978). Medicine and social control. In J. Ehrenreich (Ed.), *The cultural crisis of modern medicine* (pp. 39–79). New York: Monthly Review Press.

Emanuel, E. J., & Battin, M. P. (1998). What are the potential cost savings from legalizing physician-assisted suicide? *New England Journal of Medicine, 339*(3), 167–172.

Everett, B., & Gallop, R. (2000). *The link between childhood trauma and mental illness: Effective interventions for mental health professionals.* Thousand Oaks, CA: Sage.

Farberow, N. L. (Ed.). (1975). *Suicide in different cultures.* Baltimore, MD: University Park Press.

Farberow, N. L. (Ed.). (1980). *The many faces of death.* New York: McGraw-Hill.

Farberow, N. L. (1981). Suicide prevention in the hospital. *Hospital and Community Psychiatry, 32*(2), 99–104.

Farberow, N. L., & Shneidman, E. S. (Eds.). (1961). *The cry for help.* New York: McGraw-Hill.

Fawcett, J. (2000). The complexity of suicide. Grand rounds: Suicide: Clinical/risk management issues for psychiatrists. *CNS Spectrums Academic Supplement: The International Journal of Neuropsychiatric Medicine, 5*(2, Suppl. 1), 38–41.

Fuller, J. (1997). Physician-assisted suicide: An unnecessary crisis. *America, 177*(2), 9–12.

Furst, J., & Huffine, C. L. (1991). Assessing vulnerability to suicide. *Suicide & Life-Threatening Behavior, 21*(4), 329–344.

Goldman, S., & Beardslee, W. R. (1999). Suicide in children and adolescents. In D. G. Jacobs (Ed.), *The Harvard Medical School guide to suicide assessment and intervention* (pp. 417–442). San Francisco: Jossey-Bass.

Hatton, C., Valente, S., & Rink, A. (1984). *Suicide: Assessment and intervention* (2nd ed.). Englewood Cliffs, NJ: Appleton-Century-Crofts.

Haycock, J. (1993). Double jeopardy: Suicide rates in forensic hospitals. *Suicide & Life-Threatening Behavior, 23*(2), 130–138.

Hendin, H. (1982). *Suicide in America.* New York: Norton.

Hendin, H. (1987). Youth suicide: A psychosocial perspective. *Suicide & Life-Threatening Behavior, 17*(2), 151–165.

Hoff, L. A. (1985). [Review of the book *Suicidal women: Their thinking and feeling patterns.* By C. Neuringer & D. Lettieri (1982). New York: Gardner Press.] *Suicide & Life-Threatening Behavior, 15*(1), 69–73.

Hoff, L. A. (2000). Crisis care. In B. Everett & R. Gallop, *The link between childhood trauma and mental illness: Effective interventions for mental health professionals* (pp. 227–251). Thousand Oaks, CA: Sage.

Hoff, L. A., & Resing, M. (1982). Was this suicide preventable? *American Journal of Nursing, 82*(7), 1106–1111. (Also reprinted in B. A. Backer, P. M. Dubbert, & E.J.P. Eisenman (Eds.). (1985). *Psychiatric/mental health nursing: Contemporary readings* (pp. 169–180). Belmont, CA: Wadsworth.)

Holinger, P. C., Offer, D., Barter, J. T., & Bell, C. C. (1994). *Suicide and homicide among adolescents.* New York: Guilford Press.

Humphrey, D. (1992). Rational suicide among the elderly. *Suicide & Life-Threatening Behavior, 22*(1), 125–129.

Jacobs, D. G. (2000). The complexity of suicide. Grand rounds: Suicide: Clinical/risk management issues for psychiatrists. *CNS Spectrums Academic Supplement: The International Journal of Neuropsychiatric Medicine, 5*(2, Suppl. 1), 32–33.

Jourard, S. M. (1970). Suicide: An invitation to die. *American Journal of Nursing, 70*(2), 269, 273–275.

Kerkhof, A.J.F.M., & Clark, D. C. (1993). Stability of suicide rates in Europe. *Crisis, 14*(2), 50–51.

Leenaars, A. A., & Wenckstern, S. (1991). *Suicide prevention in schools.* Bristol, PA: Hemisphere.

Levine, S., & Kozloff, M. A. (1978). The sick role: Assessment and overview. *Annual Review of Sociology, 4,* 317–343.

Litman, R. E. (1987). Mental disorders and suicidal intention. *Suicide & Life-Threatening Behavior, 17*(2), 85–92.

Maris, R. W. (1981). *Pathways to suicide.* Baltimore, MD: Johns Hopkins University Press.

Maris, R. (1991). Assessment and prediction of suicide: Introduction [Special issue]. *Suicide & Life-Threatening Behavior, 21*(1), 1–17.

Maris, R. W. (Ed.). (with Berman, A. L., Maltsberger, J. T., & Yufit, R. I.) (1992). *Assessment and prediction of suicide.* New York: Guilford Press.

McGinnis, J. M. (1987). Suicide in America—moving up the public health agenda. *Suicide & Life-Threatening Behavior, 17*(1), 18–32.

Menninger, K. (1938). *Man against himself.* Orlando, FL: Harcourt Brace.

Moore, S. L. (1997). A phenomenological study of meaning in life in suicidal older adults. *Archives of Psychiatric Nursing, 11*(1), 29–36.

Morrell, S., Taylor, R., Quine, S., & Kerr, C. (1993). Suicide and unemployment in Australia. *Social Science & Medicine, 36*(6), 749–756.

Moscicki, E. (1999). Epidemiology of suicide. In D. G. Jacobs (Ed.), *The Harvard Medical School guide to suicide assessment and intervention* (pp. 40–51). San Francisco: Jossey-Bass.

Motto, J. A. (1980). Suicide risk factors in alcohol abuse. *Suicide & Life-Threatening Behavior, 10,* 230–238.

Motto, J. A. (1985). Preliminary field testing of a risk estimation for suicide. *Suicide & Life-Threatening Behavior, 15*(3), 139–150.

Motto, J. A. (1991). An integrated approach to estimating suicide risk. *Suicide & Life-Threatening Behavior, 21*(1), 74–89.

Motto, J. A. (1999). Critical points in the assessment and management of suicide risk. In D. G. Jacobs (Ed.), *The Harvard Medical School guide to suicide assessment and intervention* (pp. 224–238). San Francisco: Jossey-Bass.

National Center for Health Statistics. (1995). *Report of final mortality statistics.* Hyattsville, MD: Author.

Nisbet, P. A. (1996). Protective factors for suicidal black females. *Suicide & Life-Threatening Behavior, 26*(4), 325–341.

O'Carroll, P. (1993). Suicide causation: Pies, paths, and pointless polemics. *Suicide & Life-Threatening Behavior, 23*(1), 27–36.

Osgood, N. (1992). Environmental factors in suicide in long-term care facilities. *Suicide & Life-Threatening Behavior, 22*(1), 98–106.

Parent, R. B. (1998). Suicide by cop: Victim-precipitated homicide. *Police Chief, 65*(10), 111–114.

Parsons, T. (1951). Social structure and the dynamic process: The case of modern medical practice. In *The social system* (pp. 428–479). New York: Free Press.

Perrah, M., & Wichman, H. (1987). Cognitive rigidity in suicide attempters. *Suicide & Life-Threatening Behavior, 17*(3), 251–255.

Pfeffer, C. R. (1986). *The suicidal child.* New York: Guilford Press.

Philp, M. (1993, September 20). Roots of solvent abuse run deep. *Globe and Mail,* pp. 1, 4.

Recklitis, C. J., Noam, G. G., & Borst, S. R. (1992). Adolescent suicide and defensive style. *Suicide & Life-Threatening Behavior, 22*(3), 374–387.

Remafedi, G. (Ed.). (1994). *Death by denial: Studies of gay and lesbian teenagers.* Boston: Alyson.

Remafedi, G., Farrow, J. A., & Deisher, R. W. (1991). Risk factors for attempted suicide in gay and bisexual youth. *Pediatrics, 87*(6), 869–875.

Remafedi, G., French, S., Story, M., Resnick, M. D., & Blum, R. (1998). The relationship between suicide risk and sexual orientation: Results of a population-based study. *American Journal of Public Health, 88*(1), 57–60.

Rich, C. L., Fowler, R. C., Young, D., and Blenkush, M. (1986). San Diego suicide study: Comparison of gay to straight males. *Suicide & Life-Threatening Behavior, 16*(40), 448–457.

Richman, J. (1992). A rational approach to rational suicide. *Suicide & Life-Threatening Behavior, 22*(1), 130–141.

Rodin, G. M. (2000). Psychiatric care for the chronically ill & dying patient. In H. H. Goldman (Ed.), *Review of general psychiatry* (pp. 505–512). New York: Lange Medical Books/McGraw-Hill.

Rofes, E. E. (1983). *"I thought people like that killed themselves": Lesbians, gay men and suicide.* San Francisco: Grey Fox Press.

Shneidman, E. S. (1973). Suicide. *Encyclopaedia Britannica.* (Reprinted in *Suicide & Life-Threatening Behavior, 11,* 198–220.)

Shneidman, E. S. (1976). *Suicidology: Contemporary developments.* Philadelphia: Grune & Stratton.

Shneidman, E. S. (1981). Suicide. *Suicide & Life-Threatening Behavior, 11,* pp. 198–220.

Shneidman, E. S. (1985). *Definition of suicide.* New York: Wiley.

Shneidman, E. S. (1987). At the point of no return. *Psychology Today, 21*(3), 54–58.

Shneidman, E. S. (1993). Some controversies in suicidology: Toward a mentalistic discipline. *Suicide & Life-Threatening Behavior, 23*(4), 292–298.

Shneidman, E. S. (1999). Perturbation and lethality: A psychological approach to assessment and intervention. In D. G. Jacobs (Ed.), *The Harvard Medical School guide to suicide assessment and intervention* (pp. 83–97). San Francisco: Jossey-Bass.

Shneidman, E. S., & Farberow, N. L. (Eds.). (1957). *Clues to suicide.* New York: McGraw-Hill.

Smith, J. D., Mercy, J. A., & Conn, J. M. (1988). Marital status and the risk of suicide. *American Journal of Public Health, 78*(1), 78–80.

Smith, K., & Maris, R. W. (1986). Suggested recommendations for the study of suicide and other life-threatening behaviors. *Suicide & Life-Threatening Behavior, 16*(1), 67–69.

Solomon, D. A., Keitner, G. I., Miller, I. W., Shea, M. T., & Keller, M. B. (1995). Course of illness and maintenance treatments for patients with bipolar disorder. *Journal of Clinical Psychiatry, 56*(1), 5–13.

Stephens, B. J. (1985). Suicidal women and their relationships with husbands, boyfriends, and lovers. *Suicide & Life-Threatening Behavior, 15*(2), 77–90.

Stephens, B. J. (1987). Cheap thrills and humble pie: The adolescence of female suicide attempters. *Suicide & Life-Threatening Behavior, 17*(2), 107–118.

U.S. Public Health Service. (1999). *Surgeon general's call to action to prevent suicide.* Washington, DC: Author.

United Nations. (1996). *Prevention of suicide: Guidelines for the formulation and implementation of national strategies.* New York: Author.

Velting, D. M., & Gould, M. S. (1997). Suicide contagion. In R. W. Maris, S. S. Canetto, J. L. McIntosh, & M. M. Silverman (Eds.), *Review of suicidology* (pp. 96–137). New York: Guilford Press.

Workman, C. G., & Prior, M. (1997). Depression and suicide in young children. *Issues in Comprehensive Pediatric Nursing, 20,* 125–132.

Zola, I. K. (1978). Medicine as an institution of social control. In J. Ehrenreich (Ed.), *The cultural crisis of modern medicine* (pp. 80–100). New York: Monthly Review Press.

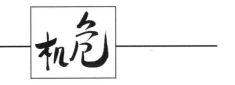

CHAPTER SEVEN

HELPING SELF-DESTRUCTIVE PEOPLE AND SURVIVORS OF SUICIDE

Several agencies or helpers are usually needed to provide distinct facets of service for suicidal people. All, however, should be aware of what constitutes comprehensive care for this at-risk population and establish linkages that actually work for clients.

Comprehensive Service for Self-Destructive People

Everyone who threatens or attempts suicide should have access to all the services the crisis calls for. Three kinds of service should be available for suicidal and self-destructive people:

1. Emergency medical treatment
2. Crisis intervention
3. Follow-up counseling or therapy

Emergency Medical Treatment

Emergency medical treatment is the obvious response to anyone who has already made a suicide attempt. Unfortunately, this is still all that is received by some people who attempt suicide. Everyone—friend, neighbor, family member, passerby—is obligated by simple humanity to help a suicidal person obtain medical treatment. First aid can be performed by police, volunteers in fire departments, rescue squads, or anyone familiar with first-aid procedures.

Any time a person is in immediate danger of death, the police should be called because police and rescue squads have the greatest possibility of ensuring rapid transportation to a hospital. If there is any question about the medical seriousness of the suicide attempt, a physician should be called. The best way to obtain a medical opinion in such cases is to call a local hospital emergency service. In large communities, a physician is always there; in small ones, a physician is on call.

Most communities also have poison control centers, usually attached to a hospital, which should be called when the lethality level of the drug is not certain. The amount of a drug necessary to cause death depends on the kind of drug, the size of the person, and the person's tolerance for the drug in cases of addiction. Sleeping pills are the most dangerous.

In general, *a lethal dose is ten times the normal dose.* In combination with alcohol, only half that amount can cause death. Aspirin is also much more dangerous than is commonly believed. One hundred five-grain tablets can cause death; less is needed if other drugs are also taken. Tylenol (acetaminophen), an aspirin substitute, is even more dangerous, as it cannot be removed from body tissue by dialysis. Tranquilizers are less dangerous; antidepressant drugs, however, can be used as a suicide weapon.

Some suicidal people have gone through hospital emergency rooms, intensive care and surgical units, and on to discharge with no explicit attention paid to the primary problem that triggered the suicide attempt. The urgency of medical treatment for a suicidal person can be so engrossing that other aspects of crisis intervention may be overlooked. For example, if a person is in a coma from an overdose or is being treated for injuries from a car crash, a careful suicide risk assessment may be forgotten after the person is out of physical danger. Great care should be taken to ensure that this does not happen.

If a person whose suicide attempt is medically serious does not receive follow-up counseling, the risk of suicide within a few months is very high. Medical treatment, of course, is of primary importance when there is danger of death. Still we should remember that the person's physical injuries are a result of the suicide attempt; treating those injuries is only a first step. The attitude of hospital emergency department staff can be the forerunner of more serious suicide attempts or the foundation for crisis intervention and acceptance of a referral for follow-up counseling. Emergency and primary care providers should also consider carefully the appropriate use of drugs for suicidal people in crisis, as discussed in Chapter Four, because prescribed drugs are one of the weapons used most frequently for suicide.

Crisis Intervention

People who threaten or attempt suicide as a way of coping with a crisis usually lack more constructive ways of handling stress. The crisis intervention principles presented in Chapters Four and Five should be used on behalf of self-destructive persons. Several additional techniques are important for a person in suicidal crisis:

1. *Relieve isolation.* If the suicidal person is living alone, physical isolation must be relieved. If there is no friend or supportive relative with whom the person can stay temporarily and if the person is highly suicidal, that individual should probably be hospitalized until the active crisis is over.

2. *Remove lethal weapons.* Lethal weapons and pills should be removed either by the counselor, a relative, or a friend, keeping in mind the active collaboration of the suicidal person in this process. If caring and concern are expressed and the person's sense of self-mastery and control is respected, he or she will usually surrender a weapon voluntarily, so it is safe from easy or impulsive access during the acute crisis. While avoiding power tactics or engaging in the heated debate regarding gun control, all human service providers should calmly inform an acutely distressed person and the family of this sobering fact: suicide risk increases fivefold and homicide risk increases threefold when there is a gun in the home (Boyd & Moscicki, 1986; Kaplan, 1998).

3. *Encourage alternate expression of anger.* If the person is planning suicide as a way of expressing anger at someone, we should actively explore with the individual other ways of expressing anger short of paying with his or her life. For example, "I can see that you're very angry with her for leaving you. Can you think of a way to express your anger that would not cost you your life?" or "Yes, of course she'll probably feel bad if you kill yourself after the divorce. But she most likely would talk with someone about it and go on with her life. Meanwhile you've had your revenge, but you can't get your life back." If anger at the crisis worker or therapist is connected to the suicide threat, a similar empathic but not indifferent response is called for: "Of course I'd feel bad, but not guilty. So I'd like to continue working with you around the pain you have even though you're disappointed right now with our progress."

4. *Avoid a final decision about suicide during crisis.* We should assure the suicidal person that the suicidal crisis—that is, seeing suicide as the only option—is a temporary state. We should also try to persuade the person to avoid a decision about suicide until all other alternatives have been considered during a noncrisis state of mind, just as other serious decisions should be postponed until the crisis is over.

A cautionary note about contracts is in order here. The *no-suicide contract* is a technique employed by some therapists, crisis workers, and primary care providers in which the client promises not to harm himself or herself between sessions and to contact the therapist if contemplating such harm. Such contracts offer neither special protection against suicide nor legal protection for the therapist (Clark & Kerkhof, 1993). No-suicide contracts may also convey a false sense of security to an anxious provider. This is because any value the contract may have flows from the *quality of the therapeutic relationship*—ideally, one in which the therapist conveys caring and concern about the client. In no way should a contract serve as a convenient substitute for the time spent in empathetic listening and in planning alternatives to self-destruction with a suicidal person. If contracts are used, they should be situated in the context of the overall service plan as discussed here and in Chapter Four, including such specifics as relieving isolation, finding substitutes for losses, and developing concrete plans and actions to control impulsive behavior—for example, calling a crisis hotline or asking a friend to join in a favorite recreation activity.

5. *Reestablish social ties.* We should make every effort to help the suicidal person reestablish broken social bonds. This can be done through family crisis counseling sessions or by finding satisfying substitutes for lost relationships. Active links to self-help groups such as Widow to Widow or Parents Without Partners clubs can be lifesaving (see Chapter Five).

6. *Relieve extreme anxiety and sleep loss.* If a suicidal person is extremely anxious and also has been unable to sleep for several days, he or she may become even more suicidal. To a suicidal person, the world looks bleaker and death seems more desirable at 4:00 A.M. after endless nights of sleeplessness. A good night's sleep can temporarily reduce suicide risk and put the person in a better frame of mind to consider other ways of solving life's problems.

In such cases, it is appropriate to consider medication on an emergency basis (Bongar, Maris, Berman, & Litman, 1992). This should never be done for a highly suicidal person, however, without daily crisis counseling sessions. Without effective counseling, the extremely suicidal person may interpret such an approach as an invitation to commit suicide. An antianxiety agent will usually alleviate the anxiety and thus improve sleep, as anxiety is the major cause of sleeplessness. Antidepressants, in contrast, are more dangerous as a potential suicide weapon. If medication is needed, the person should be given a *one- to three-day supply at most*—always with a return appointment scheduled for crisis counseling.

Sometimes nonmedical crisis counselors need to seek medical consultation and emergency medicine for a suicidal person. In such cases, the counselor must clearly advise the consulting physician of the person's suicidal state and of the recommended limited dose of drugs. This is particularly important when dealing with physicians who lack training in suicide prevention or who seem hurried and disinterested. Some practitioners accustomed to using medication in treatment programs may recommend psychotropic medication during crisis; however, these drugs are indicated only if a person is too upset to be engaged in the process of problem solving (see Chapter Four). Nonchemical means of inducing sleep should be encouraged. This assumes a thorough assessment and an effort to apply various psychosocial strategies before prescribing drugs. Crisis workers should never forget that many suicide deaths in North America are caused by *prescribed* drugs.

Crisis assessment is never more important than when working with a self-destructive person. It determines our immediate and long-range response to the individual. A person who is threatening or has attempted suicide is either in active crisis or is already beyond the crisis and is at a loss to resolve it any other way.

Not everyone who engages in self-destructive acts is in a life-and-death emergency. Anyone distressed enough to be self-destructive to any degree should be listened to and helped; however, if the suicide attempt is medically nonserious, the counselor's response should not convey a sense of life-and-death urgency. This does not mean that the person's action is dismissed as nonserious. Rather, the underlying message of the behavior—its psychosocial dynamics—should receive the greatest part of our attention. To do otherwise may inadvertently lead to further suicide attempts. A helper reinforces self-destructive behavior by a dramatic and misplaced medical response while ignoring the problems signaled by the self-destructive act. For example, while suturing a slashed wrist, the physician and nurse should regard the physical injury neutrally, with a certain sense of detachment, and focus—in an empathic tone—on the *meaning* of self-injury: "You must have been pretty upset to do this to yourself. What did you hope would happen when you cut your wrists?"

Persons at all levels of suicide risk warrant a response. The helper must differentiate between the types of response. Emergency measures are used when there is immediate danger of death from a medically serious failed suicide attempt. If the risk of death is long-range, the therapeutic approach should be long-range as well. If the attempt is medically nonserious, we should avoid using only medical treatment or a life-and-death approach. People in these risk situations need professional help to resolve crises constructively rather than by self-destructive acts.

Follow-Up Service for Suicidal People

Beyond crisis counseling, all self-destructive persons should have the opportunity to receive counseling or psychotherapy as an aid in solving the problems that led them to self-destructive behavior (Bongar et al., 1992). People who respond to life crises with self-destructive behavior often have a long-standing pattern of inadequate psychological and social coping (McLeavey, Daly, Murray, O'Riordan, & Taylor, 1987). Individual or group psychotherapy, therefore, is frequently indicated. Drug treatment for clinical depression may also be indicated.

Counseling and Psychotherapy. Psychotherapy is the proper work of specially trained people, usually clinical psychologists, psychiatric nurses, psychiatrists, and psychiatric social workers. Others qualified to do counseling may be clergy and mental health counselors. The main concern is that the counselor or psychotherapist is properly trained and supervised (Hoff & Adamowski, 1998).

Counseling should focus on resolving situational problems and expressing feelings appropriately. The person is helped to change various behaviors that are causing discomfort and that he or she usually is conscious of. Psychotherapy involves uncovering feelings that have been denied expression for a long time. It may also involve changing aspects of one's personality and deep-rooted patterns of behavior, such as an inability to communicate feelings or inflexible approaches to problem solving. People usually engage in psychotherapy because they are troubled or unhappy about certain features of their personality or behavior.

In general, counseling or psychotherapy should be made available to the suicidal person. It is particularly recommended for crisis-prone people who approach everyday problems with drug and alcohol abuse and other self-destructive behaviors. Such people have difficulty expressing feelings verbally, and self-destructive acts become an easier way to communicate. People who are extremely dependent or who have rigid expectations for themselves combined with inflexible behavior patterns are also good candidates for psychotherapy. A severely depressed, suicidal person should always have follow-up counseling or psychotherapy. When hospitalization also is indicated for seriously suicidal persons, health practitioners should observe carefully the standards of care for hospitalized people who are at risk of harming themselves (see Bongar, Maris, Berman, Litman, & Silverman, 1993).

Counseling and psychotherapy can take place on an individual or group basis, in outpatient and inpatient settings. A group experience is valuable for nearly everyone, but it is particularly recommended for the suicidal person who has underlying problems interacting socially and communicating feelings. For adolescents who have made suicide attempts, family therapy should frequently follow family crisis counseling (Richman, 1986). Marital counseling should be offered whenever a disturbed marriage has contributed to the person's suicidal crisis. These therapies can be used in various combinations, depending on the needs of the individual and family.

Whether conducted in a group or individually, counseling and psychotherapy goals should be directed toward

- Correcting psychological and social disturbances in the person's life
- Improving the person's self-image
- Finding satisfactory social resources
- Developing approaches to problems other than self-destructive behavior
- Discovering a satisfying life plan

Crisis counselors should keep in mind that a satisfying and constructive resolution of a crisis is an excellent foundation for persuading people to seek follow-up counseling or psychotherapy for the problems that made them crisis prone in the first place. However, if people in crisis are placed on waiting lists, they will find other ways to resolve their crises. If such people are suicidal, the chances of a tragic outcome are greatly increased. This is because, with or without our help, the pain of the crisis state compels one to move toward resolution—positive or negative. If waiting lists prevent people from getting help at the time they need it and later appointments are not kept, we should examine the adequacy of our service arrangements rather than conclude that the client was not motivated for therapy (Hoff & Adamowsi, 1998).

Drug Treatment for Depression. Because of the regular introduction of newly approved drugs, health providers authorized to prescribe must keep current on this topic through other sources (for example, Garcia & Ghani, 2000). Here the focus is limited to the intersection of prescription drugs with suicidal danger, especially for those without specialty training in psychopharmacology.

Antidepressants are not emergency drugs. However, these drugs may be used successfully for some suicidal persons who experience severe, recurring depression. Classic drugs for treating depression include selective serotonin reuptake inhibitors, tricyclic antidepressants, and monoamine-oxidase inhibitors. Successful response to antidepressant therapy is highly variable, and debate about the use of psychotropic drugs as a new "magic bullet" continues (Johnson, 1990, pp. 38–52). This may be due in part to the unclear demarcation between reactive depression and major depressive episodes, formerly called endogenous depression. Thus, although some people respond favorably to antidepressant treatment, research and controversy continue regarding dosage and the efficacy of such treatment in preventing suicide (Salzman, 1999, p. 373). In addition, there is no compelling evidence that antidepressant treatment, even with safer psychotropic agents, has reduced suicidal risk (Baldessarini, 2000, p. 34), whereas the risk of overdosing on antidepressants is well established (Baldessarini & Tondo, 1999, p. 356.) The success of antidepressant agents in persons with bipolar illness is significantly related to the timing of suicidal behavior, which occurs most often during the early course of illness (Baldessarini, 2000, p. 35); success is also increased when drug treatment is combined with psychotherapeutic approaches (Solomon, Keitner, Miller, Shea, & Keller, 1995). For persons with major affective disorder, especially bipolar illness, lithium is preferred for its protective effect against suicidal behaviors (Baldessarini & Tondo, p. 357).

Antidepressants should be used sparingly or not at all for a person who is going through normal grief and mourning (Worden, 1991, p. 54). They also should not be used when the person is suffering from a reactive depression; grief work and crisis counseling are indicated instead, except when the person does not respond to interpersonal interventions (Worden, p. 31). A reactive depression occurs when a person in crisis because of a loss does not express normal feelings of sadness and anger *during* the crisis and later reacts with depression (sometimes called a delayed grief reaction). Psychotherapy is indicated for such persons.

Classic symptoms, lasting at least two weeks, of a major depressive episode include weight loss, early morning wakening, loss of appetite, slowed-down body functions, sexual and menstrual abnormality, crying spells, anhedonia (lack of pleasure in life), and extreme feelings of worthlessness. The symptoms usually cannot be related to a conscious loss, specific life event, or situation. The assumption, therefore, is that the depression arises from sources within the person— that is, is biologically based; whereas in reactive depression one is aware of the loss or depressing situation (see "Loss, Change, and Grief Work" in Chapter Four). Even among people who are genetically predisposed to depression, social factors usually play a significant role in alleviating symptoms (Brown & Harris, 1978; Cloward & Piven, 1979). For example, depression in the women studied by Brown and Harris was significantly associated with their economic circumstances and large numbers of children: less money and more children meant greater depression.

Antidepressant drugs are dangerous and should be prescribed with extreme caution for suicidal persons (Bongar et al., 1992). When taken with alcohol, an overdose of drugs can easily cause death. People using these drugs can experience side effects, such as feelings of confusion, restlessness, or loss of control. Persons with symptoms of borderline personality disorder can have an increase in self-destructive behaviors while treated with antidepressants (Salzman, 1999, p. 379).

Another problem with antidepressant drugs is that they take so long to work. Ten to fourteen days elapse before depression lifts noticeably, even though the person sleeps better as a result of the sedative side effect. This delayed action should be explained carefully, because most people expect to feel better immediately after taking a drug. And during the pretherapeutic phase, a suicide could occur as a result of confusion and agitation, which are additional drug side effects.

Another danger of suicide occurs after the depression lifts during drug treatment. This is especially true for the person who is so depressed and physically slowed down that he or she did not previously have the energy to carry out a suicide plan. Because of all these factors, it is preferable to use antidepressant drugs in combination with psychotherapy or psychiatric hospitalization for a depressed person who is highly suicidal, especially if the individual is also socially and physically isolated.

Crisis counselors should always remember that antidepressants are not emergency drugs. These drugs should usually not be prescribed for a highly suicidal person during the acute crisis state unless the individual is hospitalized. The crisis counselor should routinely ask what drugs the person in crisis is taking or possesses. The prescription of *any* drug as a substitute for effective counseling is irresponsible. Not only can some of these drugs increase agitation and sometimes provoke suicidal ideation and subsequent litigation (Breggin & Breggin, 1994; Bongar et al., 1992), but the unwarranted prescription of drugs can also lead to serious drug-related problems (Duncan, Miller, & Sparks, 2000). Although conscientious therapists recognize this principle, today in the United States their best clinical judgment may be overruled by managed care policies. The results (for example, effects on developing brains) remain to be seen, especially for the young children now being treated with antidepressant and other drugs never evaluated for use with children (Zito et al., 2000). Waters (2000, pp. 42–43) describes this as a national uncontrolled experiment that portends the cruel and unnecessary outcomes similar to other mass experiments (for example, thalidomide for pregnant women) in which the gold standard of medical research, the controlled trial, was ignored.

CASE EXAMPLE: JACK

Jack, age sixty-nine, a widower living alone, had seen his physician for bowel problems. He was also quite depressed. Even after complete examination and extensive tests, he was obsessed with the idea of cancer and was afraid that he would die. Jack also had high blood pressure and emphysema. Months earlier, he had had prostate surgery. His family described him as a chronic complainer. Jack's doctor gave him a prescription for an antidepressant drug and referred him to a local mental health clinic for counseling. Jack admitted to the crisis counselor that he had ideas of suicide, but he had no specific plan or history of attempts. After two counseling sessions, Jack killed himself by carbon monoxide poisoning. This suicide might have been prevented if Jack had been hospitalized. He lived alone, and in the cultural milieu promoting "take pill, feel better," he probably expected to feel better immediately after taking the antidepressant even though the delayed reaction of the drug had been explained. An alternative might have been to prescribe a drug to relieve his anxiety about cancer in combination with a plan to live with relatives for a couple of weeks.

Intervention with Self-Destructive People: Case Examples

The following cases are continued from Chapter Six. They illustrate the resolution of ethical dilemmas regarding suicide, as well as planning for emergency, crisis, and follow-up services for self-destructive people at various levels of risk for suicide.

The Right-to-Die Dilemma

The right-to-die dilemma is illustrated in the case of Rachel.

CASE EXAMPLE: RACHEL

Rachel, age sixty-nine, is dying of cancer and feeling suicidal (see p. 177).

Rachel: This cancer is killing me. I have nothing to live for.

Nurse: You sound really depressed, Rachel.

Rachel: I am. I'm a burden to my daughter. I don't want to live like this anymore.

Nurse: You mean you're thinking of suicide, Rachel?

Rachel: Yes, I guess you could say that. At least I don't want to go on living like this. Yes, I want to die, and no one can stop me. I'm old and I'm sick. If there is a God, I'm sure I wouldn't be punished. How could any God expect me to go on living with this? Yes, I want to die. It's my right.

Nurse: I know you feel old and I know you're sick, and I agree, Rachel, that you have the right to determine your own life. But I'd feel bad if you acted on that now, Rachel, when you're feeling so depressed and like such a burden to your daughter. I'd really like to help you find some other way . . . (Rachel interrupts.)

Rachel: There's no other way that I can see. I've thought about it a lot. I don't know exactly what I'd do, but I'd figure something out. I just don't know how

things could change for me. After all, my daughter's got her own life.

Nurse: Rachel, I'd like to go back to something you said earlier. You seem to feel you're a burden to your daughter. Can you tell me some more about that? (The conversation continues.)

Other possible elements of a service plan for Rachel include the following:

1. Continue problem exploration on a one-to-one basis.
2. Talk with daughter (with Rachel's consent) after exploring the "burden" issue further with Rachel.
3. Have a joint session with Rachel and her daughter (see Chapter Five).
4. Arrange for evaluation of her pain control medication.
5. Continue weekly visits.
6. Explore home health respite service for daughter.

Some persons, many of whom are much older than Rachel, must spend their final years in long-term care facilities, either because their family may not be able to care for them or because they are the last of their family still alive. In such cases, compassionate care and ethical norms regarding the slippery slope of legally assisted suicide are crucial. Such a person may recognize and accept the sincerely given care of staff but may also "know" that the end is near and simply not want to eat anymore. Palliative care, not extraordinary lifesaving measures, should be the norm in these cases (Carson, Eisner, Kartes, & Kolga, 1999; see also Kaplan, Adamek, & Calderon, 1999).

Low-Risk Suicidal Behavior

The case of Sarah illustrates low-risk suicidal behavior.

CASE EXAMPLE: SARAH

Sarah, age forty-two, is troubled by her marriage (see p. 200).

Emergency medical intervention: Medical treatment for Sarah is not indicated because pills are absorbed from the stomach into the bloodstream within thirty minutes. The dose of five sleeping pills is not lethal or extremely toxic. Other

medical measures, such as dialysis, are therefore not indicated.

Crisis intervention: Crisis counseling should focus on the immediate situation related to Sarah's suicide attempt and decision making about her marriage.

Follow-up service: In follow-up counseling, Sarah can examine her extreme dependency on her marriage, her personal insecurity, her limited social life, and her dependency on drugs as a means of problem solving. Sarah might also be linked to a women's support group that focuses on career counseling and the midlife transition faced by women (see Chapter Thirteen).

Moderate-Risk Suicidal Behavior

Susan's case illustrates moderate-risk suicidal behavior.

CASE EXAMPLE: SUSAN

Susan, age nineteen, has a history of repeat suicide attempts (see p. 200).

Emergency medical intervention: Treatment for the overdose is stomach lavage (washing out the stomach contents).

Crisis intervention: Crisis counseling for Susan should include contacts with her parents and should focus on the situational problems she faces: unemployment, conflicts with her parents, and dependence on her parents.

Follow-up service: Because Susan has had a chaotic life for a number of years, she could benefit from ongoing counseling or psychotherapy, if she so chooses. This might include exploration of continuing her education and improving her employment prospects. Family therapy may be indicated if she decides to remain in her parents' household. Group therapy is strongly recommended for Susan.

High-Risk Suicidal Behavior

Edward, Barbara, and Shirley are all at high risk for suicide.

CASE EXAMPLE: EDWARD

Edward, age forty-one, is facing divorce and threatening to shoot himself (see p. 201).

Emergency medical intervention: No treatment is indicated as no suicide attempt has been made. Depending on level of engagement in crisis counseling, an antianxiety agent may be indicated for temporary stabilization, as discussed in Chapter Four.

Crisis intervention: Remove guns (and alcohol, if possible) or have wife or friend remove them *with* Edward's collaboration. Arrange to have Edward stay with a friend on the day his wife files for divorce. Try to get Edward to attend a self-help group, such as Alcoholics Anonymous, and to rely on an individual AA member for support during his crisis. Arrange frequent crisis counseling sessions for Edward, including daily telephone check-in during acute phase.

Follow-up service: Edward should have ongoing therapy, both individually and in a group, focusing on his alcohol dependency and his rigid expectations of himself; therapy should help Edward find other satisfying relationships after the loss of his wife by divorce.

CASE EXAMPLE: BARBARA

Barbara, age seventy-seven, is in a nursing home and is refusing to eat (see p. 202).

Emergency medical and crisis intervention: Barbara should be assigned to a nurse or other staff person she trusts, who can persuade her noncoercively to take her medication and to eat. Her daughter and son-in-law should be called and urged to visit immediately, so Barbara has some evidence that someone cares whether she lives or dies. A stable staffing arrangement should be instituted; further moving of Barbara to different wings of the nursing facility should be avoided. A trusting, caring relationship can thereby be established with at least one or two staff members, which is necessary for understanding what makes Barbara upset and suspicious.

Follow-up service: Organize problem-solving and service-planning meetings with Barbara, her daughter and son-in-law, the chaplain, and the nursing staff who have worked with Barbara most closely—her social network (see Chapter Five). Examine the rotation practices and support system for staff, which gives temporary "relief" from troublesome residents like Barbara. Frequent rotations exacerbate the underlying insecurity of an older person who has decreased ability to adjust to environmental changes and disruptions in staff-resident relationships.

CASE EXAMPLE: SHIRLEY

Shirley, age fifty-five, is acutely suicidal and psychotic in a psychiatric setting (see p. 202).

Emergency medical and crisis intervention: Institute routine precautions with regard to sharp objects, belts, and so on (see Bongar et al., 1993). Assign a staff member for one-to-one care of Shirley. Place Shirley in a bedroom arrangement with at least one other patient and that is close to the nurses' station. Engage patients or other volunteers to assist in offering support and protection to Shirley during her acute psychotic episodes. Contact relatives and encourage frequent visits.

Follow-up service: Family meetings are recommended to encourage ongoing support and help prevent future psychotic and suicidal episodes; drug therapy can help alleviate thought disorder and depression. Institute daily ward meetings in which patients' acute suicidal episodes can be discussed openly and dealt with cooperatively among all residents. Develop staff in-service training programs on suicide prevention as a means of critically examining and eliminating destructive, authoritarian, and inhumane measures such as isolation and physical restraint of suicidal people.

Suicide Prevention and Intervention with Special Populations

As noted in Chapter Six, certain groups in contemporary society are at special risk of suicide. These groups need particular service programs commensurate with their assessed needs.

Young People

The tragedy of youth suicide has commanded international attention at several levels recently. In the United States, the National Institute of Mental Health (NIMH) convened a task force on youth suicide in several locations to address the problem. The *Surgeon General's Call to Action to Prevent Suicide* (U.S. Public Health Service, 1999) affirms the continued need for attention to youth suicide. Since the occurrence of cluster suicides in recent years, a National Committee on Youth Suicide has been formed, with a focus on suicide education in schools and colleges. The American Association of Suicidology (AAS) and the Canadian Association of Suicide Prevention (CASP) have information about model school suicide prevention programs. The AAS also publishes a newsletter for survivors.[1]

In general, suicide prevention programs for young people focus on educational and support activities for the youth themselves, their parents, and their teachers (Leenaars & Wenckstern, 1991). Pastors, recreation workers, school nurses, physicians, and police officers should also receive such education. Intervention in community settings should include drop-in services, where troubled youth can receive individual help without being stigmatized and can be referred to peer support groups or family counseling services. School health programs, counseling agencies, and local crisis and suicide prevention centers usually collaborate on such programs. The reeducation and developmental approach used by Brendtro, Brokenleg, and Van Bockern (1990) is distinguished internationally for its focus on (1) recognizing (rather than pathologizing) that the troubled behavior of many youth originates from their alienation and (2) assisting them in restoring broken bonds with family and community—bonds that often are severed because of policies that are not friendly to the needs of children.

If suicidal young people are referred to mental health and psychiatric agencies, the treatment of choice should include the family in an active way (Richman, 1986). This is particularly true for an adolescent still living with parents. The adolescent's cry for help might otherwise be misunderstood; often the problem is related to family issues, or the adolescent depends on the family for necessary support during this hazardous transition state (see Chapters Five and Thirteen). In the case of suicidal college students still dependent on but not living with parents, it is crucial not only to recognize clues to suicide but also to explore the person's manifest and possible latent messages: "I don't want my parents to know" (manifest); "I'm too ashamed to tell my parents that I just can't cope with all these pressures in college" (latent). The counselor's obligations are

---

[1]Current information about these activities is available from the AAS Central Office, 4201 Connecticut Avenue N.W., Suite 310, Washington, D.C. 20008; telephone: (202) 237-2280; fax: (202) 237-2282. For CASP and other information, contact Suicide Information & Education Centre, # 201, 1615 - 10th Avenue S.W., Calgary, Alberta, Canada T3C0J7; telephone: (403) 245-3900; fax: (403) 245-0299; e-mail: siec@siec.ca; Web: http://www.siec.ca. See also www.crisisprograms.com.

threefold: (1) to form a therapeutic alliance with the young person as a context for nonauthoritarian parental involvement; (2) to facilitate engaging the person's parents in a way that honors the young person's developmental tasks around dependency; and (3) to remember that confidentiality pledges do not apply in instances of life-or-death risk among dependent persons.

Suicide prevention programs that focus their activities primarily on depression may miss their target (Motto, 1999, p. 225; Shaffer, 1993, p. 172). A study by Garrison, McKeown, Valois, & Vincent (1993) reveals a powerful relationship between suicidal behavior, aggression, and alcohol use, especially by high school males.

Suicide prevention for young people should include the following elements:

- Providing a suicide prevention information program each semester for students in junior and senior high schools and colleges, including cards listing warning signs, myths and facts about suicide, and emergency telephone numbers
- Training students in communication skills, including role playing and modeling of reaching out to others
- Developing suicide prevention curriculum packets to be used by faculty
- Conducting special information programs for parents
- Providing drop-in centers staffed by trained persons sensitive to the special needs of adolescents
- Offering information packets for gay, lesbian, bisexual, and transgendered youth

Although many communities now have such programs (Leenaars & Wenckstern, 1991; Webb, 1986), denial of suicide by school authorities and failure to provide *prevention* and *postvention* programs still occur despite the international efforts noted previously. Basic knowledge about crisis vulnerability during adolescence is also either absent or ignored. For example, the story of a highly publicized suicide of an eighteen-year-old university student revealed the university's claim that eighteen-year-olds are "adults," with no apparent recognition that late adolescence extends to the early twenties for those still in school, not married, and not yet financially independent (not to mention the fact that they are experiencing the hazardous transition from home to college). In school-based programs, students are trained to become peer counselors for classmates who feel left out, lonely, and depressed. Such programs include role playing real-life crises and exploring dramatically how to avert tragedy.

Distinct Ethnic and Sexual Orientation Groups

Besides the general principles of helping suicidal people, some other points should be kept in mind with respect to individuals in these groups.

1. *In agencies routinely serving people with language, cultural, and other differences, staff should be recruited from the distinct communities served.* This does not mean that a dis-

tressed person can only be helped by someone from the same ethnic or sexual-identity group. But by having some staff from the same community, it provides a resource for special problems related to different belief systems and lifestyles. It also helps avoid the appearance of discriminatory practices, which can be a barrier to accepting help. In cases of immigrants who speak rare languages, International Institute staff can be called on to assist (see Chapter Twelve). Communication with respect to *process, intention,* and *helping* is pivotal during suicidal crises; human bonds formed through language, culture, lifestyle, and sexual identity are therefore crucial (Blumenfeld & Lindop, 1994).

2. *The suicidal crises of people in these groups may be strongly linked to their disadvantaged social position.* When this appears to be the case, the social change strategies discussed in Chapter Two are a particularly important aspect of follow-up after crisis intervention. For example, a poor, immigrant woman with three small children became suicidal each time she was threatened with having her heat cut off because she could not pay the bill. To offer this woman only crisis counseling without linking her to social support, financial aid, and social action groups would not approach the social roots of the problem. In Boston, for example, there is an organization called the Coalition for Basic Human Needs, a welfare rights group. Gay rights organizations are also becoming increasingly visible in their advocacy work for civil rights. People in crisis because of discriminatory treatment should be linked to such groups or at least be informed that they exist on their behalf (see Chapter Six, Figure 6.1, right circle, Box 3).

People in Hospitals and Other Institutions

People in crisis, like other human beings, have a need for self-mastery and control of their lives. Sensitivity to this need is an important element of positive crisis resolution. People in crisis who are suicidal not only do not lose their need for self-determination but also frequently feel powerless to solve their problems except by the ultimate act of self-determination—suicide. As noted earlier in Shirley's case, staff members in institutions should examine various approaches to suicidal people; many approaches to protecting people from suicide may result in exactly the opposite of what is intended. Although physical restraint and isolation may prevent immediate self-injury, these methods may actually increase the long-term suicide risk. Such results are especially probable if the physical measures are carried out with authoritarian attitudes and an absence of communication, warmth, and genuine concern. People who already feel powerless may interpret such harsh, outmoded practices as another attack on their self-esteem and ability to control their lives. As Farberow (1981, p. 101) states, people in hospitals (and other institutions) "are continually impressed with a sense of powerlessness; their lives must conform to a schedule designed essentially for the convenience of the staff. Most things happen *to* them, not because of or *for* them; other people continually make the most important decisions about their lives." Ottini (1999) describes an intensive program (built on psychoanalytic and crisis concepts) designed to address the weaknesses of psychiatric inpatient services for suicidal adolescents (see also Berman, Coggins, Zibelin, Nelson, & Hannon, 1993; Osgood, 1992.)

Many people expect institutionalized people to conform to the sick role, but it is unrealistic to conduct our practice within this framework for suicidal people. The problem of expecting suicidal people to fit the traditional sick role is exacerbated if there is no systematic effort to include family or other social contacts in hospital treatment programs. Once institutionalization has taken place, a person's natural social community is often forgotten. Or if the person is suicidal because such community support is lacking, it takes a special effort by hospital staffs to help develop substitute support systems, such as transitional housing services, prior to discharge. In addition, admission to institutions is frequently the occasion of suicidal impulses based on culture shock for people not acculturated to institutions through routine work or residence.

Attention to these points can help prevent self-injury and suicides in hospitals and other institutions as well as reduce angry patients' attacks on staff and the high rate of suicide after discharge from mental hospitals. See Farberow's work (1981) and Bongar et al. (1993) for additional recommendations and standards for suicide prevention in hospitals.

Suicide prevention in holding centers and correctional institutions presents similar but even more complex problems (Haycock, 1993). A study in the Netherlands (cited in Kerkhof & Clark, 1993) revealed four types of stressors faced by prisoners: problems with relatives or the problems of relatives, legal process issues, conflicts with staff or other inmates, and issues of drug abuse. In one sense, the isolation cell is like an instrument of death. Yet relieving the physical isolation of a suicidal inmate may expose the person to possible abuse or attack by fellow inmates.

The crisis of suicide in jails and prisons is gaining attention. A unique program, Lifeline, is operated by staff of The Samaritans in Boston. Similar to the Prisoner Befriender program in several prisons in the United Kingdom, Lifeline is conducted in the county jail. Inmates—including murderers, arsonists, and rapists—receive special training to work as befrienders of the lonely and depressed. Besides reducing the number of suicides in this jail, the program is noted for its benefits to the befriending inmates: they have the satisfaction of saving others' lives and of feeling useful and appreciated for their caring (McGinnis, 1993).

Halleck's (1971) concern about chronic self-destructiveness among inmates is still relevant, as various nations, including the United States, are cited by Amnesty International for cruel and unusual treatment of prisoners. He suggests that prisoners' repeated suicide attempts are a symptom of conditions in the institution that bear examination and probable reform (see Chapter Nine). A related problem is the extensive use of psychotropic drugs on prisoners, with no psychotherapy services available for most. As crime and prison populations in the United States soar, suicide attempts are probable as long as real prison reform lags, and primary prevention of crime takes a back burner in policy circles.

Helping Survivors in Crisis

When a suicide occurs, it is almost always the occasion of a crisis for survivors: children, spouse, parents, other relatives, friends, crisis counselor, therapist, and anyone else closely associated with the person who has committed suicide. The term *survivor* in the suicidology literature properly refers to those left after *completed suicides*, not to those who survive a suicide attempt. The usual feelings associated with any serious loss are felt by most survivors of a suicide—sadness that the person ended life so tragically and anger that the person is no longer a part of one's life.

In addition, however, survivors often feel enormous guilt, primarily from two sources:

1. The sense of responsibility for not having prevented the suicide. This is especially true when the survivors were very close to the person who has died.
2. The sense of relief that some survivors feel after a suicide. This happens when relationships were very strained or when the person had attempted suicide many times and either could not or would not accept the help available.

A common tendency among survivors of suicide is to blame or scapegoat someone for the suicide. This reaction often arises from a survivor's sense of helplessness and guilt about not having prevented the suicide. Deeply held beliefs about suicide also contribute to this response. Some survivors deny that the suicide ever took place because they have no other way to handle the crisis. This often takes the form of insisting that the death was an accident.

CASE EXAMPLE: DENIAL OF SUICIDE

One couple instructed their nine-year-old daughter, who was a patient in the pediatric ward, to tell the hospital supervisor that her older brother had died of an accident. (The supervisor knew the family through the hospital psychiatric unit.) The parents had insisted that he be discharged from psychiatric care, even though he was highly suicidal and the physician advised against it. A few days later, the boy shot himself at home with a hunting rifle. These parents were apparently very guilt ridden and went to great lengths to deny the suicide.

Various authors (Dunne, Dunne-Maxim, & McIntosh, 1987; Cain, 1972) have documented problems that can occur throughout survivors' lives if they do not have help at the time of the crisis of suicide. A study by Farberow, Gallager-Thompson, Gilewski, and Thompson (1992) revealed that suicide survivors among bereaved elderly people received significantly less support than those whose spouses died by natural death; men received less support than women. Reed and Greenwald (1991) found that survivor-victim *attachment* and the quality of the relationship are more important in explaining grief reactions than the survivor's status (that is, the relationship between the survivor and the suicide, such as father and daughter or husband and wife). Problems for survivors include depression, serious personality disturbances, and obsession with suicide as the predestined fate for oneself, especially on the anniversary of the suicide or when the survivor reaches the same age.

The tragic effect of suicide is particularly striking in the case of children after a parent's suicide. In studies of child survivors, some of the symptoms found were learning disabilities, sleepwalking, delinquency, and setting fires (Cain & Fast, 1972). Crisis counseling should therefore be available for all survivors of suicide. Shneidman (1972) calls this "postvention," an effort to reduce some of the possible harmful effects of suicide on the survivors. Making such support available, however, presents a special challenge, particularly in settings such as schools (Wenckstern, 1991).

Team Analysis Following a Suicide

Some people commit suicide while receiving therapy or counseling through a crisis center, mental health agency, or private practitioner or while receiving hospital or medical care. In these cases, the counselor, nurse, or physician is in a strategic position to help survivors. Unfortunately, workers often miss the opportunity for postvention because they may be struggling with the same feelings that beset the family. It is more effective to deal with the family immediately than to wait for an impasse to develop, but if staff have not dealt with their own feelings, they may avoid approaching family survivors.

The most useful preventive measure is for helpers to learn as much as they can about suicide and about constructive ways of handling the feelings that often accompany working with self-destructive people. There will always be strong feelings following a suicide. However, a worker with a realistic concept of the limits of responsibility for another's suicide can help other survivors work through their feelings and reduce the scapegoating that often occurs.

In counseling and health care settings, a counselor or nurse should immediately seek consultation with a supervisor after a suicide occurs. Team meetings are also important, as they provide staff with an opportunity to air feelings and evaluate the total situation. For example, team analysis of John's case (Chapter Six) illustrates how easy it is to forget a person's natural place in the world and to fail to draw on social resources once the patient is in an institutional subculture. John's friends were never contacted, nor was a peer support source like AA considered. Involuntary commitment for self-protection, although well intentioned, was not enough. Analysis of this case sharpened the staff's awareness that the sense of isolation and powerlessness often experienced in mental health facilities may increase rather than decrease suicide risk. Through open discussion, staff members were able to acknowledge that John's suicide might have been prevented with a different approach to intervention, including helping him reestablish himself socially after a serious interpersonal loss (see Chapter Five). If suicide prevention efforts are based on established standards in suicidology, the staff is less likely to feel guilty, and malpractice suits are less likely (Bongar et al., 1993). In addition, self-examination and hindsight after a suicide usually yield knowledge that can be applied on behalf of others (Hoff & Resing, 1982).

Team meetings also provide a forum for determining who is best able to make postvention contact with the family. If the counselor who has worked most closely with the victim is too upset to deal with the family, a supervisory person should handle the matter, at least initially. In hospitals or mental health agencies in which no one has had training in basic suicide prevention and crisis counseling, outside consultation with suicidologists or crisis specialists should be obtained whenever possible.

Support and Crisis Intervention for Survivors

Most suicides do not occur among people receiving help from a health or counseling agency. This is one reason many survivors of suicide get so little help. In some communities, there are special bereavement counseling programs or self-help groups, such as Widow to Widow clubs, to help survivors of suicide. Ideally, every community should have an active outreach program for suicide survivors as a basic part of comprehensive crisis services (Hoff & Adamowski, 1998). Survivors are free to refuse an offer of support, but such support should be available.

A parent survivor, Adina Wrobleski, is one of the pioneers in developing survivors' grief groups, having formed such a group in 1982 following the suicide of her teenage daughter in the metropolitan Minneapolis area. Since then, many similar groups have been established. Wrobleski's work is significant in two respects: (1) following the suicide of her daughter, there were no peer support groups available to her and her husband; (2) survivors of suicide do not necessarily need professional therapy as much as they need support from people who have experienced the same kind of loss. This point has been illustrated by groups such as the SIDS Foundation and self-help groups for health and social problems, such as AA and groups for mastectomy patients (see Chapters Five, Eleven, and Thirteen).

In the absence of these avenues of help, survivors of suicide can still be reached by police, clergy, and funeral directors, if such caretakers are sensitive to survivors' needs. These key people should take care not to increase survivors' guilt and denial, recognizing how strong the suicide taboo and scapegoating tendency can be. The least one can do is offer an understanding word and suggest where people might find an agency or person to help them through the crisis. See Grollman's classic work (1977) regarding the role of clergy with survivors.

Techniques for helping survivors of suicide are essentially the same as those used in dealing with other crises. A survivor should be helped to

1. Express feelings appropriate to the event
2. Grasp the reality of the suicide
3. Obtain and use the help necessary to work through the crisis (including sometimes the survivor's own suicide crisis)

A survivor who depended on the suicide victim for financial support may also need help in managing money and housing, for example.

Helping Child Survivors of Parent Suicide

A surviving spouse with young children, including preschoolers as young as three or four, usually needs special help explaining to them that their parent has committed suicide. People tend to hide the facts from children in a mistaken belief that they will thus be spared unnecessary pain. But adults often fail to realize that children usually know a great deal more than adults think they know. Even without knowing all the facts surrounding a death, children are likely to suspect that something much more terrible than an accident has occurred. If the suicide is not discussed, the child is left to fill in the facts alone—and to do it with fantasies even more frightening than the real story would be. For example, a child may fear that the surviving parent killed the dead parent or that the child's own misbehavior caused the parent's death. The child may have unrealistic expectations that the dead parent will return: "Maybe if I'm extra good, Daddy will come back." What children do not create in their fantasy lives will often be filled in by information from neighborhood and school companions. Some child survivors also suffer from jeers and teasing by other children about the parent's suicide.

Survivors should explain the death by suicide clearly, simply, and in a manner consistent with the child's level of development and understanding. The child should have an opportunity to ask questions and express feelings. The child needs to know that the surviving parent is also willing to answer questions in the future, as the child's understanding of death and suicide grows. A child should never be left with the impression that the issue is closed and is never to be discussed again.

Parents might explain suicide to child survivors as follows:

> "Yes, Daddy shot himself. No, it wasn't an accident; he did it because he wanted to."

> "Mommy will not be coming back anymore. No, Mommy didn't do it because you misbehaved last night."

> "No one knows exactly why your daddy did it. Yes, he had a lot of things that bothered him."

Surviving parents who cannot deal directly with their children about the other parent's suicide have usually not worked through their own feelings of guilt and responsibility. In these cases, parents need the support and help of a counselor for themselves as well as for their children. Parents often do not understand that serious consequences can arise from hiding the facts from children. Counseling should include an explanation of the advantages of talking openly with children about the suicide.

In some cases, a child is completely aware that the parent committed suicide, especially if there were many open threats or attempts of suicide. Sometimes a child finds the dead parent or has been given directions by the other parent to "call if anything happens to Mommy" (Cain, 1972). If the suicidal person was very disturbed or abusive prior to committing suicide, the child may feel relief. In all of these cases, surviving children may feel guilt and misplaced responsibility for the death of their parent. They may become restless and fearful and refuse to sleep in their own beds. Parents will usually need the assistance of a crisis worker or a child guidance counselor to help a child through this crisis. Crisis intervention programs for such children are far too uncommon.

Additional Outreach to Survivors

Help for survivors of suicide has always been one of the goals of the suicide prevention movement. Such work is important but difficult to carry out. Many people, including those in some coroners' offices, tend to cover up the reality of a suicide. The suicide taboo in modern times continues, despite a growing acceptance of the morality of suicide in certain instances (Battin & Mayo, 1980; see also "Ethical Issues Regarding Suicide" in Chapter Six).

One means of reaching a large number of survivors is through coroners' offices. Every death is eventually recorded there. In Los Angeles County, all suicide deaths as well as equivocal deaths (those in which suicide is suspected but not certain) are followed up by staff from the Los Angeles Suicide Prevention Center. Suicidologists do a "psychological autopsy" (Litman, 1987)—that is, an intensive examination to determine whether the death was by suicide and if it was to uncover the probable causes. Information for the psychological autopsy is obtained from survivors and from medical and psychiatric records.

Research is the primary purpose of the psychological autopsy; however, it is an excellent means of getting in touch with survivors who are not in contact with a crisis center, physician, or mental health agency. Survivors are, of course, free to refuse participation in such postmortem examinations. Experience reveals, however, that the majority of survivors do not refuse to be interviewed and welcome the opportunity to talk about the suicide. This is especially true if they are contacted within a few days of the suicide, when they are most troubled with their feelings. Many survivors use this occasion to obtain some help in answering their own questions and dealing with suicidal inclinations following a suicide. Some people find the "official" interview an acceptable context in which to talk about an otherwise taboo subject. It thus provides an ideal opportunity for the interviewer to suggest follow-up counseling resources to the survivor. If weeks or months pass, survivors may resent the postmortem interview. By that time, they have had to settle their feelings and questions on their own and in their own way, which may include denial and resentment. A delayed interview may seem like the unnecessary opening of an old wound.

Various suicide prevention and crisis centers offer survivor counseling programs. Many communities, however, still do not have formal programs available to survivors of suicide. Obviously, a great deal of work remains to be done in this important area.

Summary

People who get help after a suicide attempt or other self-destructive behavior may never commit suicide. Much depends on what happens in the form of emergency, crisis, and follow-up intervention. However, when suicide does occur, survivors of suicide usually are in crisis and are often neglected because of cultural taboos and the lack of aggressive outreach programs for them. Children, spouses, and parents who lose a loved one by suicide are especially vulnerable if they do not receive support during this crisis. This is an area of great challenge for crisis program staff.

References

Baldessarini, R. J. (2000). The complexity of suicide. Grand rounds: Suicide: Clinical/risk management issues for psychiatrists. *CNS Spectrums Academic Supplement: The International Journal of Neuropsychiatric Medicine, 5* (2, Suppl. 1), 34–38.

Baldessarini, R. J., & Tondo, L. (1999). Antisuicidal effect of lithium treatment in major mood disorders. In D. G. Jacobs (Ed.), *The Harvard Medical School guide to suicide assessment and intervention* (pp. 355–371). San Francisco: Jossey-Bass.

Battin, M. P., & Mayo, D. J. (Eds.). (1980). *Suicide: The philosophical issues.* New York: St. Martin's Press.

Berman, A. L., Coggins, C. C., Zibelin, J. C., Nelson, L. F., & Hannon, T. (1993). Inpatient treatment planning. *Suicide & Life-Threatening Behavior, 23*(2), 162–168.

Blumenfeld, W. J., & Lindop, L. (1994). *Family, schools, and students' resource guide.* Boston: Safe Schools Program for Gay and Lesbian Students, Massachusetts Department of Education.

Bongar, B., Maris, R. W., Berman, A. L., & Litman, R. E. (1992). Outpatient standards of care and the suicidal patient. *Suicide & Life-Threatening Behavior, 22*(4), 453–478.

Bongar, B., Maris, R. W., Berman, A. L., Litman, R. E., & Silverman, M. M. (1993). Inpatient standards of care and the suicidal patient: Part I: General clinical formulations and legal considerations. *Suicide & Life-Threatening Behavior, 23*(3), 245–256.

Boyd, J. H., & Moscicki, E. K. (1986). Firearms and youth suicide. *American Journal of Public Health, 76,* 1240–1242.

Breggin, P., & Breggin, G. R. (1994). *Talking back to Prozac: What doctors won't tell you about today's most controversial drug.* New York: St. Martin's Press.

Brendtro, L. K., Brokenleg, M., & Van Bockern, S. (1990). *Reclaiming youth at risk: Our hope for the future.* Bloomington, IN: National Educational Service.

Brown, G. W., & Harris, T. (1978). *The social origins of depression.* London: Tavistock.

Cain, A. C. (Ed.). (1972). *Survivors of suicide.* Springfield, IL: Thomas.

Cain, A. C., & Fast, R. (1972). Children's disturbed reactions to parent suicide: Distortions of guilt, communication, and identification. In A. C. Cain (Ed.), Survivors of suicide (pp. 93–111). Springfield, IL: Thomas.

Carson, M., Eisner, M., Kartes, L., & Kolga, C. (1999). *A care-giving guide for seniors.* Ottawa: Algonquin Publishers.

Clark, D. C., & Kerkhof, A.J.F.M. (1993). No-suicide decisions and suicide contracts in therapy. *Crisis, 14*(3), 98–99.

Cloward, R. A., & Piven, F. F. (1979). Hidden protest: The channeling of female innovations and resistance. *Signs: Journal of Women in Culture and Society, 4,* 651–669.

Duncan, B., Miller, S., & Sparks, J. (2000, March/April). Exposing the mythmaking. *Networker,* 25–33, 52–53.

Dunne, E., Dunne-Maxim, K., & McIntosh, J. (Eds.). (1987). *Suicide and its aftermath.* New York: Norton.

Farberow, N. L. (1981). Suicide prevention in the hospital. *Hospital and Community Psychiatry, 32*(2), 99–104.

Farberow, N. L., Gallager-Thompson, D., Gilewski, M., & Thompson, L. (1992). Changes in grief and mental health of bereaved spouses of older suicides. *Journal of Gerontology, 47*(6), 357–366.

Garcia, G., & Ghani, S. (2000). Pharmacology update: Newer medications and indications used in psychiatry. *Primary Care Practice, 4*(2), 207–220.

Garrison, C. Z., McKeown, R. E., Valois, R. F., & Vincent, M. L. (1993). Aggression, substance use, and suicidal behaviors in high school students. *American Journal of Public Health, 83*(2), 179–184.

Grollman, E. (1977). *Living—when a loved one has died.* Boston: Beacon Press.

Halleck, S. (1971). *The politics of therapy.* New York: Science House.

Haycock, J. (1993). Double jeopardy: Suicide rates in forensic hospitals. *Suicide & Life-Threatening Behavior, 23*(2), 130–138.

Hoff, L. A., & Adamowski, K. (1998). *Creating excellence in crisis care: A guide to effective training and program designs.* San Francisco: Jossey-Bass.

Hoff, L. A., & Resing, M. (1982). Was this suicide preventable? *American Journal of Nursing, 82*(7) 1106–1111. (Also reprinted in B. A. Backer, P. M. Dubbert, & E.J.P. Eisenman (Eds.). (1985). *Psychiatric/mental health nursing: Contemporary readings* (pp. 169–180). Belmont, CA: Wadsworth.)

Johnson, A. B. (1990). *Out of bedlam: The truth about deinstitutionalization.* New York: Basic Books.

Kaplan, M. S. (1998). Firearm suicides and homicides in the United States: Regional variations and patterns of gun ownership. *Social Science & Medicine, 46*(9) 1227–1233.

Kaplan, M. S., Adamek, M. E., & Calderon, A. (1999). Managing depressed and suicidal geriatric patients: Differences among primary care physicians. *Gerontologist, 38*(4), 417–425.

Kerkhof, A.J.F.M., & Clark, D. C. (1993). Suicide attempts and self-injury in prisons. *Crisis, 14*(4), 146–147.

Leenaars, A. A., & Wenckstern, S. (Eds.). (1991). Suicide prevention in schools. Bristol, PA: Hemisphere.

Litman, R. E. (1987). Mental disorders and suicidal intention. *Suicide & Life-Threatening Behavior, 17*(2), 85–92.

McGinnis, C. (1993). *Lifeline: A training manual.* Boston: Suffolk County Jail.

McLeavey, B. C., Daly, R. J., Murray, C. M., O'Riordan, J. O., & Taylor, M. (1987). Interpersonal problem solving deficits in self-poisoning patients. *Suicide & Life-Threatening Behavior, 17*(1), 33–49.

Motto, J. A. (1999). Critical points in the assessment and management of suicide risk. In D. G. Jacobs (Ed.), *The Harvard Medical School guide to suicide assessment and intervention* (pp. 224–238). San Francisco: Jossey-Bass.

Osgood, M. (1992). Environmental factors in suicide in long-term care facilities. *Suicide & Life-Threatening Behavior, 22*(1), 98–106.

Ottini, J. (1999). Suicide attempts during adolescence: Systematic hospitalization and crisis treatment. *Crisis, 20*(1), 41–48.

Reed, M. D., & Greenwald, J. Y. (1991). Survivor-victim status, attachment, and sudden death bereavement. *Suicide & Life-Threatening Behavior, 21*(4), 385–401.

Richman, J. (1986). *Family therapy of suicidal individuals.* New York: Springer.

Salzman, C. (1999). Treatment of the suicidal patient with psychotropic drugs and ECT. In D. G. Jacobs (Ed.), *The Harvard Medical School guide to suicide assessment and intervention* (pp. 372–382). San Francisco: Jossey-Bass.

Shaffer, D. (1993). Suicide: Risk factors and the public health. *American Journal of Public Health, 83*(2), 171–173.

Shneidman, E. S. (1972). Foreword. In A. C. Cain (Ed.), *Survivors of suicide*. Springfield, IL: Thomas.

Solomon, D. A., Keitner, G. I., Miller, I. W., Shea, M. T., & Keller, M. B. (1995). Course of illness and maintenance treatments for patients with bipolar disorder. *Journal of Clinical Psychiatry, 56*(1), 5–13.

U.S. Public Health Service. (1999). *Surgeon general's call to action to prevent suicide*. Washington, DC: Author.

Waters, R. (2000, March/April). Generation RX: The risk of raising our kids on pharmaceuticals. *Networker,* 34–43.

Webb, N. D. (1986). Before and after suicide: A preventive outreach program for colleges. *Suicide & Life-Threatening Behavior, 16*(4), 469–480.

Wenckstern, S. (1991). Suicide postvention: A case illustration in a secondary school. In A. A. Leenaars & S. Wenckstern (Eds.), *Suicide prevention in schools* (pp. 181–196). Bristol, PA: Hemisphere.

Worden, J. W. (1991). *Grief counseling and grief therapy* (2nd ed.). New York: Springer.

Zito J. M., Safer, D. J., dosReis, S., Gardner, J. F., Boles, M., & Lynch, F. (2000). Trends in the prescribing of psychotropic medications to preschoolers. *Journal of the American Medical Association, 283*(8), 1025–1030.

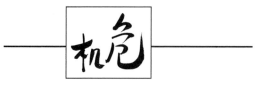

CHAPTER EIGHT

THE CRISIS OF VICTIMIZATION BY VIOLENCE

Victimization by violence knows few, if any, national, ethnic, religious, or other boundaries (Levinson, 1989; United Nations, 1996b). In the United States—with some of the highest rates of violence in the world—the homicide rate is 10 per 100,000, accounting for 25,000 deaths per year. The rate in England is one-tenth of the U.S. rate, although violence in that country is also increasing. Among African American males ages fifteen to twenty-four, homicide is the most likely cause of death (Wolfgang, 1986, p. 11). Although figures vary, about 20 percent of spouses in Canada and the United States are enmeshed in abuse; one-half of all Canadian women have experienced at least one violent incident since the age of sixteen (Johnson, 1998). Prevalence rates of intimate partner violence receiving primary care service range between 7 and 29 percent (Coker, Smith, McKeown, & King, 2000).

Of intimate partner homicides (about 50 percent of the U.S. total homicides), two-thirds are women killed by their male partners, and one-third are men killed by their female partners (Browne, 1987). Battering accounts for more injuries to women than accidents, muggings, and stranger rape combined; violence is the leading cause of injury to women between fifteen and forty-four (Novello, 1992, p. 3132). Although rape in marriage is now legally recognized as a criminal act throughout the United States and Canada, many loopholes weaken the laws. Federal crime reports estimate that over 300,000 women and 92,000 men are raped in the United States each year. A public opinion poll in Massachusetts revealed that significant numbers of ninth-grade boys and girls think that a man has a right to sexual intercourse without consent if the couple has a dating relationship. Against overwhelming evidence, a recent book asserts the biological bases of sexual coercion (Thornhill & Palmer, 2000).

Studies of acquaintance rape and date rape reveal a wide disparity between women and men on what constitutes rape; the majority of men define as "normal" what women call sexual violence (Warshaw, 1988). Even though rape victims know their attackers in the majority of cases, acquaintance rapes are reported least, probably because victims fear being blamed for the attack. Another result of victim blaming is that almost half of rape cases are dismissed before trial, and half of those convicted of rape serve less than a year behind bars.

Among children and adolescents in the United States, up to 3 million are physically or sexually abused or neglected each year, with as many as 1.3 million left homeless in a given year (Gelles & Cornell, 1985; Rivera, 1995; Powers & Jaklitsch, 1989). Surveys of women reveal that up to 50 percent report some kind of sexual encounter before the age of sixteen with an adult male (Herman, 1981, p. 12; Wolfgang, 1986, p. 12) and that abuse by stepfathers is seven times more common than by biological fathers (Russell, 1986). Developmentally disabled people are prime targets for sexual and other abuse and are often ignored, in part because of their limited ability to report or talk about the assault. While childhood sexual abuse is more common among girls than boys, the gap in prevalence rates appears to be narrowing (McManiman, 2000; Watkins & Bentovim, 1992).

National survey data in Canada and the United States reveal that about 4 percent of elderly people are abused by relatives each year, but only one in six cases is reported (McDonald, Hornick, Robertson, & Wallace, 1991; Podnieks & Pillemer, 1990). Financial exploitation of elderly people is also rising. A random survey in metropolitan Boston, with a population of more than four million, revealed between 8,646 and 13,487 abused and neglected elders (Pillemer & Finkelhor, 1987). In spite of civil rights legislation, violence originating from bias based on race, religion, and sexual identity continues. Abused immigrants usually face triple jeopardy because of social isolation, language barriers, and fear of deportation if they seek help.

Internationally, victimization is also receiving greater attention. In South Africa, for example, for every act of political violence, at least seven women are victimized at home (Dangor, Hoff, & Scott, 1998). Most research on the topic, however, has been conducted in North America and Europe (Hoff, 1992b; United Nations, 1996a). The United Nations has convened international meetings on the topic, and the United Nations Decade for Women conferences feature numerous workshops on the worldwide problem of violence against women. The last such conference was in 1995 in Beijing, People's Republic of China, with about 36,000 women attending. Beijing Plus 5 convened in New York in June 2000 to assess the progress of member nations toward the goals of the 1995 platform for action. Although progress is evident, much work remains to achieve women's equality and freedom from abuse worldwide.

Canada has demonstrated extraordinary leadership on this topic, supporting numerous projects as well as five federally funded research centers (Ross, 2001). Canada is the first country to pass a federal, mandatory arrest law for wife beaters and the first in which men in the private sector have taken national leadership in a white ribbon campaign to end violence against women and to institute training criteria for health and social service professionals on violence issues (Hoff, 1995). In Portugal, London, Massachusetts, and Toronto, an international consortium offering graduate training on violence, crisis, and gender studies is under way to better prepare educators and practitioners to confidently address this urgent topic (see www.crisisprograms.com).

In the United States, the U.S. Surgeon General's Workshop on Violence and Public Health (1986) was convened in 1985 to emphasize the fact that victims' needs, treatment of assailants, and prevention of violence should command much greater attention from health and social service professionals than it has until recently. Since then, there has been progress on many fronts (for example, the 1999 American Association of Colleges of Nursing position paper; the 1994 research of Tilden et al.), although much is left to be done. The historical neglect of victimization, especially in the domestic arena, underscores the value placed on family privacy and the myth that the family is a haven of love and security. Neglect of victimization also points to several related issues:

- Social values regarding children, how they should be disciplined, and who should care for them
- Social and cultural devaluation of women and their problems
- A social and economic system in which elderly citizens often have no worthwhile place
- A social climate with little tolerance for minority sexual orientation
- A legal system in which it is difficult to consider the rights of victims without compromising the rights of the accused
- A knowledge system that historically has interpreted these problems in private, individual terms rather than in public, social ones (Mills, 1959)

This and the following chapter address these issues in the psychosociocultural and public health perspectives that inform this book. The focus is on prevention, crisis intervention, and the interconnections of violence across the life span. The prevention and early intervention emphasis here is based on extensive interdisciplinary work with survivors, revealing the risk of serious and often long-term medical and mental health sequelae when support and crisis counseling are lacking at the time of victimization by violence (Hoff, 2000). For a discussion of comprehensive psychosocial and psychotherapeutic care beyond crisis, readers are referred to such texts as Burstow (1992), Campbell (1998), Everett & Gallop (2000), Herman (1992), and Wiehe (1998).

This chapter addresses the various categories of abuse and violence, primarily from the perspective of the victim. Chapter Nine addresses violence from the perspective of the assailant, as well as that directed against police, health and human service workers, and others. The two chapters are companion pieces, as the topics overlap; for example, many assailants have been victimized themselves.

Reflecting a major theme of crisis theory (Hoff, 1990), the term *victim-survivor* is used to acknowledge victimization but to simultaneously convey an abused person's potential for growth, development, and empowerment—a status beyond the dependency implied by *victim* (Burstow, 1992; Mawby & Walklate, 1994). The terms *violence* and *abuse* are used interchangeably.

Theories on Violence and Victimization

Earlier theories to explain violence and its prevalence fall into three categories: (1) psychobiological, (2) social-psychological, and (3) sociocultural (Gelles & Straus, 1979). Today most violence scholars reject analytical frameworks such as sociobiology, which serve to maintain violence as a private matter. Instead violence is now widely interpreted in psychological, sociological, and feminist terms (Dobash & Dobash, 1998; Gelles & Loseke, 1993). The position taken in this book is that violence is predominantly a *social* phenomenon, a means of exerting *power* and *control* that has far-reaching effects on personal, family, and public health worldwide (Dobash & Dobash, 1979; Hoff, in press; Yllo & Bograd, 1987). In addition, the book's holistic framework implies a continuum between so-called family violence and other forms of aggression. Finally, while controversy continues between feminist and mainstream theorists and activists (Gelles & Loseke, 1993), the focus here is on bridge building and the common concerns of those who teach and practice violence prevention and who work with victim-survivors and their assailants in diverse settings. An either-or position is rejected in favor of complementary feminist, sociocultural, and public health perspectives that emphasize the intersection between gender, class, race, and other social categories that may figure in the experience of particular victims or assailants. In feminist theory, this approach is called *socialist feminism*. As readers examine their own positions vis-à-vis feminist and mainstream theories of violence, it is important to note that there is no such thing as a monolithic feminism. See Boddy (1998), Breines & Gordon (1983), Hoff (1990), and Segal (1987).

Accordingly, the term *family violence* is avoided on the grounds that it obscures the fact that most perpetrators in families are men, and most victims are children and women of all ages. One of the continuing controversies about violence concerns the rates of men's and women's violence (Kurz, 1993; Straus, 1993). The argument centers on the alleged methodological flaws of the Conflict Tactics Scale used in the national surveys conducted by Straus and colleagues in 1980 and 1985 (see Johnson, 1998). The term *family violence* also deflects attention from the sociocultural roots of abuse, which extend beyond the family to deeply embedded cultural values and traditional social structures that disempower women and children particularly.

Many professionals and laypersons have accepted psychological or medical explanations of violence (see "The Medicalization of Crime and Violence in the Workplace," Chapter Nine). Common sentiments include (1) "only a sick man could beat his wife"; (2) child abuse is a syndrome calling for "treatment" of disturbed parents; (3) John W. Hinckley should have been "treated," not punished, for violently attacking President Reagan; (4) a "crazed madman" was responsible (and by implication, not accountable) for a series of fatal Tylenol poisonings in the United States; (5) "temporary insanity" sometimes excuses murder (even though juries are becoming more skeptical about this plea); and (6) women who kill their abusers are victims of the "battered woman syndrome."

Public debate about biomedical approaches to social problems is increasing (Luhrmann, 2000; Warshaw, 1989). There is growing acceptance of the view that attention to violent persons and their victims in predominantly individual terms is at best incomplete and at worst does little to address the roots of violence. This view is in accord with the crisis paradigm of this book: crises stemming from violence should be treated with a *tandem* approach, taking both individual and sociocultural factors into account. A person in crisis because of violence will experience many of the same responses as persons in crisis from other sources (Burgess & Holmstrom, 1979; Sales, Baum, & Shore, 1984, p. 131). And similar intervention strategies, such as listening and decision counseling, are called for during the acute crisis phase. However, attention to the social and cultural origins of crises stemming from violence is important in designing prevention and follow-up strategies that avoid implicitly blaming the victim (Ryan, 1971; Hoff, 1990). Indeed, the implications of a sociocultural framework are even more critical when considering crises originating from violence than when dealing with crises from other sources (see Chapter Two, Figure 2.2). For victims of violence, a strictly individual or biopsychiatric approach can compound the problem rather than contribute to the solution (Stark, Flitcraft, & Frazier, 1979).

There is no single cause of violence. Rather, there are complex, interrelated *reasons* that some individuals are violent and others are not. In cases of violence against children, wives, and elders, for example, psychological, cultural, and socioeconomic factors are often present together, forming the *context* in which violence as a means of control seems to thrive. Children, many seniors, and often wives are economically dependent on their caretakers and in most cases are physically weaker than their abusers. Caretakers of children and older people are often stressed psychologically by difficult behaviors and socioeconomically by a lack of social and financial resources to ease the burdens of caretaking (Besharov, 1990; Pillemer & Wolf, 1986; Pruschno & Resch, 1989). In cases of woman battering and sex-role stereotyping, psychological and economic factors intersect at both ends of the social class continuum: poor women are less able to survive on their own, and some women who earn more than their husbands are more vulnerable to attack in a nonegalitarian marriage.

Violence toward others, then, is one way a person can respond to stress and resolve a personal crisis at the same time. For example, a person with low self-esteem who is threatened by the suspected infidelity of a spouse may react with violence (Gondolf, 1987). A violent response is not inevitable though; it is *chosen* and may be influenced by such factors as an earlier choice to use alcohol and other drugs. The choice of violent behavior to control another person is influenced by the social, political, legal, and belief and knowledge systems of the violent person's cultural community. The element of choice implies an interpretation of violence as a moral act—that is, violence is *social action* engaged in by human beings who by nature are rational and conscious. Through socialization, humans become responsible for the actions they choose in various situations.

However, consciousness may be clouded and responsibility mitigated by social and cultural factors rooted in the history of human society. Under certain circumstances, a person may be excused from facing the social consequences of his or her behavior, as in cases of self-defense or when a violent act is considered to be irrational. This does not mean that every violent act is a result of mental illness and that the perpetrator should therefore be "treated," as suggested by a popular conception of violence. Nor does it mean that violence can be excused on grounds of racial or economic discrimination; this would suggest that the moral stature of disadvantaged groups is below the standard of responsible behavior. Given the poverty, unemployment, and other tragic results of social inequalities endured by many people—mostly racial minority groups—perhaps in no other instance is the tandem approach to crisis intervention more relevant: violent *individuals* are held accountable for their behavior, while the political and socioeconomic *context* in which much violence occurs is also addressed. In other words, an individual can be held accountable, can be restrained or rehabilitated, and at the same time the factors that have contributed to the person's vulnerability to choosing aggressive behaviors in the first place can be addressed. This principle applies regardless of gender or race.

Another troubling aspect of a simplistic interpretation of the nature of violence is the tendency toward "solutions" in the form of revenge, as suggested, for example, by U.S. voters' choice of capital punishment. To describe violence as a moral act rather than a disease does not imply support of revenge as an appropriate response. As responses to the complex problem of violence, treatment and revenge represent opposite extremes. As in the case of race or gender, excusing violent acts on the basis of psychiatric illness suggests that violent human beings are somewhat less than human, generally incapable of judging and acting according to the consequences of their behavior, and are driven by uncontrollable, aggressive impulses. In contrast, revenge—in the form of capital punishment, inhumane prison conditions, or a failure to provide economic and other opportunities for learning to change a violent lifestyle—implies a departure from the moral foundations of society.

Violence and our response to its victim-survivors and perpetrators can be interpreted in a multifaceted perspective: moral, social-psychological, legal, and medical. Violence can be defined as an infraction of society's rules regarding people, their relationships, and their property. It is a complex phenomenon in which sociocultural, political, medical, and psychological factors touch both its immediate and chronic aspects. Functioning members of a society normally know a group's cultural rules and the consequences for violating them. Those lacking such knowledge generally are excused and receive treatment instead of punishment. Others are excused on the basis of self-defense or the circumstances that alter one's normal liability for rule infractions. A moral society would require restitution to individual victims from those not excused and would design a criminal justice system to prevent rather than promote future crime. A truly moral approach to violence would also avoid or reform practices that discriminate on the basis of race, gender, class, or sexual orientation, practices that create a climate in which crime flourishes with the implicit support of society (Brown & Bohn, 1989; Dobash & Dobash, 1979; Handwerker, 1998).

Decisions about crisis and follow-up approaches to victims and perpetrators of violence demand a critical examination of the theories and research supporting such practice, an examination not undertaken until recently. This theoretical overview applies to the topics in this and the following chapter. It assumes a continuum between what happens between family members and intimates and the larger sociocultural factors affecting them. In the following discussion, social-psychological and sociocultural theories will be examined as they apply to crises stemming from violence in respect to

- Prevention
- Intervention during crisis
- Follow-up service (psychosocial care and psychotherapeutic treatment)

Each of these topics is important, but the discussion in these two chapters will focus on assessment and intervention, with general reference to the preventive and follow-up strategies necessary for a long-range political and social approach that will reduce crises stemming from violence (see Figure 8.1, right circles, Boxes 1 and 3).

Victimization Assessment Strategies

Providers in various entry points to the health and social service system should incorporate questions about possible victimization into their routine assessments. Bell, Jenkins, Kpo, & Rhodes (1994) state that protocols for such assessments should be mandated by law. Table 8.1 presents a victimization assessment scale for use by entry point workers, which is part of the Comprehensive Mental Health Assessment guide discussed in Chapter Three. Exhibit 8.1, Screening for Victimization and Life-Threatening Behaviors: Triage Questions, includes suggested questions for use with this tool as well as with the scale for assessing homicide and assault risk, which is described in Chapter Nine (see Hoff & Rosenbaum, 1994). For an abuse assessment screen designed specifically for use by health professionals working with women, see Soeken, McFarlane, Parker, & Lominack (1998).

As in the case of suicide risk assessment, *no crisis assessment is complete without ascertaining risk and trauma from victimization and assault.* Work with battered women, for example, has uncovered the repeated revelation by survivors seeking help: "No one asked." As the study by Sugg and Inui (1992) suggests, physicians, nurses, and others must move beyond their traditional fear of opening Pandora's box by inquiring about abuse. Just as health assessments now include routine questions about smoking and drinking, so should victimization and violence assessment be routine for anyone in emotional distress or whose symptoms do not readily suggest

FIGURE 8.1.   CRISIS PARADIGM.

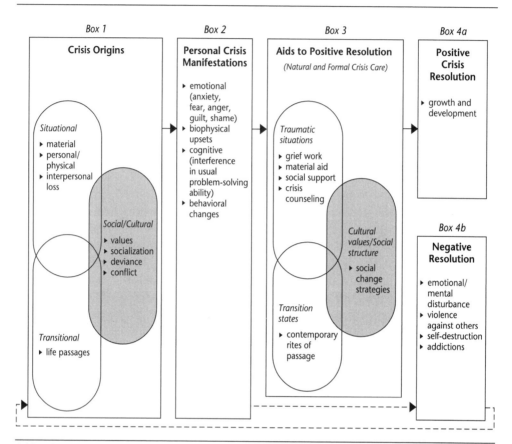

Crisis origins, manifestations, and outcomes and the respective functions of crisis care have an interactional relationship. The intertwined circles represent the distinct yet interrelated origins of crisis and aids to positive resolution, even though personal manifestations are often similar. The arrows pointing from origins to positive resolution illustrate the *opportunity for growth and development* through crisis; the broken line at bottom depicts the potential *danger of crisis* in the absence of appropriate aids. The loop between Box 4b and Box 1 denotes the *vulnerability* to future crisis episodes following negative resolution.

a medical diagnosis. Yet despite national campaigns, screening in primary care protocols for intimate partner and other types of abuse is not yet routine. Questions about suicide and assault potential and resource depletion should be included in abuse assessment protocols because these problems are often secondary to the primary problem of abuse; also, suicide and assault risk may signal the severity of trauma from victimization. As the triage questions in Exhibit 8.1 suggest, such routine inquiry could prevent suicide or murder as desperate responses to victimization trauma.

Once victimization status is identified, it should be followed by in-depth assessment (preferably by mental health professionals with backgrounds in victimology who are also sensitive to gender issues) to ascertain the extent of trauma and the victim-survivor's response (see also Burstow, 1992; Campbell & Humphreys, 1993; Everett & Gallop, 2000; Herman, 1992; van der Kolk, 1987).

TABLE 8.1. VICTIMIZATION ASSESSMENT SCALE.

Key to Scale	Level of Victimization	Typical Indicators
1	No experience of physical violence or abuse	No memory of violence recently or in the past.
2	Experience of abuse/ violence with minor physical and/or emotional trauma	Currently, verbal arguments that occasionally escalate to pushing and shoving or mild slapping. History *may* include past victimization that is no longer problematic or for which a solution is in process.
3	Experience of abuse/ violence with moderate physical and/or emotional trauma	Abused several times a month in recent years, resulting in moderate trauma/emotional distress (for example, bruises, no threat to life, no weapons). History *may* include past victimization that is still somewhat problematic (for example, a sexual abuse incident/overture by a parent or stepparent over 2 years ago).
4	Experience of abuse/ violence with severe physical and/or emotional trauma	Violently attacked (for example, rape) or physically abused in recent years, resulting in physical injury requiring medical treatment. Threats to kill, no guns. History *may* include serious victimization (for example, periodic battering, incest, or other abuse requiring medical and/or psychological treatment).
5	Life-threatening or prolonged violence/abuse with very severe physical and/or emotional trauma	Recent or current life-threatening physical abuse, potentially lethal assault or threats with available deadly weapons. History *may* include severe abuse requiring medical treatment, frequent or ongoing sexual abuse, recent rape at gun- or knifepoint, other physical attack requiring extensive medical treatment.

Child Abuse

The tragedy of child abuse continues, while public debate about related values and social issues escalates.

The Problem

Child abuse can be physical, emotional, verbal, or sexual—any acts of commission or omission that harm or threaten to harm a child (Cook & Bowles, 1980). The biblical expression "spare the rod and spoil the child" suggests a long history of child abuse. De Mause (1975) has written that the "helping mode" in caring for children is of very recent origin and was preceded historically by often widely accepted infanticide and rampant cruelty toward children. The institution of Good Samaritan laws is a legal response to those practices. Although the natural helplessness of children inspires most adults to aid and protect them, societies have

EXHIBIT 8.1.   SCREENING FOR VICTIMIZATION AND LIFE-THREATENING BEHAVIORS: TRIAGE QUESTIONS.

1. Have you been troubled or injured by any kind of abuse or violence? (for example, hit by partner, forced sex)
   Yes _____ No _____ Not sure _____ Refused _____ If yes, check one of the following:
   By someone in your family _____ By an acquaintance or stranger _____
   Describe:

2. If yes, has something like this ever happened before?
   Yes _____ No _____ If yes, when? _____
   Describe:

3. Do you have anyone you can turn to or rely on now to protect you from possible further injury?
   Yes _____ No _____ If yes, who? _____

4. Do you feel so bad now that you have thought of hurting yourself/suicide?
   Yes _____ No _____ If yes, what have you thought about doing?
   Describe:

5. Are you so angry about what's happened that you have considered hurting someone else?
   Yes _____ No _____
   Describe:

found it necessary to have specific laws to protect children. These laws also protect physicians, nurses, and social workers from prosecution for slander when they report suspected child abuse to authorities.

CASE EXAMPLE: RICHARD

A young mother with four children felt overwhelmed trying to care for her five-year-old hyperactive child, Richard. The woman's husband was employed as a hospital maintenance worker but found it difficult to support the family. The family could not obtain public assistance although their income was just above the level to qualify even for food stamps. The mother routinely spanked Richard with a strap several times during the day. By evening, the child was even more hyperactive, so the mother sometimes put him to bed without feeding him. The father and mother mutually approved of this form of disciplining Richard. A neighbor reported the parents of suspected abuse after observing the mother chase and verbally abuse Richard on the street, with a strap poised to spank him.

Child abuse happens in well-to-do families and poor families, in cities, suburbs, and rural areas. No one knows exactly how many children are abused each year because many cases are not reported. Besides the estimated 2 to 4 million abused and neglected children, 2,000 to 4,000 deaths occur annually in the United States at the hands of parents and caretakers. One or both parents or siblings may be involved. In her study of women who killed their children, Korbin (1987) uncovered a dynamic similar to the "cry for help" noted in suicidal people. If their network of relatives and professionals had responded to their behavioral pleas for help, these women would have been "secretly relieved," and perhaps fatal abuse would have been avoided.

There is disagreement on just what child abuse is. Most people agree that some kind of discipline is necessary and that a swat or controlled spanking for playing with fire or running in front of cars is not the same as child abuse. But it is difficult to persuade the average North American that a child can be brought up without physical punishment, in spite of research supporting the negative effects of such punishment (Greven, 1990).

The tragic reality of child abuse gained national attention in North America with the works of Kempe and Helfer (1980) in pediatrics and Gil (1970) in social science; work on childhood sexual abuse followed (for example, Bagley & King, 1990; Everett & Gallop, 2000; Finkelhor, 1984). Most clinicians and researchers challenge single-factor approaches, embracing instead an "ecological" interactive theory and preventive practice in response to the problem.

A tragedy related to child abuse is that of runaway children: 35 percent of these American runaways leave home because of incest and 53 percent because of physical neglect. The majority are never reported missing by their parents; 80 percent are from white, middle-class families; 150,000 disappear each year, many dying of disease, exploitation, and malnutrition (Powers & Jaklitsch, 1989; Russell, 1986).

CASE EXAMPLE: LINDA

Linda, age fifteen, had never told anyone about her father's repeated visits to her room, where he sexually abused her over a four-year period. Linda did not tell her mother because she thought her mother already knew and approved of what was happening. Linda looked forward to leaving home and marrying her boyfriend, age nineteen. One night, her boyfriend raped her; afterward she went into the bathroom and took twenty of her mother's sleeping pills. If her mother had not heard her crying and taken her to the hospital for emergency treatment, Linda would have died.

When dealing with individual cases of child abuse or neglect, especially if the parents were abused themselves or problems with alcohol are involved, it is easy to lose sight of the evidence that child abuse is rooted in the fabric of many societies:

1. Violence as an appropriate solution to problem solving is a culturally embedded value of U.S. society. There is long-standing evidence that the use of violence (such as harsh discipline) trains a person for violence (Gil, 1970; Straus, Gelles, & Steinmetz, 1980). Thus, when a parent uses violent forms of discipline while interpreting it as an act of love and concern for the child,

the child is likely to absorb the value that violence is a socially approved form of problem solving. The embeddedness of the spare-the-rod philosophy was dramatized in the 1999 acquittal of a Boston father whose strapping of his child was defended on religious grounds. More disturbing than the incident itself is the expressed view of large numbers of Americans who support such a court decision.

2. Economic hardship and stress can often be traced to unequal social opportunities in the United States. The national survey on domestic violence (Straus et al., 1980) suggests a clear association between economic disadvantage and child abuse; the difficulty of providing basic necessities as well as special medical and social services for handicapped or sick children is a source of extraordinary parental stress that continues unabated. Such stress is exacerbated by the homelessness now suffered by millions of women and children (see Chapter Twelve).

3. Child care, though necessary for the continuation of society, is socially devalued, as revealed in several practices in the United States: (a) the failure to provide adequate child care for wage-earning parents, (b) the low pay scales for those who do provide child care, (c) the continuing acceptance of child rearing as predominantly the responsibility of mothers, (d) a backlash by childless couples protesting the meager employee tax benefits afforded parents (as compared with Western Europe, for example).

Miller (1986) suggests that if men and women wish to have children, they should also figure out how to take care of them so that the children have the benefit of paternal as well as maternal upbringing (see "Birth and Parenthood" in Chapter Thirteen). However, people who choose to be childless should recognize and support in alternative ways the "work" of child rearing as a necessity that not only guarantees a society's continuity but also benefits *all* its members—including the childless.

Child Witnesses to Violence and Murder

Nationally, over three million children are at risk of witnessing violence between their caretakers. The FBI estimates that men in prison for abuse or even murder of their partners have an average of two or three children each. The adverse effects on children of witnessing violence or just living in a violent home are now viewed as a form of child abuse resulting in many of the same symptoms as if the children were directly abused themselves. A child's trauma from witnessing a parent's murder is almost beyond comprehension—not to mention retraumatization in custody cases in which the imprisoned murderer wants to see his children (see Stephens, 1999). Recent legislation in Massachusetts denies visitation rights in such cases.

Some of the symptoms of child witnesses include withdrawal from friends and activities, sleep disturbances, physical aches and pains, hypervigilance, worrying about the safety of loved ones, hyperactivity, and trouble concentrating, which may be revealed in a loss of skills learned earlier. Support and early intervention with these "silent" victims (Groves, Zuckerman, Marans, & Cohen, 1993) is central to preventing more serious problems later. A Massachusetts Department of Youth Services study of child witnesses revealed dramatic increases in their risk of suicide and abuse of alcohol and other drugs as well as committing sexual assault and other crimes (Henning, Leitenberg, Coffey, Turner, & Bennett, 1996; Moore, 1999; Taylor, Zuckerman, Harik, & Groves, 1994).

Moving from a domestic to an international arena, consider this account of trauma among Kosovo's "children of war":

> You can't see the damage in Jeton's eyes or the shy smile he gives a stranger. . . . He doesn't sleep, he is easily frightened. . . . It [a mortar shell] exploded in the garden. His grandmother, trying to find cover, was hit. The blast knocked out electricity. The family cowered in deep darkness inside their home. They heard Arifa Hasani, 57, a matriarch of five children and 10 grandchildren, gasping in the hallway. Jeton's uncle lit a lighter. In the flickering glow, Jeton saw his bloodied grandmother, dying. [Sennott, 1999, pp. A1, A31]

Though Rwanda's civil war has been less recorded for reasons of global politics, the children there probably are similarly traumatized. To those who seem to know only violence as a solution to human conflict, one could ask: Are ethnic hatred and the desire for power and control really worth the sacrifice of a nation's future—your children?

Refuges for battered women have traditionally included special support for the child witnesses of violent relationships, whether domestic or political. For children who remain in a home where violence persists and the battered parent is either unable or unready to leave, however, every effort should be made to provide special services. Primary care and emergency service personnel are in strategic positions to advocate for such services. Boston Medical Center (BMC), for example, has a publicly supported program, the Child Witness to Violence Project, that abused women should be informed about when receiving medical treatment of injuries at BMC or through public education and outreach efforts.

Big Brothers–Big Sisters programs can be part of alternative support programs. Because many of the child's symptoms may appear in school performance or behavior problems, teachers and school nurses should network with special services for child witnesses. Such collaborative community-based efforts are greatly preferred to removing a child from the home in cases of continued parental violence. Although the intention is to protect the child by such removal, to do so can leave the child with the same kind of guilt that incest survivors usually experience when they, rather than the perpetrators, are removed—that is, they may blame themselves for the disruption (Saunders, 1999).

Preventive Intervention

Preventive strategies are always important in crisis intervention, but they are particularly urgent concerning the tragedy of child abuse. A focus on the social origins of this problem is critical. Preventive intervention includes

1. Critically examining child-rearing practices and incorporating nonviolent approaches to discipline into high school curriculum courses for boys and girls (Brendtro, Brokenleg, & Van Bockern, 1990; Eggert, 1994).
2. Instituting social and political action to relieve the economic hardship and poverty of many families.
3. Instituting social and political action to address substandard child care programs and develop family policies appropriate to the resources and ideals of a nation.
4. Using consciousness raising and education to stress the advantages to individuals and to society of having children reared in an egalitarian fashion by mothers and fathers, as well as by extended family, foster grandparents, and others.
5. Examining government child welfare agencies systematically to ensure that children's problems are adequately attended to before abuse occurs.
6. Instituting public education programs on child abuse and providing in-service training programs for school nurses, teachers, and others working with children.
7. Developing hotlines and drop-in centers for children and adolescents as additional supports and outlets for troubled youth.
8. Instructing children that they own the private parts of their bodies and reassuring them that they have no obligation to satisfy the sexual desires of parents, relatives, or others. (This includes lifting the veil of denial about the sources of greatest danger: in a review of nearly seven hundred child sexual-abuse cases by the Middlesex County, Massachusetts, district attorney's office, only 4.5 percent of the abusers were strangers; 43.1 percent were related to their victims; and the remainder were other relatives, friends, or neighbors; biological fathers were the single largest group of sexual abusers. See Hart, 2000, p. B8.)
9. Renewing commitment to improving the mental health of children as an aid to resisting seduction (Conte, Wolf, & Smith, 1987)—for example, by working with police officers to teach children how to detect and resist would-be abductors.
10. Examining the societal values and economic arrangements that support the idea so many teenage mothers have absorbed—that their most important contribution to society and means of feeling valuable is to produce a baby, irrespective of their emotional, social, and economic ability to care for a child. (A related value is the near disregard of responsibility by teenage, unmarried fathers; see Eyre & Eyre, 1993.)
11. Considering the incalculable pain of children and the thoughtless sacrifice that war demands of these innocents. (Child protection needs to be undertaken on a global scale by adults who wage war on ethnic and other grounds.)

All these preventive strategies demand that we take the time to discover why so many of our children are being abused and neglected. A shift "from care to prevention" was highlighted in the U.S. Surgeon General's Workshop on Violence and Public Health (1986). The fact that Newberger's testimony (1980) before the U.S. House of Representatives is as relevant today as it was decades ago speaks to work still to be done; Newberger emphasized the need to address exploitative sex, isolation, poverty, and a cultural climate that supports violence if we are serious about preventing child abuse and neglect.

Legal and Crisis Intervention

Everyone should be aware of the signs of possible child abuse:

- Repeated injury to a child with unconcern on the part of the parent(s) or with unlikely explanations
- Aggressive behavior that implies a child's cry for help
- Neglected appearance
- Overly critical parental attitude
- Withdrawal, depression, and self-injury (especially with incest)

The serious effects of child abuse include physical handicaps, emotional crippling (an abused child may never be able to love others), homelessness, psychiatric illness, antisocial or violent behavior later in life, self-destructiveness, and death (Everett & Gallop, 2000; Helfer & Kempe, 1987).

Suspicions of child abuse must be reported to child protection authorities, although we should be cautious about making unsubstantiated accusations. A related concern, primarily in longer-term therapy situations, is the controversial "false-memory syndrome" and "therapist-induced memories." Despite this controversy, it is important to *believe* children's stories about abuse. All parents make mistakes; it is the crisis of child abuse and the pattern of abuse that must be reported. In cases of incest, the crisis for the child as well as for the entire family occurs when "the secret" is revealed (Herman, 1981). (See Chapter Thirteen regarding allegations of abuse in child custody battles.)

We can assume that most parents have the welfare of their children at heart. When parents do not appear to be concerned for the welfare of their children, they must be confronted with the reality that children as well as parents have rights. When abuse is suspected, everyone who knows the child must realize that a parent's rights are not absolute. "Minding one's own business" is inappropriate when child abuse is involved, although many people use that as an excuse for not reporting what they suspect.

Teachers are in a strategic position to help an abused child; the school is often the only recourse open to the child (Hillman & Solek-Tefft, 1988). Although teachers are not trained to deal with disturbed parents, they are responsible for reporting suspected child abuse to child protective authorities. Parents who think they are abusive or who are afraid of losing control should be encouraged to seek help on their own by contacting Parents Anonymous, a self-help organization in the United States and England. Hotlines for parents, children, and others concerned about child abuse can be contacted through any crisis or mental health agency or by simply dialing the operator. In mental health and social service settings, early signs of child abuse can often be uncovered through family-focused assessment, as discussed in Chapters Three and Five. The Child Screening Checklist (Chapter Three, Exhibit 3.3) can guide such assessment.

Child abuse is a crisis for the parent as well as for the child; the abused child is often one whose behavior or special needs cause extreme stress, even for the most forbearing parent. Parents in crisis are, unfortunately, sometimes overlooked by health personnel attending a battered child. The tragic situation of treating a helpless, beaten child makes it very difficult for nurses and physicians to recognize the equally great need of the battered child's parents. Whether parents bring the abused child to the clinic or hospital themselves or whether they are reported by nurses, teachers, or neighbors, parents are usually guilt ridden and shaken by the experience. In most cases, they are fearful for the child's life, remorseful about their uncontrolled rage, fearful of treatment at the hands of the law (including loss of custody), and fearful of future outbursts of uncontrollable anger.

If nurses, physicians, and social workers can overcome their own aversion and feelings of rejection, the crisis can become a turning point in parents' lives. Understanding the emotional needs of abusive or neglectful parents is important for doing crisis intervention with them; abusers often have the following characteristics:

- Inability to understand and communicate with children
- Emotional immaturity
- Generally disturbed lives
- Unhappy marriage
- Stress related to economic, unemployment, and housing problems
- Feelings of inadequacy in their role as parents
- Frequent life crises as well as drug and alcohol problems
- Deprived or abused childhood
- Unrealistic and rigid expectations of their children
- Minimal or inadequate parenting skills

Crisis intervention in instances of child abuse includes

1. Encouraging the parent to express feelings appropriate to the event.
2. Actively engaging the parent in planning medical care for the child—a corrective emotional experience that moves the parent in the direction of doing something constructive for the child, as would be appropriate in Richard's case.
3. Enlisting the parents' cooperation with child protection authorities, who have been appropriately informed by a health professional. This includes correcting the parents' probable perception of the government authorities as punitive.

In reality, the people representing such authorities generally are concerned and will help parents carry out their parental responsibilities. This point is important for preventing further tragedies, such as murder of the children by a father accused of incest, as is possible in the case of Linda.

4. Avoiding the removal of an incest victim instead of the assailant from the home. Removing the victim perpetuates the notion that she or he is responsible for the abuse and for the breakup of the family and also alienates the child from the mother (Herman, 1981).

5. Referring the parent to self-help groups such as Parents Anonymous or Parents in Crisis, where they can share their feelings and get help from other parents in similar situations, as would be helpful for the parents of both Richard and Linda (see Chapter Five).

6. Instituting job training and day-care services in cases of economic strain and when a mother is overwhelmed with the care of several children at home by herself, as is the case with Richard's mother.

7. Providing concrete suggestions of nonviolent alternatives to physical discipline, such as isolation or thinking time, for the child and nonviolent stress management techniques for parents. There are excellent books on this topic written specifically for parents (for example, Canter & Canter, 1988; Hillman & Solek-Tefft, 1988; McEvoy & Erickson, 1994).

Follow-Up Service

Follow-up for children abused by their parents or others should include referral of parents to a counseling agency where they can receive more extensive help concerning the underlying emotional and social problems that led to the crisis. Child protection services can facilitate parent counseling if they do not offer it themselves. Role modeling, home supervision, and parent effectiveness training are other services that should be available to these parents. Some child survivors of abuse, physical and sexual, may need extensive psychotherapeutic treatment for healing from the devastating pain of such exploitation (see Everett & Gallop, 2000).

These suggestions for prevention and referral for longer-term treatment by specialists should be incorporated into the protocols of all primary-care providers and frontline crisis workers, including complete documentation of medical examinations for possible legal action. It is never too late to consider ways to eliminate pain and the unnecessary death of our children and to reduce this tragic waste of a nation's most precious resource.

Rape and Sexual Assault

Rape is a violent crime, not a sexual act. Because of people's attitudes toward the crime of rape, the crisis of rape victims has not received appropriate attention until recently. Feminists and others who have become sensitized to the horrors of this crime against women are slowly bringing about necessary changes in a legal system that often causes double victimization of the person who has been attacked. Although most rape victims are female, male victims of rape are sometimes even more reluctant than women to report the rape and seek help.

In a widely publicized rape conviction, the defense attorney outraged the public by declaring on national television that the conviction would never have occurred if he had been allowed to enter into testimony the history of the victim's sex life. Similarly, there was public outcry against a judge who let an admitted rapist off with a light sentence for raping a five-year-old girl because of the girl's "precocious sexual behavior." If a woman is sexually abused or raped by her physician, the chances of successful prosecution are further reduced because (1) the social and political influence of the medical profession is enormous, (2) the average woman thus abused has been seduced into believing the action is part of medical practice, (3) the woman is often afraid to report the incident and cannot imagine that this could happen to anyone but herself, and (4) the woman may have absorbed the message that she invited the rape or did something wrong. This point applies to any professional who violates a position of trust and power (Burgess & Hartman, 1989).

Only recently in North America has rape in marriage been recognized legally as an offense. The cultural notion of woman as the property and appropriate object of man's violence and pleasure still lingers (Russell, 1982). Rape as a common crime of war is finally being recognized and prosecuted in the United Nations war crimes tribunal in The Hague. Fortunately, research findings by Holmstrom and Burgess (1978) and public education have changed the attitudes of most physicians, nurses, and police. This is significant when considering the threat to life accompanying many rapes and the great number of acquaintance rapes (47 percent of all rapes). In date rape, it is often assumed that if a woman says no she does not mean it and that in some way she invited the attack (Levy, 1991). This issue is complicated when women have drunk too much and are victimized by a gang of rapists. The woman's intoxication is used as an excuse to exploit her; college women are particularly vulnerable to such attacks. These are reported least often because of the continued tendency to excuse rapists on grounds of their *victims'* behavior. A survey of thousands of U.S. college students revealed that one-quarter of college women have been victims of rape or attempted rape, and almost 90 percent of the women knew their assailants (Warshaw, 1988). In discussing two campus gang rapes, women made public, victim-blaming statements—for example, "If she hadn't stayed out so late, it probably wouldn't have happened" (students in a college class on sexual assault, 1993). One interpretation of such behavior is that it is a potential victim's means of gaining some control and reducing her own vulnerability: "If *I* don't stay out too late or drink too much, I won't get raped." In Warshaw's study, 50 percent of the men had forced sex on women but did not define it as rape, and only 33 percent said that under no circumstances could they rape a woman (see also Wiehe & Richards, 1995).

We should not, however, be surprised at these responses in a culture in which women are often considered fair game. Recently, psychiatric and general health personnel have responded to the research regarding attitudes of health professionals toward rape victims. These workers are developing rape crisis intervention programs in hospital settings based on principles of equality and a rejection of popular myths about rape.

The fallacy of blaming a woman for her attack because she was "dressed too provocatively" or "out on the street alone" becomes clear in the analogy of a well-dressed man who is robbed of his wallet: no one would say he was robbed because of what he wore. Regarding women who are raped while out at night, we might attend to Golda Meir's response to the curfew proposal for Israeli women at risk of attack: let the men who are raping be curfewed instead.

Another popular myth about rape is that the victim "enjoys rape" and that the average woman entertains fantasies of being raped. This myth was evident at the dawn of a new millennium by a mental health professional at a conference when he proclaimed, "There are two kinds of rape—real rape and those who want it." This notion is reinforced by popular movies such as *Last Tango in Paris*, by hard-core and soft-core pornography, and by advertising images in which women are depicted as appropriate objects of male violence. These myths about rape stem from the persistent interpretation of rape as a sexual event (Thornhill & Palmer, 2000) rather than an act of violence.

Societal attitudes, then, play a major part in the outcome of a rape crisis experience. When rape victims are blamed rather than assisted through this crisis, it is not surprising that they blame themselves and fail to express feelings appropriate to the event, such as anger. Such attitudes also impede the process of long-term recovery (Braswell, 1989).

There is still much to be done to change public attitudes, reform institutional responses to sexual-assault victims, and dismantle the widespread belief that women and girls who are raped are "asking for it." It is instructive to note that many victims fail to report sexual assault because of fear, their perception that police are ineffective, and the threat of further victimization by authorities (Buzawa & Buzawa, 1996; Kidd & Chayet, 1984). Another study revealed that those victims who sought compensation were even more dissatisfied than those who did not, because payment was either inadequate or denied altogether (Elias, 1984, p. 113).

Rape as the Spoils of War

From a human rights perspective, rape as the spoils of war is a gender-based crime, as documented by the United Nations war crimes tribunal and by Brownmiller (1975) in her historical account. The crime of rape has continued over centuries, continues as a very visible phenomenon during wars worldwide, but only now is being addressed in the United Nations court in The Hague. During the 1990s Bosnian war, at least twenty thousand women on all sides were raped. The alleged rationale was to satisfy the sexual needs of men on the battlefield. A woman who testified in the United Nations court said that she and scores of other women were raped in classrooms and apartments, while her detained children became ill from unsanitary conditions. This woman's testimony about damage to her health included sexually transmitted disease, insomnia, severe anxiety, and reproductive dysfunction (Socolovsky, 2000).

A refugee woman from Cameroon and then Liberia, Canada, and the United States describes a triple trauma—watching her son die at the hands of soldiers, as her hands and feet were tied, then beaten to persuade her to talk about her husband, and finally placed in a corner and repeatedly raped (Hartigan, 1999). This woman suffered the additional trauma of social stigma for having been raped, because such women in her culture—as in others—are viewed as unmarriageable. As is true of many survivors of violence, this woman found meaning and healing in telling her story—another small step toward ending the worldwide plague of war in general and violence against women in particular.

Preventing Rape and Sexual Assault

Long-range strategies to prevent rape include dismantling the myths and centuries-old norms that promote the double victimization of women. Such a campaign should cover education, health, social service, and criminal justice systems worldwide, as well as the public at large.

At the individual level, a woman whose life is threatened can do little or nothing to prevent sexual assault. In some cases, however, women can lessen their chances of attack by training themselves to be street-smart—alert at all times to their surroundings when outside. Potential victims should remember that even though crime may appear to be random, the would-be criminal has a plan. That plan includes attacking a person who appears to present the greatest chance of success at the crime with the least amount of trouble. Women and children on the street who are alert and make this evident therefore have, to some extent, equalized the criminal-victim relationship. Signals of an escape plan may be as simple as looking around frequently or carrying a pencil flashlight—cues that alert a would-be attacker that you are not an easy target. The attacker does not know what else you may possess—perhaps mace or karate expertise—and generally will not take unnecessary chances with people who appear prepared to resist. Alertness at home is also important. For example, a fifty-six-year-old woman was raped in her home by a man posing as a delivery man, in spite of a highly organized neighborhood patrol on her street.

Self-defense training is also useful as an immediate protection strategy (Kidder, Boell, & Moyer, 1983). It provides physical resistance ability as well as the psychological protection of greater self-confidence and less vulnerability. However, women should not rely on self-defense excessively because (1) it may lead to a false sense of security and neglect of planning and alertness, and (2) some attackers are so fast and overpower the victim so completely that there may be no opportunity to put self-defense strategies to work.

Preventing the sexual assault of children includes not leaving children unattended, instructing them about not accepting favors—including car rides—from strangers, and keeping communication open, so that a child will feel free to confide in parents about a threat or attack. Just as important is public education about the dangers from those closest to us, a grim reality that is difficult for many to acknowledge.

Crisis Intervention

There is no question that people who have been raped are in crisis (Burgess & Holmstrom, 1979). They feel physically violated, are in shock, and are afraid to be alone. They may fear for their lives or that the rapist will return. Sometimes they feel shame and blame themselves for being attacked. They may or may not feel angry, depending on how much they feel responsible for their victimization. These feelings lead to a temporary halting of their usual problem-solving ability and often to delay in reporting the crime. Rape is sometimes accompanied by robbery and abandonment at the location where the victim was taken by the rapist. Such a series of events further reduces the victim's normal problem-solving ability. Holmstrom and Burgess (1978) have described the crisis and treatment of rape victims; Brownmiller (1975) deals with the historical and anthropological aspects of rape. Emergency and police personnel are referred to these works for more information about rape—that it is a serious crime, that the *victims* of this crime should not also be the defendants, and that medical center protocols should reflect these concepts.

If a sexual assault has occurred, friends, family, strangers, the police, and agency staff may be in a position to offer immediate crisis assistance to the victim. The rape victim is sometimes hesitant to ask family and friends for help, especially in cases of date or acquaintance rape. Helpers should actively reach out in the form of crisis intervention in every instance of sexual assault, regardless of type, the victim's gender, or the victim's sexual identity. The chance of being asked for such help and our success in offering it during crisis depend on our basic attitudes toward rape and our knowledge of what to do. Family members or friends who are unsure of how to help should seek assistance and support from a rape crisis center. The following is quoted from the public information card of the Manchester, New Hampshire, Women's Crisis Line. It contains essential information that anyone (including victims themselves) can use if someone has been raped. Similar information cards are available at hospital rape crisis intervention programs and in police departments.

What to Do If You Have Been Raped

> *Emotional considerations:* A rape is usually traumatic. Call a friend and/or Manchester Women Against Rape (MWAR) for support. A trained MWAR volunteer can provide information, support, and referral, and is willing to accompany you to the hospital, police, and court.

Medical considerations: Get immediate medical attention. Take a change of clothing along to the emergency service of a hospital or to a private physician (the police will provide transportation if you need it). The exam should focus on two concerns: medical care and the gathering of evidence for possible prosecution. You will have a pelvic examination and be checked for injuries, pregnancy, and venereal disease. Be prepared to give enough details of the attack for the exam to be thorough. Follow-up tests for venereal disease about six weeks later and pregnancy are also important.

Legal considerations: Do not bathe, douche, or change clothes until after the exam; that would destroy evidence you will need if you should later choose to prosecute. Try to recall as many details as possible. Call the police to report the crime. Be prepared to answer questions intended to help your case, such as: Where were you raped? What happened? Can you identify the man?

If the victim-survivor does come to an emergency medical facility, emergency personnel should listen to the victim and offer emotional support while carrying out necessary medical and legal procedures. Victims should be advised that there are standard protocols for these procedures that are legally required if charges are to be filed. They should be linked with crisis counseling services. Some hospital emergency departments are staffed with such counselors, and many cities have rape crisis services with crisis hotlines or women's centers. Special services are also becoming more common for rape survivors among gay, lesbian, bisexual, and transgendered groups. Where specialized services do not exist, rape victims should be offered the emergency services of local mental health agencies, which exist in nearly every community.

Crisis counseling by telephone for the rape victim is illustrated in Table 8.2, an interview example.

Follow-Up Service

Women and men who have been raped usually describe it as the most traumatic experience of their life. It should not be assumed, however, that the experience will damage the person for life. Whether permanent damage occurs depends on two factors: (1) the resources available for working through the crisis and not blaming herself or himself for the crime, and (2) the person's precrisis coping ability. A victim who has a supportive social network and a healthy self-concept will probably work through the crisis successfully, find meaning in the suffering, and go on to assist others, as did the woman from Cameroon. For victim-survivors in such circumstances, crisis counseling will usually suffice, and long-term therapy is not indicated. Without support and healthy precrisis coping, though, psychological scarring can occur—for example, becoming paranoid about all men or having difficulty with sexual intimacy. This danger is increased by a rape trial in which the defense lawyer succeeds in making the victim rather than the rapist appear to be the criminal or by one's partner and others' joining the defense in blaming the victim for the attack (Estrich, 1987). In these cases, survivors of rape will probably need longer-term therapy.

TABLE 8.2.   TELEPHONE CRISIS COUNSELING FOR A RAPE VICTIM.

Characteristics of Crisis and Intervention Techniques	Case Example: Telephone Interview Between Victim and Crisis Counselor
Establishing personal human contact	*Counselor:* Crisis Center, may I help you? *Elaine:* I just have to talk to somebody. *Counselor:* Yes, my name is Sandra. I'd like to hear what's troubling you. Will you tell me your name?
Upset, vulnerable, trouble with problem solving	*Elaine:* I'm Elaine. I'm just so upset I don't know what to do.
Identifying hazardous event	*Counselor:* Can you tell me what happened? *Elaine:* Well, I was coming home alone last night from a party. It was late (chokes up, starts to cry). *Counselor:* Whatever it is that happened has really upset you. *Elaine:* (continues to cry)
Expressing empathy, encouraging expression of feeling	*Counselor:* (waits, listens, Elaine's crying subsides) It must be really hard for you to talk about.
Self-blaming	*Elaine:* I guess it was really crazy for me to go to that party alone. I should never have done it . . . on my way into my apartment, this man grabbed me (starts to cry again).
Identifying hazardous event	*Counselor:* I gather he must have attacked you.
Self-blame and distorted perception of reality	*Elaine:* Yes! He raped me! I could kill him! But at the same time, I keep thinking it must be my own fault.
Encouraging appropriate expression of anger instead of self-blame	*Counselor:* Elaine, I can see that you're really angry at the guy, and you should be. Any woman would feel the same, but Elaine, you're blaming yourself for this terrible thing instead of him.
Self-doubt, unable to use usual social support	*Elaine:* Well, deep down I really know it's not my fault, but I think my parents and boyfriend might think so.
Obtaining factual information, exploring resources	*Counselor:* In other words, you haven't told them about this yet, is that right? Is there anyone you've been able to talk to?
Feels isolated from social supports	*Elaine:* No, not anyone. I'm too ashamed (starts crying again).
Expressing empathy	*Counselor:* (listens, waits a few seconds) I can tell that you're really upset.
Failure in problem solving	*Elaine:* (continues crying) I just don't know what to do, I feel like maybe I'll never feel like myself again.
Expressing empathy Assessing suicide risk	*Counselor:* This is a serious thing that's happened to you, Elaine. I really want to help you. Considering how upset you are and not being able to talk with your family and your boyfriend, is there a possibility that you've thought of hurting yourself?

TABLE 8.2. TELEPHONE CRISIS COUNSELING FOR A RAPE VICTIM. (*continued*)

Characteristics of Crisis and Intervention Techniques	Case Example: Telephone Interview Between Victim and Crisis Counselor	
Suicidal ideas only, is reaching out for help	*Elaine:*	Well, the thought has crossed my mind, but no, I really don't think I'd do that. That's why I called here. I just feel so dirty and unwanted—and alone—I know I'm not really a bad person, but you just can't believe how awful I feel (starts crying again).
Expressing empathy Involving Elaine in the planning	*Counselor:*	Elaine, I can understand why you must feel that way. Rape is one of the most terrible things that can happen to a woman (waits a few seconds). Elaine, I'd really like to help you through this thing. Can we talk about some things that you might do to feel better?
Feels distant from social resources	*Elaine:*	Well, yes, I know I should see a doctor, and I'd really like to talk to my boyfriend and my parents, but I just can't bring myself to do it right now.
Supporting Elaine's decision, direct involvement of counselor, exploring resources	*Counselor:*	I'd recommend, Elaine, that you see a doctor as soon as possible. Do you have a private doctor?
Decision	*Elaine:*	Yes, I'll call and see if I can get in.
	Counselor:	And if you can't get in right away, how about going to a hospital emergency service as soon as possible?
	Elaine:	OK, I'll do that.
Obtaining factual information	*Counselor:*	Elaine, I gather you didn't report this to the police. Is that right?
Helplessness, feeling isolated	*Elaine*:	I didn't think it would do any good, and besides, just like with my boyfriend, I was too ashamed.
Obtaining factual information	*Counselor:*	Were your clothes torn, and do you have any bruises from the rape?
	Elaine:	No, not that I'm aware of. I just feel sore all over, so maybe I do have some bruises I can't see. I probably shouldn't have taken a bath before going to the doctor, but I felt so dirty, I just couldn't stand it.
Reinforcing decision, suggestion to reconsider reporting	*Counselor:*	It's really important, Elaine, that you see your doctor soon. You may also want to reconsider reporting the rape to the police.
	Elaine:	I guess maybe you're right.
Exploring continued crisis counseling possibility	*Counselor:*	Elaine, considering how bad you feel about this and that you don't feel up to talking with your parents and your boyfriend yet, would you like to come in to see a counselor and talk some more about the whole thing?
Needs help in reestablishing contact with significant people in her life	*Elaine:*	Not really . . . anyway, I really feel better now that I've talked with you. But I still can't really face my parents and boyfriend.

**TABLE 8.2. TELEPHONE CRISIS COUNSELING FOR
A RAPE VICTIM. (*continued*)**

Encouraging further expression of feeling with significant others, paving way for this through crisis counseling	*Counselor:*	This is a lot to handle all at one time. I'm sure you're going to continue feeling upset, especially until you're able to talk with your boyfriend and parents about it. That's one of the things a counselor can help you with. A counselor can also help you take a second look at the pros and cons of reporting or not reporting the rape to the police.
Mutually agreed-on plan	*Elaine:*	I guess maybe it's a good idea. I do feel better now, but I've been crying off and on since last night, and maybe I'll start crying all over again after I hang up. Besides, I called in sick today because I couldn't face going to work. So I guess I'll stay home tomorrow too and come in and talk to somebody. What time?
Establishing concrete plan mutually arrived at by Elaine and counselor	*Counselor:* *Elaine:* *Counselor:* *Elaine:*	How about 10 o'clock? That's OK, I guess. How are you feeling right now, Elaine? Like I said before, quite a bit better.
Reinforcing of plan	*Counselor:* *Elaine:*	Elaine, I'm really glad you called and that you're going to see a doctor and come here to see someone too. Meanwhile, if you get upset and feel you want to talk to someone again, please call, as there's always someone here, OK? OK, I will. Thanks so much for listening.

In an era of cutbacks in funding for social services, vigilance and advocacy are indicated to ensure the continuation of special services to rape victims. In fact, with the current AIDS crisis, additional services are needed to assist the victim through not only the trauma of rape but also the additional crisis of the threat of infection by HIV (see Chapter Eleven). Peer support groups of others who have been abused are also helpful. The difficulty of undoing the damage of sexual assault highlights the importance of preventing rape in the first place.

Finally, in regard to child victims, it is important not to project our own shock and horror about the crime onto the child. The child should be treated and supported in proportion to her or his own trauma and perception of the event, physical and psychological, not in proportion to our adult view of the attack. Protection, sympathy, and anger are in order but should not be expressed in a way that might cripple a child's future development and normal interaction with others.

Woman Battering

Abused women say they do not expect us to rescue them. Rather, they want health and crisis workers to be there for them and offer support as they seek safety, healing, and a life without violence. They want us to listen to their terror and dilemmas, as the following vignettes depict.

Vignettes from the Lives of Battered Women

One time when he beat me I started to fight back. . . . He threw kerosene
around me and threatened to put a match to it. . . . I never fought back
again . . . just kept trying to figure out what I was doing wrong that he would
beat me that way. There were some good times together, like when we talked
about going to college, and somehow I just kept hoping and believing he
would change.

Before I came to this shelter, I had no idea so many other women were going
through the same thing I was. . . . I used to think the only way out of my situation would be a tragic one—to kill either myself or him. I'd go to my friend's or
mother's house, but I just couldn't make ends meet. I didn't have a baby-sitter,
money, or the physical and mental strength. . . . I was depressed about everything. My mother stuck it out for forty years. I didn't believe in divorce; I believed in marriage. Basically, it was my religion and need for financial support
[that kept me from leaving earlier]. [Hoff, 1990, pp. 31, 69]

Traditionally, it was often assumed that a woman was beaten because the man
was drinking, unemployed, or otherwise under stress or that the woman provoked
his behavior by saying the wrong thing or failing to meet his whimsical demands.
If, for example, a man beat his wife while she was pregnant, it was because
"women are so emotional during pregnancy." It was also claimed that women did
not leave violent relationships because they were not sufficiently motivated and ignored the resources they had. Such conclusions were drawn in spite of the fact
that when the same women sought help from the police, family, friends, or health
or social service professionals, they received little assistance or were blamed by
their confidants. A "resource" is hardly a resource if it provides a negative response
to a woman in crisis.

Now, works such as Dobash & Dobash (1979), Hoff (1990), Schechter (1982),
and Stark and Flitcraft (1996) reveal that legal, health care, and religious institutions have supported and given tacit approval to woman battering by such actions
as the following:

1. *Defining assault on one's wife as a misdemeanor, whereas the same assault on a stranger is
   a felony* and then failing to hold violent men accountable even at this level. This
   situation is changing with better police training. Several class action suits
   brought against large police jurisdictions for failure to arrest and act on abuse
   prevention laws have also helped to effect change (Gee, 1983).
2. *Diagnosing a battered woman as mentally ill and psychiatrically excusing a violent man.*
   This practice was uncovered in 1979 by Stark et al. in a study of 481 battered
   women using the emergency service of a metropolitan hospital. In this study,
   "medicine's collective response" to abuse was found to contribute to a
   "pathological battering syndrome," actually a socially constructed product in
   the guise of treatment (pp. 462–463). Problems such as alcoholism and

depression were treated medically, masking the political aspects of violence. The abused woman was psychiatrically labeled, suggesting that she was personally responsible for her problems, and violent families were treated to maintain family stability. The researchers state that medical and psychiatric agencies have played a major role in the violence related to the political and economic constraints of a patriarchal authority structure (see also Hilberman, 1980; Warshaw, 1989).

3. *Counseling a woman to stay in a violent relationship for the sake of the children,* instead of examining the damaging effects of the violence on the children as well (see Bograd, 1984).

4. *Failing to enforce laws that require equal pay and job opportunities,* making it very difficult for women to support themselves and their children alone.

5. *Failing to provide enough refuge facilities and emotional support for battered women in crisis,* claiming that battering is a private matter between the woman and her husband.

6. *Failing to consider the powerful and complex obstacles a woman faces* when she tries to free herself from violence and blaming the victim instead (Hoff, 1992a, 1993).

Thanks to massive public and professional education campaigns, today most medical and mental health professionals have abandoned the traditional search to uncover what the woman is doing to "provoke" her husband, although the inclusion of effective protocols in primary care is by no means routine.

Although traditional responses to wife battering are damaging enough to women, they are not complimentary to men either. Maintaining simplistic explanations of this complex problem implies that men are less than moral beings. It suggests that they are essentially infants, driven largely by impulse and not responsible for their actions. Hoff's (1990) study supports earlier research (Dobash & Dobash, 1979; Stark et al., 1979) and provides new insights into the *process* of violence between spouses. It suggests that violence occurs not merely as a stress response but as a complex interplay between conditions of biological reproduction and economic, political, legal, belief, and knowledge systems of particular historical communities. These interacting systems produce a *context* in which cultural values, the division of labor, and the allocation of power operate to sustain a climate of oppression and conflict. In such a climate, violence against women flourishes, suggesting a link between the *personal* trouble of individual battered women and the *public* issue of women's status.

Prevention

This sociocultural interpretation of why men are violent with their mates and why many women stay in abusive relationships aids our understanding of the problem. How, though, can this understanding help us deal constructively with the woman who repeatedly calls police and repeatedly receives emergency medical treatment but does not leave the relationship? This cyclic aspect of violence is one of the most complex issues facing police, nurses, physicians, and others trying to help abused women. There is probably nothing more frustrating for a concerned helper than the situation illustrated in the following example.

CASE EXAMPLE: STAYING IN AN ABUSIVE RELATIONSHIP

A woman calls a hotline, afraid for her own life and worried that she might kill her husband if he returns. She says she wants to come to the shelter and wants to know how she can get there, as she has no money. She agrees to a plan to have police come and bring her to a designated place to meet the shelter staff member. The woman never shows up. On follow-up, the shelter volunteer learns that when the police arrived, the woman had changed her mind.

Even people who are sympathetic to the plight of women and eager to help are ready to give up in the face of such apparent resistance to being helped. Such situations make it tempting to blame the victim and assume that if a woman did not like to be beaten, she would take advantage of available help. A helper can avoid falling into this trap by (1) remembering that the issue is much larger than the immediate crisis of a particular woman and (2) realizing that the woman has reasons for staying, whether or not the helper understands or agrees with those reasons. Some of these reasons might be (1) fear of the unknown and how she can manage without her husband's financial support, (2) continued hope and belief that the man will act on his frequent promises and stop beating her, and (3) fear of retaliation—even murder—after she leaves the shelter unless she leaves the area permanently. The experience of women in shelters reveals that some men employ elaborate detective strategies to find a woman who has left. Some who find a woman in a shelter threaten to harm all the shelter residents unless the woman returns. This is why many shelters maintain a secret location.

The complexity of the problem is illustrated further by an analysis of what happens after the first time a woman is beaten. She faces a difficult situation: the first violent incident usually is very shocking to her ("How could he do this to me?") and is followed by the man's elaborate promises never to do it again. The woman believes him and decides not to leave. This apparently rational decision is reinforced by positive, valued aspects of the relationship that the woman wishes to salvage. When the man beats her a second time, he not only has broken his promise but also has distorted her trust and belief in his word into justification for beating her again ("If she didn't think it was all right for me to beat her, she'd leave"). The cycle is reinforced by the man's blaming his behavior on the woman—she doesn't cook right, dress right, or respect him—which she increasingly absorbs and believes and which eventually takes an enormous toll on her self-esteem. This complex interactional process underscores the importance of preventing violence in the first place. Once this cycle begins, it is very difficult to interrupt. Our prevention efforts therefore should focus on the following:

1. *Reinforcing and educating police, health, and social service workers about abuse protection acts,* which in some countries define partner abuse as a crime punishable by law. Through the battered women's movement, these laws have been updated in North American states and provinces. Recent crime legislation in the United States also describes battering as a gender-based civil rights violation. Legal information about battering can be obtained from local shelters, the police, and government offices concerned with this issue.

2. *Examining educational, social, and religious programs for their implicit support of violence* through socialization of boys and men to aggressive behavior and girls and women to passive, dependent behavior (Broverman, Clarkson, Rosenkrantz, & Vogel, 1970; Sadker & Sadker, 1994). This process reinforces the view of wives as appropriate objects of violence.

3. *Instituting campaigns to end the marketing of pornography* and other products of popular culture that portray women as objects and glorify violence against them.

4. *Enforcing the Equal Pay Act,* passed in the United States in 1967, and *improving child care and economic and educational services for women,* so that financial and educational disadvantages do not prevent them from leaving violent relationships.

5. *Instituting communitywide consciousness-raising groups for men and women* and focusing on ways to promote egalitarian marriage or other partnerships and break out of dominant or excessively dependent behavior patterns.

These and other "upstream" preventive strategies should be carried out in tandem with immediate intervention for women in acute crisis (see Figure 8.1, Box 3). (For a detailed discussion of the obstacles faced by abused women and ways these can be removed, see Campbell, 1998; Hoff, 1992a, 1993.)

Crisis Intervention

Assistance during crisis should be available to women from family and friends. However, relatives and friends often view marital violence as a private issue and are reluctant to get involved. They may also be afraid of getting hurt themselves or making things worse.

Vignette from the Life of a Battered Woman

Until I found out about and came to the shelter, I kept thinking I was the only one. I didn't have any idea so many other women were in the same boat. I was so ashamed and kept thinking that it somehow must have been my fault. He told me it was my fault and I believed him—though I still don't know what I did wrong because I was always trying to second-guess and please him so I wouldn't get beaten. [Hoff, 1990, p. 112]

The least a relative or friend can do is to put a woman in touch with local crisis hotlines, which have staff prepared to deal with the problem. Because many battered women call the police and contact emergency medical resources, putting these women in touch with crisis workers is the first and most important thing emergency workers can do after providing medical treatment and safety planning.

Two factors, however, may impede the accomplishment of this task: some women do not acknowledge the cause of their physical injuries, or they provide a cover-up story. There are several reasons for this: (1) the woman may have been threatened by her mate with a more severe beating if she reveals the beating; (2) she may simply not be ready to leave for her own reasons; (3) she may sense the judgmental or unsympathetic attitude of a physician or nurse and therefore not confide the truth. Because of social isolation, prejudice, and fear of deportation, immigrant minority and refugee women who are abused usually face additional impediments to receiving help (Bui & Morash, 1999; Jang, Lee, & Morello-Frosch, 1991; Perilla, 1999). (See also Campbell, 1998, "Part VI: Culturally Specific Clinical Interventions.")

Sensitivity to these factors will help us interpret a woman's evasiveness about her injuries and recognize the implausibility of a cover-up story. Besides physical injuries, a battered woman will show other signals of distress or emotional crisis, as discussed in Chapter Three, and may present with aches and pains or vague symptoms not traceable to specific medical causes (Sugg & Inui, 1992) (see Figure 8.2). Medical and nursing staff who use a crisis assessment tool can more accurately identify and appropriately respond to a battered woman in crisis (see Exhibit 8.1 and the "Service Forms" section in Chapter Three). As is true in dealing with a person at risk of being suicidal, it is appropriate to question a woman directly, which will probably result in her being relieved to know that someone is caring and sensitive enough to discern her distress. And as with suicidal people, if a woman refuses to acknowledge the battering, her refusal may have more to do with our attitude than with her willingness to disclose (Hoff, 1992a).

The important techniques to remember in these situations are (1) withhold judgment, (2) offer an empathic, supportive response, (3) assist the woman with safety planning, and (4) provide the woman with information—a card or brochure with the numbers of hotlines and women's support groups. This seemingly small response is central to the process of the woman's eventual decision to leave the violent relationship (Hoff, 1993). The reason to have confidence in the value of such a response is that a woman feels empowered if she believes others respect her decision, even if it is to stay in the violent relationship for the time being. She also needs explicit recognition from us that ultimately it is her decision that makes the difference and that she can take credit for the decision. Because abused women often feel powerless and unrespected, we should convey to them that they are in charge of their lives (see next chapter and Pence & Paymar, 1986, for details regarding the *power and control wheel*). When a woman *believes* this, it becomes a premise for her eventual action. Thus, although a woman may not be ready for more than emergency medical treatment, she at least has the necessary information if she decides to use it in the future. These principles apply to police officers as well as health workers.

FIGURE 8.2. INTERACTIVE RELATIONSHIP BETWEEN STRESS, CRISIS, AND POSSIBLE ILLNESS IN A BATTERING SITUATION.

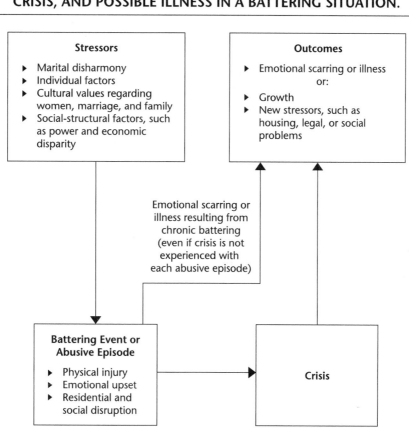

The arrows suggest the interactional relationship between *stress, crisis,* and *illness.* Trouble and stressors in a marriage can lead to positive or negative outcomes through several different routes, depending on personal, social, and economic circumstances.

It is also important to assure abused women that they are not responsible for their victimization, no matter what the person who battered them says to the contrary (see Chapter Two, Figure 2.2). In order to do this, we must be convinced that except in self-defense, violence is not justified no matter what happens in the interaction or the relationship. Even when used in self-defense, a return of violence often escalates rather than decreases the violence (see "Assessing the Risk of Assault and Homicide" in Chapter Nine). In addition, we should not assume that battered women are routinely in need of therapy; this could add a psychiatric label to an already heavy burden (Stark et al., 1979). If a woman is suicidal, the principles and techniques discussed in Chapters Six and Seven apply.

Once a woman is treated for physical trauma and resolves the dilemma of what to do next, she may be faced with the crises of finding emergency housing, caring for her children, and obtaining money. If a community does not have a safe home network or emergency shelter, if a woman cannot stay with relatives, and if she has no money, she may have little choice but to return to the violent situation. In such instances, crisis care providers should assist her in developing a survival plan that includes, for example, having a bag packed and getting a key to a friend's house in case of acute danger. When a woman decides to leave, up-to-date abuse prevention laws require police to accompany her to her home to get her children, legal documents, and whatever possessions she can bring to an emergency housing situation. Once the woman is in a shelter or linked to a support group network, further assistance is available to deal with legal, housing, and other aspects of the crisis (NiCarthy, 1989). In many countries, such assistance has been made possible by national coalitions. The 1995 Beijing Women's Conference and the 2000 Beijing Plus 5 Conference proceedings are valuable sources for organizing such coalitions and action groups (see United Nations, 1996b).

When a woman is battered, her children are affected as well (as discussed in the child abuse section). An important element of helping a mother in crisis, as well as her children, is making child care services available. The mother needs time away from her children to deal with housing and other problems. The children are often highly anxious and in need of a stable, calming influence as well as appropriate physical outlets and nonviolent discipline (see Ericksen & Henderson, 1992; Gary & Campbell, 1998; Humphreys, 1998; Jaffe, Wolfe, and Wilson, 1990).

Follow-Up Service

When an abused woman has successfully dealt with the crisis aspect of her situation, the biggest decision she faces is whether or not to leave her partner permanently. Some women take months, even years, to make this decision, even after living in a safe environment for some time. Peer support groups of other women who have been battered and have broken out of violent relationships are probably the most valuable resource for a woman at this time. Such groups are important for several reasons:

1. If a woman decides to return to her partner, hoping for a change, and the battering continues, it is important that she knows there are people who will not judge her for her decisions.
2. Many women come to shelters convinced that they are psychologically disturbed and in need of a therapist. They have absorbed the message that the battering occurred because of something wrong with them. When they begin to feel strong and in charge of their lives, they may discover that a therapist is not needed after all and that other women can help them in ways they had not imagined. This discovery is a significant contrast to the traditional

view of other women as "competition" in what many perceive as the all-important life task of catching and holding a man. Finding alternatives to therapy occurs most often in shelters or support groups that actively encourage women to assume charge of their lives. It also happens through the process of decision making and taking action to obtain housing, money, and legal services. Observing women in responsible, independent, collaborative, and caring roles in shelter staffing also seems to help. After feeling powerless for so long, a woman does not need a program that dictates every hour and detail of her life.

3. These support experiences may provide the basis for abused women to join, if they wish, a wider network of women working on the larger social, political, and economic aspects of stopping violence against women. A woman's positive experience of support while in crisis is the best preparation for possible involvement in such social change activity.

If women request therapy, referrals should be made to therapists working from a woman's perspective (for example, Burstow, 1992; Everett & Gallop, 2000; Mirkin, 1994). Therapy may be indicated if, after crisis intervention and social network support, a woman continues to be depressed and suicidal or finds herself unable to make decisions and break out of patterns of dependency and self-blame (see Counts, 1987; Stephens, 1985). When the violent marriage and abuse of the children have left damaging scars, family therapy is indicated.

Other aspects of follow-up include

- An opportunity for the woman to grieve and mourn the loss of a relationship if she finally decides to leave (see "Loss, Change, and Grief Work" in Chapter Four)
- For women who wish to marry again, a group in which to examine and share with others the complex aspects of avoiding relationships that may lead to a repeat of excessive dependency and violence
- Parent effectiveness groups to explore nonviolent ways of dealing with children

Crisis Counseling with an Abused Woman

The preventive, crisis, and follow-up aspects of helping abused women should be practiced with a view to their vital connectedness. This triple approach to the problem may not only help end the pain and terror of women who are attacked but may also remove the negative consequences of violence for children, men, and the entire society (Hoff, 1990). The following case is an example of how crisis counseling with a battered woman might proceed.

CASE EXAMPLE: SANDRA LE CLAIRE

Sandra Le Claire is a twenty-two-year-old woman who is currently separated from her abusive husband of five years. She is the mother of two small children, ages two and five. She does not work for pay and is in the process of applying for welfare. Her husband has been her sole source of financial support, and since their separation nine months ago, his support has been sporadic at best. Sandra's visit today is one of several she has made to an emergency department. She presented with cuts and bruises about her face and across her chest and two black eyes, which are swollen shut—all as a result of a beating by her husband. Sandra says this beating was the culmination of an argument over her husband's lack of financial support to her and her children. She has never been willing to press charges against her husband out of fear, as he has threatened to kill her; nor has she ever retaliated with violence herself. She has been drinking more frequently and heavily and is becoming increasingly depressed and despondent about her situation. Sandra has suicidal ideation but denies having a specific plan, although in the past she has thought about taking an overdose of Tylenol when upset with her husband. She says her children have not witnessed any of the abusive episodes.

Sandra became pregnant at age sixteen. She quit high school to get married. She grew up in poverty, the youngest of five children with an alcoholic father and a born-again, church-going mother. She viewed her marriage as a way out.

Although her father worked steadily, he did not earn enough money to support both his family and his drinking. Her mother did not believe in divorce. She raised the children and largely ignored her husband's drinking, sustaining many beatings herself at his hands. Though Sandra feels supported by her mother, who helps her with child care, she does not feel understood. Her mother believes God will provide. She tells Sandra it is just a phase that men go through and that things will improve for Sandra, as they have for her, since Sandra's father has grown less violent over the years. Sandra is not sure she can wait.

Sandra's first language is Haitian Creole; her second is English. She has problems with getting welfare because she cannot complete the forms. Her abusive husband is also a drinker. Sandra had no drinking problem prior to abuse.

Session One

Using the Comprehensive Mental Health Assessment form presented in Chapter Three, the problems and issues Sandra faces could be summarized as follows:

- Safety
- Suicidality
- Problem solving
- Financial support
- Substance use and abuse
- Goals and decisions regarding marriage
- Social support

Exhibit 8.2 illustrates these issues and the action plan that Sandra and the crisis worker developed as a service contract (as presented in Chapter Four) in her first crisis counseling session. Such a session would occur following initial assessment and referral by a triage nurse and the physician or nurse practitioner treating Sandra's injuries. Typically, the full crisis assessment is done by a crisis team member, usually in liaison with triage nurses and physicians. At Boston Medical Center, for example, this function is carried out by psychiatric nurses; at the Ottawa General Hospital, crisis counseling is done by social workers. Crisis counseling as illustrated here is also done by family practice physicians and advanced practice nurses across specialties. Although session one focuses on assessment and developing a service contract, it does not conclude without an explicit plan around safety issues (items 14, 20, and 21) that might need implementation between sessions one and two.

The following are illustrations of how crisis counseling might proceed on behalf of Sandra. In general, the sessions are balanced between structure, an aid to making order out of the chaos of trauma, and openness, which facilitates compassionate regard and empowerment. Typically, there would be six to ten sessions, with attention to the interface between crisis and chronic problems, as discussed in Chapter Five.

Session Two

In the second session, the counselor would set out these plans and goals:

- Explore feeling state and urgent issues, including effects of abusive climate on children
- Review safety and progress with action planned from last session
- Examine barriers to progress with planned action
- Identify any new problems
- Negotiate new or revised action plan for problem solving

The following progress notes and action plan might come out of the session:

Progress Notes

- Feels less despondent and suicidal
- Does not want to go to a shelter, at least not now
- Discussed women's support group as alternative
- Feels ambivalent about restraining order on husband
- Drinking about the same
- Did not call substance abuse treatment source
- Did not go to welfare office; would like someone to go with her

Action Plan

- Continue crisis intervention plan for suicide prevention
- Continue journal regarding drinking pattern; rethink calling AA or other treatment source
- Call advocate and arrange visit to welfare office; also discuss nature of battered women's support group during outing to welfare office with advocate

EXHIBIT 8.2. SERVICE CONTRACT: A BATTERING SITUATION.

Date: _____

Code: _____

1. Physical health	8. Decision-making ability
2. Self-acceptance/self-esteem	9. Problem-solving ability
3. Vocational/occupational	10. Life goals/spiritual values
4. Immediate family	11. Leisure time/community involvement
5. Intimate relationship(s)	12. Feelings
6. Residential/housing	13. Violence/abuse experienced
7. Financial security	14. Injury to self

15. Danger to other(s)	
16. Substance use/abuse	
17. Legal	
18. Agency use	
19. Relationship with abuser	
20. Safety—self	
21. Safety—children	

Stress Rating Code: 1 = low stress/very high functioning   5 = high stress/very low functioning

Item/Stress Rating	Problem/Issue Specification	Strategies/Techniques (planned actions of client and health provider)
20. Safety—self (5)	Husband threatened to kill her	*Explore* (a) shelter option, (b) changing locks, (c) restraining order, (d) feelings regarding use of these options.
13. Violence/abuse experienced (4)	Does not seem clear about extent of danger	*Provide information about* (a) shelter number and admission process (brochures/cards), (b) emergency phone number.
14. Injury to self (3)	Suicidal ideation/no specific or past attempts	*Discuss/listen* to feelings of hopelessness and reluctance to confide in close friend. *Provide* number of suicide prevention/crisis hotline.
12. Feelings (4)	Increasingly depressed	*Sandra agrees to* (a) call/reconnect with friend within 3 days, (b) dispose of her supply of Tylenol, (c) call hotline if very despondent and feeling impulse to take pills.

Need (priority)	Assessment	Intervention
7. Financial security (4)	Husband/abuser is sole source of support	*Explore* Sandra's ambivalence regarding financial aid versus continued attempt to obtain support from husband.
	Has language trouble with welfare forms	*Review* the welfare application forms to ascertain Sandra's understanding.
16. Substance use/abuse (3)	Never drank before battering	*Discuss* feelings about referral to substance abuse treatment program.
	Now drinking more frequently	*Provide* names, dates, places of local accessible programs.
		Sandra agrees to (a) choose and phone one source, (b) keep a journal record of drinking context and other possible options when upset.
9. Problem-solving ability (3)	Uses alcohol and considers drug overdose in response to abuse	*Agree to discuss* other 2 priority items (goals/decisions about marriage and social support) during second or later session.
		Engage Sandra in decision counseling around abuse and safety issues.
		Explore alternative coping devices.
21 Safety—children (3)	No direct witnessing but living in climate of violence	*Protect* children from witnessing conflict situation.
		Discuss adverse effect of domestic violence on healthy development.
		Identify protective measures for children in conflict situations.

Signatures: Client _____

Crisis Worker _____

Remaining Sessions

Each of the remaining sessions would include

- Identification of any urgent issues, particularly safety of self and children
- General review of mood
- Review of progress with previous action plan
- Identification of any new problems and barriers to progress
- Decision counseling around any issues identified
- Negotiated plan for next steps, strategies, and actions regarding problems, including time and place of next appointment

Possible Problems, Issues, and Barriers to Progress

As crisis counseling proceeds with Sandra, new problems and issues may emerge— for example,

1. *Indecision and ambivalence about divorce.* Sandra may say, "I don't want to be one of those welfare mothers," or "if only he'd get some help for his drinking," or "maybe if I were just more patient when he gets angry."

Action plan: Listen to feelings and fears; discuss pros and cons regarding separation, divorce, and future safety; explore level of financial support (husband, welfare, self); consider possibility of job training; discuss self-blame and issue of accountability for violence.

2. *Need for social support.* Sandra feels lonely, wishes her mother were more understanding; advocate gave her information about a battered women's support group, but she does not feel like going; would rather be able to communicate better with her mother; feels ashamed to have her problem known beyond her family.

Action plan: Explore feelings of shame; reconsider calling AA as an alternative source of support; explore possibility of a joint session with mother to air issues, goals, and possible further support.

Husband Beating

This discussion is incomplete without attention to the controversial issue of husband beating. Women as well as men can be violent; not to acknowledge this fact is equivalent to viewing women as less than moral beings, in the same way that excusing male violence implies that men are less than moral beings. Women, like men, should be held accountable for their behavior.

It has been suggested that the "real" domestic problem is husband battering and that the reason it is still hidden is because it is too much of an assault on the male ego to acknowledge the shame of having been beaten by a woman. A national survey in the United States on domestic violence revealed that in *numbers* of violent acts—*not in quality or context*—women and men were approximately equal (Straus, 1993; Straus et al., 1980). This statistical finding, however, needs to be qualified: when women are violent, it is primarily in self-defense, and their attacks are not as dangerous or physically injurious as those of men (Kurz, 1993). Since then, survey research has been refined (for example, Johnson, 1998), and there is progress in undertaking nonexploitative research on this topic. In addition, when women kill their mates, it is usually after years of abuse, and they do so less frequently than men kill their wives (Browne, 1987; Jones, 1980). Considering also the fact that at least 25 percent of pregnant women have a current or past history of being battered, the contrast is even more dramatic (McFarlane, Parker, Soeken, & Bullock, 1992).

The pattern of injustice and violence used primarily in self-defense should be kept in mind in trials of women who kill abusive husbands. Rather than medicalizing the woman's case by using a contrived insanity plea, women should have a fair trial on self-defense grounds when the evidence points in that direction. The suggestion that husband beating is more rampant than wife battering covers up the roots of violence against women in traditional social structures and the low socioeconomic status of women that allows violence to flourish. To claim an equal problem of husband battering belies reality, especially as it is revealed in emergency settings and in the differences in physical strength between most men and women. The majority of men are physically more capable of inflicting injury than are women. In addition, men who are beaten have much more freedom to leave because of their socioeconomic advantage in society and relative freedom from child care. Men who are abused by their partners should nevertheless receive the same medical care and social support as recommended for women.

Battering of Lesbian, Gay, Bisexual, and Transgendered Partners

Prevention and intervention strategies for abused heterosexual partners apply to those in lesbian, gay, bisexual, or transgendered relationships. Additional factors to be considered arise from the bias and social isolation faced by most of these couples; individuals in these relationships usually rely more heavily than others on their partners for emotional support and companionship. As discussed in Chapter Five, excessive dependency in any intimate relationship may be the source of additional stressors that constitute the context in which abuse occurs. In addition, gay men are more vulnerable than lesbian women to violence from strangers or associates who are motivated explicitly by antigay bias or homophobia.

The extraordinary stress experienced by couples in alternative lifestyles is compounded by stereotypes and the bias that keeps them isolated in the first place. One such stereotype is that all lesbians are feminists, and because a battering lesbian partner has violated the feminist agenda of nonviolence, she is thereby deemed less deserving of help. Another stereotype is that women become lesbians because they have been victims of sexual abuse. In reality, not all lesbian women are feminists, and some feminists are just as homophobic as others are. In fact, many women have been sexually abused as children; most of them are heterosexual. Finally, because lesbian, gay, bisexual, and transgendered people are members of a larger cultural community just as others are, why would they be exempt from having absorbed the pervasive message of violence as a control strategy and a solution to conflict resolution? Their disadvantaged social position may result in greater sensitivity to issues of abuse generally, but they face even greater odds in avoiding violence than the general population.

To provide appropriate service for victims in alternative lifestyles, it is imperative that crisis workers examine attitudes that can prevent battered lesbian, gay, bisexual, or transgendered partners from disclosing their plight and receiving the help needed. In general, the legacy of victim-blaming experienced by battered women is exacerbated with regard to those in sexual orientation minority groups (Renzetti, 1992). Major cities in Canada and the United States now have publicly established groups addressing violence among these minority groups—for example, in Boston, the Violence Recovery Program at the Fenway Community Health Center. State and provincial offices for victim assistance can provide information about local services for these groups (see also the World Wide Web in English and Spanish).

Abuse of Older Persons

Attention to abuse of older people is gaining increasing international attention (MacLean, 1995; McDonald et al., 1991; Pillemer & Wolf, 1986).[1] Elder abuse includes willful infliction of physical injury or debilitating mental anguish, financial exploitation, and unreasonable confinement or deprivation of necessary care and services. Earlier, public attention was focused on abuse and substandard care in nursing homes. In spite of the prevalence of institutional care of some older people in the United States, the majority of seniors (95 percent) live alone or with family or other caretakers. The victims are overwhelmingly female, with 58 percent of women victims naming their spouse as the attacker and 24 percent naming a son or daughter as the aggressor (Pillemer & Finkelhor, 1987). Although abuse and neglect may occur in institutions, legal protections limit such abuse. In private settings, legal protections are more difficult to enforce because of civil rights and family privacy issues (Advocacy Centre for the Elderly and Community Legal Education Ontario, 1991). This discussion is particularly relevant to community health nurses, home health aides, pastors, and other professionals offering consultation and supervision on behalf of older people cared for at home.

---

[1] The terms *older persons, elders,* and *seniors* are used interchangeably.

Why are elders abused? As already noted, there are parallels between battered children and abused seniors: (1) they are in a dependent position for survival; (2) they are presumed to be protected by love, gentleness, and caring; (3) they are a source of emotional, physical, and financial stress for the caretaker, particularly if the older person is physically or mentally impaired (Sommers & Shields, 1987).

Several other factors can be identified in tracing the roots of elder abuse. Inattention to these factors can form obstacles to prevention, crisis intervention, and follow-up service for older people at risk.

1. *Social factors.* In the contemporary nuclear family structure, there is often no social, physical, and economic room for elders. For example, death rituals in traditional African societies include transfer of social responsibility held by the deceased (Goody, 1962; see Chapter Thirteen). In modern societies, an older person's body may linger long after social death occurs. Responsibility for the care of older people is complicated by the trend of women working outside the home while maintaining their traditional home responsibilities.

2. *Cultural factors.* U.S. society is noted for idolizing youth. The cultural emphasis on economic productivity tends to eclipse elders' contributions of wisdom, life experience, and often continued work. Consequently, seniors often lack status, respect, and similar rewards that are taken for granted in other societies. The culture of violence as it affects children and women flows over to seniors as well; older, abused women are referred to as "forgotten victims." In spite of elders' increasing political influence, ageism is still rampant, particularly with respect to older women (Doress & Siegal, 1987).

3. *Economic factors.* The poverty of many old people is an almost inevitable result of the social and cultural factors noted previously. Strong economic motives for protecting children often do not extend to seniors. In addition, spiraling inflation for caretakers and inadequate home care services increase further the risk of elder abuse (Estes, 1986).

4. *Psychological factors.* One of the normal features of growing old is a decreased capacity to control impulses and adjust to change. A lifelong pattern of inflexibility can result in a demanding, unpleasant personality in old age. Considering also the interaction between physical dependence and fear of retaliation, elder abuse can remain hidden for some time. Elders abused by adult children—not unlike battered women—will feel deep shame and try to account for the abuse in terms of their own failure as parents. They say, in effect, "What kind of a parent am I that my own child would turn on me in my helplessness and old age?"

5. *Legal factors.* Civil liberties in democratic societies protect one's right to privacy, self-determination, and the refusal of services. Although most jurisdictions now have adult protective service authorities, not all require mandatory reporting of suspected elder abuse cases, as they do in cases of suspected child abuse. These factors, combined with an abused elder's shame and fear of retaliation, constitute formidable barriers to dealing effectively with elder abuse.

Prevention, Crisis Intervention, and Follow-Up Service

As with other crises, prevention, crisis intervention, and follow-up are interrelated and demand awareness of the origins of the crisis. Preventive measures related to the sociocultural and economic aspects of elder abuse suggest an examination of values regarding old people. Social and political changes affecting seniors are also needed, such as provision of tax and insurance benefits for families who would care for an older person at home if they could add a room to their house and obtain home health care assistance without serious financial hardship. Psychologically, we can reduce the risk of elder abuse by preparing for the social, economic, and physical realities of later life (see Chapter Thirteen for a detailed discussion). As we prepare for old age, it is wise to remember that old people with unpleasant personalities are the same as young people with unpleasant personalities, except that changing undesirable habits can be more challenging as we grow older.

Crisis intervention for older people at risk of abuse demands careful application of the assessment, planning, and intervention strategies discussed in Chapters Three, Four, and Five, with particular attention to social network approaches. Emergency medical care and crisis intervention for abused elders are complicated for two reasons:

1. *Mental incapacity or confusion on the part of the elder.* State and provincial departments of mental health and elder affairs have standard protocols for these cases. Involuntary commitment or appointment of a legal guardian requires clear and convincing evidence that the adult in question is cognitively impaired and that an emergency exists. When these legal actions are taken, they should be based on the principle of *least-restrictive alternative* and the guarantee of civil liberties.

2. *Misplaced emergency care or crisis intervention.* Carelessness in this area of care for older people or the use of inappropriate savior tactics can alienate family members, who may be needed in the long term. Considering shame, possible retaliation, and the dynamics of family loyalty, follow-up after the emergency as well as future crisis intervention will be very difficult if family members are alienated. Unless foster care is readily available, great care must be taken to prevent complicating further an already difficult situation. Thus, although laws now exist for reporting elder abuse—similar to the Good Samaritan laws protecting children—overzealous action on these laws should not become the occasion for precipitating more trouble.

In both situations, primary care providers treating older persons in crisis or presenting with mental confusion need to carefully ascertain whether neuropsychiatric symptoms and cognitive incapacities can be traced to drug reactions or the interactive effects of the medications prescribed for some. In these complex cases, consultation should be sought from gerontology and psychopharmacology specialists.

Application of Intervention and Follow-Up Principles

The following example reveals the intersection of caretaker stress and elder abuse. It also shows the importance of careful teamwork in responding to such abuse.

CASE EXAMPLE: MARTHA

Martha, age eighty-two, suffered from crippling arthritis and heart disease. She was visited regularly in her daughter's home by a home health aide, who bathed her three times a week. The rest of the time her daughter, Jane, age fifty-five, gave her medicine and helped Martha out of bed into a chair when she had time. Jane worked full-time as a legal secretary. Jane's husband, Robert, age sixty-three, was home most of the day. He had been on disability support for ten years, after seriously injuring his back doing construction work. For the most part, Robert felt useless, although he did help with shopping and laundry. The disabilities of both her mother and husband left Jane feeling very stressed.

The home health worker discovered black and blue marks on Martha's chest and back and suspected that abuse was occurring. Her attempts to talk to Martha about this were met by silence. The aide reported her observation to the visiting nurse, who in turn consulted a social worker. (The nurse had known this family for over a year and visited the home approximately once a month in a supervisory, coordinating, and teaching capacity). The nurse then called Jane and suggested she be seen by the social worker to discuss the problems of taking care of her mother. Even though the nurse did not directly mention the suspicion of abuse, Jane felt threatened, refused to act on the suggestion, dismissed the nurse and home health aide, and hired a private nurse to care for Martha around the clock to "prove" she was not neglectful of her mother. This move was a great financial burden for the family. Three months later, Jane again requested service for her mother from the home health agency.

Several things seem very clear in this example: (1) everyone concerned appeared to be well intentioned; (2) Jane was alienated by the approach used by the nurse; (3) the problem was complicated by an inappropriate intervention strategy. The nurse seemed to lack confidence in her ability to take on a key role in intervention; she assumed that a social worker was the more appropriate person to act, in spite of her own yearlong relationship with the family.

Success in dealing with sensitive issues like these depends very much on the quality of the relationship between the caregiver and the recipient. If the nurse had recognized this, she would not have suggested what Jane interpreted as an accusation that she neglected her mother. Instead the nurse might have used other intervention and follow-up strategies:

1. After hearing the aide's report, the nurse could have planned an extra visit to the home to spend some time with Martha and Jane individually to further assess the situation. To facilitate communication about the issue, the nurse might

have bathed Martha herself once as a way of gaining her confidence. A concerned rather than an accusatory approach to Jane might have resulted in Jane's revealing voluntarily the stress and exasperation she experienced in carrying out her multiple responsibilities. Their conversation might have proceeded as follows:

Nurse: How are things going, Jane, with all the things you have to juggle these days? I know that Terri, the aide, has been coming in three times a week. Do you think you're getting all the help you need?

Jane: Well, it's hard, but somehow I'm managing. On the days I have to get mother out of bed myself, I sometimes feel like a nervous wreck. She screams with pain when I touch her. I can't stand the thought of putting mother in a home, but sometimes I don't know.

Nurse: So it seems things are pretty rough for you, Jane? I was in to see your mother this week while Terri was bathing and dressing her, and I noticed several black and blue marks. *[Nurse tries to keep the aide's relationship with the family intact.]* She wouldn't talk about it though, so I'm wondering whether things are getting too difficult for you and if maybe we could be of more help to you.

Jane: If you're thinking I hit my mother, well, I didn't. A couple of times I might have handled her kind of roughly; she's really frail and thin, you know. But I certainly never hit her. After all, she's my mother.

Nurse: This is a really touchy thing to talk about, Jane, and I don't mean to accuse you of anything. I know it must be very difficult at times. What I'm suggesting is that we work on this together to be sure both you and your mother get what you need. I know that you want the best possible care for your mother, and it seems like Robert's disability might wear on you, too. Can you tell me more about the problems you have in taking care of your mother?

Problem exploration continues in this vein; the session ends with agreement to talk again the next week to work on the problem that had been uncovered. It never becomes explicit whether Jane did or did not abuse her mother. It is not a good strategy to try to prove that abuse occurred when the old person is refusing to talk and the caretaker is denying it. It is more important to focus on the underlying issues related to abuse.

2. If, after this, the nurse still does not feel confident about proceeding, she might consult the social worker but not turn the problem over to her.

3. The nurse might also talk with Jane's husband to see whether he might become more helpful with household tasks.

4. After exploring the problem with everyone concerned, a social network conference might be indicated (see Chapter Five). This would include Martha, Jane, Robert, Terri, and possibly a social worker consultant and a representative from respite services, which should be discussed as one avenue of relief for Jane.

As the proportion of elders in the population increases, there is hope for favorable political change for elder affairs. With increasing public sensitivity to the problems of seniors, we may devise more creative ways to foster the conditions for peace, safety, and health and for social services during the later years. Changes are already occurring with New Age families, the foster grandparent program, intergenerational housing experiments, and comprehensive health and other services delivered in home settings. The latter include, for example, around ten people of various ages, with 60 percent over sixty, living in a large, ordinary family home. Each person has a separate room; other areas and general tasks are shared communally. Elders who participate in these programs feel socially useful, with beneficial effects for physical and mental health and less chance of violence directed against them.

Battering of Parents and Teachers by Children

The abuse of infirm and dependent elders by adult children differs from another aspect of violence in families—the physical abuse of parents by their minor children. A national survey by Straus et al. (1980) revealed that almost 10 percent of children ages three to eighteen attacked their parents. Clinicians and others note the increasing number of parents and teachers who fear attacks by children and adolescents. Parricide, the most extreme form of parental assault, is usually associated with severe parental sexual and physical abuse of the child (Mones, 1993). Some abusive teenagers may be responding to parents who are excessively permissive and indulgent. Some parents act from the misguided belief that acceding to a child's demands for extra privileges and material things will result in the child's improved behavior. A common example is paying children for performing tasks that should be a normal contribution to the common good by every household member who benefits from the whole. A more extreme example is buying an adolescent a luxury car for the good behavior that should be expected without elaborate rewards. Experience in mental health practice with out-of-control adolescents suggests just the opposite result of what parents anticipate from their indulged children. The probable reason is that the adolescent feels insecure and entrapped when forced, through lack of parental authority and leadership, to assume an independent role before feeling developmentally ready.

Parents experiencing abuse by their children are in a catch-22 dilemma: as with their elder counterparts, confronting the situation implies an admission of failure at parenting; not confronting it reinforces the child's misplaced sense of omnipotence and need to control others (Harbin & Madden, 1979, p. 1290).

Preventive strategies are similar to those discussed for child and elder abuse: at the societal level, fostering nonviolent solutions to child rearing and greater respect for seniors can reinforce parental authority. Crisis and follow-up strategies include parent effectiveness training or if necessary family therapy. In addition, parents should have access to help during crisis without shame or denial of the problem. Crisis intervention planning with such families should feature nonviolent tactics that a child can use when angry at a parent. Parents, too, need alternatives to giving in to children who behave like dictators (Charney, 1993).

Parents, however, are not the only ones abused by violent children. For years, teachers have been terrorized, raped, knifed, and attacked in other ways (Walker, 1993). The same issues are at play here: social and cultural approval of violence, poverty, racism, loss of respect for parental and other authority, and the need to listen to children. The widespread neglect of inner-city public schools and the disadvantages to students who attend them must also be remedied if we wish to stem the large-scale loss of disaffected, traumatized, and burned-out teachers. Poorly supported schools cannot be solely responsible for the intellectual and moral training of children (Long & Wilder, 1993).

In many communities, a violence prevention curriculum has been instituted (Eggert, 1994). Teens are taught nonviolent approaches to conflict resolution, and troubled teens and their families are referred to hotlines and other crisis intervention services (see Brendtro et al., 1990, for an educational and developmental approach to troubled youth).

Other Sources of Victimization

In addition to abuse from one's own family or spouse, there are many other sources of violent crime. Public opinion polls reveal continued concern about crime (especially the dramatic incidents of school shootings), even though the U.S. Justice Department crime statistics show declining rates. People are angry and afraid. They blame their unease on the media, the courts, television, stressed families, pornography, the economy, drugs, poor housing conditions, indifference to the poor, racial tension and discrimination, poverty, youth gangs, the police, handguns, and the disintegration of the American family. In the United States, there are nearly as many firearms as there are people, along with widespread denial of scientific evidence showing that the presence of guns *decreases* rather than increases safety. The significantly lower rates of homicide and other assaults in Canada and Western European countries are attributed to stringent gun control laws and related cultural factors. As Jackson (1994, p. 13) notes, nothing will come of public outrage over children killing children "unless the grownups have had enough of guns."

No doubt, each of the factors mentioned plays some part in this complex problem. Fear of crime seems to generate chronic stress, worry, paranoia, and a sense of helplessness. If no arrests are made or criminals receive light sentences or acquittals, victims and the general public often feel that no one cares or that there is no justice. These feelings can lead to alienation, revenge, and a sense of callousness and insensitivity to others. This may account for the popularity among Americans of the death penalty and for the support of prosecuting violent adolescents in adult courts. However, there is a beginning reconciliation movement among the relatives of some murder victims—for example, Crime Victims for a Just Society. Although generally shunned by survivors who seek solace in the death penalty, those seeking alternatives to the death penalty point out that vengeance is a dead end that does not deal with anger and grief (Latour, 2000).

Victim Assistance After a Crime

What is the ordinary citizen's role in assisting victims of crime? In France, such assistance is mandated by law; in the United States, it is not. Should we intervene on the victim's behalf or ignore a crime? In a frequently cited case in New York City, Kitty Genovese was attacked decades ago late one night while people in at least a dozen households listened to her screams. Nobody went to help or even bothered to call the police from the safety of their own homes. In contrast today, many groups of people are organizing neighborhood patrols and other means of coming to the aid of people victimized by crime. Every would-be helper faces the dilemma of whether and how to intervene in a crime. A basic principle of crisis intervention is to protect oneself from getting hurt while assisting others. Although some people voluntarily sacrifice their lives for others, such a sacrifice is neither expected nor demanded. Not intervening out of fear for one's own safety is fair enough. But not to mobilize police on behalf of a victim is a failure to meet the obligations implicit in our common humanity.

There is now a specialty field called *victimology*, complete with journals and professional conferences. Yet at the practical level, many victims of crime still seem cruelly shortchanged in the criminal justice, emergency medical, and crisis service systems. Through federal task forces and the advocacy and lobbying of the National Organization for Victim Assistance (NOVA), many communities now have victim assistance programs, as do some crisis centers. In general, however, there are no constitutional protections for victims, nor is there much special training for police and emergency medical personnel in meeting the special needs of victims. NOVA has been instrumental in improving this situation, particularly through its crisis response team, which offers service in instances of community-wide trauma.

Funding of victim assistance programs is a continuing struggle, as funds are often focused on programs that try to understand and reform the criminal. This is not to say that criminals' needs should be ignored, but the rights of victims should be no less protected than the rights of defendants in a fair justice system. Indeed, the visibility of victims and their needs should benefit even the criminal.

Since the task forces on violence and victimization, federal legislation has supported the development of victim witness and assistance programs in the states. These include the development of self-help groups, the training of victim advocates, and a plan for financial assistance to victims. The U.S. government executive branch even established a national toll-free hotline number for domestic violence victims, 1-800-799-7233. Similar programs have been instituted in Canada, England, and other countries.

Greater attention, meanwhile, should be focused on the needs of victims in emergency medical, police, and criminal justice systems. Victims are people in crisis who should have the advantage of being listened to and helped by workers who are sensitive, knowledgeable, and skilled in crisis intervention. However, emphasizing crisis service does not mean that we should neglect lifesaving physical treatment in a hospital trauma unit. While medical and legal needs are met, psychosocial needs can be addressed as well. Victims therefore need a bill of rights—for example, the right to

- Be informed of the release of a prisoner who has previously harmed them. Most jurisdictions now oblige psychotherapists, for example, to warn potential murder victims of would-be assailants' plans for release (VandeCreek & Knapp, 1993).
- Receive information about protection services.
- Be secure in a court waiting room that is separate from defendants.
- Receive restitution of stolen or damaged property.
- Receive social and psychological support in working through the crisis.

The international attention currently focused on this problem is a hopeful sign for this facet of crisis care.

Summary

People in crisis because of the violence of others suffer emotional and physical injury and are disrupted from their place in society if the violence is from a family member or intimate. In addition to assistance for individual victims of violence, social change strategies are paramount in addressing the culturally embedded values and social practices from which so much violence originates worldwide. Such a tandem approach may eventually reduce the tragic effects of violence for individuals, their family, and society as a whole.

References

Advocacy Centre for the Elderly and Community Legal Education Ontario. (1991). *Elder abuse: The hidden crime.* Toronto: Author.

American Association of Colleges of Nursing. (1999). *Position paper: Violence as a public health problem.* Washington, DC: Author.

Bagley, C., & King, K. (1990). *Child sexual abuse: The search for healing.* New York: Routledge.

Bell, C. C., Jenkins, E. J., Kpo, W., & Rhodes, H. (1994). Response of emergency rooms to victims of interpersonal violence. *Hospital and Community Psychiatry, 45*(2), 142–146.

Besharov, D. (1990). *Recognizing child abuse: A guide for the concerned.* New York: Collier Books

Boddy, J. (1998). Violence embodied? Circumcision, gender politics, and cultural aesthetics. In R. E. Dobash & R. P. Dobash (Eds.), *Rethinking violence against women* (pp. 77–110). Thousand Oaks, CA: Sage.

Bograd, M. (1984). Family systems approaches to wife battering: A feminist critique. *American Journal of Orthopsychiatry, 54*(4), 558–568.

Braswell, L. (1989). *Quest for respect: A healing guide for survivors of rape.* London: Pathfinder Press.

Breines, W., & Gordon, L. (1983). The new scholarship on family violence. *Signs: Journal of Women in Culture and Society, 8,* 490–531.

Brendtro, L. K., Brokenleg, M., & Van Bockern, S. (1990). *Reclaiming youth at risk.* Bloomington, IN: National Educational Service.

Broverman, I. K., Clarkson, F. E., Rosenkrantz, P. S., & Vogel, S. R. (1970). Sex-role stereotypes and clinical judgments of mental health. *Journal of Consulting and Clinical Psychology, 34,* 1–7.

Brown, J. C., & Bohn, C. R. (1989). *Christianity, patriarchy, and abuse: A feminist critique.* New York: Pilgrim Press.

Browne, A. (1987). *When battered women kill.* New York: Free Press.

Brownmiller, S. (1975). *Against our will.* New York: Simon & Schuster.

Bui, H. N., & Morash, M. (1999). Domestic violence in the Vietnamese immigrant community: An exploratory study. *Violence Against Women, 5*(7), 769–795.

Burgess, A. W., & Hartman, C. (Eds.). (1989). *Sexual exploitation of patients by health professionals.* New York: Praeger.

Burgess, A. W., & Holmstrom, L. L. (1979). *Rape, crisis and recovery.* Englewood Cliffs, NJ: Brady.

Burstow, B. (1992). *Radical feminist theory: Working in the context of violence.* Thousand Oaks, CA: Sage.

Buzawa, E. S., & Buzawa, C. G. (1996). *Domestic violence: The criminal justice response.* Thousand Oaks, CA: Sage.

Campbell, J. C. (Ed.). (1998). *Empowering survivors of abuse: Health care for battered women and their children.* Thousand Oaks, CA: Sage.

Campbell, J. C., & Humphreys, J. H. (1993). *Nursing care of survivors of family violence.* St. Louis: Mosby-Year Book.

Canter, L., & Canter, M. (1988). *A proven step-by-step approach to solving everyday behavior problems* (Rev. ed.). Santa Monica, CA: Lee Canter & Associates.

Charney, R. (1993). Teaching children nonviolence. *Journal of Emotional and Behavioral Problems, 2*(1), 46–48.

Coker, A. L., Smith, P. H., McKeown, R. E., & King, M. J. (2000). Frequency and correlates of intimate partner violence by type: Physical, sexual, and psychological battering. *American Journal of Public Health, 90*(4), 553–559.

Conte, J. R., Wolf, S., & Smith, T. (1987, July). *What sexual offenders tell us about prevention: Preliminary findings.* Paper presented at the Third National Family Violence Conference, Durham, NH.

Cook, J. V., & Bowles, R. T. (Eds.). (1980). *Child abuse.* Toronto: Butterworths.

Counts, D. A. (1987). Female suicide and wife abuse: A cross-cultural perspective. *Suicide & Life-Threatening Behavior, 17*(3), 194–204.

Dangor, Z., Hoff, L. A., & Scott, R. (1998). Woman abuse in South Africa: An exploratory study. *Violence Against Women: An International Interdisciplinary Journal, 4*(2), 125–152.

De Mause, L. (1975). Our forebears made childhood a nightmare. *Psychology Today, 8,* 85–88.

Dobash, R. P., & Dobash, R. E. (1979). *Violence against wives: A case against the patriarchy.* New York: Free Press.

Dobash, R. E., & Dobash, R. P. (Eds.) (1998). *Rethinking violence against women.* Thousand Oaks, CA: Sage.

Doress, P. B., & Siegal, D. L. (1987). *Ourselves, growing older.* New York: Simon & Schuster.

Eggert, L. L. (1994). *Anger management for youth: Stemming aggression and violence.* Bloomington, IN: National Educational Service.

Elias, R. (1984). Alienating the victim: Compensation and victim attitudes. *Journal of Social Issues, 40,* 103–116.

Ericksen, J., & Henderson, A. D. (1992). Witnessing family violence: The children's experience. *Journal of Advanced Nursing, 17,* 1200–1207.

Estes, C. L. (1986, June 30). *Older women and health policy.* Paper presented at the Women, Health, and Healing Summer Institute, University of California, Berkeley.

Estrich, S. (1987). *Real rape: How the legal system victimizes women who say no.* Cambridge, MA: Harvard University Press.

Everett, B., & Gallop, R. (2000). *Linking childhood trauma and mental illness: Theory and practice for direct service practitioners.* Thousand Oaks, CA: Sage.

Eyre, J., & Eyre, R. (1993). *Teaching your children values.* New York: Simon & Schuster.

Finkelhor, D. (1984). *Child sexual abuse: New theory and research.* New York: Free Press.

Gary, F. A., & Campbell, D. W. (1998). The struggles of runaway youth: Violence and abuse. In J. C. Campbell (Ed.), *Empowering survivors of abuse: Health care for battered women and their children* (pp. 156–173). Thousand Oaks, CA: Sage.

Gee, P. W. (1983). Ensuring police protection for battered women: The Scott v. Hart suit. *Signs: Journal of Women in Culture in Society, 8,* 554–567.

Gelles, R. J., & Cornell, C. P. (1985). *Intimate violence in families.* Thousand Oaks: Sage.

Gelles, R. J., & Loseke, D. R. (Eds.). (1993). *Current controversies on family violence.* Thousand Oaks, CA: Sage.

Gelles, R. J., & Straus, M. A. (1979). Determinants of violence in the family: Toward a theoretical integration. In W. R. Burr et al. (Eds.), *Contemporary theories about the family* (Vol. 1, pp. 549–581). New York: Free Press.

Gil, D. (1970). *Violence against children.* Cambridge, MA: Harvard University Press.

Gondolf, E. (1987). *Man against woman: What every woman needs to know about violent men.* Bradenton, FL: Human Services Institute.

Goody, J. (1962). *Death, property, and the ancestors.* London: Tavistock.

Greven, P. (1990). *Spare the child: The religious roots of punishment and the psychological impact of physical abuse.* New York: Knopf.

Groves, B. M., Zuckerman, B., Marans, S., & Cohen, D. (1993). Silent victims: Children who witness violence. *Journal of the American Medical Association, 269*(2), 262–264.

Handwerker, W. P. (1998). Why violence? A test of hypotheses representing three discourses on the roots of domestic violence. *Human Organization, 57*(2), 200–208.

Harbin, H. T., & Madden, D. J. (1979). Battered parents: A new syndrome. *American Journal of Psychiatry, 136,* 1288–1291.

Hart, J. (2000, May 30). Statistics say abuse hits close to home: Most young victims know their molester. *Boston Globe,* pp. B1, B8.

Hartigan, P. (1999, June 16). "It's like I had this war in me." *Boston Globe,* pp. E1, E4.

Helfer, R., & Kempe, R. S. (1987). *The battered child* (4th ed.). Chicago: University of Chicago Press.

Henning, K., Leitenberg, H., Coffey, P., Turner, T., & Bennett, R. T. (1996). Long term psychological and social impact of witnessing physical conflict between parents. *Journal of Interpersonal Violence, 11,* 35–51.

Herman, J. (1981). *Father-daughter incest.* Cambridge, MA: Harvard University Press.

Herman, J. (1992). *Trauma and recovery: The aftermath of violence.* New York: Basic Books.

Hilberman, E. (1980). Overview: The "wife-beater's wife" reconsidered. *American Journal of Psychiatry, 137,* 1336–1347.

Hillman, D., & Solek-Tefft, J. (1988). *Spiders and flies: Help for parents and teachers of sexually abused children*. San Francisco: New Lexington Press.

Hoff, L. A. (1990). *Battered women as survivors*. London: Routledge.

Hoff, L. A. (1992a). Battered women: Understanding, identification, and assessment—a psychosociocultural perspective (Part 1). *Journal of American Academy of Nurse Practitioners, 4*(4), 148–155.

Hoff, L. A. (1992b). Review essay: Wife beating in Micronesia. *ISLA: A Journal of Micronesian Studies, 1*(2), 199–221.

Hoff, L. A. (1993). Battered women: Intervention and prevention—a psychosociocultural perspective (Part 2). *Journal of American Academy of Nurse Practitioners, 5*(1), 34–39.

Hoff, L. A. (1995). *Violence issues: An interdisciplinary curriculum guide for health professionals* [in English and French]. Ottawa: Health Canada, Health Services Directorate.

Hoff, L. A. (2000). Interpersonal violence. In C. E. Koop, C. E. Pearson, & M. R. Schwartz (Eds.), *Critical issues in global health* (pp. 260–271). San Francisco: Jossey-Bass.

Hoff, L. A. (in press). International consortium on crisis, violence, and gender studies. *Distance Learning, 1*(3).

Hoff, L. A., & Rosenbaum, L. (1994). A victimization assessment tool: Instrument development and clinical implications. *Journal of Advanced Nursing, 20*(4), 627–634.

Holmstrom, L. L., & Burgess, A. W. (1978). *The victim of rape: Institutional reaction*. New York: Wiley.

Humphreys, J. (1998). Helping battered women take care of their children. In J. C. Campbell (Ed.), *Empowering survivors of abuse: Health care for battered women and their children* (pp. 121–137). Thousand Oaks, CA: Sage.

Jackson, D. Z. (1994, September 7). Handguns in our homes put children at risk. *Boston Globe*, p. 13.

Jaffe, P., Wolfe, D., & Wilson, S. (1990). *Children of battered women*. Thousand Oaks, CA: Sage.

Jang, D., Lee, D., & Morello-Frosch, R. (1991). Domestic violence in the immigrant and refugee community: Responding to the needs of immigrant women. *Response to the Victimization of Women and Children, 13*(4), 2–7.

Johnson, H. (1998). Rethinking survey research on violence against women. In R. E. Dobash & R. P. Dobash, (Eds.), *Rethinking violence against women* (pp. 23–51). Thousand Oaks, CA: Sage.

Jones, A. (1980). *Women who kill*. Austin, TX: Holt, Rinehart and Winston.

Kempe, H., & Helfer, R. E. (Eds.). (1980). *The battered child* (3rd ed.). Chicago: University of Chicago Press.

Kidd, R. F., & Chayet, E. F. (1984). Why do victims fail to report? The psychology of criminal victimization. *Journal of Social Issues, 40*(1), 39–50.

Kidder, L. H., Boell, J. L., & Moyer, M. M. (1983). Rights consciousness and victimization prevention: Personal defense and assertiveness training. *Journal of Social Issues, 39*(2), 155–170.

Korbin, J. E. (1987, July). *Fatal child maltreatment*. Paper presented at the Third National Conference on Family Violence, Durham, NH.

Kurz, E. (1993). Physical assaults by husbands: A major social problem. In R. J. Gelles & D. R. Loseke (Eds.), *Current controversies on family violence* (pp. 88–103). Thousand Oaks, CA: Sage.

Latour, F. (2000, June 8). Victims against vengeance. *Boston Sunday Globe*, pp. E1, E5.

Levinson, D. (1989). *Family violence in cross-cultural perspective*. Thousand Oaks, CA: Sage.

Levy, B. (1991). *Dating violence: Young women in danger*. Seattle: Seal Press.

Long, N. J., & Wilder, M. T. (1993). From rage to responsibility: A massaging numb values life space interview. *Journal of Emotional and Behavioral Problems, 2*(1), 35–40.

Luhrmann, T. M. (2000). *Of two minds: The growing disorder in American psychiatry*. New York: Knopf.

MacLean, M. (Ed.). (1995). *Abuse and neglect of older Canadians.* Toronto: Thompson Educational Publishing.

Mawby, R. I., & Walklate, S. (1994). *Critical victimology.* London: Sage.

McDonald, P. L., Hornick, J. P., Robertson, G. B., & Wallace, J. E. (1991). *Elder abuse and neglect in Canada.* Toronto: Butterworths.

McEvoy, A., & Erickson, E. (1994). *Abused children: The educator's guide to prevention and intervention.* Holmes Beach, FL: Learning Publications.

McFarlane, J., Parker, B., Soeken, K., & Bullock, L. (1992). Assessing for abuse during pregnancy. Severity and frequency of injuries and associated entry into prenatal care. *Journal of the American Medical Association, 267*(23), 3176–3178.

McManiman, J. (2000). The invisibility of men's pain. In B. Everett & R. Gallop, *The link between childhood trauma and mental illness* (pp. 253–270). Thousand Oaks, CA: Sage.

Miller, J. B. (1986). *Toward a new psychology of women* (Rev. ed.). Boston: Beacon Press.

Mills, C. W. (1959). *The sociological imagination.* Oxford: Oxford University Press.

Mirkin, M. P. (Ed.). (1994). *Women in context: Toward a feminist reconstruction of psychotherapy.* New York: Guilford Press.

Mones, P. (1993). Parricide: A window on child abuse. *Journal of Emotional and Behavioral Problems, 2*(1), 30–34.

Moore, S. Y. (1999, December 26). Adolescent boys are the underserved victims of domestic violence. *Boston Sunday Globe,* p. E7.

Newberger, E. (1980). *New approaches needed to control child abuse.* Presented before the Subcommittee on Select Education of the Committee on Education and Labor. Washington, DC: U.S. House of Representatives.

NiCarthy, G. (1989). *You can be free: An easy-to-read handbook for abused women.* Seattle: Seal Press.

Novello, A. C. (1992). From the Surgeon General: U.S. Public Health Service. *Journal of the American Medical Association, 267*(23), 3132.

Pence, E., & Paymar, M. (1986). *Power and control: Tactics of men who batter.* Duluth: Minnesota Program Development.

Perilla, J. L. (1999). Domestic violence as a human rights issue: The case of immigrant Latinos. *Hispanic Journal of Behavioral Sciences, 21*(2), 107–133.

Pillemer, K. A., & Finkelhor, D. (1987). The prevalence of elder abuse: A random survey. Durham, NH: Family Violence Research Program.

Pillemer, K. A., & Wolf, D. W. (1986). *Elder abuse: Conflict in the family.* Westport, CT: Auburn House.

Podnieks, E., & Pillemer, K. (1990). *National survey on abuse of the elderly in Canada: The Ryerson study.* Ottawa: Health and Welfare Canada. National Clearinghouse on Family Violence.

Powers, J., & Jaklitsch, B. (1989). *Understanding survivors of abuse: Stories of homeless and runaway adolescents.* San Francisco: New Lexington Press.

Pruschno, R., & Resch, N. (1989). Husbands and wives as caregivers: Antecedents of depression and burden. *Journal of Gerontology, 29,* 159–162.

Renzetti, C. M. (1992). *Violent betrayal: Partner abuse in lesbian relationships.* Thousand Oaks, CA: Sage.

Rivera, C. (1995, April 26). U.S. child abuse report declares health crisis. *Boston Globe,* p. 3.

Ross, M. (2001). *Nursing education and violence prevention, detection, and intervention: Report.* Ottawa: Health Canada, Family Violence Prevention Unit.

Russell, D.E.H. (1982). *Rape in marriage.* New York: Collier Books.

Russell, D.E.H. (1986). *Secret trauma: Incest in the lives of girls and women.* New York: Basic Books.

Ryan, W. (1971). *Blaming the victim.* New York: Vintage Books.

Sadker, M., & Sadker, D. (1994). *Failing at fairness: How America's schools cheat girls.* New York: Scribner.

Sales, E., Baum, M., & Shore, B. (1984, February 14). Victim readjustment following assault. *Journal of Social Issues, 40*(1), 117–136.

Saunders, C. I. (1999). Finding a better way. *Boston Sunday Globe*, pp. D1–D2.

Schechter, S. (1982). *Women and male violence*. Boston: South End Press.

Segal, L. (1987). *Is the future female? Troubling thoughts on contemporary feminism*. London: Virago Press.

Sennott, C. M. (1999, April 18). For Kosovo's children of war, the wounds of trauma run deep. *Boston Sunday Globe*, pp. A1, A31.

Socolovsky, J. (2000, April 26). Rape victim testifies against Serb soldiers. *Boston Globe*, p. A17.

Soeken, K. L., McFarlane, J., Parker, B., & Lominack, M. C. (1998). The abuse assessment screen: A clinical instrument to measure frequency, severity, and perpetrator of abuse against women. In J. C. Campbell (Ed.), *Empowering survivors of abuse: Health care for battered women and their children* (pp. 195–203). Thousand Oaks, CA: Sage.

Sommers, T., & Shields, L. (1987). *Women take care: The consequences of caregiving in today's society*. Gainesville, FL: Triad.

Stark, E., & Flitcraft, A. (1996). *Women at risk: Domestic violence and women's health*. Thousand Oaks, CA: Sage.

Stark, E., Flitcraft, A., & Frazier, W. (1979). Medicine and patriarchal violence: The social construction of a "private" event. *International Journal of Health Services, 9,* 461–493.

Stephens, B. J. (1985). Suicidal women and their relationships with husbands, boyfriends, and lovers. *Suicide & Life-Threatening Behavior, 15*(2), 77–90.

Stephens, D. L. (1999). Battered women's views of their children. *Journal of Interpersonal Violence, 14*(7), 731–746.

Straus, M. A. (1993). Physical assaults by wives: A major social problem. In R. J. Gelles & D. R. Loseke (Eds.), *Current controversies on family violence* (pp. 67–87). Thousand Oaks, CA: Sage.

Straus, M. A., Gelles, R. J., & Steinmetz, S. K. (1980). *Behind closed doors: Violence in the American family*. New York: Anchor Books.

Sugg, N. K., & Inui, T. (1992). Primary care physicians' response to domestic violence: Opening Pandora's box. *Journal of the American Medical Association, 267*(23), 3157–3160.

Taylor, L., Zuckerman, B., Harik, V., & Groves, B. M. (1994). Witnessing violence by young children and their mothers. *Developmental and Behavioral Pediatrics, 15*(2), 120–123.

Thornhill, R., & Palmer, C. (2000). *A natural history of rape*. Cambridge, MA: MIT Press.

Tilden, V. P., Schmidt, T. A., Limandri, B. J., Chiodo, G. T., Garland, M. J., & Loveless, P. A. (1994). Factors that influence clinicians' assessment and management of family violence. *American Journal of Public Health, 84*(4), 628–633.

United Nations. (1996a). *Report on the world's women 1995: Trends and statistics*. New York: Author.

United Nations. (1996b). *The Beijing declaration and the platform for action*. New York: Author.

VandeCreek, L., & Knapp, S. (1993). *Tarasoff and beyond: Legal and clinical considerations in the treatment of life-endangering patients* (Rev. ed.). Sarasota, FL: Professional Resource Press.

U.S. Surgeon General. (1986). *Surgeon General's workshop on violence and public health: Report*. Washington, DC: U.S. Department of Health and Human Services.

van der Kolk, B. A. (1987). *Psychological trauma*. Washington, DC: American Psychiatric Press.

Walker, H. M. (1993). Anti-social behavior in school. *Journal of Emotional and Behavioral Problems, 2*(1), 20–24.

Warshaw, C. (1989). Limitations of the medical model in the care of battered women. *Gender and Society, 3*(4), 506–517.

Warshaw, D. (1988). *I never called it rape*. New York: HarperCollins.

Watkins, B., & Bentovim, A. (1992). The sexual abuse of male children and adolescents: A review of current research. *Journal of Child Psychology and Psychiatry, 33*(1), 197–248.

Wiehe, V. R. (1998). *Understanding family violence: Treating and preventing partner, child, sibling, and elder abuse.* Thousand Oaks, CA: Sage.

Wiehe, V. R., & Richards, A. L. (1995). *Intimate betrayal.* Thousand Oaks, CA: Sage.

Wolfgang, M. E. (1986). Interpersonal violence and public health care: New directions, new challenges. In *Surgeon General's workshop on violence and public health: Report* (pp. 9–18). Washington, DC: U.S. Department of Health and Human Services.

Yllo, K., & Bograd, M. (Eds.). (1987). *Feminist perspectives on wife abuse.* Thousand Oaks, CA: Sage.

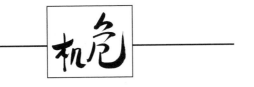

CHAPTER NINE

THE VIOLENT PERSON: INDIVIDUAL AND SOCIOCULTURAL FACTORS

The theoretical overview in Chapter Eight introduced the concept of a continuum between violence against intimates and family members and the violence pervading the larger sociocultural milieu. For example, violence against female partners is no longer regarded as a private matter between the couple but is now recognized as a major public health issue. One of the reasons for connecting what happens behind closed doors to the public domain is to avoid transferring the legacy of individual victim blaming to the level of family blaming. As noted in the last chapter, much personal misery can be traced to family dynamics, neglect, and patterns of harsh discipline or outright abuse and violence. But families do not exist in a social or cultural vacuum. In families, children absorb from their parents values that support aggression and violence as solutions to problems. The parents' behavior has been reinforced by policies and media celebrations that nourish—if they do not condone outright—aggression as a norm in social life.

Aggression and Violence: A Contextual Versus Adversarial Approach

It has been an axiom of victims' rights organizations that victims deserve the same justice as their accusers and assailants. The last chapter amply supports this position. Yet in addition to academic debates about "family" versus "feminist" research, there are polarizations, even within advocacy and feminist communities, that do not advance the common goal of reducing violence and caring for victims. For example, women are portrayed *either* as victims *or* as having "made it" on equal terms with men. Of course, many women have made it, but the fact remains that millions of women worldwide are victimized and most of the assailants are men (Pan American Health Organization, 1994; Yllo, 1993).

This chapter focuses on the perpetrators of violence—the crises of assailants and their sociocultural underpinnings—and suggests that attention to perpetrators forms part of a comprehensive program to reduce violence. Some would argue that programs for perpetrators deflect from the more urgent need of refuge for victims. Violence is a major public health problem as well as a criminal justice issue. At worst, an either-or position damages both victim-survivors and assailants; at best, it constitutes empty polemics. It is therefore not a question of whether we (1) *either* provide refuge and care for battered women *or* provide treatment programs for their batterers, (2) *either* hold parents accountable for the violent and abusive behavior of their children *or* offer parent effectiveness training and socioeconomic support to parents unduly burdened with the task of parenting, or (3) *either* teach inner-city youth anger management skills *or* address the sociocultural and economic roots of their anger. Essentially, either-or debates are adversarial and reflect the power component of violence itself. These counterproductive arguments have surfaced anew just as progress appeared in respect to treatment programs for batterers. Criminal justice and mental health professionals argue about who should direct these programs. The arguments assert that such programs should be directed *either* by criminal justice professionals *or* by mental health professionals (Bennett & Piet, 1999).

From the perspective of health and human service providers who deal with such crises, it is clear that a contextual *both-and* approach offers more than an either-or polarity. A long history of human service organizations reveals that when staff are divided along ideological and programmatic lines, clients are the ones who suffer the most severe consequences by falling through the cracks in a system. One group cannot do everything; a particular discipline or person cannot be all things to all survivors or perpetrators of abuse. But greater coordination could mend some of the serious systemic problems that can trigger crisis responses. And in the case of violence and victimization, the life-and-death consequences as well as the long-term health, financial, and social consequences are enormous in both human and financial terms.

Accordingly, assessment for the risk of assault and homicide is integral to a complete crisis assessment, as well as to follow-up treatment of survivors. When the indicators of dangerousness described in Table 9.1 and the assessment tool described in Chapter Three were introduced routinely in crisis and counseling clinics in western New York, staff were astounded at how many clients were entertaining violent fantasies. But crisis workers in that public mental health system also noted the clients' openness to receiving help in dealing with their anger and violent impulses. The next section discusses safety issues for police and crisis workers as well as criteria for such assessment, followed by elaboration of these themes with respect to two major categories of abusive and violent assailants: (1) the international increase in violence and antisocial behavior among young people and (2) programs for men who batter their women partners.

TABLE 9.1.   LETHALITY ASSESSMENT SCALE: OTHER.

Key to Scale	Immediate Dangerousness to Others	Typical Indicators
1	No predictable risk of assault or homicide	Has no homicidal ideation, urges, or history of same; basically satisfactory support system; social drinker only
2	Low risk of assault or homicide	Has occasional assault or homicidal ideation (including paranoid ideas) with some urges to kill; no history of impulsive acts or homicidal attempts; occasional drinking bouts and angry verbal outbursts; basically satisfactory support system
3	Moderate risk of assault or homicide	Has frequent homicidal ideation and urges to kill but no specific plan; history of impulsive acting out and verbal outbursts while drinking and otherwise; stormy relationship with significant others with periodic high-tension arguments
4	High risk of homicide	Has homicidal plan; obtainable means; drinking history; frequent acting out against others, but no homicide attempts; stormy relationships and much verbal fighting with significant others, with occasional assaults
5	Very high risk of homicide	Has current high-lethal plan; available means; history of homicide attempts or impulsive acting out, plus feels a strong urge to control and "get even" with a significant other; history of drinking; also with possible high-lethal suicide risk

Violence Against Police Officers and Health, Mental Health, and Crisis Workers

One of the first principles in crisis work is safety—for ourselves, our clients, significant others, and the general public. Violence as an occupational health hazard is only now gaining public attention (Levin, Hewitt, & Misner, 1992; Lipscomb & Love, 1992); police officers, health, mental health, crisis, and other workers make up a special category of victims. Among women who died as a result of workplace trauma, 41 percent were homicide victims (Jenkins, Layne, & Kisner, 1992). The killing of police officers is particularly demoralizing and frightening because it shows disrespect for the very people dedicated to ensuring public safety. The issue is compounded when officers are victims of violence but there is no certainty that a crime has been committed. This potentially dangerous situation in crisis work embroils us in the controversy introduced in Chapter Eight, the relationship between crime and mental illness (Daniels, 1978; Gove, 1975; Scheff, 1975). Despite numerous debates on this topic, the distinctions between crime and mental illness overlap with relevance to life crises and our response to them; police and mental health professionals are often caught in the middle and become victims of violence. In many cases, their victimization could have been avoided (see the case example of Robert in Chapter Four).

Why, then, is there an apparent increase in the number of crisis workers and others who are injured, killed, or threatened on the job? In considering this question, the focus is not on what to do if attacked but on why known crisis intervention strategies are not used or why they are ineffective. Research by Melick, Steadman, & Cocozza (1979) suggests that three factors are related to this issue: (1) the lack of crisis intervention training, (2) the widespread absence of appropriate collaboration between police and mental health professionals, and (3) the social trend toward the medicalization of life's problems. Several strategies could reduce the hazard of workplace violence: (1) routine application of danger assessment techniques, (2) implementation of the principles and strategies for creating a therapeutic milieu, and (3) use of social network techniques to defuse highly anxious and hostile behavior by nonchemical means. Staff in these highly charged situations also need to reserve time and energy for considering the impact of managed care policies on treatment of the seriously and persistently mentally ill. Some of the results of these policies include the current focus on pharmacological and very brief hospital care and reduced staffing by skilled professionals; in response, staff may then resort to more authoritarian approaches to disruptive behavior, which in turn escalates tension and violence potential among patients.

Crisis Intervention Training

Traditionally, nurses and psychiatric professionals have been taught that if they get hurt by mentally disturbed people, it is probably because they missed cues to rising anxiety levels or they antagonized or otherwise dealt inappropriately with the disturbed person. For example, using chemical or physical restraint before time-tested interpersonal approaches have been tried by trained mental health professionals often results in retaliative attacks on the staff. Over the years, mental health professionals have worked to dispel the myth that all mental patients are dangerous; only a small percentage are. Psychiatric facilities usually have precise protocols for preventing and responding to violence among mental patients (Engel & Marsh, 1986; Morton, 1986). Police procedures are also precise and comprehensive. A basic principle in both disciplines is to avoid force and physical restraint except for protecting oneself and others. This interpretation is strongly supported by the research of Bard (1972) and his precedent-setting training for New York City police officers. The number of police injuries and deaths on the job were significantly reduced as a result of the application of crisis intervention techniques, especially in family disturbance calls. These techniques have been expanded to deal with terrorists through hostage negotiation strategies.

Details of hostage negotiation are beyond the scope of this book or the skills expected of an ordinary crisis worker. The highly sophisticated developments in this field, however, point to the importance of collaborative use of knowledge between police and behavioral science fields in responding to certain crises. Everyone who is even remotely involved with hostage situations—such as when a mentally ill relative holds a child hostage and threatens to commit murder and then suicide if a rescue is attempted—must recognize that offers by civilians to "handle him because I know him better than anyone" can backfire and need thorough investigation. Even police officers chosen for hostage negotiation are carefully screened on several counts, including their professional success in handling general crisis situations. Everyone should also be familiar with ways to reduce the chances of injury or murder.

Besides their usefulness in standard criminal justice and police work, the criteria for assessing the degree of danger and the risk of assault apply in a number of situations:

1. In crisis, emergency, mental health, and forensic services
2. In the event that a worker is threatened with violence or is being taken hostage
3. In all domestic disputes

The third situation in this list would apply, for instance, when an abused woman is in imminent danger of being taken hostage or murdered. Such danger is heightened in relationships in which a man acts as though he owns his wife, as when he says, "If I can't have you, no one can." Most battered women are already aware of the danger they face, but for those who are not, for whatever reason, a crucial part of safety and crisis intervention planning for her includes a frank discussion of the potential for assault or homicide. While acknowledging that violent people can learn other ways, past violent behavior is still a powerful indicator of future behavior. And as the triage questions in Exhibit 8.1 in Chapter Eight indicate, routine screening for assault and homicide potential is gender neutral; therefore, the abused woman's own potential for assaulting or killing her assailant following abuse must also be ascertained.

Assessing the Risk of Assault and Homicide

As emphasized in Chapter Three, crisis intervention training includes assessment for risk of assault and homicide. As in the case of suicide risk assessment, there is no absolute prediction of homicide risk. The topic itself is highly controversial; Monahan (1981, p. 6), for example, cites three criticisms regarding prediction in forensic work:

1. It is empirically impossible to predict violent behavior.
2. If such activity could be forecast and averted, it would, as a matter of policy, violate the civil liberties of those whose activity is predicted.
3. Even if accurate prediction were possible without violating civil liberties, psychiatrists and psychologists should decline to do it, since it is a social control activity at variance with their professional helping role.

Whereas prediction of violence is an issue in forensic work, assessment of violence potential can be a matter of life or death in domestic, occupational, and clinical settings. The clinical assessment of risk for assault and homicide is an inherent aspect of police officers' and health and crisis workers' jobs. And the average citizen is always calculating safety maneuvers when in known risk areas. This is not the same as making an official prediction of risk as part of the court-requested psychiatric or psychological examination of persons who are detained for crimes and who plead insanity (Halleck, 1987). Although assessment of dangerousness by crisis workers is far from an exact science, it can be based on principles and data, not merely on guesswork. Based on Monahan's (1981) research, these include

1. *Statistics*—for example, men between the ages of eighteen and thirty-four commit a much higher percentage of violent crimes than older men or women of any age. Statistical indicators, however, should be viewed with the same caution as in suicide risk assessment (see Chapter Six).
2. *Personality factors,* including motivation, aggression, inhibition, and habit.
3. *Situational factors,* such as availability of a weapon or behavior of the potential victim.
4. *The interaction* between these variables.

Toch (1969) claims that the interaction factor is a crucial one influencing violence. There are several stages in the interactional process. First, the potential victim is classified as an object or a potential threat—essentially, a dehumanization process. Based on this classification, some action follows, after which the potential victim may make a self-protective move. Whether or not violence occurs depends on the interaction of such variables as the effectiveness of the victim's self-protection or the would-be attacker's interpretation of resistance as an "ego" threat demanding retaliation. Establishing a bond, therefore, between victim and terrorist can counteract dehumanization and thus serve to prevent an attack, although that strategy should not be relied on in all cases. This is the basis for a widely held principle in crisis intervention and hostage negotiation: *time* and keeping *communication* channels open—rather than precipitous action, taunts, or threats—are to the benefit of the negotiator and can save the lives of victims, terrorists, and suicidal persons.

Clearly, assessing danger is no simple matter, but lives can be saved by taking seriously the fact that only potentially dangerous people make threats of assault or homicide. A careful read of newspaper accounts of murders reveals almost invariably the assailant's verbal and other cues that were either ignored or misinterpreted as not being serious. Thorough training in crisis assessment and intervention is paramount, therefore, for professionals and others who work with disturbed or potentially violent people. This includes always inquiring about the *meaning* of verbal threats that too many times are dismissed by family, friends, and associates. Health and social service providers should educate their clients and the general public about this safety issue.

CASE EXAMPLE: MARGIE

Margie, age thirty-five, had filed for divorce on grounds of her husband's jealousy and abusive behavior. In the parking lot where she worked, he took her hostage and threatened to first kill her and then himself. As Margie's estranged husband, armed with a revolver, drove her across the state for several hours, she accommodated his desire to "talk," to the point that he trusted her when she asked to go to the ladies' room while they were in a restaurant. On her way to the rest room, she was able to whisper her plight to a waitress, who quickly called the police. As she cowered beneath a stairwell, the police arrested her husband at the restaurant table. The time and communication principle that Margie so astutely applied most likely saved her life.

Police–Mental Health Collaboration

Crisis intervention alone is not enough to prevent violence. Another critical aspect of preventing victimization concerns collaboration between police and mental health professionals, especially when the boundaries of these institutions overlap (Baracos, 1974). The following case example illustrates the tragic results of failure in such collaboration.

CASE EXAMPLE: ARTHUR

A mentally disturbed man, Arthur, age sixty-one, was brought to a hospital emergency department by two police officers for psychiatric examination at the request of his wife. Arthur had a history of paranoid delusions and at this time was accusing his wife of infidelity, though he threatened no harm to her. Arthur's wife had committed him three times before when he refused to seek treatment. This time, as he was getting out of the car, Arthur grabbed the gun of one of the officers and shot him. The other officer in turn shot Arthur, who died instantly. The police officer died a few hours later. Although Arthur had a history of mental disturbance, he had no lethal weapons at the time of the police investigation. It was also learned after the deaths that this man's history of mental disturbance had never included violence, although he did get very angry each time his wife had him hospitalized.

This case suggests that if police officers had not been required to perform the tasks of mental health professionals—assessing danger and performing crisis intervention with an acutely disturbed mental patient—two deaths might have been avoided. As it was, the community in which this double tragedy occurred had no mobile crisis outreach capacity. The same situation prevails in other communities, to the point that police are often performing by default and alone the high-risk mental health work that should be carried out in collaborative arrangements with mental health professionals. Many officers resent this situation, and with justification, as mental health professionals are often unavailable for such collaboration with police in cases such as Arthur's. If mobile crisis outreach teams are not available, police officers should have twenty-four-hour access to telephone consultation regarding mental patients. Such arrangements between police and mental health professionals skilled in crisis intervention should exist in every community (Hoff & Adamowski, 1998). The need has become more urgent because of managed care and deinstitutionalization of mental patients, often with inadequate community support (Hoff, 1993; Johnson, 1990). Mental patients are at great risk for all sorts of crises, often with no one available to help but police officers.

In addition, crisis intervention training for police should be routine. Some officers may resist such training, claiming that a police officer should spend more time preventing crime. However, 80 percent of an average officer's time is spent in service or domestic calls. Ignoring this reality is foolhardy and can cost officers' lives. In England, where police officers are not armed, and gun availability to laypersons is much more stringent than in the United States, the "service" orientation of officers is more easily promulgated and upheld (P. Sully, Society, Violence and Practice Program at City University, London, personal communication, 2000).

Even if officers are not physically injured in hostage or other crisis situations, they and their families can suffer psychological trauma that may require weeks or months for recovery. Reactions similar to those of disaster victims are common (see Chapter Ten). Recognizing these reactions and the need for support, the FBI and police departments are making special services available to officers who are involved in shooting and other highly traumatic incidents.

Application of Assault and Homicide Risk Assessment Criteria

Translated into everyday practice, the following criteria are helpful as guidelines to assess the risk of assault or homicide:

- History of homicidal threats
- History of assault
- Current homicidal threats and plan, including on the Internet
- Possession or easy availability of lethal weapons
- Use or abuse of alcohol or other drugs
- Conflict in significant social or clinical relationships—for example, infidelity, threat of divorce, labor-management disputes, authoritarian approaches to mental patients
- Threats of suicide following homicide

Assault and homicide risk assessment is illustrated in a variation of Arthur's case (see Table 9.1). This assessment is based on the risk criteria cited in the Comprehensive Mental Health Assessment tool presented in Chapter Three. Suppose that Arthur had been seen at home by two crisis outreach specialists and no guns were available. According to the criteria cited, Arthur was a low risk for assault or homicide, with a rating of 2 at most. His anxiety level increased as he was forcibly taken to a hospital; guns were available; the risk of homicide increased dramatically. It seems reasonable to suggest that both Arthur and the officer might be alive today if Arthur and his wife had had the advantage of skilled crisis assessment and intervention from mental health professionals, preferably in their home. Similar dynamics can operate in psychiatric settings when a show of force is used before other measures are exhausted; staff (most often nurses) risk being injured by mental patients who already feel disempowered by rigid hospital rules or forced chemical restraint. In Margie's case, the homicide risk was very high, 5 on the scale, and the necessity of collaboration with police was obvious because the husband was armed.

The Medicalization of Crime and Violence in the Workplace

It is true that the standards of crisis intervention training among health and mental health workers are far from being met. The Life Crisis Institute and the American Association of Suicidology recommend a minimum of forty hours of training for all frontline and specialty crisis workers—nurses, physicians, police, and mental health professionals (Hoff & Adamowski, 1998; Hoff & Wells, 1989). Still, the level of exposure to risk is probably not much higher than it was ten or fifteen years ago, and in many instances workers have had some training in crisis intervention. Yet health and mental health professionals and others seem to be assaulted in the course of their work more often than in the past. Why?

A health or mental health professional could be a paragon of perfection in crisis intervention practice and still be injured or killed on the job. Mental patients are probably no more violent than they were in the past, but nurses and others may be getting hurt more often by patients who should never have been admitted to a mental health facility in the first place. This assertion is based on overwhelming evidence that life is becoming increasingly medicalized. Nowhere are the consequences of medicalization potentially more dangerous than when this social trend is applied to violent behavior—for example, when a violent criminal is classified as mentally ill and assigned to medical rather than penal supervision. Research findings (Melick et al., 1979, p. 235) during early phases of community mental health development in the state of New York are still relevant today: "The reason that a case does not reach trial [for criminal justice versus mental health dispositions] probably has as much to do with the strength of the prosecutor's case as it does with the mental state of the defendant."

The medicalization of crime may also be related to overcrowded prisons and empty mental hospitals, conditions that have been created through the process of deinstitutionalization (Johnson, 1990). The replacement of state-owned space in mental hospitals by private hospital psychiatric units, buttressed by managed care and support of the biomedical approach to treatment (Luhrmann, 2000), exacerbates the argument for medicalizing criminal behavior. But apart from the public debate on this topic, health professionals and others should critically examine the trend to interpret life's problems in an "illness" framework (Hoff, 1993). For example, it is still common to refer to a man who has sexually molested dozens or even hundreds of children as "sick," despite a record of stellar job performance and stable family life.

It is certainly true that some people who commit crimes are mentally deranged, therefore entitling them to leniency before the law. Many insanity pleas, however, leave much room for doubt. Insanity is a legal, not a mental health, concept. Our difficulties in dealing with this issue in the United States are complicated by a criminal justice system that often denies a decent standard of treatment to criminals. The humanitarian impulse of most people is to spare even a violent person an experience that seems beyond the deserts of the crime. It is paradoxical, then, that the tendency to treat a person rather than hold him or her responsible for violent behavior exists in concert with the movement to assert the rights of mental patients (Capponi, 1992). We cannot have it both ways. One cannot, on the one hand, exercise the freedom to reject treatment and hospitalization for behavioral disorders and, on the other hand, plead temporary insanity when one then fails to control violent impulses and commits a crime (or in psychiatric settings, assaults a staff member who may or may not press criminal charges). The following cases illustrate this point, as well as the need for mental health professionals to examine their misplaced guilt feelings when they hold clients accountable for their violent behavior.

CASE EXAMPLE: CONNIE

Connie, age fifty-one, was being treated in a private psychiatric facility for a drinking problem and depression following a divorce. A mental status examination revealed that Connie was mentally competent and not suffering from delusions or other thought disorders, though she was very angry about her husband's decision to divorce her because of her drinking problem. When Connie, therefore, decided to check out of the residential treatment facility against medical advice, there was no basis for confining her involuntarily, according to any interpretation of the state's mental health laws. A discharge planning conference was held, at which follow-up therapy sessions were arranged through a special program for alcoholic women. Connie failed to keep her counseling appointments. One week after leaving the psychiatric unit, Connie attempted to demolish her former husband's car by crashing her own car into it. She endangered the lives of other people by driving on sidewalks, where pedestrians successfully managed to escape her fury. Connie was arrested and taken to jail. Two mental health professionals involved with her case were called to testify. The defense attorney was incredulous that the mental health professionals (both female) did not plead with the judge to commit Connie to a mental health facility rather than to jail. The judge clearly seemed to prefer committing Connie to the psychiatric unit where she had been treated but was assured (against the protests of the defense attorney) that her mental status and physical capacity provided no basis on which to keep her from being a further menace to society.

CASE EXAMPLE: ERIC

Eric, age twenty-eight, was employed but distressed over interpersonal relationships on the job. He came to a group therapy session, and shortly after the session began, he got up and swung his clenched fists, first at one of the therapists. Then he swung at other clients, while making threatening statements. Eric had apparently had something to drink, as the smell of alcohol was on his breath. But as he swung his fists at people, he seemed very controlled; he came just an inch or so from their noses. The therapists and other clients were unable to persuade Eric to stop his violent, threatening behavior and therefore called the police. Eric was taken to the nearby jail. The senior therapist meanwhile, feeling overwhelmed with guilt about her client being in jail, reviewed the mental health laws to ascertain grounds for having Eric transferred from jail to a mental health facility. She reported the incident to the executive director (a psychiatrist) and explored with him the idea of having Eric committed for treatment. The psychiatrist replied, "Treated for what? Threatening you and the other clients?" The therapist revised some of her traditional ideas about "treating" people for violent behavior rather than holding them accountable for it.

These cases suggest a spillover of violence from home to workplace, as well as its sociocultural context. A biomedical versus public health response to workplace violence may help perpetuate the problem if the larger social ramifications of the issue remain unaddressed. Obviously, this takes us well beyond the individual crisis worker's responsibility. Yet our safety in the work setting and our common humanity in a violent society demand such a two-pronged approach to this serious issue (see Arnetz & Arnetz, 2001).

As already noted regarding danger assessment, too often the signs of impending assault or homicide are either not recognized or are ignored until it is too late, as documented in widely publicized massacres at schools and worksites. Crisis and violence-prevention specialists should extend their expertise to human resource personnel in public and private institutions. The layperson needs to know that murder does not occur in a cultural or social vacuum; it does not "just happen." Rather, it is planned, although impulse may play a part. The humane treatment of workers when delivering news of discipline or layoff is another violence-prevention measure needing attention, if for no other reason than self-interest.

Fortunately, the days of assaulted health workers' having to absorb their injury and emotional trauma as "part of the job" appear to be coming to an end. Research has uncovered the relationship of workplace injury to gender, race, and class factors, as well as to the work environment itself—for example, inadequate staffing and lack of structured supervisor support. Guidelines from the Occupational Safety & Health Administration and labor union action portend the prospect of redressing the neglect of many victimized workers who have been largely on their own in the process of recovering from the trauma of such mostly preventable violence (Jenkins et al., 1992; Levin et al., 1992; Lipscomb & Love, 1992; Miller, 1999).

The Crisis of Youth Violence

Aggressive, antisocial, and violent behavior among children and adolescents is gaining international attention. Overall crime rates in the United States and Western Europe have declined sharply for several years, while dramatic shootings by school children have captured international attention. Bullying and mobbing—usually child-on-child aggression—continue to create terror in schools and have even been associated with suicide (Hoover & Juul, 1993). Youth violence has moved parents, social scientists, journalists, legislators, and others to debate and earnest soul-searching about the cultural climate and other factors that have spawned these tragedies. Research on bullying in Europe traces such behavior to a combination of factors in the home (for example, inconsistent discipline, abuse, alcohol), the school (more antisocial behavior in the worst schools), and the individual victims and perpetrators, underscoring this book's premise of the *interactional* character of aggression and its sequelae. Paralleling adult patterns, the majority of bullying and antisocial behavior is perpetrated by males against both males and females (Ellickson, Saner, & McGuigan, 1997; Hoover & Juul, 1993, p. 28; Walker, 1993, p. 21). As Sadker and Sadker (1994, p. 198) point out, however, families begin the process by raising boys according to the cultural ideal of being active, aggressive, and independent; schools inadvertently collude in rewarding their aggressiveness by "going the extra mile" with attention and resources for the nation's future male leaders, as destined by tradition.

Factors Contributing to Youth Violence

In the United States, behavioral specialists assert that antisocial behavior by children should be viewed as a national emergency. For example, young children who bring weapons to school today may become future school dropouts, batterers, and rapists. Given the cultural norms, perhaps the most surprising thing is that there is not more violence. As a paradoxical commentary on the influence (or failure?) of the women's movement, many young girls and women use their newly found "freedom" to adopt the aggressive and violent norms of men, including arming themselves in the illusion of self-protection (Morgenstern, 1997; Webster, Vernick, Ludwig, & Lester, 1997; Wright, Wintemute, & Rivara, 1999). The incidence of violence by teenage girls is rising (one of every four juveniles arrested is female), although female rates of homicide are far behind those for boys (Buzawa & Buzawa, 1996; Chesney-Lind, 1997; Cotten et al., 1994). While some men are discovering the pleasures and growth potential of assuming the parenting and nurturing roles traditionally dominated by women, some women choose violence. They have yet to learn from the plight of battered women that violence begets more serious violence (Hoff, 1990). Educators and youth workers Brendtro,

Brokenleg, and Van Bockern (1990, pp. 6–7) trace the discouragement and alienation of youth at risk to four ecological hazards:

1. *Destructive relationships,* as experienced by the rejected or unclaimed child, hungry for love but unable to trust, expecting to be hurt again
2. *Climates of futility,* as encountered by the insecure youngster, crippled by feelings of inadequacy and a fear of failure
3. *Learned irresponsibility,* as seen in the youth whose sense of powerlessness may be masked by indifference or defiant, rebellious behavior
4. *Loss of purpose,* as portrayed by a generation of self-centered youth, desperately searching for meaning in a world of confusing values

These hazards are intertwined with contemporary parenting and family life—among poor families, inadequate time and resources for effective parenting; among some privileged families, excessive material indulgence and permissiveness that leave a child with few boundaries and skills to control behavior and a vacuum around life's larger meaning beyond consumerism.

In the United States, in view of such factors as racism, the powerful gun lobby, and the pauperization of mothers who are raising children alone in an inequitable labor market, not only must "teachers, parents, and peers" (Walker, 1993, p. 23) influence antisocial children, but policymakers, church leaders, and all who care about the future of humanity must look "upstream" to discover why children are lost to violence and despair (DuRant, Cadenhead, Pendergast, Slavens, & Linder, 1994; Holinger, Offer, Barter, & Bell, 1994; Way, 1993; West, 1994). As Marian Wright Edelman (1994, p. 6) said following a survey commissioned by the Children's Defense Fund and the Black Community Crusade, "This poll confirms what black leaders already know—that we have a major black child crisis, the worst since slavery."

In response to the crisis of youth violence that is primarily sociocultural in origin, will we invent yet another medicalized explanation like "urban stress syndrome" to excuse assailants and neglect victims? Or will we examine social environments we have created or allowed to fester as a plague that threatens the lives of all who dwell there? Jenkins and Bell (1992, p. 82) note, for example, that in a study of five hundred elementary school children, 24 percent had witnessed a murder. Many youthful offenders have had no support in healing from childhood trauma (Holinger et al., 1994; Mendel, 1994). Will people make a connection between values (Dionne, 1999; Eyre & Eyre, 1993), the proliferation of guns, and the shocking increase of children killing children—and others? Again, this is not an either-or dichotomy. Mitigating circumstances must be considered in judging individual cases, but excusing violent action does nothing to facilitate the growth and resiliency that distressed people, including alienated youth, are capable of when supported through crisis. DiNapoli's research (2000) supports this point; findings revealed previous victimization (such as by gang-related violence) as the strongest predictor of youth violence. While facing the enormous challenge of youth violence, it is crucial to remember that we are *influenced* by our past, not *determined* by it. Further, with social support, individuals who have endured almost unimaginable cruelty have lived to tell their stories of endurance and survival. Paul Mones (1993, p. 32), an attorney specializing in the defense of children who have killed their parents, notes that the most common trigger event before parricide is the child's despair after receiving no help when they finally report abuse to an adult.

Clearly, youth violence cuts across class, race, and gender boundaries. Despite continued disparity in educational and other resources between racial minority groups and the white majority, it is noteworthy that in the vast majority of recent school shooting tragedies, the assailants were white boys from a range of socioeconomic classes. These highly publicized instances of youth violence tend to obscure the statistical decline in youth crime rates, including school-based violence, over the past several years. But nonstatistical examination of these dramatic examples of youth violence reveals the complexity of factors influencing each case; in many instances, social alienation, harassment by classmates, and mental health problems were evident but not attended to with preventive measures such as recognizing and responding to the meaning of supposedly "idle" verbal threats or unusual behaviors.

Crisis Prevention and Intervention Programs

Despite this grim picture, the tide may be turning; crisis intervention and anger management programs are being developed in many schools and special treatment settings for disturbed youth. Leona Eggert (1994), for example, has developed a guide for teachers, school nurses, and others working with adolescents and young adults. Fritz Redl developed the Massaging Numb Values Life Space Interview to help aggressive students, many with histories of abuse, who become overwhelmed with guilt and remorse about their destructive behavior (Long & Wilder, 1993). Holden and Powers (1993) describe a therapeutic crisis intervention program developed at Cornell University. The four phases in this model—*triggering, escalation, crisis,* and *recovery*—correspond roughly to the phases of crisis development originally put forth by Caplan (see Chapter Two), with a particular focus on observing behavioral cues in young people. At the institutional or ecological level, Watson, Poda, Miller, Rice, & West (1990) offer step-by-step guidelines to prevent and manage a range of school emergencies, including violence. Such ecological approaches include the active involvement of parents and the entire community to provide safety and a hopeful future for its most vulnerable citizens.

In their hope-inspiring book, *Reclaiming Youth at Risk,* Brendtro et al. (1990) draw on values of a traditional Native society of North America, the Lakota Sioux, in their application of the medicine wheel, with its four spokes depicting *belonging, mastery, independence, and generosity.* To many Native peoples, the number four has sacred meaning. They see the person standing in a circle (a symbol of life) surrounded by the four directions—the requisites for a child to feel whole, competent, and cherished as a member of the community.

The tradition in which the entire community assumes responsibility for its children is highlighted by a widely publicized case of tribal justice. Two seventeen-year-old boys of the Tlingit Nation in Alaska, who were convicted of robbing and beating a man, were turned over to their village by a judge in Washington state. Village elders meted out justice in the form of a year to eighteen-month exile on Alaska's uninhabited islands. The intent was for the boys to reflect on their behavior, observe the power of natural beauty, and emulate the basic skills taught by their elders—something offenders rarely learn in a locked cell. Holland (1994) shares similar hopeful themes among the people of Soweto, South Africa, who are trying to reclaim their heritage after the devastating effects of apartheid.

A central theme in these programs is that controlling, authoritarian responses by adults to aggressive behavior is part of the problem, not the solution. This is because much of youth violence springs from a history of abuse, neglect, and behaviors that control rather than nurture, direct, and foster growth through love and consistent nonviolent discipline. Inconsistent discipline—or conflicting messages from parents and other adults—leaves children confused, directionless, and anxious.[1] Many young people act out aggressively because they feel disempowered and alienated in a society that does not meet their needs. But as frightening as youth aggression and violence can be, it is crucial to remember that *violence begets violence* (Charney, 1993; Tierney, Dowd, & O'Kane, 1993). There are many models of effective intervention with troubled youth, and many professionals and others are skilled at using them. Outcome studies of programs such as skills training in anger management are not yet available, though preliminary results suggest that youthful participants respond positively to them (Ferrell & Meyer, 1997; Jenkins & Bell, 1992, p. 79). Certainly, at-risk youth can learn and benefit from nonviolent responses to conflict situations. But if they see no hope of escape from racism and a neglected social milieu, their individual tactics to avoid violence may be very short-lived. The greater challenge, then, is in the primary prevention domain of changing the socioeconomic and other factors—including a cultural climate glorifying violence—that severely shortchange young people, a nation's most precious resource (see Chapter Eight, Figure 8.1, Box 3).

Men Who Batter Women

The programs that are now being developed and implemented for dealing with batterers are possible because of the evolution in thinking about how we view these offenders. The most successful programs combine community intervention with criminal justice efforts.

[1]For practical manuals and videos dealing with prevention of aggression and violence among youth, readers are referred to National Educational Service at 800-733-6786 or 812-336-7700. Readers can also call the National Youth Violence Prevention Resource Center toll-free hotline at 1-866-SAFEYOUTH (723-3968) or see their Web site at www.safeyouth.org.

Views on Battering and Batterers

Early work in the violence literature depicted wife battering as the norm in marriage and batterers as incorrigible, with character disorders or a problem with alcohol that excused them from accountability. Gondolf's research (1987) with violent men reveals four types of batterers—sociopathic, antisocial, chronic, and sporadic. Gondolf suggests that sociopathic batterers need continual restraint to stem their violence, whereas those with antisocial behaviors need a variety of coordinated interventions. In a controversial experimental study, Sherman and Berk (1984) found that arrest had the greatest impact on reducing recidivism (repeat battering) as compared with mediation and crisis intervention. Edleson and Tolman (1992, p. 132), citing later studies, note that community intervention such as the Minneapolis Intervention Project *combined* with criminal justice efforts may offer more protection to women. Similar findings have been reported in Canada, despite its aggressive arrest laws (MacLeod, 1989).

This view is supported by Klein's (1994) study of 664 men who were issued civil restraining orders by the Quincy, Massachusetts, court. Reliance on such orders alone did not prevent more abuse, especially among younger, unmarried abusers with prior criminal records who also abused alcohol. Klein, chief probation officer of the Quincy court, asserts, "These male batterers look like criminals, act like criminals, and re-abuse like criminals" (p. 111). The majority of men in this study who reabused were not arrested and if arrested were not sentenced to jail or probation supervision. Another finding with particular relevance for those who ask, "Why doesn't she leave?" was that many of the victims had either divorced or physically separated from their abusers—suggesting how little control women have in preventing reabuse (p. 113). Klein's study supports earlier critiques of the criminal justice system that has failed to treat domestic violence as criminal behavior. Newspaper accounts also reveal that restraining orders have not prevented the murders of women. In fact, clinical work with abused women reveals that they are perhaps in greatest danger after filing for a restraining order, particularly in cases in which the woman's partner feels that he owns her and is now confronted with an external force threatening his need to control her. This underscores the need for caution in persuading a woman to seek court protection and for trusting the woman's own judgment of the man's potential for violence and the contextual factors that may inflame him.

Programs for Violent Men

Moving beyond the debate about whether batterers should receive treatment or serve time in jail, the both-and approach discussed earlier should generally be the norm, even when the women who have been battered—especially those intent on salvaging their relationship and marriage—just want the violence to stop, by whatever means. To carry out that approach, the health and criminal justice aspects of domestic violence must be synchronized. In the public health and crisis prevention framework of this book, any program for men who batter must include two key facets:

1. The need to assess and reassess their potential for further assault or homicide, as suggested in Table 9.1
2. The importance of holding the perpetrator accountable for his violent behavior, regardless of mental pathology and any excuses, such as the woman's behavior provoked him to violence

These program elements imply regular supportive contact with the woman who was abused and is possibly still at risk, particularly if she has filed a restraining order and in instances when men present themes of jealousy, desperation, and ownership of their partner (Meloy, 1992).

Court-mandated counseling has led to a proliferation of batterer programs illustrating a variety of intervention systems (Gondolf, 1999; Lee, Green, & Rheinscheld, 1999). Despite progress in evaluating the effects of these programs, results are still mixed (Babcock & Steiner, 1999). However, those who have developed standards for and researched batterer programs assert that accountability and victim safety are central, regardless of competing perspectives (Austin & Dankwort, 1999; Bennett & Piet, 1999). Outcome measures of effectiveness across four programs that Gondolf evaluated included reassault rates (recidivism), rates of men making threats, and victims' assessment of quality of life since the abuser completed a treatment program. The longest, most comprehensive program demonstrated the lowest reassault rate; this nine-month program of weekly group counseling also includes an extensive clinical evaluation, in-house substance abuse treatment, individual psychotherapy for emotional and mental problems, and casework with women partners (Gondolf, 1999, pp. 44–45).

Some mental health professionals object to the standardization and certification of these programs, based on their view of domestic abuse as a psychiatric disorder or a biologically based dysfunction (Bennett & Piet, 1999). The flaw in this argument is similar to that held until recently regarding mental patients' assaults against health workers. Interpreting the assaults as the expected expression of aggression originating from the patient's psychopathology led to this conclusion: assaulted workers are not entitled to justice; rather, they should accept their victimization as part of the job.

There is nevertheless a move toward certification and regulation of batterer programs across the United States and Canada; standards have been enacted in twenty-one states and three provinces, and several more (five states and three provinces) have drafts of standards. Groups establishing these programs acknowledge the need for mental health service such as cognitive-behavior therapy, but they define battering as a learned behavior—*not* pathology—which is used to intimidate and control the victim (Bennett & Piet, 1999). The polarizing arguments between mental health and criminal justice professionals appear as a microcosm of the larger debate regarding biomedical and psychotherapeutic approaches to therapy (Luhrmann, 2000). The American Psychological Association asserts that psychologists should set standards (Bennett & Piet, p. 12). Meanwhile, in Massachusetts, the batterers certification program is under jurisdiction of the Department of Public Health, in keeping with the global definition of violence as a public health problem.

Today in the United States and Canada, most programs are modeled after the Domestic Violence Intervention Project developed by Ellen Pence and colleagues in Duluth, Minnesota. This model is informed primarily by profeminist principles that define woman battering and sexual violence in terms of power and control (Kurz, 1993; Pence & Paymar, 1986; Yllo, 1993). In the *power and control wheel* central to this model, eight spokes depict the ways in which men use violence to maintain power and control of women:

- Intimidation—smashing things, displaying weapons
- Emotional abuse—putting the woman down, making her think she is crazy
- Isolation—controlling what she does, where she goes
- Minimization of abuse—denying, blaming, making light of the abuse, saying she caused it
- Exploitation of children—using visitation to harass her
- Assertion of male privilege—treating her like a servant
- Economic abuse—giving her an allowance, taking her money
- Coercion and threats—threatening to leave or commit suicide

In most programs for men who batter, group counseling is the preferred mode (Edleson & Tolman, 1992), usually including other men who have been violent in the past but are no longer violent. This approach underscores the premise that violence is not inevitable but is learned and reinforced through parenting practices and its pervasiveness in the sociocultural milieu. Couples counseling and family systems approaches are highly controversial (Bograd & Mederos, 1999), as they tend to obscure violence as the primary problem in the use of such terms as *transaction* and imply the counselor's "neutrality" in regard to criminal behavior. If couples counseling is used, safety, ownership of responsibility for violence, and a *prior* intention of reconciliation must first be established (Edleson & Tolman, 1992, pp. 88–107).

Although programs for batterers and refuges for victims must be supported, these are only secondary and tertiary measures; essentially they are our reactive approaches to a problem that would be much less costly in financial and human terms if primary prevention were more valued and promoted, as discussed later in this chapter.

Crises of People Prosecuted for Violence

Many people believe that the perpetrators of crime have a clear advantage over their victims. Aside from the issue of accountability for violent behavior, we should remember that violent people or those who are apprehended for a crime, especially if they go to jail, are also in crisis—the parents who have beaten their child to death; the rapist; the woman batterer; the eighteen-year-old who goes to jail after his first offense of breaking and entering with intent to rob; the middle-class man who has sexually abused a child; the mother who loses custody of her children when she goes to prison for a minor drug offense, shoplifting, or prostitution; and the murderer. In addition to the trauma of being arrested and incarcerated, the prisoner may experience extreme shame, desertion by family, or panic over homosexual advances. Or the prisoner may suffer from chronic mental illness and if awaiting the death penalty may lack adequate legal council because of poverty. For mothers of young children, imprisonment may also result in permanent loss of custody of their children. With the increased number of women prisoners, space and other conditions are often more deplorable than they are in overcrowded men's prisons. Suicides are more likely in short-term detention facilities during the height of crisis when there is great uncertainty about one's fate; in long-term holding centers, they are often related to prison conditions.

Let us consider the crises of those prosecuted for crimes in the context of public policy and statistical data on U.S. prisoners. Between 1970 and 1999, the number of inmates in federal and state prisons and jails increased fivefold to nearly two million; 94 percent are male, 25 percent are there for drug offenses, a majority have not completed high school, 33 percent were unemployed prior to sentencing, and over half had been under the influence of alcohol or other drugs at the time of their offense. There are similar dramatic increases in the number of persons on probation or parole, with a disproportionate number (48 percent) being young black males. Rates of incarceration in the United States are the second highest in the world, behind Russia. Women are more likely than men to be in prison for nonviolent crimes (68 percent), as sentencing becomes harsher. The newborns of pregnant prisoners are separated from their mothers within twenty-four hours of birth (Chicago Legal Aid to Incarcerated Mothers, 1997).

Crisis Intervention with Assailants and Those Threatening Violence

All of the principles of crisis intervention apply to the violent or potentially violent person in prison, the home, or the workplace. The application of these principles to aggressive, antisocial, or violent people can help ensure safety of self and others. They are summarized as follows:

1. Keep communication lines open. As long as a person is communicating, violence usually does not occur.
2. Facilitate communication between a disgruntled employee or patient, for example, and the person against whom he or she is threatening violence.
3. Develop specific plans—*with* the dangerous person—for nonviolent expression of anger, such as time-out, jogging, punching a pillow, or calling a hotline.
4. Communicate by telephone or behind closed doors whenever possible when dealing with an armed person, especially until rapport is established and the person's anxiety subsides.

5. If dangerous weapons are involved, collaborate with police for their removal whenever possible; implement emergency procedures for appropriate application of force, such as calling security or police or mobilizing a team effort to warn fellow workers. Failure to work in teams can be life threatening.

6. Insist on administrative support and emergency backup help; refuse any assignment that requires working alone in high-risk settings—for example, psychiatric wards or crisis outreach visits.

7. Make hotline numbers and emergency call buttons readily available.

8. Examine social and institutional sources of violent behavior—for example, harsh authoritarian approaches to employee relations, which may trigger violence by an upset patient or a disgruntled worker; failure to help disturbed persons seek professional help as an alternative to violence; and rigid structures and rules for geriatric and psychiatric patients.

9. Warn potential victims of homicide, based on risk assessment and the principles of the Tarasoff case (see *Tarasoff* v. *The Regents of the University of California*, 1976; VandeCreek & Knapp, 1993).

10. Remember that a violent person who is also threatening suicide is a greater risk for homicide.

11. Conduct follow-up. Engage in social and political activity to prevent violence.

Several factors, however, may become obstacles to providing aid to these people in crisis: (1) the sense of contempt or loathing one may feel toward a criminal or patient who has threatened a health worker, (2) the fear of the prisoner or other person threatening violence, and (3) the need to work within the physical and social constraints of the detention setting or workplace where one does not anticipate interaction with disturbed or violent persons. People working in these settings, therefore, must assess and deal with crises according to the circumstances of their particular situations. The works of McGinnis (1993), Meloy (1992), and Tavris (1983) are particularly recommended.

Follow-Up Service

Specialists in criminal justice cite the problem of recidivism among people convicted of crimes. The ex-offender is stripped of status and community respect and often has been exposed to conditions that harden and embitter rather than rehabilitate. Considering the dire financial straits of the ex-prisoner—a situation that frequently was present before incarceration—along with a lack of job skills, discrimination in employment, and the absence of follow-up programs, it is not difficult to understand why crime becomes a career for some.

Advocates of prison reform and various church groups are working to bring about long-term change in the conditions that seem to breed rather than prevent crime. For the nonviolent offender (more than half the American prison population), alternatives to jail sentencing are being tried in many states—a penalty system used in Native communities and in Europe for years. These less costly and more effective options include (1) community service, such as working in parks and public buildings, (2) restitution, a sanction that is particularly appealing because it takes into account the person most directly affected by the crime—the victim, (3) intermittent confinement, a strategy that spares total disruption of work and family, and (4) intensive probation—that is, no more than twenty-five persons per officer. These humane approaches should be weighed against the thousands of dollars spent each year to keep a person in prison.

The mandatory minimum drug sentencing laws of 1986 have played a major role in the 400 percent increase of incarcerated women in the United States (Cooper, 1999). This law, the widening gap between the privileged and the disadvantaged, and policies emanating from the legacy of slavery and racism in the United States contribute to the counterproductivity of punitive versus rehabilitative measures. Instead of a criminal justice system emanating from revenge and punishment, as in "three strikes and you're out," which often does not fit the crime, let us consider the principles and Signposts of Restorative Justice. As Zehr and Mika (1997) state, "Crime wounds. . . . Justice heals." We are working toward restorative justice when we

1. focus on the *harms* of wrongdoing more than the rules that have been broken,
2. show equal concern and commitment to *victims and offenders,* involving both in the process of justice,
3. work toward the restoration of *victims,* empowering them and responding to their needs as they see them,
4. support *offenders* while encouraging them to understand, accept, and carry out their obligations,
5. recognize that while *obligations* may be difficult for offenders, they should not be intended as harms and they must be achievable,
6. provide opportunities for *dialogue,* direct or indirect, between victims and offenders as appropriate,
7. involve and empower the affected *community* through the justice process, and increase its capacity to recognize and respond to community bases of crime,
8. encourage *collaboration* and *reintegration* rather than coercion and isolation,
9. give attention to the *unintended consequences* of our actions and programs,
10. show *respect* to all parties, including victims, offenders, and justice colleagues.
    [Reprinted with permission from the Mennonite Central Committee]

These issues regarding violence, its prevention, and restorative justice speak to the social change strategies in Box 3 of the Crisis Paradigm.

The Families of Prisoners

Inmates and ex-offenders are not alone in their distress. Historically, their families, especially children, are also neglected. Although there are generally fewer women than men in prison, at least a quarter of a million U.S. children have mothers who are incarcerated. Families not only lose a spouse, parent, or child to prison but may also lose a source of income and status in the community. Poverty, loneliness, and boredom are just a few of the problems faced by these families. Those who attempt to sustain relationships find that prison regulations (such as body searches of visitors and lack of privacy) or societal pressure and personal circumstances thwart their efforts. Children of imprisoned parents feel sadness, anxiety, guilt, and anger. If a divorce occurs during or following imprisonment, the postrelease problems of the ex-offender are increased.

To address the crises of prisoners' families, more self-help groups such as Families and Friends of Prisoners in Dorchester, Massachusetts, are needed. This group provides moral support, counseling, information, and inexpensive transportation to state and federal prisons. Similar groups, such as Aid to Incarcerated Mothers, focus on the special needs of mothers and children. Information about these groups is available through public health departments and coalitions for abused women.

Primary Prevention of Crime and Antisocial Behavior

Chapter One presented a general picture of primary prevention as it pertains to life crises, emphasizing the public health and communitywide action necessary if we are to prevent stressful events and situations from escalating into full-blown crises. Here this approach is explicated with particular reference to crises of both victims and perpetrators of violence and antisocial behavior. Clearly, as long as loopholes exist in the criminal justice system's response to battering, refuges are no less than lifesaving for many women. Similarly, residential treatment programs for out-of-control youth are necessary. But the very fact that an entire system of residential programs for battered women has been established speaks to the tendency, especially in the United States, toward *reactive* rather than *preventive* approaches. History reveals that all societies establish rules for how to treat deviant members.

Criminal justice system loopholes and refuges for victims beg for an alternative approach. Instead of forcing victims to live like fugitives, with the additional burden of single parenting, what if *perpetrators* were required to leave and receive counseling in alternative housing as an incentive to stop their violent behavior? Perhaps when the cultural milieu and would-be offenders are saturated with the message of zero tolerance for violence—in the next generation, we hope—the present refuges for victims might be retrofitted for perpetrators instead. The fruits of such a policy recommendation (Hoff, 1990) are underscored by a study in twenty-nine cities documenting that the lives saved by the shelter system are mostly those of men—that is, murders are prevented because women receive help through hotline, shelter, and legal services before reaching the point of using deadly force against their abusers. However, if the male partners do not receive help, they are more likely to kill the women (Dugan, Nagin, & Rosenfeld, 2001; Masters, 1999). In other words, refuges for abused women are just that—an emergency resource, not primary prevention.

But how do we get beyond emergency measures? We certainly will not get there without the communitywide endeavors generally intrinsic to the primary approach to health care. Such measures have already been suggested in the section on youth violence; more strategies follow.

Personal and Social-Psychological Strategies

When sincerely addressing the issue, individuals may become overwhelmed by the pervasiveness of violence and withdraw out of a sense of helplessness, self-protection, or both. It is important therefore to focus on selected actions and obtainable goals. These may include

1. Adopting nonviolent language in everyday social interaction
2. Using nonviolent ways of disciplining children; attending parent effectiveness training groups to assist with difficult child-rearing challenges
3. Attending self-defense courses as a means of bolstering self-confidence and providing a substitute for arming oneself; avoiding violence as a response to violence
4. Reading about and attending continuing education courses on nonviolent conflict resolution in personal relationships
5. Avoiding sex-role stereotyping in child rearing and other interactions with children
6. Organizing neighborhood patrols and systematic ways of watching out for one another
7. Providing employees with violence prevention information and emergency protocols, including how to recognize and respond humanely to an upset or disgruntled worker with antisocial tendencies

Sociopolitical Strategies

These strategies are most successful when combined with personal and social-psychological approaches on the premise that people need grounding in information and self-confidence in order to stand firm against obstacles in the political arena. Among the most obvious are these:

1. *Educating the public through schools, community organizations, and churches.* How many people who have attended church, synagogue, or mosque, for example, have heard a sermon condemning violence against women and children or have sponsored programs to explicitly address such issues? Probably not many have done so. Abused people often turn to clergy for help, and many religious leaders are now responding to the unique opportunity they have in preventing violence (Fortune & Hertze, 1987). And how many nurses, for example, who conduct childbirth and parenting classes routinely include strategies to deal nonaggressively with a demanding, finicky, or special-needs infant?

2. *Contacting legislators and organizing for a change in laws that may be outdated or otherwise do not address the issues local people confront.* In the United States, this includes addressing the powerful gun lobby.
3. *Using advocacy and systematic organizing around racial and economic justice.* This includes seeking equality in educational opportunities and addressing the media influence on violence (see Sorenson, Peterson, & Berk, 1998).

Professional Strategies

In the United States, the Surgeon General's report (U.S. Department of Health and Human Services, 1986) recommended that all licensed professionals be required to study and pass examination questions in violence prevention and the treatment of various victims of violence. As a complement to this public policy statement, individual professionals can exert leadership and advocacy within their own groups for curriculum and in-service program development to systematically address this topic. At present, such educational endeavors are incidental at best (Ross, Hoff, & Coutu-Wakulczyk, 1998, Tilden et al., 1994; Woodtli & Breslin, in press). In Canada, the federal government has published a document entitled *Violence Issues: An Interdisciplinary Curriculum Guide for Health Professionals* (Hoff, 1995), which covers education about violence prevention and service for victims and assailants in a life-span perspective. This document is addressed to the following disciplines: dentistry, medicine, nursing, occupational therapy, pharmacy, physical therapy, psychology (clinical), and social work. The American Association of Colleges of Nursing (1999) has produced a position paper underscoring the need for inclusion of violence content in all nursing education programs. Similar programs have been developed for criminal justice professionals in North America and other countries.

The vast knowledge already available to professionals must be combined with personal strategies in order to

- Widely disseminate new knowledge about this poignant topic to the public
- Change the values and attitudes that have served as fertile soil for nurturing violent and antisocial behavior
- Effect broad policy and functioning of social institutions through the political process necessary to bring about needed change

Summary

The crisis of increasing violence, especially among the young, is gaining international attention, while more and more health professionals and educators are joining grassroots community groups to address the crisis. Because children and youth are a nation's most precious resource, few crises command more urgent attention, not only for the sake of the assailants and their victims but also for the future of a nation. Sociopolitical responses must be joined with assistance to the individuals and families affected by violence.

References

American Association of Colleges of Nursing. (1999). *Position paper: Violence as a public health problem*. Washington, DC: Author.

Arnetz, J. E., & Arnetz, B. B. (2001). Violence towards health care staff and possible effects on the quality of patient care. *Social Science and Medicine, 52*, 417–427.

Austin, J. B., & Dankwort, J. (1999). The impact of a batterers' program on battered women. *Violence Against Women, 5*(1), 25–42.

Babcock, J., & Steiner, R. (1999). The relationship between treatment, incarceration, and recidivism of battering: A program evaluation of Seattle's coordinated community response to domestic violence. *Journal of Family Psychology, 13*(1), 46–59.

Baracos, H. A. (1974). Iatrogenic and preventive intervention in police-family crisis situations. *International Journal of Social Psychiatry, 20*, 113–121.

Bard, M. (1972). *Police, family crisis intervention, and conflict management: An action research analysis*. Washington, DC: U.S. Department of Justice.

Bennett, L., & Piet, M. (1999). Standards for batterer intervention programs: In whose interests? *Violence Against Women, 5*(1), 6–24.

Bograd, M., & Mederos, F. (1999). Battering and couples therapy: Universal screening and selection of treatment modality. *Journal of Marital and Family Therapy, 25*(3), 291–312.

Brendtro, L. K., Brokenleg, M., & Van Bockern, S. (1990). *Reclaiming youth at risk: Our hope for the future*. Bloomington, IN: National Educational Service.

Buzawa, E. S., & Buzawa, C. G. (1996). *Domestic violence: The criminal justice response*. Thousand Oaks, CA: Sage.

Capponi, P. (1992). *Upstairs in the crazy house*. Toronto: Penguin Books.

Charney, R. (1993). Teaching children nonviolence. *Journal of Emotional and Behavioral Problems, 2*(1), 46–48.

Chesney-Lind, M. (1997). *The female offender: Girls, women, and crime*. Thousand Oaks, CA: Sage.

Chicago Legal Aid to Incarcerated Mothers. [http://www/c_l_a_i_m.org/factsheet.htm]. 1997.

Cooper, K. (1999, Spring). Mandatory sentencing. *Behind the Wall, 4*.

Cotten, N. U., Resnick, J., Browne, D. C., Martin, S. L., McCarraher, D. R., & Woods, J. (1994). Aggression and fighting behavior among African-American adolescents: Individual and family factors. *American Journal of Public Health, 84*(4), 618–622.

Daniels, A. K. (1978). The social construction of military psychiatric diagnosis. In J. G. Manis & B. N. Meltzer (Eds.), *Symbolic interaction* (3rd ed., pp. 380–392). Needham Heights, MA: Allyn & Bacon.

DiNapoli, P. (2000). *A Contextual analysis of adolescent violence using the interaction model of health behavior*. Unpublished doctoral dissertation, University of Massachusetts, Lowell.

Dionne, E. J. (1999, September 20). Our exceptionally violent nation. *Boston Globe*, p. A13.

Dugan, L., Nagin, D., & Rosenfeld, R. (2001). *Explaining the decline in intimate partner homicide: The effects of changing domesticity, women's status, and domestic violence resources*. Paper presented at the 1997 meeting of the American Society of Criminology.

DuRant, R. H., Cadenhead, C., Pendergast, R. A., Slavens, G., & Linder, C, W. (1994). Factors associated with the use of violence among urban black adolescents. *American Journal of Public Health, 84*(4), 612–617.

Edelman, M. W. (1994, May 27). Poll finds pervasive fear in blacks over violence and their children. *Boston Globe,* p. 6.

Edleson, J. L., & Tolman, R. M. (1992). *Intervention for men who batter: An ecological approach.* Thousand Oaks, CA: Sage.

Eggert, L. L. (1994). *Anger management for youth: Stemming aggression and violence.* Bloomington, IN: National Educational Service.

Ellickson, P., Saner, H., & McGuigan, K. A. (1997). Profiles of violent youth: Substance use and other concurrent problems. *American Journal of Public Health, 87*(6), 985–991.

Engel, F., & Marsh, S. (1986). Helping the employee victim of violence in hospitals. *Hospital and Community Psychiatry, 37*(2), 159–162.

Eyre, J., & Eyre, R. (1993). *Teaching your children values.* New York: Simon & Schuster.

Ferrell, A. D., & Meyer, A. L. (1997). The effectiveness of a school-based curriculum for reducing violence among urban sixth-grade students. *American Journal of Public Health, 87*(6), 979–984.

Fortune, M., & Hertze, J. (1987). A commentary on religious issues in family violence. In M. Pellauer, B. Chester, & J. Boyajian (Eds.), *Sexual assault and abuse: A handbook for clergy and religious professionals* (pp. 67–83). New York: HarperCollins.

Gondolf, E. (1987). *Research on men who batter.* Bradenton, FL: Human Services Institute.

Gondolf, E. (1999). *A comparison of four batterer intervention systems: Do court referral, program length, and services matter? Journal of Interpersonal Violence, 14*(1), 41–61.

Gove, W. (1975). *The labeling of deviance.* New York: Wiley.

Halleck, S. L. (1987). *The mentally disordered offender.* Washington, DC: American Psychiatric Press.

Hoff, L. A. (1990). *Battered women as survivors.* London: Routledge.

Hoff, L. A. (1993). Review essay: Health policy and the plight of the mentally ill. *Psychiatry, 56*(4), 400–419.

Hoff, L. A. (1995). *Violence issues: An interdisciplinary curriculum guide for health professionals* [in English and French]. Ottawa: Health Canada, Health Services Directorate.

Hoff, L. A., & Adamowski, K. (1998). *Creating excellence in crisis care: A guide to effective training and program designs.* San Francisco: Jossey-Bass.

Hoff, L. A., & Wells, J. O. (Eds.). (1989). *Certification standards manual* (4th ed.). Denver: American Association of Suicidology.

Holden, M. J., & Powers, J. L. (1993). Therapeutic crisis intervention. *Journal of Emotional and Behavioral Problems, 2*(1), 49–52.

Holinger, P. C., Offer, D., Barter, J. T., & Bell, C. C. (1994). *Suicide and homicide among adolescents.* New York: Guilford Press.

Holland, H. (1994). *Born in Soweto.* Harmondsworth, England: Penguin Books.

Hoover, J. H., & Juul, K. (1993). Bullying in Europe and the United States. *Journal of Emotional and Behavioral Problems, 2*(1), 25–29.

Jenkins, E. J., & Bell, C. C. (1992). Adolescent violence: Can it be curbed? *Adolescent Medicine: State of the Art Reviews, 3*(1), 71–86.

Jenkins, L., Layne, L. A., & Kisner, S. M. (1992). Homicide in the workplace: The U.S. experience, 1980–1988. *American Association of Occupational Health Nursing Journal, 40*(5), 215–218.

Johnson, A. B. (1990). *Out of bedlam: The truth about deinstitutionalization.* New York: Basic Books.

Klein, A. (1994). *Re-abuse in a population of court-restrained male batterers after two years: Development of a predictive model.* Unpublished doctoral dissertation, Law, Policy, and Society Program, Northeastern University, Boston.

Kurz, D. (1993). Physical assaults by husbands: A major social problem. In R. J. Gelles & D. R. Loseke (Eds.), *Current controversies on family violence* (pp. 88–103). Thousand Oaks, CA: Sage.

Lee, M., Green, G. J., & Rheinscheld, J. (1999). A model for short-term solution-focused group treatment of male domestic violence offenders. *Journal of Family Social Work, 3*(2), 39–57.

Levin, P. F., Hewitt, J. B., & Misner, S. T. (1992). Female workplace homicides: An integrative research review. *American Association of Occupational Health Nursing Journal, 40*(5), 229–236.

Lipscomb, J. A., & Love, C. C. (1992). Violence toward health care workers: An emerging occupational hazard. *American Association of Occupational Health Nursing Journal, 40*(5), 219–228.

Long, N. J., & Wilder, M. T. (1993). From rage to responsibility: A Massaging Numb Values LSI. *Journal of Emotional and Behavioral Problems, 2*(1), 35–40.

Luhrmann, T. M. (2000). *Of two minds: The growing disorder in American psychiatry.* New York: Knopf.

MacLeod, L. (1989). *Wife battering and the web of hope: Progress, dilemmas, and visions of prevention.* Ottawa: Health and Welfare Canada. National Clearinghouse on Family Violence.

Masters, B. A. (1999, March 15). Women's shelters save mostly men. *Boston Globe,* p. A3.

McGinnis, C. (1993). *Lifeline: A training manual.* Boston: Suffolk County Jail.

Melick, M. E., Steadman, H. J., & Cocozza, J. J. (1979). The medicalization of criminal behavior among mental patients. *Journal of Health and Social Behavior, 20,* 228–237.

Meloy, R. (1992). *Violent attachments.* Northvale, NJ: Aronson.

Mendel, M. P. (1994). *The male survivor.* Thousand Oaks, CA: Sage.

Miller, L. (1999). Workplace violence: Prevention, response, and recovery. *Psychotherapy, 36*(2), 160–169.

Monahan, J. (1981). *Predicting violent behavior: An assessment of clinical techniques.* Thousand Oaks, CA: Sage.

Mones, P. (1993). Parricide: A window on child abuse. *Journal of Emotional and Behavioral Problems, 2*(1), 30–34.

Morgenstern, H. (1997). Editorial: Gun availability and violent death. *American Journal of Public Health, 87*(6), 899–900.

Morton, P. G. (1986). Managing assaultive patients. *American Journal of Nursing, 86*(10), 114–116.

Pan American Health Organization. (1994, November 16 and 17). *Inter-American Conference on Society, Violence, and Health.* Washington, DC: Author.

Pence, E., & Paymar, M. (1986). *Power and control: Tactics of men who batter.* Duluth: Minnesota Program Development.

Ross, M., Hoff, L. A., & Coutu-Wakulczyk, G. (1998). Nursing curricula and violence issues: A study of Canadian schools of nursing. *Journal of Nursing Education, 37*(2), 53–60.

Sadker, M., & Sadker, D. (1994). *Failing at fairness: How America's schools cheat girls.* New York: Scribner.

Scheff, T. J. (Ed.). (1975). *Labeling madness.* Englewood Cliffs, NJ: Prentice Hall.

Sherman, L. W., & Berk, R. A. (1984). The specific deterrent effects of arrest for domestic assault. *American Sociological Review, 49*(4), 261–272.

Sorenson, S. B., Peterson, J. G., & Berk, R. A. (1998). New media coverage and the epidemiology of homicide. *American Journal of Public Health, 88*(10), 1510–1514.

Tarasoff v. *The Regents of the University of California.* (1976). 551P. 2d 334. Also in 131 California Reporter 14. Supreme Court of California.

Tavris, C. (1983). *Anatomy of anger.* New York: Simon & Schuster.

Tierney, J., Dowd, T., & O'Kane, S. (1993). Empowering aggressive youth to change. *Journal of Emotional and Behavioral Problems, 2*(1), 41–45.

Tilden, V. P., Schmidt, T. A., Limandri, B. J., Chiodo, G. T., Garland, M. J., & Loveless, P. A. (1994). Factors that influence clinicians' assessment and management of family violence. *American Journal of Public Health, 84*(4), 628–633.

Toch, H. (1969). *Violent men.* Hawthorne, NY: Aldine de Gruyter.

U.S. Department of Health and Human Services. (1986). *Surgeon General's workshop on violence and public health: Report.* Washington, DC: Author.

Vande Creek, L., & Knapp, S. (1993). *Tarasoff and beyond: Legal and clinical considerations in the treatment of life-endangering patients* (Rev. ed.). Sarasota, FL: Professional Resource Press.

Walker, H. M. (1993). Anti-social behavior in school. *Journal of Emotional and Behavioral Problems, 2*(1), 20–24.

Watson, R. S., Poda, J. H., Miller, C. T., Rice, E. S., & West, G. (1990). *Containing crisis: A guide to managing school emergencies.* Bloomington, IN: National Educational Service.

Way, D. W. (1993). I just have a half heart. *Journal of Emotional and Behavioral Problems, 2*(1), 4–5.

Webster, D. W., Vernick, J. S., Ludwig, J., & Lester, K. J. (1997). Flawed gun policy research could endanger public safety. *American Journal of Public Health, 87*(6), 918–921.

West, C. (1994). *Race matters.* New York: Vintage Books.

Woodtli, A., & Breslin, E. (in press). Violence-related content in the nursing curriculum: A follow-up national survey. *Journal of Nursing Education.*

Wright, M. A., Wintemute, G. J., & Rivara, F. P. (1999). Effectiveness of denial of handgun purchase to persons believed to be at high risk for firearm violence. *American Journal of Public Health, 89*(1), 88–90.

Yllo, K. (1993). Through a feminist lens: Gender, power, and violence. In R. J. Gelles & D. R. Loseke (Eds.), *Current controversies on family violence* (pp. 47–62). Thousand Oaks, CA: Sage.

Zehr, H., & Mika, H. (1997). *Restorative justice signposts.* Akron, PA: Mennonite Central Committee.

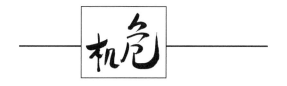

CHAPTER TEN

VIOLENCE AND CRISIS FROM DISASTER

The natural world is both a nurturing home and a source of potential destruction. The sun warms us. The beauty of foliage, seacoasts, forests, plains, and mountains satisfies our aesthetic needs and inspires us to write, sing, and love one another. Yet these same elements have the capacity to destroy us if we do not protect ourselves from nature's violent forces. For example, we must build shelters to prevent freezing in a snowstorm. We are also in danger if we misuse or destroy nature's resources, for instance, by the uncontrolled burning of coal, which causes acid rain and destroys lakes and the creatures that live in them.

As human beings, we can see and respond to the differences and connections between natural elements and ourselves. Our ability to rationally construct our social and material world allows us to contain the forces of nature for our own protection. The natural world yields much of what we need for survival; yet the victims of fires, floods, tornadoes, tidal waves, earthquakes, and snowstorms provide ample evidence of nature's destructive potential in spite of great technological attempts to decipher nature's mysteries and direct them for human ends.

> "I managed to drag myself out, but my mother and father were buried. My mother was unrecognizable. She was all burnt."

> For 97 hours and 33 minutes, Er meditated, thought, and prayed. And then his prayers were answered. Before dawn Saturday, he was pulled from beneath 15 feet of debris by a Turkish Rescue team. By Sunday, the elation of his rescue had faded. He learned of the deaths of his wife and daughter as he listened to his son being interviewed on television. . . . Surrounded by friends

and family, Er said, "I'm going to try to make the most of it. I want to deserve a happy life with the people I love."

Harlan [an elementary school janitor] thrived on the children, and he was a humble and special man, the closest thing to a saint that anyone would know. . . . [Three days after the flood] Harlan hanged himself in his home, itself damaged by the flood.

"I saw deaths, devastation, agony and misery of a magnitude I have never seen before. . . . The bodies were decomposed and the stench was unbearable."

"Our people have learned to resist difficulties, and consider the national disaster to be a divine test."

Dulal Biswas gave thanks that his 5-year old daughter was safe [with her grand-parents]. A few days later on his way to where Shanti had gone, he stumbled upon a child's body on the bank of the Pasur River. He peered in disbelief at the bloated, decomposing body. Then he screamed, beat his chest, and cried, "Shanti, my little doll, Shanti." Biswas' wife had died a year earlier of cholera, and Shanti was his only child. As he related his story to the Red Crescent Society worker, he was incoherent with grief.

These are a few of the reactions of victims and survivors of floods in North Dakota in 1997, Central America in 1998, Columbia in 1999, Mozambique in 2000; the 1991 cyclone in Bangladesh; and the 1999 earthquake in Turkey. Similar disasters occurred in India, Manila, Armenia, Los Angeles, Iran, and Japan. The number of dead, injured, and homeless from these disasters is staggering—for example, 138,000 dead from a Bangladesh hurricane, 100,000 dead and a half million homeless in Armenia, 40,000 dead in Iran. In the worst natural disaster in Colombia's history, the 1985 eruption of a volcano in Armero killed more than 22,000 people, with another 20,000 injured or homeless and 200,000 evacuated. Hurricane Mitch in Central America left 10,000 dead (7,000 in Honduras alone), 1,000 buried alive, and 1,000,000 uprooted from their homes. A relative who flew from the United States to survivors in Honduras said that it was like the country had stepped back in time about a hundred years. Children as young as thirteen suddenly became the head of their little nuclear family.

Human Potential for Catastrophic Violence

Yet nature's potential for violence seems small beside the destructive possibilities for disaster caused by human beings. In Bhopal, India, a gas leak at a chemical plant killed 2,000 and disabled tens of thousands more. Besides the 300 dead and 10,000 evacuated from the Chernobyl nuclear accident in the former Soviet

Union, radioactive fallout affected people and animals thousands of miles away, and illness and death from the accident are still being counted, even as the plant is finally being dismantled. Survivors of the underground gold mine explosion near Yellowknife in the Northwest Territories, Canada, cite the tragedy as proof of the need for reform of labor-management relations. Famines in Ethiopia, Mozambique, and Somalia, though apparently "natural," can also be traced to human origins (Wijkman & Timberlake, 1984). By most accounts, the inferno that killed at least eighty people in Waco, Texas, could have been avoided. Ethnic cleansing and tribal wars in the former Yugoslavia and Rwanda are the most recent man-made disasters creating incalculable misery and loss of life; the systematic slaughter of people in Rwanda is being compared with the Nazi Holocaust in the war crimes category. *Environmental racism,* a term applied to placing toxic waste dumps in communities where ethnic minority groups live, and in poor countries, surely takes its toll—with cleanup and restitution yet to occur in many places.

Human potential for both good and evil seems limited only by the technology we create. For example, a child can be saved through a liver transplant; amputated hands can be replaced; energy from the sun can be collected and stored; but technology also made it possible for the Nazis to perform inhuman experiments on Jews and others in concentration camps and for most of the population of Hiroshima and Nagasaki to be destroyed. While many enjoy the benefits of scientific knowledge, others suffer. For example, in the United States, the Love Canal disaster was a prototype for the 1980 Superfund Law enacted by Congress as the public health response to hazardous waste sites (Logue, 1996). As Lois Gibbs (1982, p. 1), a Love Canal resident turned activist, wrote,

Ask Those Who Really Know!

Ask the Victims of Love Canal why they need immediate permanent relocation, and why some will refuse to leave their motel rooms once funds are cut off.

Ask the innocent victims of corporate profits.

The reasons are simple. We cannot lead a normal life, we:

Cannot go in our basements because of contamination from Love Canal.

Cannot eat anything from our gardens because of soil contamination.

Cannot allow our children to play in our yards because of contaminated soils.

Cannot have our children attend school in the area—two have been closed due to Love Canal contamination.

Cannot breathe the outside air—because of air contamination we are now in hotels.

Cannot become pregnant—miscarriage rate is state defined: 45%. Homeowners' survey: 75%.

Cannot have normal children—because of 56% risk of birth defects.

Cannot sell our homes. Love Canal was not mentioned in our deeds; who wants a contaminated house?

Cannot get a VA or FHA loan in Love Canal; even the government is reluctant.

Cannot have friends or relatives visit us on holidays; they're scared it's unsafe.

Cannot have our pregnant daughters, or our grandchildren visit: it's unsafe for them.

We need your support and your help to end the suffering of men, women, and especially children of Love Canal. We have lost our constitutional rights of life, liberty and the pursuit of happiness. Justice for all but not Love Canal Victims. We cannot live at Love Canal—we cannot leave Love Canal.

The disastrous effects of violence from natural and human sources can be described in both personal and social terms. Although people have now moved back to Love Canal, this highly publicized disaster holds lessons for other communities still struggling against toxic waste. How do people respond to disasters of natural origin, as compared with those of human origin? Why are disasters of human origin, such as Love Canal and Hiroshima, not usually viewed as a form of violence? What can individuals and groups do to reduce our vulnerability to disasters from natural and human sources? Our answers to these questions could affect

- What happens to disaster victims
- The quality of our everyday lives
- The quality of life on earth that we can realistically anticipate
- Whether we ultimately destroy ourselves and our planet

Natural and Accidental Disaster: Prevention and Aid

One can only guess at the extent to which a disaster such as a flood, fire, or earthquake affects the people who experience it. Although global media networks beam a disaster's devastating effects to our television screens, the depth of the tragedy is private and immeasurable. Although the negative consequences of disaster are not always clear, some research suggests long-term stress responses (Baum, Fleming, & Singer, 1983; Erikson, 1994; Gist & Lubin, 1989). Preventive measures and help for survivors are therefore of great importance. What do we need to know about disaster and its victims in order to help? The nature and duration of a disaster, plus individual factors such as age, general personality stability, and religion, affect the victim's response. Disaster is a perilous event that for most falls outside the range of everyday life experience or challenges. A disaster usually occurs rapidly and is therefore completely unexpected and shocking. It shatters one's assumptions about the order and security of daily life, depending on type of loss: home, country, intact family, memorabilia, health, and means of livelihood.

The following excerpts from the Doolin and Collins (1998) account portray vividly the depth of loss and destruction of life and property that resulted from Hurricane Mitch in Central America, the deadliest storm there in over two hundred years.

Face to Face with the Suffering in Central America

Arriving the day after the rains from Hurricane Mitch stopped, our five-person Archdiocese of Boston delegation . . . witnessed the aftermath of the most destructive event in Central America in recent memory. More than 1 million people uprooted from their homes in Honduras and Nicaragua, tens of thousands dead or missing, crops and food inventories lost to the storm.

The scale of human suffering in these two poor countries cannot adequately be described. . . . Beyond the immediate devastation, millions of people face a public health crisis for lack of potable water and because of fatal diseases that are incubating and ready to break out.

Diarrheal illness caused by drinking polluted water has already begun. Skin infections and scabies are prevalent. And perhaps neglected for now, but equally important, is the mental health of the victims. There is the potential for widespread psychiatric illness and depression as people deal with the trauma of their losses.

The victims arrive at shelters and tent cities on foot, their meager remaining possessions transported like so many shipments of Mayan misery in the backs of huge open trucks. The faces of these proud peoples are haunting. High cheekbones uplifted in pain, smooth, copper-olive skin, clear dark eyes glint in the drying sun, betraying both shame and despair.

Yesterday, their home was a modest dwelling, though coarse by our standards. Today, their home is a sheet of plastic on a stick. They have nothing and are surrounded by thousands of other families with nothing in spaces capable of accommodating a few hundred people. No electricity, toilets, running water, cooking facilities. Nothing.

Children without schools to go to frolic in fetid rivers of waste, bathing in the novelty of flood waters that hadn't been there for several years. Parents huddle in hospital emergency rooms, exhausted and watchful. A child wrenches in excruciating pain because his mother hasn't got $2 to buy medication. Young, stern-faced militiamen enforce the curfew behind Jeeps and machine guns. There's no order to the crowds, with lines so tight the people almost seem to be snuggling for the security of each other despite the heat.

The Pan-American Highway in many spots has become a shallow river or even a broad lake. In Nicaragua, stalled buses and vans are filled with people trying to get to higher ground. The roadway is lined with mattresses to sleep on, sewing machines to work on, and kitchen tables to eat on.

Resignation and patience mark the endless rosary of mostly female faces that make up the water queues. They hold . . . containers of all kinds. Ironically, it is water that has brought their lives to ruin; it is water that will help them survive to struggle another day.

We greet hundreds of downtrodden and tired people in a little church outside Managua. Tired and disheartened, they expect to hear words of reassurance, solidarity, and hope. They were not disappointed when their own bishop, Cardinal Obando y Bravo, was joined by [Boston's] Cardinal Law. . . . What cannot be underestimated . . . is the importance of church-to-church aid—the Boston to Central America assistance that Cardinal Law has been able to make happen.

In fact, the response of churches and social service agencies is just as critical as the U.S. government's official response. Their values and experience are grounded in the commitment of helping others in time of dire need.

Assistance comes in other ways. The U.S. ambassador to Honduras, James Creagan, became a local hero by arranging for the evacuation of an orphanage in Tegucigalpa at the height of the hurricane. His quick action saved the lives of more than 40 youngsters and staff.

Why should we help? As a nation and people blessed with so much, our assistance can lessen the victims' suffering. Food will feed the hungry. Water will quench their thirst. Medicine will aid the sick. But, most important, our assistance will bring what is most needed, and that is hope.

Albeit from different perspectives, both the Truman-era "Good-Neighbor" policy for Central America and the parable of the Good Samaritan ask the question: Who is my neighbor? Last week, we saw their faces. This week they still need us. Next week they will need us even more. [Doolin & Collins, 1998, p. A19]

Fortunately, tragedies like this happen rarely—or not at all—to most people. Most of our expectations of disaster are formed in the abstract; while observing on television the tragedies of others, denial often serves to tell us, "This couldn't happen to me." Public consciousness and public health efforts are promising, however, since the 1990s were declared the International Decade for Natural Disaster Reduction (Logue, 1996). Overall, our lack of experience with disaster, along with the suddenness, lack of preparation, and unexpectedness with which most disasters strike, greatly reduces the opportunity for escape and effective problem solving. Yet in a poor country, Turkey, the bulk of the devastation caused by the 1999 earthquake that left 13,000 dead and 200,000 homeless was attributed largely to substandard housing and lax regulation of building codes. As Ahmet Mete Isikara, director of the Bosphorus University's earthquake research center said, "Earthquakes don't kill, badly constructed buildings kill" (Marcus, 1999, p A26).

Technological and Political Factors Affecting Aid to Victims

Rescue operations and assistance with physical necessities occur in disaster-stricken communities throughout the world. Foreign countries, the International Red Cross, religious and other organizations assist in such relief work: millions of dollars in aid were sent to Iran, Colombia, India, Mexico, and Central America following their devastating disasters. A country's ability to respond is also related to the amount and quality of its resources, technological developments, and the bureaucratic functioning of its government.

The uncontrolled forces of nature may not seem to differentiate between rich and poor, north and south, or between white people and those of color. But the effects of these forces differ. Widespread flooding in the United States, for example, is less frequent and results in fewer lives lost than it did years ago because of the resources and technology available for good prevention programs—building dams, for example. But a poor country like India still has difficulty preventing massive floods that take thousands of lives. A poor nation also has fewer government resources for assisting survivors. Similarly, fires of the proportion of the Cocoanut Grove disaster, which claimed 492 lives in Boston in 1942, are rare today because political action has facilitated enforcement of building safety regulations. Federal aviation policy has likewise been tightened to prevent jetliner crashes due to faulty technology or nonenforcement of safety codes.

However, news accounts of disasters worldwide repeatedly emphasize the difference between rich and poor countries' access to resources for preventing, or at least warning of, impending disaster. Presidents of poor countries often plead for technical assistance to warn people of impending disaster, so they can take measures to avoid injury. Natural disasters, of course, should always be expected. However, the effects of population growth and land use management are illustrated in this difference in disaster mortality over a hundred-year period: the 1876 Bay of Bengal typhoon killed 100,000 people, whereas the 1970 East Bengal cyclone killed 200,000 (Logue, 1996, p. 1208). The devastation wreaked by Hurricane Mitch in Central America can properly be defined as an ecological disaster in that its greatest damage in floods and mud slides occurred in deforested areas (Goldoftas, 1998). Absent economic policies regarding globalization, the debts of poor countries payable to the World Bank, and the widening gap between rich and poor, Central America's poor people who are vulnerable to future disasters will nevertheless out of necessity eke out a living from the remaining forested areas.

Consider also the contrast in flood damage and compensation in a rich nation, the United States, and a poor nation, Bangladesh. As Fauzia E. Ahmed, SouthAsia coordinator of Oxfam America, wrote,

Hurricane Andrew claimed 20 lives. Last year, a hurricane with no name struck Bangladesh, killing 138,000 people. Both hurricanes had winds of 140 miles per hour. But why was one hurricane approximately 7,000 times more lethal? The answer is poverty. Bangladesh has 300 shelters for hurricanes. It needs 5,000, which could be built for less than the cost of one C-17 military cargo aircraft.

When Hurricane Andrew came to Miami, it found a ghost town. Most people had fled to shelters. In Bangladesh, hundreds of thousands of people tried to run as a huge wall of water advanced on them. Abdul, a survivor, told me, "My two children could not run fast enough. The wave caught up with them and they died. The roar of the sea was so great I could not even hear their cries for help."

There was also tremendous psychological devastation. In Miami, a business-man died of a heart attack after seeing his business reduced to rubble. In Bangladesh, mothers were forced to choose which children to save. They will somehow have to go on living with the consequences of this choice. "I had four children," one mother told me. "But I only have two hands. With one hand I grasped a tree and held my 6-month-old baby with the other. I had to watch my three other children drown because I could not save them."

In Florida, there was insurance for homeowners. The Federal Emergency Management Agency dispensed money for the cleanup. In Bangladesh, there was no compensation for people who lost their livestock—which was often the sum total of all their worldly possessions.

Bangladesh is a nation where there are more riverways than dirt tracks and more dirt tracks than paved roads. In good times, fishermen live off the water. In hurricanes, the water drags them to their death. The overall lack of quality roads makes it impossible for relief supplies to reach people in remote areas.

In Florida, the warning system and evacuation plan worked. Bangladesh's 80 percent illiteracy rate makes it difficult for many citizens to understand storm warnings. In Bangladesh, illiteracy runs highest among women. The majority of the dead in the hurricane with no name were women. Despite all this, people were resilient and struggle to help one another. Women talked of searching for food and finding some rice buried in the sand. A 13-year-old boy found his father's body and gave him proper burial rites. He felt proud that he was able to do his duty toward his father. The media did not report this. In Florida, pictures were shown on TV of neighbors helping each other. Reporters interviewed survivors, asking them how they hoped to return to normal lives. But in Bangladesh, the media showed only dead bodies and masses of dark-skinned people begging for food. Fourteen million people were made homeless, but the media left them as nameless as the hurricane.

This sort of coverage led to absurd queries. Why do these stupid people live in a disaster-prone area? Are there too many people in Bangladesh already? Nobody is asking why 44 million people crowd into hurricane-prone counties from Texas to Maine.

The truth is, death like this does not have to be inevitable in the developing world. What is more important: One C-17 airplane or enough shelters to keep 138,000 people from floating away? [Ahmed, 1992, p. 15]

Material, financial, and human resources, then, play an important part in preventing disasters from natural or accidental causes. These economic, political, and technological conditions highlight the continued need for international programs of aid and cooperation in the distribution and use of natural and human resources. Bureaucratic and political rivalries can result in further tragedy and loss of life. Technology, public health, and effective political organizations are central to controlling nature, responding to health hazards during disaster, and aiding disaster victims with material and other resources. The social and behavioral sciences also have contributed to the reduction in human error and accidental disaster through, for example, research on perception and reaction times of pilots and air traffic controllers.

Psychological and Other Factors

In the psychological realm, confronting the unhealthy mechanism of denial is central to preventing victimization by natural disaster. Because a natural disaster is a dreaded experience, most people deny that it could happen to them, even when they live in high-risk areas for floods, tornadoes, or earthquakes. People use denial as a means to go on living normal lives while under more or less constant threat of disaster. Escape and problem solving are also affected by the extent of a person's denial, although some may be in special circumstances that prevent them from hearing the warnings.

CASE EXAMPLE: MARTIN AND EVELYN SCHONER

Martin Schoner, age seventy, and his wife, Evelyn, age sixty-eight, had lived all their lives in a valley neighborhood. The Schoners had both been retired for several years; Martin as a men's clothing merchant, Evelyn as a nurse. They enjoyed the activities of their retirement years, including occasional baby-sitting for their five grandchildren. They and their two children exchanged visits frequently.

The evening before the flood, Martin was admitted to the hospital for chest and stomach discomfort. When Evelyn left her husband at the hospital that evening, they still did not know his diagnosis, nor did they have any suspicion that disaster was imminent. Meanwhile, flood warnings, were being broadcast by radio and television. Evelyn, however, heard none of these. She went to bed as usual, only to be awakened at 5:00 A.M. by a telephone call from a friend advising her of the flood and the need to leave her house quickly. She immediately packed a bag and drove to her friend's house. A few hours later, she learned on the radio that houses in her neighborhood were filled with water up to the second floor. She was unable to reach her husband; the hospital was also flooded and the patients were evacuated. Both Martin and Evelyn were beside themselves with fear and worry, for each had no idea of the whereabouts of the other.

One of Evelyn's special concerns was Martin's medical condition. She still did not know if his symptoms signaled heart trouble. As it turned out, Martin's symptoms were from food poisoning. He had been moved to a local college that was converted into a temporary shelter; seriously ill patients were moved to another hospital. Martin, however, was so upset and worried about his wife that rescue workers finally sent a hospital chaplain to talk with him. Martin stated afterward that he found it a tremendous relief to pour out his worry to a sympathetic listener, who helped him through a good cry without embarrassment or shame. Evelyn had no way of knowing these facts because public communication networks were not operating.

Two days later, Evelyn finally learned from a friend that Martin was at the college emergency shelter. Evelyn went to pick him up; they stayed for a few days together at their friend's house before returning to their neighborhood to assess the damage. When they returned, they were grief stricken over the loss of their possessions and the destruction of the home they had treasured. Evelyn was particularly upset.

She kept repeating, "If only I had known that this was going to happen, I would have moved at least some of our precious things upstairs or packed them up to take with me."

Martin and Evelyn, with the help of their friend, decided to stay in the neighborhood and rebuild their home with federal aid. In the aftermath of the crisis, Martin gained a new lease on life despite the tragedy. He no longer had any empty hours in his days; he single-handedly took the job of repairing the flood damage and refinishing the house. He became a source of support and encouragement for others in the neighborhood. Evelyn felt the flood left an indelible mark on her. She seemed unable to stop grieving over the loss they had suffered. Evelyn also stated, "If only our minister hadn't been out of town at the time, I would have had someone to talk to when it happened." Martin and Evelyn did not know that specially trained crisis counselors were available to survivors of the disaster. This highlights the fact that communication in a disaster-stricken community is often inadequate.

Martin, Evelyn, and their neighbors live in fear of another flood; they have no assurance that adequate pre-cautionary measures have been taken to prevent a recurrence. They decided, however, to take a chance and live their last years in the neighborhood they love, with the resolution that should another flood occur, they will move away once and for all.

In contrast to the Schoners, there was little time to prepare for Hurricane Mitch in Central America. A Honduran woman and her family were quickly swept away in their house by the merged sea and river created by the hurricane. When the river tore through the house, it also tore away her entire family, leaving her as the sole survivor after being rescued from a makeshift raft she had constructed out of tree roots, branches, and a piece of scrap. A woman in Mozambique also responded to imminent danger by flight to a tree, where she lived above raging waters for four days and gave birth to her baby. She and her daughter were rescued by helicopter; the rescue team included a medic who cut the umbilical cord.

It is difficult for anyone who has not experienced a flood to imagine that heavy rain alone can produce enough water to break a dam, merge a river and sea into a single body of water, and flood a whole city or region. People are used to associating certain results with certain causes. When cause and effect are unfamiliar, denial is likely. But when reality strikes, and some survive, reckoning with profound loss is the next ordeal.

Preventive Intervention

It is impossible to prepare for the crisis of disaster the way one can prepare for transition states such as parenthood, retirement, or death. However, we can act on a communitywide basis before disaster strikes. This is particularly important in communities at high risk for natural disasters. Such preparation is a form of psychological immunization. There are several things a community can do to prepare for possible disaster:

1. Make public service announcements during spring rains or tornado seasons, urging people not to ignore disaster warnings.
2. Broadcast educational programs on television, dramatizing techniques for crowd control and for helping people who are panic-stricken or in shock.
3. Review public safety codes to ensure adequate protection against fire in public gathering places such as restaurants, theaters, and hospitals.
4. Make public service announcements, urging people to take first-aid courses with local Red Cross and fire departments.
5. Broadcast educational programs on radio, television, and the Internet to acquaint people with social agencies and crisis services available to them in the event of disaster.
6. Offer crisis intervention training for mental health and social service workers as an addition to their traditional skills.
7. Institute an upgraded program of disaster preparation by medical, public health, and welfare facilities, including mechanisms for community coordination of disaster rescue services. (In communities with an excellent medical disaster plan, survivors had adequate medical and health care during and after floods.)
8. Develop plans for support of disaster relief workers, who themselves usually are shocked and numbed from the experience. For example, workers assigned to recover human remains from an airplane wreckage (typically emergency medical and fire-fighting personnel) can tolerate only a few hours at a time confronting the horror. They need time-out and an opportunity to process what they have witnessed with a crisis or mental health counselor.
9. Ensure that local authorities for disaster prevention and response have up-to-date copies of field manuals and other resources available through Web sites

of federal offices—for example, in the United States, the Public Health Service and the National Institute of Mental Health (NIMH).

These preparations will not prevent the devastating effects of a disaster, but they may reduce the impact of the trauma and help people live through the experience with less physical, social, and emotional damage than they might otherwise suffer.

Individual Responses to Disaster

Reactions to the stress and trauma of a disaster are not unlike reactions to transition states such as migration or loss of a loved one through death. They also resemble responses to victimization by crime (see Chapter Eight). Tyhurst's classic works (1951, 1957a, 1957b) identify three overlapping phases in disaster reaction. These are similar to the four phases in the development of a crisis state noted by Caplan (see Chapter Two).

1. *Impact.* In this period, the person is hit with the reality of what is happening. In catastrophic events, the impact period lasts from a few minutes to one or two hours. The concern of disaster victims during the impact phase is with the immediate present. An automatic stimulus-response reaction occurs, with the catastrophe as stimulus. Victims are struck later with wonder that they were able to carry on as well as they did, especially if they finally break down under the full emotional impact of the experience. During the impact phase, individual reactions to the disaster fall into three main groups:

a. Ten to 25 percent of the victims remain calm and do not fall apart. Instead they assess the situation, develop a plan of action, and carry it through.
b. Seventy-five percent of the victims are shocked and confused. They are unable to express any particular feeling or emotion. The usual physical signs of fear are present: sweating, rapid heartbeat, upset stomach, and trembling. This is considered the normal reaction to a disaster.
c. Another 10 to 25 percent become hysterical or confused or are paralyzed with fear. These victims may sit and stare into space or may run around wildly. The behavior of this group is of most concern for rescue workers and crisis counselors who may be on the scene during emergency operations.

Evelyn Schoner, caught in the Wilkes-Barre flood because she did not hear the warnings, had the first type of reaction during the impact phase. When she finally received the warning telephone call, she packed her bag and drove to safety. She had no difficulty doing this, even though she ordinarily depended heavily on her husband when in distress, and he was in the hospital. Evelyn stated, "It really only hit me afterward, that everything I treasured was lost. I just had to drive away and leave everything behind. You don't know what that's like—saving precious things all your life, then all of a sudden they're gone, even the photographs of our family." We cannot accurately predict which people will fall into the third group of reactors to disaster. However, prediction criteria (see Chapter Three) indicate that the following types of people are particularly vulnerable to crisis or emotional disturbance following acute stress from a disaster:

- The elderly who have few physical resources and a reduced capacity to adapt to rapid change
- Those who already are coping with stress in self-destructive or unhealthy ways, such as taking solace in alcohol
- Those who are alone and friendless and who lack physical and social resources that they can rely on in an emergency

During the San Fernando Valley earthquake, mental health staff at the Los Angeles County–Olive View Medical Center observed that some acutely disturbed mental patients reacted more rationally than usual during the acute phase of the quake. For example, they helped rescue fellow patients (Koegler & Hicks, 1972). In Mozambique, a couple and their three children were perched in a tree for a day and night before the water subsided. In Armero, Colombia, rescue workers dug with their bare hands and bailed out water with tin cans to save a thirteen-year-old girl trapped beneath a cement slab. These incidents reveal the commonly observed heroism and humanity of disaster victims, despite personal pain and loss. People rise dramatically to the occasion and mobilize resources to help themselves and others.

2. *Recoil.* During this phase, there is at least a temporary suspension of the initial stressors of the disaster. Lives are no longer in immediate danger, although other stressors such as cold or pain from injury may continue. Often, however, more floods follow the first one, and aftershocks follow earthquakes. During the recoil phase, survivors are typically en route to friends' homes, or they have found shelter in community facilities set up for the emergency. They may look around for someone to be with. They want to be taken care of, to receive a cup of coffee or a blanket. Chilled survivors of an earthquake, for example, huddle in makeshift camps and tent cities, lighting fires to keep warm. The disaster experience leaves some survivors with a childlike dependency and need to be with others. At this phase, survivors gradually become aware of the full impact of what they have been through. Both women and men may break down and weep. Survivors have their first chance to share the experience with others. Their attention is focused on the immediate past and how they managed to survive. This phase has the greatest implication for crisis workers helping the survivors.

However, mental health professionals trained in assessment of psychopathology must be very careful not to pathologize what is essentially a normal response to an event that is beyond the range of events experienced by most people (see Zunin & Zunin, 1991). Caution is also in order around formalized debriefing, known as Critical Incident Stress Debriefing (CISD), after disaster, especially for survivors who might interpret ritualized debriefing as a sign they are going crazy. The focus should be on practical help, listening, problem solving, and sincere presence for those who may wish to share their experience with a stranger (that is, a "debriefer") rather than with fellow survivors and members of their own community—in essence, the basics of crisis care. There are no studies documenting that CISD is more effective than traditional crisis care; in fact, it could be experienced as intrusion, or another form of "ambulance chasing."

3. *Post-trauma.* During this period, survivors become fully aware of the losses they have sustained during the impact phase: loss of home (for some, even country), financial security, personal belongings, and particularly loved ones who may have died in the disaster. In this phase, much depends on a person's age and general condition. As Jane Cantor, a Wilkes-Barre survivor put it, "A disaster can bring out the best and the worst in a person." Those who are too old to start over again find their loss of home and possessions particularly devastating. Older people who prize the reminders of their children and their earlier life feel robbed of what they have worked for all their lives. Anger and frustration follow. If loved ones have died in the disaster, grief and mourning predominate. Murphy (1986, p. 339) cites studies of bereavement suggesting that the recovery period varies from several months to several years and is subjectively defined. Murphy found that among survivors who lost a loved one in a close relationship to the Mount Saint Helens volcanic eruption, bereavement was intense and prolonged, especially if they perceived the disaster as preventable. Some survivors of the Rapid City, South Dakota, flood felt overwhelming guilt over the death of loved ones: "Why me? Why was I spared and not she?" Many survivors describe the horror of listening to screams, of watching people being swept past them to their deaths, and of being helpless to save them. Lifton and Olson (1976) have described this reaction as "death guilt." Survivors somehow feel responsible for the death of their relatives or others they were unable to save. They cannot quite forgive themselves for living, for having been spared. At the same time, they may feel relief at not being among the dead. This, in turn, leaves them feeling guiltier.

During this third phase, survivors may have flashbacks, reactive depressions, anxiety reactions, and dreams in which they relive the catastrophic experience. Some agencies report increased numbers of hospital admissions for emotional disturbances following disaster. Staff of the Child Guidance Center in the San Fernando Valley counseled hundreds of parents and children following the earthquake. Children typically were afraid to be alone and afraid to go to sleep in their own beds. Lifton and Olson (1976) report that when survivors perceive a disaster as a reflection of human callousness, rather than an act of God or nature, the psychological effects are more severe and long lasting.

This post-traumatic phase may last for the rest of a person's life, depending on that individual's predisaster state, the extent of loss, the help available during the disaster, and whether the disaster was natural or from human origins (Richman, 1993). Evelyn Schoner said, "I don't think I'll ever be the same. I just can't get over it. I live in constant fear that there might be another flood. There's just no guarantee that there won't be another one." (See Leon, Poole, & Kloner, 1996; and Epstein, 1995, who cite increased morbidity and mortality figures following disaster.)

A small group of disaster survivors give up. These people remain despondent and hopeless for the rest of their lives. Most survivors, however, gather together and reconstruct their lives, their homes, and their community. Although a number of people in flood-prone areas move to higher elevations, many others rebuild their homes on the same location, even though there is no guarantee against further flooding. This is particularly true for older people, who find it too costly to start over and who want to keep the comfort of a familiar neighborhood, even though they have lost everything else.

Rescue and crisis workers have the most influence during the impact and recoil phases (Joseph, Yule, Williams, & Andrews, 1993), whereas mental health workers may play a key role during the post-traumatic phase for the small percentage who manifest severe depression, for example, or who may have a recurrence of previous psychiatric illness (see Tucker, Pfefferbaum, Nixon, & Foy, 1999). As noted throughout this book, crisis intervention—available at the right time and in the right place—is the most effective means of preventing later psychiatric disturbances. As Evelyn Schoner said, "If only I would have had someone to talk to when it happened." The availability of crisis assistance to individuals, however, is intricately tied to the community response to disaster.

Community Responses to Disaster

The most immediate social consequence of a disaster is the disruption of normal social patterns on which all community members depend (Tyhurst, 1957a). The community suffers a social paralysis. People are separated from family and friends and spontaneously form other groups out of the need to be with others.

When disaster strikes, large numbers of people are cut off from public services and resources that they count on for survival. These can include water—one of the first resources to go in the event of a flood—electricity, and heat. People scramble for shelter, food, and water. Traffic controls are out, so accidents increase. In flooded areas, many people fall in the slippery mud and break limbs, thus placing more demands on hospital staff. Often hospitals are flooded out, and all patients must be transferred to other facilities. Schools and many businesses close, creating further strain and chaos in homes and emergency shelters.

Disaster can bring out the worst in people. Some take advantage of the disorder to loot and steal; some business owners take advantage of the occasion to profit from others' misfortune by inflating the prices of necessary supplies.

Because normal communication networks are either destroyed or are very limited, rumors abound and panic and chaos increase. Communication problems and physical distance also make information about relief benefits difficult to disseminate. This causes resentment among those who feel they did not receive a fair share of the benefits. Assisting survivors through the bureaucratic maze of many relief organizations is one of the most helpful things crisis workers can do. Residents who are not even on the scene of the disaster can be affected by media generalizations and sensationalistic reports.

In most instances, disasters are instrumental in bringing the people of their neighborhood closer together. During the impact period of a disaster, there is greater cohesion among community members; later, people focus on their individual concerns. People must rely on one another for help and support during a disaster in a way that was not necessary before. During the Rapid City flood, for example, a group of professionals were attending a conference on death and dying. A call was put out to the conference participants to assist families who had lost loved ones. The helpers reported that many friends had already turned out to help the bereaved families and that there was no special need for mental health professionals.

During the impact and recoil stages of a disaster, community control usually passes from elected government officials to professionals who direct health, welfare, mental health, and public order agencies. Elected officials have the important function of soliciting assistance for the community from state, federal, and sometimes international resources. The community's priorities are rapidly defined by professional leaders, and an emergency health and social service system is quickly established. This emergency network focuses on

- Preservation of life and health—rescue activities, inoculations, treatment of the injured
- Conservation and distribution of resources—organization of emergency shelters and distribution of supplies such as water, food, and blankets
- Conservation of public order—police surveillance to prevent looting and accidents from arising out of the chaos and the scramble for remaining resources
- Maintenance of morale—dispatching mental health, welfare, and pastoral counselors to assist the panic-stricken and bereaved during the acute crisis phase

Material, social, and psychological services should be available for as long as they are needed.

In summary, a community's response to disaster is poignantly revealed in the following description by Kizzier (1972) of Rapid City and is repeated many times over in other communities.

> With all of this help from private, city, county, state, and federal funds and with the compassion and support offered from an entire nation, Rapid City is restoring and rebuilding with a new appreciation for life. It has pulled together for a purpose before, but never before has it become a pulsating, throbbing being as it is now, in the aftermath of a flood.

Not one person has been untouched by the drama of recovery. Through the silent heartache and compassion, we again remember what it is like to be patient with each other. There is a need for the comfort of physical contact as we greet each survivor with a thankful hug.

We are more aware of the things we take for granted like the utility companies, bridges, and the National Guard. We now look at the police with new respect, feel thankful for the closeness of the air force base and vow never again to pass the ringing Christmas bells of the Salvation Army without dropping in a coin.

We go to the citywide memorial service on Sunday, feeling sad and empty and discouraged after being threatened by another torrent of rain the night before. We see people there who have lost far more than we have, bearing their burden with surprising spirit. We want to cry with all the pent-up emotion, but we are being told that we must overcome our grief, rejoice, and sing and carry on with life. And so we will, just like everyone around us will, because people need to laugh or they will break. We come from the memorial service feeling renewed and we try laughing and it makes us feel warm inside and a little lightheaded.

Factors Affecting Recovery of Survivors

Tyhurst (1957a) notes that the nature and severity of reactions to disaster and the process of recovery are influenced by several factors:

1. *The element of surprise.* If and when warnings are given, they should be followed by instructions in what to do. Warnings followed by long silences and no action plan can heighten anxiety and lead to the commonly observed denial of some residents that a disaster is imminent.

2. *Separation of family members.* Children are particularly vulnerable to damaging psychological effects if separated from their families during the acute period of a disaster (Durkin, Khan, Davidson, Zaman, & Stein, 1993). Families should therefore be evacuated as a unit whenever possible.

3. *Outside help.* Reasonable recovery from a disaster requires aid from unaffected areas. Because military forces have the organization, discipline, and equipment necessary for dealing with a disaster, their instruction should include assisting civilians during disaster.

4. *Leadership.* As in any crisis situation, a disaster demands that someone have the ability to make decisions and give direction. The police, the military, and physicians have leadership potential during a disaster. Their training should include preparation to exercise this potential appropriately.

5. *Communication.* Because failures in communication give rise to rumors, it is essential that a communication network and public information centers are established and maintained as a high priority in disaster work. Much impulsive and irrational behavior can be prevented by the reassurance and direction that a good communication network provides.

6. *Measures directed toward reorientation.* Communication lays the foundation for the reidentification of individuals in family and social groups. A basic step of reorientation is the registration of survivors, so that they can once again feel like members of society. This also provides a way for relatives and friends to find one another.

7. *Evacuation.* In any disaster, there is a spontaneous mass movement to leave the stricken area. Planned evacuation will prevent the panic that results when people find their escape blocked or delayed. Failure to attend to the psychological and social problems of evacuation can result in serious social and interpersonal problems.

Resources for Psychological Assistance

Federal aid for reconstruction has been available to communities stricken with disaster for many years. Since 1972 in the United States, aid for victims' psychological needs is also routine. The significance of the NIMH policy to offer crisis services is twofold. First, it demonstrates the need for outside mental health assistance in times of disaster to supplement local resources. Local mental health workers may be disaster victims themselves and may be temporarily unable to help others in distress. Second, it confirms that the ability of people to help others in crisis is strongly influenced by their prior skill or training in crisis intervention.

In most communities, the special federal aid for crisis intervention supplements crisis services offered by other groups. For example, Catholic, Jewish, Mennonite, and various Protestant denominations traditionally offer help to disaster-stricken communities.

It is probably impossible to have an oversupply of crisis intervention services for people struck by a disaster. However, community mental health agencies must have prior crisis intervention skills in order to mobilize the resources necessary when a disaster occurs. Health and mental health workers, along with other community caretakers, must know how to put these crisis intervention skills to use when a disaster strikes. As there is little or no time to prepare for the disaster, there is no time to prepare as a crisis worker once a disaster is imminent. Workers must be ready to apply their knowledge, attitudes, and skills in crisis intervention.

In spite of much progress in this area and the United Nations declaration of the 1990s as the International Decade for Natural Disaster Reduction (Logue, 1996), more long-term planning is needed to better meet the psychological needs of disaster victims, many of whom suffer from severe shock.

Help During Impact, Recoil, and Post-Trauma Phases

The helping process during disaster takes on distinctive characteristics during the disaster's impact, recoil, and post-trauma phases. Table 10.1 illustrates the kind of help needed and who is best suited to offer it during the three phases of a disaster. The table also suggests the possible outcomes for disaster victims if help is not available in each of the three phases.

TABLE 10.1.   ASSISTANCE DURING THREE PHASES OF NATURAL DISASTER.

	Help Needed	Help Provided by	Possible Outcome if Help Unavailable
Phase I: Impact	Information on source and degree of danger	Communication network: radio, TV, public address system	Physical injury or death
	Escape and rescue from immediate source of danger	Community rescue resources: police and fire departments, Red Cross, National Guard	
Phase II: Recoil	Shelter, food, drink, clothing, medical care	Red Cross	Physical injury
		Salvation Army	Delayed grief reactions
		Voluntary agencies such as colleges to be converted to mass shelters	Later emotional or mental disturbance
		Local health and welfare agencies	
		Mental health and social service agencies skilled in crisis intervention	
		Pastoral counselors	
		State and federal assistance for all of the above services	
Phase III: Post-trauma	Physical reconstruction	State and federal resources for physical reconstruction	Financial hardship
	Social reestablishment	Social welfare agencies	Social instability
	Psychological support concerning aftereffects of the event itself; bereavement counseling concerning loss of loved ones, home, and personal property	Crisis and mental health services	Long-lasting mental, emotional, or physical health problems
		Pastoral counselors	

Crisis Intervention and Follow-Up Service

The basic principles of crisis intervention should be applied on behalf of disaster victims. In disaster situations, however, crisis care should be embedded in the natural context of practical problem solving, not in a formal counseling framework. During and after a disaster, people need an opportunity to

- Talk out the experience at their own pace and express their feelings of fear, panic, loss, and grief
- Become fully aware and accepting of what has happened to them
- Resume activity and begin reconstructing their lives with the social, physical, and emotional resources available

To assist victims through the crisis, the crisis worker should

- Listen with concern and sympathy; ease the way for the victims to tell their tragic story, weep, and express feelings of anger, loss, frustration, and despair
- Help the survivors accept the reality of what has happened a little bit at a time—perhaps by simply staying with them during the initial stages of shock and denial, accompanying them to the scene of the tragedy, and supporting them when they are faced with the full impact of their loss
- Assist victims in making contact with relatives, friends, and other resources needed to begin the process of social and physical reconstruction—perhaps by making telephone calls to locate relatives, accompanying people to apply for financial aid, and giving information about social and mental health agencies for follow-up services

In group settings where large numbers are housed and offered emergency care, those who are panic-stricken should be separated from the rest and given individual attention to avoid the contagion of panic reactions. Assigning these people simple, physical tasks will move them in the direction of constructive action. Any action that helps victims feel valued as individuals is important at this time. Yet in spite of massive efforts to help survivors of disaster, it may be impossible to prevent lifelong emotional scarring—depending on age, predisaster emotional stability, and so forth—among those who live through the experience. Crisis and bereavement counseling can at least reduce some negative effects and should be available to all victims.

No local community can possibly meet all of the physical, social, and emotional needs of its residents who are disaster victims. In the United States, it is now routine to provide federal funds for crisis services and physical reconstruction in communities that are struck by disaster. This is necessary even when local mental health, welfare, and health workers are trained in crisis intervention. In most disasters, the need is too great for the local community to act alone, especially because some of its own human service workers (police officers, nurses, clergy, and counselors) will themselves be among the disaster victims.

In summary, individual responses and the needs of natural disaster victims, as in other crisis situations, vary according to psychological, economic, and social circumstances. Natural disaster victims seem to have something in common for coping with this kind of crisis: they interpret these tragedies as acts of God, or fate, or bad luck—and thus beyond anyone's control. Accounting for an event from a common viewpoint is an important aspect of constructive crisis coping at the cognitive level. Emotional coping can then occur through grief work and can be followed by behavioral responses to rebuild lives. The victims' interpretation of these crises as natural and beyond their control is the basis for the hope felt by survivors of natural disasters in spite of enormous suffering. It is the reason they can rise from the rubble and begin a new life; it lets them move beyond the emotional pain and gain new strength from the experience. This element of disaster response and recovery constitutes the greatest distinction between natural disasters and those occurring from human indifference, neglect, or design.

Disasters from Human Origins

The world knows about the atomic bombs dropped in Japan, the Nazi Holocaust, and the destruction of Love Canal. War and environmental pollution are planned disasters that bring about physical, social, and emotional destruction of immeasurable proportions. Some survivors of Hiroshima describe the horror:

> People who were laying there and dying and screaming and yelling for help and the people who were burned were hollering, "I'm so hot, please help me, please kill me" and things like that and . . . it was terrible. (Mary)

> We had a hospital near our place and many, many hundreds of injured people came to the hospital and there weren't too many adequate medical supplies and there were some doctors there, some nurses there, but they didn't have enough medicine to take care of all the people. And these people were thirsty and hurt and dying and all night long I could hear them calling, "mother, mother," and it sounded to me like ghosts calling out in the middle of the night. (Mitsuo)

> In the Japanese tradition, you're supposed to look for your family. I walked for three weeks, every single day, looking for my grandparents and my brother. It was a feeling of real loneliness and looking at the devastation of the whole city wondering why God left me here alone. You know, why didn't he take me too. At the time, yeah, I did want to go too. I felt they should have . . . I should have gone too instead of being left alone. (Florence) [WGBH Educational Foundation, 1982, pp. 4–6]

On August 6, 1945, the first atomic bomb was dropped on Hiroshima. Three days later, Nagasaki was bombed. Six days later, World War II was over. Over 80 percent of the people within one kilometer of the explosion died instantly or soon afterward. By December 1945, the number of dead in Hiroshima and Nagasaki was over 200,000. By 1950, another 140,000 people had died from the continuing effects of radiation exposure; since then, 100,000 more people have died from radiation-related cancer. Before and during the same war, millions of Jews, gypsies, homosexuals, mentally retarded people, and others viewed as undesirable by the Nazis were systematically exterminated in what many consider the most horrible crime in the history of the world.

When Japanese-American victims of the atomic bomb declared themselves as survivors, insurance companies withdrew their health and life insurance policies, and employers discriminated against them. Nightmares, flashbacks, and fear for themselves and their children are common today among these survivors. Finally, these survivors formed the Committee of Atomic Bomb Survivors in the United States to gain medical benefits from the U.S. government. Now, in the new millennium, a memorial to Japanese-American survivors is being erected to signify publicly the sacrifice and unjust suffering of these people.

Vietnam War veterans also finally succeeded in gaining veterans' benefits for health damage they believe resulted from exposure to the defoliant Agent Orange, damage affecting at least 250,000 U.S. families. For many Vietnam veterans, America's most unpopular war still rages; many still feel that the loss of life and limb, accepted as necessary in earlier wars, was not justified in a war that most believe should never have been fought. Veterans of the Gulf War (Desert Storm) have had a much shorter struggle. They have been given compensation for damages that they believe to have resulted from exposure to as-yet-unidentified agents during warfare, based on testimony in Congress from sick veterans and their advocates.

In Buffalo Creek, West Virginia, a mining corporation carelessly dumped coal waste, which formed artificial dams that eventually broke and caused dozens of deaths. Buffalo Creek residents knew that the dam was considered dangerous and that the mining corporation had neglected to correct the problem (Lifton & Olson, 1976). When loved ones, homes, and the natural environment were destroyed, survivors concluded that the mining company regarded them as less than human. In fact, one of the excuses offered by the company for not correcting their dangerous waste disposal method was that fish would be harmed by alternative methods. The survivors' feelings of devaluation were confirmed by their knowledge of the coal company's proposal of hasty and inadequate financial settlements. The physical damage to the community was never repaired, either by the company or through outside assistance. Residents are constantly reminded of the disaster.

Unlike the Rapid City community described earlier, Buffalo Creek survivors did not respond to the disaster with community rejuvenation borne of the tragedy. Lifton and Olson (1976) attribute this tremendously different response to the disaster's human (rather than natural) origin. Even though the mining company was forced to pay $13.5 million in a psychic damage suit, Buffalo Creek residents seem to feel that they and their community will never be healed. Considering genetic, health, and material damage such as that suffered by Love Canal residents, monetary compensation becomes practically meaningless. Money cannot repair such losses. *Prevention of* and *learning from* such tragic neglect seem the only reasonable responses.

The reactions of Buffalo Creek and Love Canal survivors are similar to those observed among survivors, including children, of Hiroshima, the Nazi Holocaust, and other wars (Apfel & Simon, 1994b; Lifton, 1967). Quoting Luchterhand (1971), Lifton and Olson (1976) state, "As the source of stress shifts from indiscriminate violence by nature to the discriminate oppression by man, the damage to human personality becomes less remediable" (p. 10). Survivors of planned disaster—including war—feel that their humanity has been violated. Their psyches are bombarded to such a degree that their capacity for recovery is often permanently damaged.

In a related category are victims and survivors of technological disaster, an increasing occurrence worldwide. As people demand more goods and energy, technical errors occur, and more toxic wastes are produced. The most outstanding international examples are the Bhopal and Chernobyl disasters. At least seven thousand people died in the Bhopal industrial calamity; it took years for the half million survivors to negotiate compensation and to bring to trial the plant officials, who were charged with manslaughter. On a less dramatic scale are the increasing numbers of people exposed to occupational hazards, as evidenced by increasing rates of infertility, especially among low-paid workers (predominantly people of color) in the least protected environments. Central to the emotional recovery of persons exposed to such hazards are the concepts of *meaning* and *control*.

Preventing Post-Traumatic Stress Disorders

As discussed in Chapter Two, emotional recovery seems to require that traumatized people be able to incorporate events into their meaning system and to maintain at least some perception of control. If a situation seems beyond one's control, self-blame may be used as a way to cope with the event (Baum et al., 1983, p. 134). Thus, if the origin of trauma or prolonged distress is external—that is, if people are exposed to occupational hazards or are victims of disasters traced to negligence—it is important that victims attribute responsibility to its true sources rather than to themselves. Interpreting a person's anger and demand for compensation as a "dependency conflict" or in other psychopathological terms is a form of blaming the victim (Schottenfeld & Cullen, 1985). Instead, such traumatized people should be linked to self-help and advocacy groups through which they might channel their anger into constructive action for necessary change—in this case, improved safety standards on the job (Chavkin, 1984) or social change regarding toxic waste (Grossfeld, 1993; Hoff & McNutt, 1994). (See also Chapter Eight, Figure 8.1, Box 3, right circle). This is not to say that prior psychopathologies do not play a role in some injury claims, but these should not be used to obscure the fact that injurious exposure reduces some people to joblessness, ill health, and poverty.

Many of these ideas are now being examined in studies of *post-traumatic stress disorder* (PTSD), a controversial concept describing a chronic condition that may occur years after an original trauma that falls outside the normal range of life events, such as during a war or in a concentration camp or from terrorist bombings (McCarroll, Ursano, & Fullerton, 1993; Peterson, Prout, & Schwarz, 1991; Schottenfeld & Cullen, 1985). When the DSM-IV diagnostic criteria of PTSD are relevant to those with histories of childhood abuse (physical or sexual) or other interpersonal violence, it is termed *complex PTSD* (Everett & Gallop, 2000). Although PTSD has some features common to clinical depression, panic disorder, and alcoholism, its increasing prevalence underscores the importance of crisis intervention for all traumatized people in addition to renewed efforts to prevent abuse and trauma in the first place (see Miller, 1999).

Maintaining or regaining health (*salutogenesis*) and avoiding illness are greater challenges when the crisis originates from sociocultural sources—in this case, disasters of human origin. This is because the emotional healing process requires, among other things, that people answer for themselves the question, "Why did this happen to me?" If the answer is, "It was fate," "It was God's will," or "That's life; some bad things just happen," people are able to recover and rebuild their lives, especially with social support. But if the answer can be traced to one's gender, race, sexual identity, or other prejudice; to neglect or hatred from individuals, groups, or corporations (as in environmental pollution); to ethnic cleansing; or to any other human origin, the persons affected must receive a message of caring and compensation to counteract the devastating effects of such malevolent actions. Otherwise a person's sense of coherence, including comprehensibility, meaning-fulness, and manageability (Antonovsky, 1987, pp. 17–19), is shaken; the person tends to absorb the blame and devaluation implied by others' neglect or outright damage. This process is similar to the downward spiral to depression and possible morbidity discussed in Chapter Two (Figure 2.2), which can occur when survivors of violence are blamed for their plight. Follow-up service for *individual* survivors of man-made disaster includes particular attention to the meaning of these traumas in cross-cultural perspective. Those meanings are often associated with social and political action, especially prevention efforts, that can benefit other people.

Follow-Up and Prevention

Vietnam veterans are still trying to rebuild their lives after a generation of being made scapegoats for a nation's guilt and shame about a war they were not per-sonally responsible for starting. Holocaust survivors have formed awareness groups as resources for support and the preservation of history. Atomic bomb survivors say their sacrifice was worthwhile if only the bomb is never used again. First Nations people are fighting for their cultural survival as well as against the destruction of the environment, which they view as a crime against the harmony that should exist between nature and human beings (Mousseau, 1989). Lois Gibbs's story (1982) about the Love Canal tragedy moved a nation to awareness of similar hazards in numerous other communities. Not unlike the parent survivors of teenage suicide, these survivors are trying to find meaning in their suffering by sharing the pain and tragedy of their lives to benefit others. The survivors of human malice, greed, and prejudice tell us something about ourselves, our world, and the way we relate to one another and the environment.

Yet more than a hundred years after the American Civil War, over a half century after the Holocaust, and decades after the Vietnam War, we still have

- Racially motivated violence and institutionalized racism across the United States
- Crimes with apparent anti-Semitic and other ethnic, religious, and political motives, from Boston to Ireland, Bosnia, Haiti, Rwanda, and the Middle East
- A systematic attempt to declare the Holocaust a "myth"
- Repeated famines in African countries that can be traced to war and to the widening gap between the haves and have-nots of the world (Wijkman & Timberlake, 1984)

- An international nuclear capacity for destruction more than one million times the power of the atomic bomb dropped on Hiroshima

To meet the challenges of these potentially destructive forces, there are now national and international debates about nuclear proliferation, regional wars, and arms trade that are unparalleled in the history of the human race in their importance to our ultimate survival. But the social, political, religious, and psychological ramifications of national and international crises and chronic problems are complex, controversial, and passionately debated. People are deeply divided, for example, in their views about

- Whether or how ethnic cleansing should be stopped
- What the division of government spending should be between domestic and defense needs
- Whether the environmental crisis is as serious as some claim

These issues will probably be argued for a long time. The following facts remain nevertheless.

- Many crises can be traced to social, economic, and political factors of local and global origins.
- Children are pressing their teachers for answers about crime and environmental threat.
- Fear about nuclear accidents and environmental pollution has increased since the Chernobyl disaster.
- Effective crisis intervention cannot be practiced without considering the sociocultural context of the crisis.

It is imperative that individual and public crises be understood in terms of their human meaning (Mills, 1959). Public issues should be debated and acted on, not abstractly, but in terms of their impact on each of us—you, me, our families and friends, and others. Not only is there a dynamic interplay between public and private life, but in both realms our sensitivity to others' perceptions and value systems regarding controversial issues can foster cooperation and prevent conflict.

Each person's unique perception of traumatic events is central to understanding and resolving a crisis. Without communication, we cannot understand another's interpretation of an event or issue, and we may become a hindrance to constructive crisis resolution. The differences in interpretations of personal, social, and political problems are as diverse as community members themselves. Unquestionably, communication is the key to uncovering these interpretations and thus understanding people in crisis and instituting appropriate care. A person tells of a traumatic experience through emotional display, behavior, and verbal communication—Hansell's "crisis plumage" (1976). Responses are often embedded in cultural differences. If there is no caring and supportive listener, the chances of a constructive crisis outcome are diminished.

But although listening is necessary, it is not sufficient if the crisis did not originate from individual circumstances. Social and political action are pivotal to a positive crisis outcome if the origin of the crisis is social and political (see Crisis Paradigm, Box 3, right circle). Individuals traumatized from these sources are more real than the casualty figures reported on the evening news make them seem.

- Richard, a refugee from Rwanda with recurrent nightmares, is someone's husband, father, son, and brother. He is forty-eight years old and lives on Locust Street in a town of forty-five thousand people.
- Shigeko is an atomic bomb survivor who has had twenty-six operations on her face and lips and is glad that she is alive and that her son is not ashamed of her appearance.
- Jane, age five, lives near a hazardous waste site and has toxic hepatitis.

These people and many others like them tend to get lost in statements of "statistically significant" incidences (of cancer, deformed children, or other medical problems), scientific jargon, and "investigative procedures" for determining whether corrective action is in order. This process of generalizing does not seem to apply to real people. The abstractness, along with the grossness of the figures—10 million victims of the Holocaust, nearly 500,000 dead from atomic bomb blasts—contributes to denial and psychic numbing for the average person. The numbers, the destruction, and the sheer horror are unimaginable for most of us. To defend ourselves against the terror, we deny and try to convince ourselves that there is nothing we personally can do about these global issues.

Although the Cold War is officially over, there are still stockpiles of nuclear arms sufficient to destroy the planet several times over, and additional nations are testing nuclear devices even as the United Nations Security Council debates how to deal with one regional crisis after another in which thousands of innocent civilians (many of them children) are slaughtered or wounded by warring factions. As Apfel and Simon (1994a, p. 72) note, "If we decide it is the responsibility of the enemy's leadership to take care of its own children, then we can more easily go ahead with our bombing program. If we decide children anywhere in the world are also our children, we can less easily bomb. We distance ourselves and say that children who are far away are not our children, and if they suffer it is because their leaders and their parents are irresponsible." In the spirit of violence prevention and Ruddick's thesis (1989) regarding "maternal practice," it is reasonable to suggest that if men and women shared equally in the everyday tasks of caring for children and learned the conflict resolution tactics demanded by nonviolent parenting, they would insist that more resources be spent to promote peace and conserve lives and resources than are presently spent on war and destruction (Goodman & Hoff, 1990).

From a safe distance, it is relatively easy to think of our enemies as less than human and therefore worthy of destruction. As in our attitudes toward the homeless, deinstitutionalized mental patients, and unwed mothers, our enemies are distant; they belong to groups and are the responsibility of the state or church.

When they are thus objectified, we do not have to think of them as someone's sister, father, mother, or friend.

Our worst enemies are people like ourselves: they eat; sleep; make love; bear children; feel pain, fear, and anger; communicate with one another; bury their dead; and eventually die. Statistics and machines will never be a substitute for human interaction, just as rating scales can aid but not displace clinical judgment in evaluating individual suicide risk. As Albert Einstein said, "Peace cannot be kept by force. It can only be achieved by understanding."

In a particular crisis situation, if we do not *communicate*, for example, with a suicidal person, we will not understand why death is preferable to life for that individual and therefore may be ineffective in preventing suicide. If we take the time to *talk* with and *listen* to a person in crisis, we are less likely to suggest or prescribe a drug as a crisis response. Similarly, at the national and international levels, if we keep communication open and foster political strategies to handle crises, there is less likelihood of resorting to physical force for solving problems. Human communication, then, is central to our survival—as individuals and as a world community.

Our ethnocentrism is nevertheless often so strong, and greed and power motives are often so disguised that the average person may find it difficult to think of disasters occurring from human design as a form of violence. Victims of disasters and other traumas of human origin, however, feel violated. They have experienced directly the destruction of their health, their children, their homes, their sense of security, their hopes for the future, and their sense of wholeness and worth in the human community.

In many ways, the poignant testimonies and tragic lives of the victims of ethnic, class, and political conflicts speak for themselves. Still, two of the most painful aspects of their crises are that they feel ignored and often cannot receive even material compensation for their enormous losses. People suffering from these policies feel denied. A hopeful sign of policy change is the international response to the Central American devastation wrought by Hurricane Mitch. The United States put a hold on deporting immigrants back to their devastated countries, and some countries reduced the debt burden of these poor countries. Another hopeful sign is advocacy for forgiving these debts altogether, in that they accrued around global economic policies developed with the major advantage going to rich countries.

If we have not listened, or if we have been silent when we should have spoken, convinced that we have nothing to say about public issues, perhaps we should reexamine what Nobel Peace Prize recipient Albert Schweitzer said in 1954: "Whether we secure a lasting peace will depend upon the direction taken by individuals—and, therefore, by the nations whom those individuals collectively compose." Survival is too serious to be confined to partisan politics, the government, or liberal versus conservative debates. Every citizen—and certainly crisis workers—should be informed on the critical issues confronting the human race (see Ekins, 1992; Foell & Nenneman, 1986; Hoff & McNutt, 1994). Therapist neutrality is a concept that will not do in cases of crisis originating in sociocultural and political sources. People traumatized by violence need explicit public acknowledgment that what happened to them is wrong.

When confronted with the enormity and horror of disaster from human sources, denial is understandable. Although we may feel helpless and powerless, in fact, we are not. The opinions of officials and professionals are not necessarily wiser or more lifesaving than those of ordinary citizens. Lois Gibbs (1982), in describing why she wrote *Love Canal: My Story*, emphasizes the fact that as an average citizen with limited education and almost no funds, she was able to fight city hall and the White House and win! Every country has someone or many like Lois Gibbs, who, in the face of unnecessary and preventable suffering, join with others to make a difference for themselves, their families, and the world.

Murray Levine, a community psychologist, wrote, in his introduction to Gibbs's story (1982, pp. xii–xviii), reasons why her story and others like it should be told; he also illustrated crisis and preventive responses to a disaster of human origins:

1. Lois Gibbs is in many respects a typical American woman—a mother of two children and a housewife. In response to crisis and challenge, she courageously "transcended herself and became far more than she had been."
2. Her story informs us of the relationship between citizens and their government and shows that the government's decisions about a problem are not necessarily in the interests of ordinary people whose lives are threatened by these decisions.
3. Lois Gibbs's story is one of "inner meanings and feelings of humans," a story that "provides a necessary and powerful antidote to the moral illness of those cynics and their professional robots who speak the inhuman language of benefit-cost ratios, who speak of the threat of congenital deformities or cancers as acceptable risks."

In conclusion, the differences between disasters of natural and human origin are striking: the uncontrolled, violent forces of nature (fire, water, wind, and temperature), destructive as they are, are minuscule in comparison with disasters from human sources. The possible crisis outcomes for the victims are also markedly different, with enormous implications for prevention. As discussed, technology has been a double-edged sword, sometimes the cause of disaster, sometimes the cure. Through technology and public health planning, much has been done to harness some of the destructive potential of nature. Natural disaster–control technology, land management policies, and resources for aid to victims should now be shared more widely in disaster-prone areas of the world. Concerning disaster from human sources, however, we have been much less successful in directing and controlling conflict and indifference toward the health and welfare of others. This is unfortunate but not hopeless. Violence is not inevitable (Lifton, 1993); it results from our choices, action, and inaction (see Crisis Paradigm, Box 3, right circle).

In the discussion of understanding people in crisis in Chapter Two, emphasis was placed on the examination of crisis origins. In the case of disasters of human origin, such an examination inevitably leads us into the most pressing social, political, and economic questions facing humankind. After hearing the voices of survivors of nuclear bombs, of the downwind fallout in Utah, of Love Canal, of the concentration camps, or of still another war or ethnic cleansing, the crisis worker may well begin to question the social and political choices that led to these disasters. The broad view suggested by these questions is important for the crisis worker to develop, in tandem with individualized crisis intervention strategies. Without it, the helper may begin to perceive the task of helping victims of man-made disasters as an exercise in futility. Frustration, loss of effectiveness, and burnout may replace the understanding, sensitivity, and problem-solving ability that the crisis worker should bring to this task.

Summary

Disaster is experienced as a crisis unlike any other that a person will ever live through. Victims may face a threat to their lives and may lose loved ones, homes, and personal belongings in a single stroke. Many spend the rest of their lives mourning these tragic losses and trying to rebuild their homes and lives. Rescue services, crisis intervention, and follow-up care for physical, emotional, and social rehabilitation are necessary for all survivors. Although financial aid for physical restoration and rehabilitation has been available for years, crisis counseling services are a newer phenomenon on the disaster scene. Communities will be better equipped to handle the emotional crisis related to the disaster experience when health and social service workers, as well as other caretakers, are prepared in advance with skills in crisis management. The urgency of preventing disasters of human origin is self-evident.

References

Ahmed, F. E. (1992, September 1). The Bangladesh hurricane has no name. *Boston Globe,* p. 15.

Antonovsky, A. (1987). *Unraveling the mystery of health: How people manage stress and stay well.* San Francisco: Jossey-Bass.

Apfel, R. J., & Simon, B. (1994a, February 13). Children in the cross-fire. *Boston Globe,* pp. 69, 72.

Apfel, R. J., & Simon, B. (Eds.). (1994b). *Minefields in the heart: Mental life of children of war and communal violence.* New Haven, CT: Yale University Press.

Baum, A., Fleming, R., & Singer, J. E. (1983). Coping with victimization by technological disaster. *Journal of Social Issues, 39*(2), 117–138.

Chavkin, W. (Ed.). (1984). *Double exposure: Women's health hazards on the job and at home.* New York: Monthly Review Press.

Doolin, J., & Collins, M. (1998, November 10). Face to face with the suffering in Central America. *Boston Globe,* p. A19.

Durkin, M. S., Khan, N., Davidson, L. L., Zaman, S. S., & Stein, Z. A. (1993). The effects of a natural disaster on child behavior: Evidence for post-traumatic stress. *American Journal of Public Health, 83*(11), 1549–1553.

Ekins, P. (1992). *A new world order: Grassroots movements for global change.* New York: Routledge.

Epstein, P. R. (1995). Emerging diseases and ecosystem instability: New threats to public health. *American Journal of Public Health, 85,* 168–172.

Erikson, K. (1994). *A new species of trouble.* New York: Norton.

Everett, B., & Gallop, R. (2000). *Linking childhood trauma and mental illness: Theory and practice for direct service practitioners.* Thousand Oaks, CA: Sage.

Foell, E., & Nenneman, R. (1986). *How peace came to the world.* Cambridge, MA: MIT Press.

Gibbs, L. (1982). *Love Canal: My story.* Albany: State University of New York Press.

Gist, R., & Lubin, B. (Eds.). (1989). *Psychosocial aspects of disaster.* New York: Wiley.

Goldoftas, B. (1998, December 11). Hurricane Mitch's deadly ally. *Boston Globe,* p. A35.

Goodman, L. M., & Hoff, L. A. (1990). *Omnicide.* New York: Praeger.

Grossfeld, S. (1993, March 28). The exhausted earth: Life in the poison zones. *Boston Sunday Globe,* pp. 1, 24–27.

Hansell, N. (1976). *The person in distress.* New York: Human Sciences Press.

Hoff, M. D., & McNutt, J. G. (Eds.). (1994). *The global environmental crisis.* Aldershot, England: Avebury.

Joseph, S., Yule, W., Williams, R., & Andrews, B. (1993). Crisis support in the aftermath of disaster. *British Journal of Clinical Psychology, 32*(Part 2), 177–185.

Kizzier, D. (1972). *The Rapid City flood.* Lubbock, TX: Boone.

Koegler, R. R., & Hicks, S. M. (1972). The destruction of a medical center by earthquake. *California Medicine, 116,* 63–67.

Leon, J., Poole, W. K., & Kloner, R. A. (1996). Sudden cardiac death triggered by an earthquake. *New England Journal of Medicine, 334,* 413–419.

Lifton, R. J. (1967). *Life in death.* New York: Simon & Schuster.

Lifton, R. J. (1993). *The protean self: Human resilience in an age of fragmentation.* New York: Basic Books.

Lifton, R. J., & Olson, E. (1976). The human meaning of total disaster: The Buffalo Creek experience. *Psychiatry, 39,* 1–18.

Logue, J. N. (1996). Disasters, the environment, and public health: Improving our response. *American Journal of Public Health, 86*(9), 1207–1210.

Luchterhand, E. G. (1971). Sociological approaches to massive stress in natural and man-made disasters. *International Psychiatry Clinic, 8,* 29–53.

Marcus, A. (1999, August 19). Amid din of heavy equipment, rescuers strain to hear voices of the trapped. *Boston Globe,* p. A26.

McCarroll, J. E., Ursano, R. J., & Fullerton, C. S. (1993). Symptoms of post-traumatic stress disorder following recovery of war dead. *American Journal of Psychiatry, 150*(12), 1875–1877.

Miller, L. (1999). Treating posttraumatic stress disorder in children and families: Basic principles and clinical applications. *American Journal of Family Therapy, 27*(1), 21–24.

Mills, C. W. (1959). *The sociological imagination.* Oxford: Oxford University Press.

Mousseau, M. (1989). *The medicine wheel approach to dealing with family violence.* Dauphin, Manitoba, Canada: West Region Child and Family Services.

Murphy, S. A. (1986). Status of natural disaster victims' health and recovery 1 and 3 years later. *Research in Nursing and Health, 9,* 331–340.

Peterson, K. C., Prout, M. F., & Schwarz, R. A. (1991). *Post-traumatic stress disorder: A clinician's guide.* New York: Plenum.

Richman, N. (1993). After the flood. *American Journal of Public Health, 83*(11), 1522–1523.

Ruddick, S. (1989). *Maternal thinking: Toward a politics of peace.* Boston: Beacon Press.

Schottenfeld, R. S., & Cullen, M. R. (1985). Occupation-induced post-traumatic stress disorders. *American Journal of Psychiatry, 142*(2), 198–202. (See also "Reply" in Letters to the Editor, *142*(9), 35–42, 93–95.)

Tucker, P., Pfefferbaum, B., Nixon, S. J., & Foy, D. W. (1999). Trauma and recovery among adults highly exposed to a community disaster. *Psychiatric Annals, 29*(2), 78–83.

Tyhurst, J. S. (1951). Individual reactions to community disaster. *American Journal of Psychiatry, 107,* 764–769.

Tyhurst, J. S. (1957a). Psychological and social aspects of civilian disaster. *Canadian Medical Association Journal, 76,* 385–393.

Tyhurst, J. S. (1957b). The role of transition states—including disasters—in mental illness. In *Symposium on preventive and social psychiatry.* Washington, DC: Walter Reed Army Institute of Research and the National Research Council.

WGBH Educational Foundation. *Survivors* [Public television documentary]. (1982). Boston: Author.

Wijkman, A., & Timberlake, L. (1984). *Natural disaster: Acts of God or acts of man?* London: International Institute for Environment and Development.

Zunin, L. M., & Zunin, H. S. (1991). *The art of condolence: What to write, what to say, what to do at a time of loss.* New York: HarperCollins.

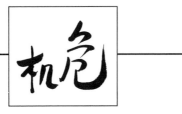

PART THREE

CRISES RELATED TO SITUATIONAL AND TRANSITION STATES

Hazardous life events, both anticipated and unanticipated, are traditionally defined as transitional and situational state crises (see Crisis Paradigm). In presenting crises associated with various transitions, the first two chapters of Part Three address the theme of passage from health to illness (including the paradigmatic crisis of AIDS in global perspective), from employed to unemployed status, and from one residence or country to another. Chapter Thirteen highlights rites of passage and life crises arising from status and role changes through developmental phases of the life cycle. It concludes with the final crisis for all—passage from life to death—and how we can help ourselves and others through this last developmental task.

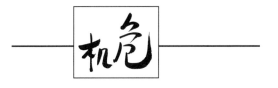

CHAPTER ELEVEN

THREATS TO HEALTH STATUS AND SELF-IMAGE

Many have said that if their health is intact, they can endure almost anything else. This is because a change in health status is not only hazardous in itself and potentially life threatening, but poor health status leaves one more vulnerable than otherwise to hazardous events. To avoid a crisis state, all of us need to have

- A sense of physical and emotional well-being
- An image of self that flows from general well-being and acceptance of one's physical attributes
- Some control in everyday life functions and the activities of daily living

These aspects of life are acutely threatened by illness, accidents, surgery, physical or mental handicap, and the uncontrolled use of alcohol and other drugs. Several of our basic needs are in jeopardy when events that are hazardous to health occur. A full crisis experience can be avoided if the threatened person is supported by family, friends, and health workers and receives necessary treatment regardless of financial status. Self-defeating outcomes such as suicide, assault or homicide, mental illness, and depression can also be avoided if appropriate treatment and emotional support are available when threats to health status occur.

People in emotional crisis related to illness, injury, surgery, or handicap rarely come to the attention of crisis specialists or mental health workers in the acute crisis stage. Mental health workers often see people *after* a crisis episode, when they may have become dependent on alcohol or other drugs, lapsed into depression, or experienced other emotional disturbance. This pattern underscores the pivotal role of general health workers such as physicians and nurses in the crisis care process, especially at various entry points to the health care system. In addition, many frontline workers such as police, rescue teams, firefighters, and Travelers Aid caseworkers are the first to confront a person injured or in emotional shock from an accident, violent attack, or fire.

Centuries ago, Hippocrates said that it is more important to "know the man who has the disease than the disease the man has." More recent research, along with the human potential movement, documents the intrinsic relationship between mind, body, and spirit (Borysenko, 1987; Edmands, Hoff, Kaylor, Mower, & Sorrell, 1999). The congressional document *Action for Mental Health* (Congressional Joint Commission on Mental Health and Illness, 1961) and federal legislation that led to pioneering efforts in the community mental health movement in the United States also documented the fact that many distressed people *first* visit physicians or clergy, *not* mental health professionals.

These data underscore a premise of this book, that the crisis response is a *normal*, not pathological, life experience. Yet crisis assessment and intervention in general health care practice are by no means routine. As Sugg and Inui (1992) report, physicians are afraid of opening Pandora's box by inquiring about the possibility of abuse. Similarly, Moore and Schwartz (1993) report that emergency nurses may not be delivering the psychosocial support that they believe they are. In contrast, many health and frontline workers are already doing crisis intervention but may lack self-confidence because they have no formal training in the field. They often need reinforcement and confirmation from crisis specialists for work they are doing with distressed people (Adamowski, Dickinson, Weitzman, Roessler, & Carter-Snell, 1993; Hoff & Adamowski, 1998).

This chapter addresses the crisis care process as applied in *general* health care situations when a person is in a status change from health to illness or from physical intactness to handicap. It includes illustrations of how to synchronize rapid assessment and social support with appropriate use of psychotropic drugs for clients who present with high anxiety but who refuse a mental health referral. The strategies apply in doctors' offices; emergency, intensive care, and other hospital departments; primary care settings such as prenatal clinics—in virtually all health and human service settings, including long-term care facilities. The discussion here assumes the underpinnings of general assessment and intervention strategies and life-threatening situations addressed in other chapters, including the use of psychotropic drugs for suicidal persons.

Crisis Care in Primary Health Care Settings

Since the essential features of formal crisis intervention have not changed much since the era when it was deemed a mere Band-Aid, we have a paradoxical situation. On the one hand, mental health care and crisis intervention are being increasingly cited in health reform policy statements (for example, Fiedler & Wight, 1989). On the other hand, a mind-body split is still evident as many general health practitioners hesitate to deal with emotional issues, citing either discomfort with them or lack of time. Understandably, most nonpsychiatric physicians and nurses do not think of themselves as psychotherapists, yet the psychosocial facet of treatment and care is a given whether the primary health problem is physical or emotional. And therein may lie insight into the paradox. As already discussed, although crisis intervention shares certain techniques with psychotherapy and may have *psychotherapeutic* outcomes if aptly applied, it is not psychotherapy. The social construction of crisis intervention as therapy within a decade of having discounted it as a Band-Aid may partially explain the continued reluctance of general health practitioners to incorporate the model into routine health care practice. The medicalization of crisis intervention is one facet of the tradition, especially in North America, where equating "health" care with "medical" care is common (Rachlis & Kushner, 1994; Smith, 1994). There is a need to reclaim the primary prevention model espoused by Caplan (1964) and recast crisis intervention within the public health model, rather than the biomedical model (Feingold, 1994; Hoff & Adamowski, 1998; Navarro, 1994).

The increasing emphasis on primary care and concerns about the escalation of health care costs underscore the inclusion of crisis intervention as an essential element of comprehensive health care. As the book's Crisis Paradigm illustrates, prevention (including through crisis intervention) is less costly than treatment, especially in residential facilities. But crisis and quick-fix drug approaches must not be used as *financially expedient* substitutes for the longer-term care and rehabilitation that some problems require (Hoff, 1993; Johnson, 1990). In many of these primary care situations, crisis assessment, social support, and a referral to a peer support or self-help group, as discussed in Chapter Five, will do. For example, one woman said that her physical and emotional recovery after a mastectomy might have been much more precarious if a nurse had not comforted her when she broke down crying the first time she looked in the mirror. This was the beginning of her grief work around the loss of her breast. It was facilitated by a surgical nurse who was not a psychotherapist; the nurse simply understood and responded to the crisis dimensions of the woman's transition in health status and potentially her self-image. Pappano (1998) writes movingly about the "Thursday Group," a cancer support group whose members say their shared strength is what keeps them going as they struggle with the side effects of treatment and, for some, the reality of their final loss.

Hazards to Physical and Emotional Health

Physical illnesses or accidents are often the beginning of a series of problems for an individual as well as for that person's family. If struck by a potentially fatal illness such as cancer, the person may experience the same sense of dread and loss that death itself implies. A person's self-image is also threatened by serious physical alteration resulting from a mastectomy, amputation of an arm or leg, scars from an accident or extensive burns, AIDS, or genital herpes. If injury and illness result from a disaster of human origins, crisis resolution that avoids despair, revenge, or violence is especially challenging. People with sexually transmitted diseases (STDs) are also particularly crisis prone; shame, revulsion, ignorance, and fear about such diseases can precipitate marriage breakups, suicidal tendencies, social isolation, self-loathing, and depression. And if a person realizes that an STD may be a forerunner of AIDS and was caused by having unprotected sex, the potential for crisis is increased. This is also true when HIV is transmitted through rape.

In addition to facing the illness or accident itself, the person acutely or chronically ill often faces another crisis—institutionalization in a hospital or nursing home. As noted in Chapter Three, hospital admission in itself may precipitate a crisis. Hospitals and other institutions can be considered as subcultures in which the longest-term occupants—the staff—know the procedures and rules that prevent chaos and help them do their jobs. The sick person, however, especially one who has never been hospitalized, may experience culture shock, a condition that can occur when the comfort of familiar things is missing. Because the staff of these institutions become enculturated to their work environment, they often forget that a hospital admission is a temporary detour in the sick person's normal, everyday existence.

Without support, in the "foreign" institutional environment a person's usually successful response to life's ups and downs may be weakened. In extreme cases, a person in culture shock feels too surprised and too numbed by a new culture's unfamiliarity to proceed with the successful management of everyday life tasks. Add the fear of the unknown regarding the outcome of treatments, and it is easy to understand why some patients lash out at staff in what may appear to be unreasonable outbursts or manifest other classic signs of culture shock or crisis. Even in transitional or long-term care placements, attention to these crisis manifestations, especially upon admission, can avoid much pain for both client and staff. Complicating this scenario is the potential crisis response of a patient who feels unready for discharge. In this era of cost containment and concern about dependency issues, timely discharge may seem cost-efficient. But premature discharge does not save money and may eventually cost more through readmission or result in extreme responses such as suicide (Hoff, 1993).

In some instances, people's illnesses and the crisis of hospitalization are complicated further by negligence, mishandling, or unethical medical practice. Millman (1978) discusses the systematic cover-up of iatrogenic illness and death (that is, caused by the health care provider). In addition to the original illness, the patient (or survivor) must contend with the personal damage inflicted by the people he or she trusted. Despite progress in the women's health movement, some women are still dying prematurely from illnesses that were dismissed as manifestations of their "neurotic personalities" (Ehrenreich & English, 1979). In one 1993 case, a forty-three-year-old woman died of ovarian cancer within a year of diagnosis after spending six months trying to persuade her physician to take her symptoms seriously. When he finally examined her, she already had nine metastatic sites.

Patients and families, however, are not the only ones in crisis around these issues. Nursing and medical colleagues face the moral dilemma of collusion in cover-up of negligence. If lawsuits occur, a new series of crises may unfold: joblessness, financial loss, and damage to professional status.

A related issue concerns unnecessary surgery. A historical account of surgery (Dally, 1992) documents experimentation on women and black slaves. Although unnecessary elective surgery is under scrutiny for ethical and cost containment reasons, cosmetic surgery such as breast implants continues despite highly controversial results such as disfigurement and immune system breakdown. Without the profits to be made and the cultural component of women's general concern (and sometimes obsession) with body image, some of the crises related to these health issues might be avoided. Among those surgeries with the highest unconfirmed rates (those in which the second opinion did not support the initial recommendation) are breast surgery, hysterectomy (removal of the uterus), and in men removal of the prostate gland. Women have the majority of unnecessary operations and also receive 50 percent more prescription drugs than men (Hamilton, Jensvold, Rothblum, & Cole, 1995). This practice is especially significant in view of women's emotional and physical assets: on average, women in industrialized societies live seven years longer than men and are assumed worldwide to be the emotional and social caretakers of society. But many women have insufficient access to care. These facts are linked to the political economy of medicine and to cultural values about women that portray them as less valuable than men and when sick in need of medical intervention and control (Becktell, 1994; Ehrenreich & English, 1979; Lugina, 1994).

The issue of surgery as a crisis point is particularly poignant in the case of breast surgery. Preparing a woman for a mastectomy and explaining alternative treatments can help her live through this crisis (Bredenberg, 1991). Offering support through self-help referrals after surgery is equally important. Yet in one state, the legislature had to pass a law requiring physicians to make nonsurgical options known to women with breast cancer. Increasingly, women who have had mastectomies are referred to self-help groups such as Reach for Recovery, which offer emotional support during this crisis-prone period. However, in many communities, advocacy is needed to ensure such referrals. As the rates of breast cancer steadily grow and research begins to examine possible environmental causes, such as contamination of the food chain by pesticides, it is important to link this personal traumatic event with broader social concerns.

Hoskins and Haber (2000) highlight the key role of nurses in education and counseling to reduce the risk of crisis for women and their families during the four phases of adjustment: diagnostic, postsurgical, adjuvant therapy, and ongoing recovery. For each phase, they suggest specific techniques for talking with patients and their partners—for example, for partners in the postsurgical phase: "Many partners of women who have had breast surgery are concerned, as are the women themselves, about how they'll respond to the loss. How have you felt about your partner's losing [part of] her breast?" (p. 29).

Men having surgery on sex organs also need supportive communication and accurate information. Although radical surgery (prostatectomy) has increased dramatically in recent years, there is no proof that this surgery saves lives, whereas there is evidence of incontinence and impotence following the operation. Nurses are in especially strategic positions to encourage male patients to communicate their feelings regarding this sensitive issue and to assist them in making informed decisions about surgery (see O'Rourke, 1999). The crisis for men having such surgery is heavily tinged by the threat to male potency and self-image that is signaled by cancer or surgery affecting sex organs. The hazards of such a diagnosis are compounded because males have been socialized not to cry or to express feelings readily. Together these factors become barriers to early diagnosis of prostate cancer, which is very important in improving survival rates. This is especially important for African American men who have the highest prostate cancer rates. Although there were only a handful of prostate cancer support groups until recently, several hundred such groups exist now, according to the American Foundation for Urologic Disease, which has helped organize them. Some physicians recommend that men begin routine screening for prostate cancer at age fifty, although the issue is still controversial. Education, as well as communication with the man's sex partner, is important (Shipes & Lehr, 1982). Crisis prevention and intervention can also prevent later problems by timely support during medical and surgical care (Shalev, Schreiber, Galai, & Melmed, 1993).

Physicians and advance practice nurses play a pivotal role in such crisis situations. Alex, for example, was upset with the news that his wife intended to divorce him. When his physician diagnosed his cancer of the testicle, he was even more distressed. The physician simply told him to check into the county hospital's psychiatric unit thirty miles away if he continued to feel upset. Instead Alex went home, told his wife what the physician had said, and shot himself in his front yard.

Alex had been discussing the impending divorce with a crisis counselor who lived in Alex's community; the physician also practiced there. Even if the physician had no time to listen to Alex, he should have made a local referral. This case illustrates how local crisis specialty services may go unused if effective linkages with health and other frontline professionals are lacking (Hoff & Adamowski, 1998).

If illness, surgery, and hospitalization are occasions of crisis for most adults, they are even more so for children and their parents (Kruger, 1992). Research has revealed the traumatic effects of hospitalization on children, and a new organization has emerged, the Association for the Care of Children in Hospitals. Professionals with special training in child development now work in child life departments of many hospitals. They arrange preadmission tours and listen to children's questions and worries:

- Sam, age four, has been told by his doctor that a hole will have to be made in his stomach to make him well again. Because the doctor neglected to mention that the hole will also be stitched up again, Sam worries that "the things inside me will fall out."

- Cindy, age nine, sees an intravenous bottle and tubes being wheeled to her bedside. She had once seen the same apparatus attached to her cousin Jeffrey, who later died. As the needle is being inserted, she wonders if she is as sick as Jeffrey was.
- Ken, a junior high school football player, is confined to a traction frame. Unable to dress or wash himself each morning, he suffers acute embarrassment in front of the nurses.

If a child is going to the hospital, child life workers offer the following advice to parents:

1. Accept the fact of the hospitalization.
2. Be honest with your child.
3. Prepare yourself; for example, find out about procedures.
4. Prepare your child, for example, through preadmission get-acquainted tours.
5. Whenever possible, stay with your child.

In addition to these general health care situations, frontline health workers need to increase their vigilance on behalf of victims whose first contact after injury is a health care professional or emergency medical technician (Hoff & Rosenbaum, 1994; U.S. Department of Health and Human Services, 1986).

Crisis Response of People in Health Status Transition

To better understand the responses of those who are in pain, are ill, or are hospitalized, some questions must be addressed, such as, How do sick and hospitalized people feel? How do they perceive their illness and its relationship to their beliefs and lifestyle? How do they behave in the "sick role" (Brody, 1988)? The person whose physical integrity, self-image, and social freedom are threatened or actually damaged by these hazards to health shows many of the usual signs of a crisis state (see Chapter Three).

As noted in Chapter One, a majority of distressed people present first in health clinics, emergency departments, or offices of primary care providers. Health care workers' pivotal role in detecting and preventing florid crises therefore cannot be overstated. There are parallels in general medical and psychosocial care. For the client presenting with acute pain, general physical discomfort, or impairment of normal functioning, common responses and questions include, "Tell me where it hurts. When did it begin? Have you taken any medication to relieve the pain? When are the symptoms most bothersome?" Some clients present with symptoms suggesting *Generalized Anxiety Disorder* (GAD)—a DSM-IV Axis I diagnosis. This diagnosis requires three or more of the following symptoms: worry and apprehension, restlessness, easily fatigued, poor concentration, irritability and frustration, muscle tension, sleep disturbance, and mild to moderate transient physical symptoms (Oakley & Potter, 1997, pp. 92–95).

Most of these symptoms overlap with the classical manifestations (biophysical, emotional, cognitive, behavioral) of a person in crisis (see Chapter Three). In addition, given the undisputed connections between stress, crisis, and illness (physical and mental), physicians and advanced practice nurses are challenged with differentiating acute crisis responses (that is, duration of a few days to six weeks) from the longer-standing Generalized Anxiety Disorder (GAD) symptoms (that is, symptoms that are present more days than not over a six-month period). The importance of this differentiation underscores the key role of primary care providers in *preventing* the negative resolution of acute crisis in the form of emotional and mental illness without the hazard of a psychiatric diagnosis (see Chapter Three regarding DSM-IV diagnosis and managed care; Des Jarlais, 2000; Link, Struening, Rahav, Phelan, & Nuttbrock, 1997).

In the holistic preventive approach presented in this book, primary care providers are therefore advised as follows regarding clients presenting with acute or chronic anxiety or physical complaints that diagnostic tests rule out as biologically based: instead of concluding with a psychiatric diagnosis of GAD in the biomedical paradigm, assume that the presenting symptoms designate *emotional pain* (from loss, threat, abuse, and so on) and proceed with comments such as, "You seem to be very upset. Can you tell me what's happening?" To the client asking for a tranquilizing prescription: "Of course I can write you a prescription; that will help you feel less anxious, but it won't really solve whatever is troubling you. I think I'd be helping you more if we talked a bit before giving you a tranquilizer to see if maybe a referral for counseling would be the most helpful." This approach avoids pathologizing essentially *normal* responses to life's ups and downs and sometimes life-threatening events. As evidence of the biomedical versus public health emphasis in the United States, legislative language in states that require parity in health insurance defines all persons benefiting from mental health care as having a "disease." While recognizing that insurance reimbursement may require a DSM-IV diagnosis, it should be remembered that the original intent of the DSM was for use by mental health professionals trained in psychopathology and its treatment. Current pressures on primary care providers to use it portends the need for advocacy and policy change for insurance coverage for *preventive* psychosocial care, an essential component of which is crisis intervention in primary care settings. Let us review the classical crisis manifestations in reference to health status loss or threat of loss:

1. *Biophysical response.* Besides enduring the pain and discomfort from the disease or injury itself, the person losing health and bodily integrity suffers many of the biophysical symptoms experienced after the loss of a loved one (see "Loss, Change, and Grief Work" in Chapter Four). For example, Parkes (1975) compares the "phantom limb" experience with the "phantom husband" of widows, noting the influence of connections between psychological factors and the nervous system.

2. *Feelings.* After an amputation or a diagnosis such as heart disease, AIDS, herpes II, diabetes, or cancer, people respond with a variety of feelings:

- Shock and anger: "Why me?"
- Helplessness and hopelessness in regard to future normal functioning: "What's left for me now?"
- Shame about the obvious scar, handicap, or reduced physical ability and about dependence on others: "What will my husband think?"
- Anxiety about the welfare of spouse or children who depend on them: "How will they manage at home without me?"
- Sense of loss of bodily integrity and loss of goals the person hoped to achieve before the illness, accident, or trauma from abuse: "I don't think I'll ever feel right again."
- Doubt of acceptance by others: "No one will want to be around me this way."
- Fear of death, which may have been narrowly escaped in an accident or a violent attack by one's partner, or which now must be faced, in the case of cancer: "It was almost the end," or "This is the end."
- Fear that one's sex life is over after diagnosis with prostate cancer: "Am I condemned to lead a celibate life now?"

3. *Thoughts and perceptions.* The fears raised by a serious illness, an accident, or a changed image from the trauma of abuse or from a surgical operation usually color the person's perception of the event itself—the understanding of the event and how it will affect the future. For example, a young woman with diabetes assumed that she would be cut off from her cocktail party circuit, which she felt was necessary in her high executive position. She lacked knowledge about how social obligations might be synchronized with diabetes.

A person with heart disease may foresee spending the future as an invalid; the reality is that he or she must only change the manner and range of performance. The woman with a mastectomy may perceive that all men will reject her because of the bodily alteration; in reality only some men would do so. A woman who does not have a secure relationship with a man before a mastectomy may experience rejection; we can help such a woman consider the value of a relationship with a man who accepts her primarily for her body. Women with stable relationships are seldom rejected by their husbands or lovers following a mastectomy.

4. *Behavior.* The behavior of people who are ill or suffering from the physical effects of an accident, surgery, or other trauma is altered by several factors. First, hospitalization enforces a routine of dependency, which may be necessary when people are weak, but the routine also keeps the hospital running according to established rules of hierarchy. This hierarchy has little or nothing to do with patient welfare. In fact, rigidity in the hierarchy often defeats the purpose for which hospitals exist—quality care of patients.

The environment of an intensive care unit—the tubes, lights, and electrical gadgets—is a constant reminder to the patient and family members of proximity to death (Kleeman, 1989). Furthermore a patient's fears, anger, and lack of knowledge about illness, hospital routines, and expectations can elicit the worst behavior from a person who is otherwise cooperative and likable. The rules and regulations governing visitors to these settings present a further hazard to people already in a difficult situation.

To understand and respond appropriately to the emotional, perceptual, and behavioral responses of people to illness, pain, and hospitalization, we must be sensitive to cultural differences. The role of culture and value systems in the development of and response to crisis was discussed in the first four chapters; the cultural component becomes even more important in the face of illness, pain, and hospitalization. For example, Zborowski's classic study (1952) of Jewish, Italian, Irish, and other Americans revealed that (1) similar *reactions* to pain by different ethnocultural groups do not necessarily reflect similar *attitudes* to pain and (2) similar reactive patterns may have different functions in various cultures. For instance, typically, Jews' responses to pain elicit worry and concern, whereas Italians' elicit sympathy. Standard texts on health, illness, and healing in cross-cultural perspective offer further discussion of this topic (Conrad & Kern, 1990; Loustaunau & Sobo, 1997).

Nurses, physicians, social workers, chaplains, and others familiar with the common signs of patients in crisis can do much to relieve unnecessary stress and harmful outcomes of the illness and hospital experience. The patient in crisis needs an opportunity to

- Express the feelings related to his or her condition
- Gain an understanding of the illness, what it means in terms of one's values, what limitations it imposes, and what to expect in the future
- Have the staff understand his or her behavior, how it relates to feelings and perceptions of the illness, and how the behavior is related to the attitudes and behavior of the primary care provider or the entire hospital staff

---

CASE EXAMPLE: MICHAEL AND MARIA FRENCH

Michael French, age fifty-five, had suffered from prostate cancer for several years. During the past year, he was forced to retire from his supervisory job in a factory. The cancer spread to his bladder and colon, causing continuous pain as well as urinary-control problems. Michael became very depressed and highly dependent on his wife, Maria, age fifty-one. Stress for both of them increased. Michael began to suspect Maria of infidelity.

Maria was scheduled to go to the hospital for a hysterectomy for fibroids of the uterus but repeatedly cancelled the surgery. Her husband always protested her leaving, and at the last minute, she would cancel. Finally, her doctor pressed her to go through with the operation. Because Maria did not look sick to Michael, he felt she was abandoning him unnecessarily. Along with the ordinary fears of anyone facing a major operation, Maria was very worried about her husband's condition when she went to the hospital. However, she was too embarrassed by Michael's accusations of infidelity to discuss her fears with the nurses or with her doctor.

After going to the hospital, Maria received a message from her friend that her husband was threatening to kill her when she came home. He had dismissed their tenants without notice and changed the locks on the doors. The friend, who was afraid of Michael in this state, also called a local community health nurse who, in turn, called a nearby crisis clinic. The nurse had been making biweekly visits to supervise Michael's medication.

Crisis intervention took the following form:

1. The crisis counselor called Maria in the hospital to talk about her concerns and to determine whether Michael had any history of violence or whether guns were available. Michael's accusations of infidelity—which, according to Maria, were unfounded—may have been related to his concern about his forced dependency and to feelings of inadequacy, as he had cancer of the sex gland.

2. The crisis counselor called Michael and let him know that the counselor, Maria, and the neighbors were all concerned about him. Michael accepted an appointment for a home visit by the counselor within the next few hours. He expressed his fears that people were trying to take advantage of him during his wife's absence. This was his stated reason for dismissing the tenants and changing the locks. Further exploration revealed that he felt inadequate to handle household matters and the tenants' everyday requests, which Maria usually managed (Maxwell, 1982).

3. Michael agreed to the counselor's recommendation for a medical-psychiatric-neurological evaluation to determine whether his cancer might have spread to his brain. The counselor explained that brain tumors can contribute to acute emotional upsets or paranoid ideation such as Michael was experiencing.

4. As Michael had no independent means of visiting Maria in the hospital, the counselor arranged for such a visit. The counselor also scheduled a joint counseling session between Michael and Maria after they had had a chance to visit. This session revealed that Michael and Maria each had serious concerns about the welfare of the other. In their two telephone conversations during Maria's stay in the hospital, Michael and Maria had been unable to express their fears and concern. The joint counseling session was the highlight in successful resolution of their crisis. Michael's threat to kill Maria was a once-in-a-lifetime occurrence, triggered by his unexpressed anger at her for leaving him and for the troubles he had experienced during her absence.

5. When Maria returned from the hospital, a joint session was held at the Frenches' home, which included the two of them, the community health nurse, and the friend who had made the original calls (see the "Social Network" sections in Chapter Five). This conference had several positive results: (a) it calmed the

neighbor's fears for Michael; (b) it broadened everyone's understanding of the reactions people can have to the stress of illness and hospitalizations; (c) the community health nurse agreed to enlist further home health services to relieve Maria's increasingly demanding role of nurse to her husband (Halldorsdottir & Hamrin, 1997); and finally, (d) Michael and Maria agreed to several additional counseling sessions to explore ways in which Michael's excessive dependency on his wife could be reduced. Michael and Maria had never discussed openly the feelings they both had about Michael's progressive cancer (Pruchno & Potashnik, 1989). In future sessions, the Frenches dealt with ways they could resume social contacts with their children and friends, whom they had cut off almost completely.

Preventive Intervention

This case history reveals at least three earlier points at which crisis intervention should have been available to the Frenches:

1. At the time Michael received his diagnosis of cancer
2. When Michael was forced to retire
3. Each time Maria delayed her operation, as well as at the point of Maria's hospitalization

In each of these instances, nurses and physicians were in key positions to help the Frenches through the hazardous events of Michael's illness and Maria's operation. Sessions with the crisis counselor confirmed the fact that the Frenches, like many other people facing illness, received little or no attention regarding the fears and social ramifications of their illnesses and hospitalization.

When Maria expressed to the community nurse her original concern about Michael's early retirement, the nurse might have extended her ten-minute visits to a half hour, thus allowing time for Maria to express her concerns. For example, the nurse might have said, "Maria, you seem really concerned about your husband being home all the time. Can we talk about what's bothering you?" Or the nurse might have made a mental health referral after observing Michael's increasing depression.

The gynecologist attending to Maria's health problems might have explored the reason for her repeated cancellations of the scheduled surgery, saying, "Mrs. French, you've cancelled the surgery appointment three times now. There must be some serious reason for this, as you know that the operation is necessary. Let's talk about what's at the bottom of this." Such a conversation might have led to a social service referral.

The nurse attending Maria before her operation, as well as the community health nurse visiting the home, might have picked up on Maria's concerns about the effect of her absence on Michael. Such a response requires listening skills and awareness of psychological cues given by people in distress.

The nurse might then explain the hospital resources, such as social services or pastoral care—ways of helping Maria explore the problem further.

CASE EXAMPLE: INTERVIEW WITH MARIA

Hospital nurse: Mrs. French, you've been very quiet, and you seem tense. You said before that you're not particularly worried about the operation, but I wonder if something else is bothering you.

Maria: Well, I wish my husband were here, but I know he can't be.

Nurse: Can you tell me more about that?

Maria: He's got cancer and isn't supposed to drive. I hated leaving him by himself.

Nurse: How about talking with him by phone?

Maria: I've done that, but all we talk about is the weather and things that don't matter. I'm afraid if I tell him how worried I am about him, he'll think I'm putting him down.

Nurse: Mrs. French, I understand what you're saying. A lot of people feel that way.

But you know there's really no substitute for telling people honestly how we feel, especially those close to us.

Maria: Maybe you're right. I could try but I'd want to be really careful about what I say. There's been a lot of tension between us lately.

Nurse: Why don't you start by letting him know that you wish he could be here with you and that you hope things are OK with him at home. (Pause) You said there's been a lot of tension. Do you have anyone you can talk to about the things that are bothering you?

Maria: No, not really.

Nurse: You must feel pretty alone. You know, we have counseling services here in the hospital that could be very useful for you and your husband. I could put you in touch with someone, if you like.

In this brief interaction about a hazardous event such as surgery, the nurse has (1) helped Maria express her fears openly, (2) conveyed her own understanding of Maria's fears, (3) helped Maria put her fears about not communicating with her husband in a more realistic perspective, (4) offered direct assistance in putting Maria in touch with the person most important to her at this time, and (5) made available the resources for obtaining counseling service if Maria so desires.

This type of intervention should be made available to everyone who has a serious illness or who experiences the traumatic effects of an operation, burns, or an accident. Putting people in touch with self-help groups, as discussed in Chapter Five, is another important means of reducing the hazards of illness and hospitalization. Such groups exist for nearly every kind of illness or operation a person can have: heart disease, leukemia, diabetes, mastectomy, amputation, and others. Many hospitals also hold teaching and discussion groups among patients while they are still in the hospital. This is an excellent forum in which people can air their feelings with others who have similar problems, gain a better understanding of an illness or operation and how it will affect their lives, and establish contacts with people who may provide lasting social support in the future.

People with AIDS: Personal, Community, and Global Perspectives

"Working with Ted changed my life. I'll never be the same." [hospice volunteer]

"It's so humiliating [to be so dependent on people]. I think I'll kill myself." [twenty-three-year-old man with Kaposi's sarcoma, dying of AIDS]

"The nurses really want to be here [a hospital AIDS unit in Boston]. Lance [who had no appetite] forced himself to eat one of the chocolate chip cookies I made because, 'You made it just for me.' I almost cried, there was such a bond there." [psychiatric liaison nurse]

"I can't move my legs at night, but if I touch even one person, then maybe it will help them be good to my boy, who lost his mother to this horrible disease." [woman dying of AIDS]

These statements from people with acquired immunodeficiency syndrome (AIDS) and those who help them dramatize the *opportunity* and the *danger* of a crisis that more than any other may symbolize a much larger crisis of the modern world—the persistent and growing inequalities that leave the poor, people of color, and women disproportionately at risk for AIDS. Of all health-related experiences and potential for crisis, HIV-AIDS is one of the most illustrative of intersections between clinical and public health perspectives in crisis care.

The Crisis Paradigm informing this book describes the experience of people in crisis and the process of using the opportunities a crisis provides and avoiding its dangers. Earlier chapters have shown that success in crisis work requires understanding the origins of a particular crisis experience and tailoring intervention strategies to these distinct yet interrelated sources. AIDS is not only a crisis of global proportions. It also typifies life crises as a whole and cuts across the ramifications of crises already discussed: loss, grief, and mourning; suicide by despairing people with AIDS; antigay violence; social network support; family and community crises; status changes in health, residence, and occupation; and finally, life cycle transitions and death.

The traumatic event of being diagnosed with a fatal disease reverses the natural progression of life-span development, forcing the person with AIDS to face death at a life phase when energy, independence, sexuality, and community involvement are at their peak rather than in decline. A person who tests positive for the virus (HIV) that causes AIDS may feel similarly overwhelmed. Add to this the prevalence of AIDS among groups already despised or disadvantaged because of sex-role prejudice and the effects of racism and poverty, and AIDS can be viewed not only as the most tragic epidemic of this century but also as the paradigmatic or typical life crisis—for those suffering from AIDS, for those caring for them, and for the global community. In the United States, prevalence rates are most prominent among gay and bisexual men, blacks, Hispanics, and intravenous drug users. In Africa and Asia, HIV-AIDS is concentrated among heterosexual persons. However, racism and poverty as risk factors cut across populations in wealthy and poor countries. Not only for the individuals confronting AIDS, but for all of us, perhaps no other crisis will present greater danger or opportunity for the human community.

As AIDS progresses into its third decade, rates of new infections continue unabated. Infected persons in the United States, Canada, and Western Europe are living longer, and the death toll from AIDS in these countries has declined dramatically for those treated early (the financially and racially advantaged), and for many of these, infection can be controlled as a chronic disease (Fleming, Wortley, Karon, DeCock, & Janssen, 2000). But in sub-Saharan Africa alone, the death toll exceeds the combined forty million deaths caused by the fourteenth-century bubonic plague and the 1917 flu epidemic, and rates of infection are spreading in Asia, Eastern Europe, and Russia (Thea, Rosen, and Simon, 1999). The bulk of the transmission in these regions is by heterosexual contact, with women bearing the brunt of responsibility for protected sex, stigma attached to infection (including shunning by the community), and care of a couple's children, along with the burden of her own illness (Lloyd, 2000, p. A2). In the countries most affected, a third of all children are orphans, most hospital beds are occupied by AIDS patients, and life expectancy has fallen by a third (Thea et al., 1999).

With no vaccine on the horizon and a widening gap between rich and poor nations, public health officials and activists are focusing on prevention, especially among the disadvantaged groups in which the rates are highest (Auerbach & Coates, 2000). However, even as dire statistics are cited, there appears to be a paradigm shift to the view that AIDS is not primarily a medical-scientific issue but rather an issue of *justice:* factors placing people at risk of chronic immunodeficiency are primarily *social* and *political* (Murphy, 1994). Citing the work of immunologist Root-Berstein (1993), Murphy, a Canadian activist and policy analyst, declares that AIDS itself is not a disease, but a medical construct including a growing list of almost thirty associated diseases. Murphy asserts that as such, it is not an epidemic but a by-product of poverty, malnutrition, and chronic exposure to such diseases as malaria and tuberculosis.

In essence, AIDS is endemic, a view supported in mainstream analysis at international AIDS conferences. The late Jonathan Mann of the International AIDS Center at the Harvard School of Public Health (1993, p. 1379) was prophetic in his statement, which now expresses the dominant analysis of this global crisis: "The central insight gained from over a decade of global work against AIDS is that societal *discrimination* [emphasis added] is fundamentally linked with vulnerability to HIV. The spread of HIV in populations is strongly influenced by an identifiable societal risk factor: the scope, intensity, and nature of discrimination practiced within the particular society. The HIV pandemic flourishes where the individual's capacity to learn and to respond is constrained. Belonging to a discriminated-against, marginalized, or stigmatized group reduces personal capacity to learn and to respond."

Mann stressed that curtailment of AIDS is also in a nation's economic interest (given the cost of caretaking and loss of productive workers), though many now recognize the intrinsic connection between health status and human rights issues. Fortunately, AIDS is now commanding "front burner" attention by the United Nations and health professionals worldwide. So profound is the pandemic of AIDS that even groups upholding traditional sex roles and norms regarding men's sexual conduct are acknowledging the need for fundamental change on combined fronts: (1) individual responsibility in sexual behavior and (2) social, political, and economic measures directed to the global inequalities affecting the poor and women (predominantly people of color), who are most at risk of infection and its sequelae (Fuller, 1996; Lloyd, 2000).

Illustration of the Crisis Paradigm

These perspectives provide support for the overall message that AIDS as a crisis for individuals is intertwined with the sociocultural origins depicted in the Crisis Paradigm informing this book. Let us examine this crisis from the perspective of people with AIDS and those who help them, keeping in mind the link between their personal pain and the underlying social and cultural factors that leave them disempowered and vulnerable. (See standard texts for historical overview and medical and nursing facets, such as Shilts, 1987; Durham & Lashley, 2000; Barth, Pietrzak, & Ramler, 1993; Hughes, Martin, & Franks, 1987; Sande & Volberding, 1995).

CASE EXAMPLE: DANIEL

Daniel is a thirty-eight-year-old bisexual man who has been diagnosed with AIDS for eighteen months and is now living in a hospice managed by the local AIDS Action Committee (AAC). Pneumocystis pneumonia was the occasion for Daniel's several hospitalizations in the past eighteen months. He is down from his usual 185 pounds to 130, has periodic bouts of nausea and diarrhea, and has some neurological involvement that affects his gait. Once a successful health care worker and artist, Daniel lost his human service job because of federal cuts in domestic programs and could not find another. Getting AIDS further reduced his employability. He is now without a paid job, receives Social Security disability payments, and is eligible for food stamps.

Daniel says that he was "cancelled by Medicaid three times for no reason. When

I left the hospital, I had no money, no job, no apartment. I'm still struggling with the VA for the benefits coming to me. If It weren't for AAC, I would have been out on the street. With the trouble I've had getting care, especially an awful case worker, I got a dose of what the elderly and the homeless go through. You know, I say 'forget your cure.' What would I ever want to come back [from death] for? Homelessness? Poverty? I have no regrets. I used to be seen as a pillar of strength, then people saw me as sick and no longer there for them, but slowly they're coming back. So I don't have a regular job anymore, but now I'm a teacher and counselor [helping other people with AIDS], and I work three hours volunteering at a local men's shelter. I also do liaison work at the hospital where I was a patient. Yes, I get weak, but now I do what I can when I can and as much as I can. There's not the same pressure as before. As long as I don't set expectations, there's no disappointment."

CASE EXAMPLE: SOPHIA

Sophia, age thirty, has a four-year-old son whom she placed with relatives as an infant because she could not care for him properly as long as she was addicted to drugs. Although she had symptoms for about four years, Sophia was diagnosed with AIDS only two years ago. She suffers from night sweats, thrush, shingles, chronic fatigue, abscesses, a platelet disorder, and central nervous system involvement, including seizures and memory loss. Through her twelve years of addiction, Sophia worked as a waitress and a prostitute to support her drug habit. "It's hard to realize that all the things I dreamed about if I was drug free can't be now because of AIDS. I thought having a baby would help me get my act together. I was wrong, but I would never hurt my son. I don't take pride in too many things I've done, but I spared Mickey by putting him in a stable environment. I'm not sorry I had Mickey because he's what keeps me going now. If it weren't for him, I probably would have killed myself already. I'm not through doing what has to be done—helping other drug users and letting my son know me better. And I do a lot of talks for doctors and nurses about AIDS.

Mickey and I spend every weekend together. I'm making some videos for him, so he will remember who I was and how much I love him. He knows to say no to drugs. Behind every addict, you know, there is a child, a lover. It's people's responsibility to set aside their biases, to take care. I have my problems, but at least I can care for someone else's pain, maybe because I've been close to pain. Some say they should lock up prostitutes, but don't tell me it's my fault that a man rides around in his Mercedes-Benz looking for sex instead of being faithful to his wife. I have wonderful friends. When the memory problems get worse, I'll give one of them power of attorney because my family judges me very harshly—for my addiction, prostitution, and now AIDS, plus I'm a lesbian—and if I left it to them, they would put out all the people who care about me when I'm dying. None of my family come to see me when I'm in the hospital. It's sad. I've spent half my life finding myself, and now I'm going to die, but I have an opportunity to plan my time and get closure, and that's good."

Daniel and Sophia are at peace; indeed, talking and being with them is an inspiration.[1] Both are doing meaningful work. At his young age, Daniel feels he has accomplished much of his life's work, though he still wants to write his memoirs. Daniel does not seem to be afraid of death. When asked if he would commit suicide if his symptoms included a new crisis point, dementia, he said "No. It could be tough, though, because I've always been very independent and self-sufficient. I had to fight like hell to get what I have now, but if it came to the point where I needed more care and they don't respond, well, I'm going anyway." As Daniel's neurological symptoms progressed, his struggle to remain at peace intensified. He also was stressed by the fact that some of his friends could not face the reality of his approaching death, but instead of expressing their pain and impending loss, they either avoided him or made fleeting visits, stating they "didn't have time" to talk. Daniel's occasional angry outbursts toward his friends may also be displacements of the anger he feels about dying, but that is difficult to express because it implies a contradiction to his "caretaker" and "nice guy" image of self. Sophia readily expresses her sadness and pain but says her work is not done yet, so she keeps going and no longer feels like killing herself.

How did Daniel and Sophia arrive at the peace and acceptance they experience in spite of constant physical pain and the knowledge that they are dying? By what process did Daniel win his "fight like hell" to get where he is? How did Sophia come to manage her ultimate life crisis in a constructive manner and finally give up her addiction to drugs? The Crisis Paradigm illustrates the process of dealing with the crisis of AIDS and how people with AIDS can capitalize on the opportunity of this tragic unanticipated event to arrive at positive resolution and avoid the danger inherent in crisis. The following discussion elaborates on the paradigm, using the AIDS crisis experience and illustrations from the lives of Sophia and Daniel. It shows what people with AIDS have in common with others, such as victims of violence or man-made disaster, whose crises originate primarily from the sociocultural milieu.

Crisis Origins. Although AIDS was initially viewed as a "gay" disease, people now generally recognize that HIV makes no distinction based on race, class, sex, age, religion, or sexual identity. For those it strikes, a diagnosis of AIDS is an unanticipated, traumatic event of overwhelming proportions. With the growing belief that more than half of HIV carriers will eventually develop AIDS unless new treatments are found, we may only have seen the tip of the iceberg, particularly if the endemic conditions of poverty, malnutrition, and widening disparities between rich and poor nations are not alleviated. Individuals, of course, can modify behaviors such as drug use or unprotected sex that place them at greater risk, especially if a person's cultural heritage is considered in prevention programs

---

[1]Daniel and Sophia are now dead, but they live on because in spirit they are everyman and everywoman.

(Bayer, 1994; Haygood, 1999; Neufeld, 1999; Singer, 1992; Watson, 2000). However, as in the case of other epidemics, history reveals that *public health* measures—not medicines—have had the greatest impact in saving and lengthening lives. Thus, even among groups in the wealthy United States, in the so-called outerclass, education in risk reduction behaviors must be combined with economic and other change; in other words, the intertwined origins of the problem must be addressed simultaneously.

Given the lack of a vaccine or cure for AIDS, only a few years ago, death was the almost certain prediction, and it still is for those uninsured or too poor to afford the expensive treatment and support services for living with AIDS—an increasingly reasonable option for people in wealthy countries. Progress in the United States and Canada with civil rights of the gay community has also alleviated the additional stress affecting sexual minority individuals who are not "out" or whose communities are unfriendly or openly hostile toward such groups. Figure 11.1, Box 1, depicts the intersecting origins of crisis for people with HIV-AIDS, which may apply to the diagnosis of any serious illness in which such factors as stigma (for example STDs) or sociocultural disadvantage play a key role.

Once a person is diagnosed as having AIDS, other events often follow: loss of job, home, friends, and sometimes family. But these losses are closely tied to sociocultural factors and differ from losses such as temporary homelessness due to a fire or the unexpected death of a loved one from an illness that is not stigmatized (Sontag, 1978). Certainly, individual behaviors are part of the picture, but attention to those outside of family and cultural context will have limited success (Bayer, 1994). And the more socially disadvantaged the people targeted for prevention are, the less chance there is for individualistic approaches to be applied successfully (Mann, 1993).

Personal Crisis Manifestations. The person afflicted with AIDS will experience most of the common emotional responses to a traumatic life event. Anger springs not simply from being stricken by the ultimate misfortune of facing an untimely death but also from unfair or violent treatment by a society with limited tolerance for anyone who is different or is perceived as receiving deserved punishment for a deviant lifestyle. Besides feeling angry, persons who get AIDS through a blood transfusion may feel self-righteous as they compare their misfortune with those they perceive as afflicted because of their own behavior. Anxiety is felt not only for one's own health and welfare but also for one's lover or previous partners whom one may have infected. *Survivor guilt,* as noted for Holocaust survivors in Chapter Ten, may also surface for those who have lost partners and loved ones to AIDS. Some may also feel guilt or shame over their gay lifestyle, having incorporated societal homophobia (Blumenfeld, 1992). Sophia says, for example, "I can't take pride in too many things I've done," but she does not wallow in guilt, nor is she ashamed of being a lesbian even though her family condemns her for it.

Denial of the medical facts and the need for behavioral change, especially if accompanied by free-floating anger at being infected, may result in irresponsible

FIGURE 11.1.   CRISIS PARADIGM.

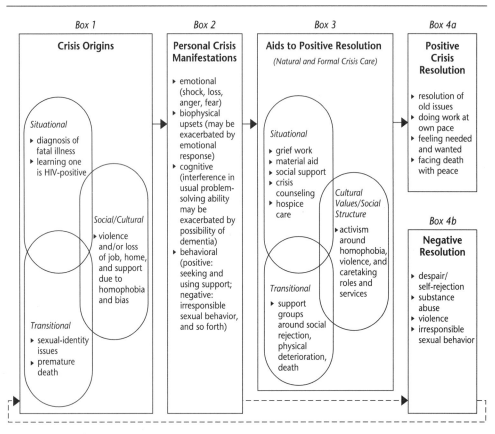

Crisis origins, manifestations, and outcomes and the respective functions of crisis care have an interactional relationship. The intertwined circles represent the distinct yet interrelated origins of crisis and aids to positive resolution, even though personal manifestations are often similar. The arrows pointing from origins to positive resolution illustrate the *opportunity for growth and development* through crisis; the broken line at bottom depicts the potential *danger of crisis* in the absence of appropriate aids. The loop between Box 4b and Box 1 denotes the *vulnerability* to future crisis episodes following negative resolution.

sexual behavior and the risk of infecting others. But in some cases, people are not even informed of the facts. When Sophia was told she had AIDS (after being tested without her consent), no one told her about cleaning her needles with bleach or practicing safer sex. She regrets that she may have infected others, but if she did, it was out of ignorance, not malice. In general, the most ethical approach is to inform a sex partner of one's infection status. Crisis counseling and support are clearly indicated for infected persons who act out their anger by placing others at risk. Sexual decision making is a complex process often not amenable to a simplistic, "just say no" approach. Sadness over loss of health and impending death is compounded by fear of losing friends or lovers and the necessary support to face early death.

Anxiety's usual interference in cognitive functioning during crisis may be exacerbated with AIDS because of the fear of dementia. For example, normal forgetting may be interpreted as a first sign. AIDS Dementia Complex may sometimes be the only sign of AIDS. Sophia is clearly planning for this possibility by arranging for a friend to act with power of attorney on her behalf. In the case of Charlie, another person dying with AIDS, flashes of awareness and clarity pierced his general comatose state, so that he could convey his wish not to be kept alive with heroic measures.

In general, the emotional and biophysical stress responses common during any life crisis are exaggerated here because of sociocultural facets of the crisis that are usually beyond the control of an individual to manage alone. In addition, the physical toll that the disease exacts usually includes drastic energy reduction, which in turn increases stress because of inability to engage in physical stress reduction activities. Table 11.1 summarizes effective and ineffective coping with AIDS and forms the foundation for planning crisis care strategies with the affected person and his or her family, lover, and other network members.

Aids to Positive Crisis Resolution. In spite of Daniel's spirit of independence, he recognized his need for support and accepted it. He said that the hospital nurses were wonderful and that friends and his overall attitude helped the most. Daniel also said that he was greatly strengthened by helping his friends face death, an experience common among many people with cancer. One buddy of Daniel's with Boston's AAC said, "Sometimes I feel guilty because it seems like I get more than I give." He also said of standing by a man dying of AIDS, "I've never been so compelled by anything in my whole life. What a gift it was to be able to be with him. Nothing I've done since has been as honest."

What about Sophia? Precisely what did she have or receive that assisted her along the path of constructive coping with AIDS? Sophia tells of being hospitalized for abscesses, violating hospital rules by shooting up drugs on the ward, and leaving the hospital only to collapse shortly afterward. She knew that without treatment she would probably die, but having a drug fix at the time seemed more important. Later she checked back into the hospital and was confronted by the head nurse, who said, "You ruined my day. I can help you, but here are the rules. Are you willing to keep them?" Sophia said, "You know, that nurse did me a real favor. She was furious with me and I don't blame her, but instead of burying her anger, she confronted me and I could tell that she did it because she cared."

These responses highlight the point repeatedly made by people with AIDS and others facing a life-threatening illness: they are not victims and do not want to be treated as victims. For those of us less ready for death than Daniel is, it is important to remember that emotional healing from life's traumatic events requires the individual in crisis to make sense out of the experience and to process it within his or her personal meaning system. For example, when Daniel's immune system became weaker and weaker, he was advised to discontinue volunteer work at the men's shelter to protect himself from further infections. He then replaced

TABLE 11.1.   EFFECTIVE AND INEFFECTIVE CRISIS COPING BY PERSON WITH AIDS AND FAMILY MEMBERS.

Person in Crisis	Personal Crisis Manifestations	Crisis Coping	
		Ineffective	Effective
Person with AIDS	Emotional	Denial of medical facts and probability of death	Grief work
		Repression	Communication of feelings with caring persons
		Depression	
		Hatred of self	
	Biophysical	Additional stress symptoms of emotional origin	Physical symptoms limited to opportunistic infections
			Resistance to additional stress symptoms
	Cognitive	Conviction that one is being punished for lifestyle or sexual orientation	Recognition and acceptance of the reality and horror of the disease and all that it implies
		Failure to accept reality of illness	
	Behavioral	Irresponsible sexual behavior placing others at risk	Safer sex practices
		Violence	Preventive health practices: diet, rest, exercise, relaxation
		Substance abuse	Acceptance of love and necessary assistance
			Preparation for death
Family member of person with AIDS	Emotional	Denial of medical facts	Grief work
		Inappropriate self-blame for child's sexual orientation	Unconditional acceptance regardless of sexual orientation or lifestyle
	Biophysical	Additional stress symptoms of emotional origin	Resistance to additional stress symptoms and burnout through self-care and acceptance of support and respite
		Burnout from failure to care for self	
	Cognitive	Perception of AIDS as a "gay" disease	Recognition and acceptance of medical facts about AIDS
		Clinging to myths about contagion, and so forth	
	Behavioral	Judgment and blaming of person with AIDS	Expression of caring through communication, hugging, and so forth
		Avoidance and withholding of support and love	Material support and assistance with activities of daily living

his on-site volunteering with a monthly monetary donation out of his meager welfare funds.

Similarly, Sophia finds meaning in her suffering and a reason to keep going for the sake of her child as well as for the influence she can have on the drug problem and the help she can give health professionals as they learn about AIDS. Her lifelong proximity to suffering and pain has apparently heightened her sensitivity to the needs and pain of others. Assistance to Daniel, Sophia, and many like them during crisis is available primarily through groups like the AAC in Boston. They provide housing and hospice care as well as neighborhood people who help as needed with mowing the lawn, keeping the sidewalks clear, and tending the garden. With this kind of assistance, Daniel and others in his hospice house are able to live a normal life in the community and face their impending deaths with greater comfort than institutional care would provide. This is the kind of care that should be available everywhere, but it is rare in poor countries where the toll is greatest.

Positive Crisis Resolution. The crisis care strategies that have helped Daniel correspond to the interrelated origins of his crisis in situational, transitional, and sociocultural factors. Together they have led to growth and development; for example, he says that getting AIDS has been the occasion for him to resolve with his ex-wife old issues around his bisexuality. He is no longer rushed and overworked. He feels needed and wanted by the homeless men and others with AIDS and has a healthy circle of friends, including a cadre of mental health professionals who enjoy chatting with him. His adjustment to a healthy interdependence allows him to maintain as much independence as he can, but he does not hesitate to ask for the help he needs. Daniel says that AIDS has forced him to take a "closer, more intense look at life, so now I'm more ready to leave it."

For Sophia, in addition to her educational work with health professionals and the importance of being there for her son as long as possible, she says, "There's a reason for this. I went on the radio and made $53,000 for the AIDS Action Committee. It makes it meaningful. I feel robbed by this disease, but it's an opportunity to plan my time and get closure, and that's good.

Avoiding Negative Crisis Outcomes. For Jesse, one of Daniel's friends with AIDS, things did not go as well, at least temporarily. Jesse had Kaposi's sarcoma. His skin was dying; he was being eaten away. Jesse also had neurological involvement and some beginning symptoms of dementia. He found it humiliating to have people do things for him that he was used to doing for himself. Daniel helped out by putting reminders up around the house to compensate for Jesse's growing mental impairment. One day, Jesse declared to Daniel that he just could not go on any more: "I want to kill myself." Daniel's response was, "Jess, no matter how bad this hits us, let's face it together. I'm in pain, too. You know where I'm at. Let's share it. You're strong. Look at what you've done for others." Jesse did not commit suicide but died in the hospital a few weeks later.

As we examine the interchange between Daniel and Jesse, it is clear that Daniel did not simply talk Jesse out of suicide. First of all, the issue of suicide for people dying of AIDS raises all the ethical issues discussed in Chapter Six. In the case of AIDS, it might be easier for people to favor "rational suicide" than in other crisis situations. Many would argue therefore for the right of people dying with AIDS to commit suicide rather than suffer the horrors of physical and mental deterioration. However, as tragic as AIDS is, Daniel, Sophia, and thousands like them tell us that life can be meaningful and worthwhile in spite of great suffering. If those afflicted with AIDS experience insult added to injury through scorn and violence and then decide to commit suicide, those of us left can well ask whether we have in some sense "manipulated" such suicides (Battin, 1980), even those considered to be rational, through our failure to respond to them with the necessary, nonjudgmental care. If a person with AIDS or another terminal illness requests assistance in committing suicide, the caretaker or friend must not only be familiar with ethical and legal issues regarding suicide but should consider hidden messages as well. One of those messages may be the inability or unwillingness to tolerate chronic severe pain. Most people dying of cancer do not wish to kill themselves, although some individual and couple suicides have occurred. Perhaps the greatest challenge for supporters of people with AIDS is to help create a milieu that will make it unnecessary for them to choose suicide. It is altogether remarkable and inexcusable that some people in excruciating pain in modern medical facilities still do not receive adequate medication and information about nonpharmacological treatment of chronic pain (Bral, 1998; Caudill, 1994; Fishbain, 1996). And in a global human rights perspective, it is morally reprehensible that for the vast majority of people with AIDS, medications are either unavailable or unaffordable, even if health professionals are there to administer them. An appropriate environment and care, either at home or in a hospice house, would underscore the love and caring that helps dying people put their material affairs in order; say good-bye to lovers and family after reconciliation and, it is hoped, healing; and be recognized and valued for their place on this earth and thus be ready for life's final stage.

Women and Children with AIDS

Sophia and Daniel illustrate commonalities among people with AIDS: shock, anger, loss, and mourning a shortened life. But women, whether sick with AIDS or as caretakers, face several special issues. For example, because of cultural messages regarding body image, women may experience greater stress around appearance as they deteriorate physically. Women have the additional stress of worrying about becoming pregnant and possibly transmitting the virus to offspring. Fortunately, having her child infected with the AIDS virus was not one of Sophia's many stressors. Women who are HIV-positive generally are advised not to become pregnant. However, although there is support for a sperm-washing procedure for men who wish to have children, there is no corollary support for women with the same desire. Because of the general inattention to women in research, this pattern of neglect influences AIDS prevention as well, in the limited research on chemical and barrier methods women might use to protect themselves (Stein, 1995). Research and prevention trends have also slighted the fact of women's unequal power at personal, family, and social levels worldwide (Bianco, 1992). Women's continued inequality has major implications for risk not only of contracting AIDS from their male partners demanding sex but also of violence if they urge the use of condoms.

Female prostitutes, perhaps more so than gay men, are scorned by most in society, as Sophia's case amply illustrates. It is therefore easy to scapegoat them for spreading AIDS. In Africa, where AIDS is distributed equally between women and men in the heterosexual population, female prostitutes in particular have been blamed for its transmission, whereas male promiscuity is rarely mentioned. Prostitutes who have AIDS or are HIV-positive already receive discriminatory treatment. Blaming them for AIDS also reveals the double standard regarding prostitution—arresting the women, but rarely their patrons—and the economic disadvantages of women that drive many of them into prostitution in the first place. Similar dynamics operate in regard to the traffic in sex—for example, women who are kidnapped, raped, and sent to places like Japan or Europe and forced into prostitution to service tourists (Barry, 1979). Women like this who get AIDS are in crisis not only because of a fatal illness but primarily because of the worldwide sexual and economic exploitation of women (Bianco, 1992). In other words, their crises around AIDS are primarily of social and cultural origin; essentially, AIDS is a human rights issue calling for structural change (Gollub, 1999).

A problem faced by those prostitutes and many other women who attempt to have safer sex by using condoms is that many men refuse to cooperate. When that happens, a woman is at a disadvantage not only because of inadequate female barrier methods but also because she may be physically abused if she asserts herself—a contemporary version of the traditional responsibility for contraception being borne primarily by women. This issue highlights the additional danger presented by AIDS if people ignore the imperative to change stereotypical sex roles and accept equal responsibility for safer sex.

An additional hazard for women with AIDS is linked to the pregnancy risk. If they are also intravenous drug users (the largest group of U.S. women with AIDS) and fail to prevent pregnancy, their ability to take care of a child will be even more limited because the problems connected with drug use are added to the debilitating effects of AIDS. Sophia's foresight in this area (and access to resources not available to many poor women) moved her to place her child with a stable family when she was unable to overcome her addiction. In addition, a woman whose child has AIDS will probably feel guilty and angry whether she does or does not have AIDS herself. The millions of orphans in AIDS-devastated countries underscore the double burden of illness and caretaking as AIDS affects women.

Lesbian women, although in the lowest-risk group for AIDS, are nevertheless at risk for the same reasons other women are, and the number of lesbians with

AIDS is rising (Hollibaugh, 1994). Sophia, for example, traces her infection to dirty needles to support her drug habit, not to her lesbian status. Lesbian women are affected by the crisis in other ways as well. As significant others for gay men, some lesbians will suffer the loss of friendships through the deaths of these men. They are similarly affected by antigay discrimination and violence, primarily because of inaccurate portrayals by the media and public ignorance about how AIDS is spread. Lesbians are also concerned if they are considering artificial or self-insemination. Finally, lesbians in the United States are among the majority of AIDS caretakers.

The tragedy of AIDS is even more poignant with respect to children. While an adult with AIDS can come to terms with the inevitability of death and work through the crisis, including its implications for previous and future sexual behavior, children with AIDS obviously cannot. This implies an additional challenge for people with AIDS to prevent pregnancy and for caretakers to treat and care for children with AIDS with extraordinary compassion. Attention should also be paid to the disenfranchised parents who brought them into the world.

Similarly poignant and tragic is the fear of HIV infection following rape. Although this double crisis also affects male victims of rape, the majority of rape victims are women. The emotional trauma for such victims is overwhelming, particularly in the face of continuing public attitudes of blaming the crime of rape on its victims and prosecuting very few assailants. If these attitudes prevail, rape victims may continue to blame themselves not only for the rape but also for contracting AIDS; in addition, they must face all that any other person with AIDS confronts in an untimely death.

The Worried Well, Prevention, and HIV Testing

The challenge in this area is to unbundle realistic concern about AIDS from anxiety about various other issues, such as sexual practice or sexual identity. Krieger (1988, pp. 263–264) suggests five steps in a counseling approach to persons with heightened anxiety about AIDS and fears about sexual transmission of AIDS: (1) obtain accurate information, (2) assess fear of prior exposure, (3) learn to protect oneself and others, (4) gather strong peer support, and (5) address related issues, such as homophobia, addictive attachments to dangerous sex, or guilt over sexual or drug use behavior. Everyone working with the worried well and people in high-risk groups for AIDS should be thoroughly familiar with the clues to suicide, risk assessment techniques, and strategies of suicide prevention discussed in Chapters Six and Seven. Of particular note here is the trend among a minority in the U.S. gay community toward laxity in HIV prevention measures since the decline in death rates due to drug therapy. The behavior of the few who intentionally seek HIV infection can best be interpreted as a cry for help not unlike that of the self-destructive persons described in Chapter Six, who lack other ways of communicating their need for attention. In the gay community, the AIDS epidemic galvanized a sense of community and mutual assistance that was rare before the appearance of AIDS.

This leads to consideration of the controversial issue of testing for HIV infection. If testing were more definitive than it is, opinion might be less divided. Testing reveals infection with the virus but not whether a person has AIDS. Because it takes some time for antibodies to form, even if a person were exposed yesterday, tests might be negative today, thus potentially conveying false reassurance. In general, opinion is equally divided between the advantages and disadvantages of testing. Because a positive test can send psychologically unstable people into panic and possible suicide, testing should be carefully considered in each case. Counseling and ongoing support services for those who either are considering testing or have been tested are therefore essential. Such services are available through groups like the AAC and health centers. Self-testing kits are also available now, although their use is controversial because of concern about access to emotional support when receiving results.

Although the issue of testing will probably remain controversial as long as we lack a vaccine and adequate drugs to treat AIDS-related diseases, testing is definitely indicated when pregnancy is being considered for one who has symptoms and a differential diagnosis is needed. In all cases, however, individuals should have a choice about being tested (Galea, Lewis, & Baker, 1988). Those who are psychologically healthy enough to deal with the unknown and who have greater tolerance for ambiguity may choose not to be tested. Conversely, some people embarking on a new relationship may decide jointly to be tested before engaging in sex. The situation is similar to that faced by people at risk for various genetically transmitted diseases.

Caretakers of People with AIDS: Support and Self-Care

We have seen from our examples that Daniel and Sophia have come through the first crises of AIDS to the point of peace and acceptance of eventual death. They managed to do so with a combination of natural and formal crisis care strategies. We have also seen that their personal coping abilities compensated in part for the extra stress they endured because of less than ideal approaches by some health care providers and that they understand and accept those around them who cannot understand.

Others with fewer resources, however, may not come through life's final passage to death with peace, fulfillment, and the comfort of family and friends without extraordinary assistance from various caretakers. Families and lovers in crisis over the impending loss of loved ones and the emotional cost of caring need similar help. In short, providing for others whose needs are very great also demands caring and understanding for the caretakers. In the family network, it is not uncommon for mothers of gay or bisexual men to know about their sons' sexual identity while fathers remain unaware. This results in a large emotional burden for these women that they have not been able to share with their husbands. In hospitals as well, women provide most of the care for the acutely ill and dying; in addition, they face the stress of overwork because of fiscal constraints and health reform measures that leave nurses and low-wage workers vulnerable because of their historical disempowerment within the system (Rachlis & Kushner, 1994). As so often in the past, so now with AIDS, the cost of caring is borne dispropor- tionately by women, regardless of sexual orientation.

In caring for people with AIDS, extraordinary stressors must be dealt with: fear of contagion (though this is decreasing with increased education); danger of needle stick infection for nurses and physicians; stigmatization stemming from association with devalued members of society (Goffman, 1963); confrontation with issues of sexual identity, one's own risk of AIDS, and death; assuming power-of- attorney roles; dealing with suicide issues; and finally, simple overload from asso- ciation with the depths of pain and tragedy surrounding people with AIDS, their families, and lovers. Meisenhelder's study (1994) of 114 randomly selected regis- tered nurses revealed homophobia, fear of the unknown, and lack of emotional involvement as the strongest predictors of their fear of contagion; adequate knowl- edge and extended contact with a person with AIDS were suggested as the most effective interventions for decreasing nurses' fear of contagion. When nurses and other workers are accidentally exposed to possible infection through needle pricks or contact with body fluids, counseling should be readily available, as for any "worried well."

The principle of providing ongoing support for all AIDS crisis workers and family members must be applied in order to prevent burnout, compassion fatigue, and the eventual loss of needed staff (Hoff & Adamowski, 1998). Among fami- lies as well, the ability to care for a dying loved one varies, requiring that pro- fessionals provide what families may not be able to. Caring for an AIDS patient includes the need for a comprehensive system of respite service for families offering care at home, in addition to skilled home nursing assistance. This is par- ticularly important in view of the Centers for Disease Control and Prevention and the World Health Organization projections of future AIDS cases. The chal- lenge of facing great numbers of new cases in the United States and worldwide will probably not be met if the general caretaking issue and national health insurance crisis are not addressed at a societal level. One response to this chal- lenge is the increased employment of nurse practitioners as primary care providers (Aiken et al., 1993).

Groups in the forefront of the AIDS crisis (SHANTI in San Francisco, Gay Men's Health Crisis in New York City, AIDS Action Committee in Boston) have recognized the stressors on caretakers and have provided support groups and staffing arrangements that offer respite from the stress of caring for dying people. Those working with persons with AIDS cite the following factors as most signifi- cant for self-care and the prevention of burnout from the constant giving and confrontation with loss and death:

- Participating in support groups
- Being connected to a community of caring people
- Reading, taking time to smell the roses and watch the sunset

- Calling people "when I need them, when they need me"
- Accepting love on both sides unconditionally
- Realizing there is more to life than material riches

These support and coping strategies apply to both formal and informal care-takers: volunteers, nurses, physicians, family members, friends, lovers, and anyone caring for people with AIDS. As one volunteer says, however, "Caretaking is very painful. Don't go into it if you don't want to grow. By seeing other people's pain, you grow yourself." Fortunately, with public education the attitudes of church representatives and others are changing toward compassion. For example, ecumenical healing services in various churches are becoming common. People who might otherwise despair under the weight of the AIDS crisis are finding new meaning and community support in these ritual gatherings—examples of con-temporary rites of passage (see Figure 11.1, Box 3, lower circle).

Whereas some have the choice of volunteering to work directly with people with AIDS, most families and those in the health and social service professions do not. The global nature of the AIDS crisis and its embeddedness in social disad-vantage mean that practically everyone is affected, at least indirectly, and the enor-mous demands of caretaking require that the burden be shared within the human community. This will probably not happen, however, without learning all we can about AIDS, without attention to caring for ourselves to prevent burnout, and without acceptance of the challenge to grow from humane involvement with the AIDS crisis. Concern about these needs of the caretakers of people with AIDS is expressed in the AAC requirement that volunteers attend support group meetings at least twice a month. As the numbers of people with AIDS increase, necessary care must increasingly be absorbed by mainstream health and social services and not be left primarily to alternative agencies such as the AAC. Similarly, sup-port services for caretakers should become a routine part of the total service program if we are to meet the challenge of providing all the care demanded by this ongoing crisis.

One mark of a humane and civilized society is its ability to care for the sick, the "different," and the suffering and dying in a compassionate manner. There is evidence of a paradigm shift that Bianco (1992, p. 61) suggested in her address to the international AIDS conference: "Despite repeated calls and protests by women all over the world, despite international conferences and the United Nations Convention on Elimination of All Forms of Discrimination Against Women, inequality is still ignored when political and social decisions are made. Will AIDS be the detonator needed to end this inequality?"

And Jonathan Mann's visionary statement (1993, p. 1379) seems to have inspired the approach many now accept as the most promising: "We are all Berliners—because to the extent that societies can reduce discrimination, they will be able to uproot the HIV/AIDS pandemic, rather than addressing only its surface features. . . . The world needs—and is now ready for—a far-reaching transfor-mation of our approach to the global epidemic of AIDS."

Rarely has the world community had such an opportunity through the paradigmatic crisis of AIDS to mobilize together, combine efforts, and reconsider policies and the distribution of national and international resources. Yes, there is danger of compassion fatigue in the face of this crisis. But aside from the horrors of this crisis, AIDS can be viewed as a catalyst to address issues that we might otherwise continue to ignore, such as universal health care, widening inequality between rich and poor nations, the caretaking crisis, and advocacy of equal rights for all (see Farmer, 1999). As the AIDS crisis unfolds into the next millennium for the individuals and families affected around the world, our attempts to understand people with AIDS and communicate compassionately with them and their families can increase the opportunities for personal and community growth and forestall such dangers as suicide, violence, bigotry, and the creation of scapegoats for societal problems and global inequalities.

Crisis Intervention in Mental Institutions, Transitional Housing, and Hostels

As noted in Chapters Two and Three, admission to a psychiatric facility is often a sign that crises have not been constructively resolved at various points along the way. Whenever possible, crisis hostels and other alternatives to psychiatric hospitalization should be used if a person cannot be helped in the home environment (Polak, 1976). Although mental hospitals are intended to relieve acute breakdowns or stress situations, they, like general hospitals, can create another kind of crisis.

CASE EXAMPLE: ANGELA

Angela, age eighteen, highly suicidal, upset, and dependent on her family, was admitted to the psychiatric service of a private hospital on the advice of a psychiatrist whom the mother had called a few hours earlier. Angela and her mother arrived at the hospital at 3:00 P.M. The admitting nurse stayed with them until 3:30 P.M., when she was scheduled to go off duty. Angela was just beginning to calm down but became very upset again when the nurse left. The nurses were unable to reach the physician to obtain an order for tranquilizing medication. Visiting hours ended meanwhile, and Angela's mother was asked to leave. At this point, Angela became even more upset. The nurse on the evening shift was unable to quiet or console her. By the time an order for tranquilizing medication arrived, Angela's behavior had become uncontrollable, and she was placed in a high-security room, as she became more suicidal. During the process of administering the medication, Angela screamed that she wanted to see her mother. After being told her mother was no longer in the unit, she became more upset; Angela struck and injured the attending nurse and was then placed in four-point restraints.

In this case, the rules and regulations of the hospital and the absence of an efficient call system to obtain doctor's orders for emergency medication clearly contributed to Angela's crisis state, which reached the point of panic. Richardson's study (1987) of inpatients' perceptions of the seclusion-room experience revealed that in 58 percent of the cases, patients experienced negative interaction with the staff before being secluded; 50 percent said that seclusion protected them; 58 percent perceived seclusion as a form of punishment, and 50 percent said that a different approach would have averted the need for seclusion.

In general, the same principles of crisis intervention discussed in earlier chapters apply in mental institutions and residential settings. The worker should (1) help people express their feelings, (2) help them understand their situation and develop new ways of problem solving, and (3) help them reestablish themselves with family and community resources. The staff in residential facilities should examine their programs and routines to determine whether people become even more upset than they were originally as a result of the rules, thus defeating the purpose of the residential program (Hoff, 2000; Kavanagh, 1988).

For example, most psychiatric facilities routinely search patients on admission for dangerous articles, contraband, and anything that might be used as a weapon. Considering the number of dangerous people now admitted to psychiatric centers instead of prisons and the frequency of attacks on staff (see Chapter Nine), such searches seem reasonable. They should not, however, be done without a full explanation to the patient as to the reasons. A person's psychotic condition does not preclude the prospect of experiencing culture shock or eliminate the need for respect and personal integrity, including for those committed involuntarily to a mental institution (Farberow, 1981).

The constraints of managed care, including sometimes the excessive use of chemical restraint as a substitute for longer psychotherapeutic approaches not covered by insurance, may account for the increased rates of violent outburst by psychiatric patients. Such system-produced crisis episodes are compounded if staff use rigid authoritarian approaches—in essence, engage in power struggles with persons already disempowered and vulnerable instead of skilled crisis prevention strategies that are primarily interpersonal. Once health care or other human service workers become enculturated into the minisocieties of bureaucratic agencies, they can easily forget that others may experience culture shock when entering them—not unlike the shock an anthropologist or tourist may feel when entering a foreign country.

Physical and Mental Handicap

Becoming a parent can be a crisis, even if everything occurs as expected. The birth of a handicapped child, however, presents a serious threat to the parents' image of themselves as successful parents. Frequently, the parent asks, "What did I do wrong?

What have I done to deserve this?" Parents conclude mistakenly that something they did or failed to do is responsible for their child's handicapped condition.

Because of the strength of the parent-child bond, the child's physical or mental handicap is, in a sense, the parent's handicap as well (Childs, 1985). The intergenerational and family aspects of handicap suggest that initial and successive crisis points related to birth and the continued care of a handicapped person extend well beyond childhood. The degree of handicap and the level of parental expectation of a normal child are key factors influencing the likelihood of crisis for concerned parents. Handicaps vary greatly. Down syndrome is a mental deficiency with distinctive physical signs: slanting, deep-set eyes that are close together and often crossed; flattened nose; loose muscles; thick, stubby hands; and short stature. Hydrocephalus is characterized by an enlarged head containing excessive fluid. In addition to Down syndrome and hydrocephalus, the range of handicaps varies from gross deformity to minor physical deformity, to developmental disabilities that surface later, such as a learning disability or hypothyroidism.

Initial Crisis Point

In many cases, birth defects are obvious immediately after birth. Sometimes, however, the handicap is not noticed until the child is obviously lagging in normal development. Whenever the handicap becomes known to the parents, the usual response includes anger, disbelief, a sense of failure, numbness, fear for the child's welfare, guilt, and an acute sense of loss—loss of a normal child, loss of a sense of success as parents. The parents' initial reactions of disbelief and denial are sometimes compounded unnecessarily by medical personnel who withhold the truth from them. Seventy to 80 percent of developmentally disabled children also have physical disabilities, but parents should not be encouraged to believe that when these physical conditions are remedied, the mental condition will be cured as well.

CASE EXAMPLE: ANNA

Edgar and Jean took their six-year-old girl, Anna, for kindergarten evaluation. They were told bluntly that she required special education. They were shocked by the news. No psychological or social services had been made available to these parents. Edgar and Jean had tried to ignore their daughter's obvious differences and had not questioned their physician, who was noncommittal. Finally, the grandparents and a sister convinced them to seek guidance from the local Association for Retarded Children.

A child's physical or mental handicap can be a source of crisis for a parent even before the child is born. When medical tests reveal a fetal handicap, parents face the decision of whether or not to abort the fetus. An infant born with devastating brain damage can now be kept alive through advanced medical technology. Like the spouse and children of an elderly parent who is dying, parents of a handicapped infant are caught in the middle of passionate public debates on life-and-death issues such as whether it is morally justifiable to sustain physical life by extraordinary means when brain death is certain (Lynn & Childress, 1991; Solomon et al., 1993). Parents of unborn children who are certain to die now face another moral dilemma—whether to carry the infant to term in order to donate healthy organs to other infants. Sensitive health care workers will make themselves available to parents who need to work through these dilemmas.

Successive Crisis Points

Parents of children who are developmentally disabled or otherwise handicapped can experience crisis at many different times, the most common of which are

- When the child is born
- When the child enters school and does not succeed in a normal classroom
- When the child develops behavior problems peculiar to the handicap
- When the child is ridiculed or sexually abused
- When the child becomes an adult and requires the same care as a child
- When the child becomes an intolerable burden and parents lack the resources to care for him or her
- When it is necessary to institutionalize the child
- When institutionalization is indicated and parents cannot go through with it out of misplaced guilt and a sense of total responsibility
- When the child is rejected by society and parents are reminded once again of their failure to perform as expected
- When parents decide on home-based care instead of the publicly funded institutional care that their child was entitled to, only to discover they are now ineligible for such funds as they plan for the continued care of their adult child after their own deaths

The classic signs of crisis are easily identified in most parents of handicapped children.

1. *Feelings.* They deny their feelings and may displace their anger onto doctors, nurses, or each other. They feel helpless about what to do. Essentially, they feel they have lost a child as well as their role as successful parents.
2. *Thoughts.* Expectations for the child are often distorted. The parents' problem-solving ability is weakened; they lack a realistic perception of themselves as parents and sometimes expect the impossible. In short, they deny reality.
3. *Behavior.* Sometimes parental denial takes the form of refusing help. Sometimes help is not readily available, or parents are unable to seek out and use available help without active intervention from others.

The following case illustrates these signs of crisis and the manner in which a maternal health nurse successfully intervened.

CASE EXAMPLE: MONA ANDERSON

Mona Anderson, age thirty-one, had been married for ten years when she finally became pregnant after many years of wanting a child. Her baby girl was born with Down syndrome. When Mona was tactfully informed of this by the physician and nurse in the presence of her husband, she became hysterical. Initially, she refused to look at the baby. Whenever the nurse attempted to talk with her about the baby's condition, she denied that she could give birth to a "defective child." The nurse allowed her this period of denial but gradually and consistently informed her of the reality of her child's condition. During this time, Mona's husband was also very supportive. Neither he nor the nurse insisted that Mona see the baby before she was ready.

When she felt ready and the nurse brought the baby in, Mona broke down, crying, "All I wanted was a normal baby. I didn't expect a genius." Mona continued to grieve over her loss of a normal child. Gradually, she was able to talk with the nurse about her hopes for her child, her sense of loss, and what she could and could not expect of her baby girl. Although the nurse could not answer all of Mona's or her husband's questions, she referred them to a children's institute for genetic counseling. They were also given the name and number of a self-help group of parents of children with Down syndrome.

The nurse was also helpful to other members of Mona's family who were drawn into the crisis. Mona's sister had had a baby two months previously. She concluded, wrongly, that she could not come to visit Mona with her normal baby because such a visit would only remind Mona again of her "abnormal" baby. The nurse counseled the family members against staying away, as it would only support Mona's denial of the reality of her child's condition.

The nurse, in the course of her usual work in a maternity ward, practiced successful crisis intervention by supporting Mona through her denial and mourning periods, offering factual information about the reality of Down syndrome, and actively linking Mona to her family as well as to outside resources that could continue to help in the future. Because hospital stays after delivery now average only twenty-four to forty-eight hours, a visiting nurse would also be a key figure in a situation like Mona's. An important source of continued help for these families is the availability of respite care (Ptacek, 1982). Other crises associated with birth and parenthood are discussed in Chapter Thirteen.

Besides crises around parenting a handicapped child, any person, child or adult, with a handicap is more vulnerable than others to additional stressors, trauma, and potential crises. For example, physical limitations may prevent one from protecting oneself in cases of domestic dispute, rape, or robbery; lack of access to public transportation and buildings affects one's mobility, financial security, and other requisites for a healthy self-image. Another vulnerability of people with mental handicaps is that their grief following the loss of a loved one often goes unnoticed. Luchterhand and Murphy (1998) offer guidelines for families and service providers to assist this special population through the grieving process. The alienation and feelings of powerlessness associated with such stressors can also lead to unhealthy coping, such as excessive drinking (Seeman & Seeman, 1992). Recent federal legislation in the United States has facilitated addressing some of these issues that affect the health, crisis vulnerability, and general welfare of people with disabilities.

Substance Abuse and Other Chronic Health Problems

The abuse of alcohol, other drugs, or food is not a crisis in itself. A common view of these problems is that they are diseases; another view is that they are possible negative outcomes of crisis that leave one with greater vulnerability to future crisis episodes. In either case, the person who abuses substances is engaging in a chronic form of self-destructive behavior (see Chapter Six). The abuse of food by excess eating is sometimes accompanied by bulimia, compulsive gorging followed by self-induced vomiting to avoid weight gain. This is related to excess dieting, which may result in anorexia nervosa, a life-threatening condition of severe weight loss. Because eating disorders are most common among young women, they are increasingly linked to female identity issues and the pressure on young women to conform to cultural images of women's roles and body size (Chernin, 1985). Crises arising from these chronic problems can bring about lasting change in the tendency to abuse food. It can be assumed that when people were in crisis at earlier points in their lives, they lacked the social support and personal strength to resolve the crisis in a more constructive manner. People abusing food, drugs, and alcohol commonly avoid getting help for their problem until another crisis occurs as a result of the addiction itself. Frequently, a crisis takes the form of a family fight, eviction from an apartment, loss of a job, or trouble with the law. Depending on the attitude and skill of helpers at such times, later crises can be the occasion of a turning point.

CASE EXAMPLE: ANITA

Anita was abused physically and verbally by her husband for years. Her way of coping with the abuse was by overeating to the point of gaining over a hundred pounds. When her husband threatened her life, she finally left the violent marriage and sought refuge in a shelter for abused women. This crisis was a turning point, leading Anita to seek help for her compulsive overeating in Overeaters Anonymous, a peer support group similar to Alcoholics Anonymous.

Chronic Self-Destructive Behavior and Crisis Intervention

The opportunity to change a self-destructive lifestyle is often missed. This is due in part to the lack of appropriate long-term treatment facilities and in part to the negative attitudes some hospital and clinic staff hold toward self-destructive people. Careful application of crisis intervention techniques can greatly reduce the sense of defeat experienced by client and staff alike. Crisis principles that apply especially to the person dependent on alcohol or other drugs include the following:

1. Crisis represents a turning point—in this case, a turning away from drugs or food as a means of coping with stress. For example, intravenous drug users are at high risk for AIDS and therefore are offered clean needles, in a nonjudgmental manner, to reduce the risk of transmitting HIV. Users might reach a turning point in their lives through this constructive interaction with health and social service workers.

2. In crisis intervention, we avoid doing things *for* rather than *with* people. Proposed solutions to problems are mutually agreed on by client and staff person. The substance-dependent person will often act helpless and try to get staff to do things for him or her unnecessarily, thus increasing dependency even more. While expressing concern, staff should avoid falling into this rescue trap (see Chapter Four, Figure 4.2, the Victim-Rescuer-Persecutor Triangle).

3. Basic social attachments that have been disrupted must be reinstated or a substitute found to help avoid further crises and more self-destructive behavior. Usually, people who abuse drugs, alcohol, and food are more isolated than most.

4. For all of these reasons, the principles and techniques of social network intervention (see Chapter Five) are particularly helpful in assisting the person in repeated crisis because of chronic underlying problems. Although other approaches often yield little progress, clinicians skilled in network techniques point to impressive results (Garrison, 1974; Hansell, 1976; Polak, 1971).

Failure to observe these points leads to greater dependency of the client and increasing frustration of the staff. These crisis intervention techniques should be practiced in hospitals, transition facilities, primary care offices, and by police and rescue services—wherever the substance-dependent person is in crisis. The use of these techniques would be a first step for many persons toward a life free of these harmful addictions.

CASE EXAMPLE: EMMA JEFFERSON

Emma Jefferson, age forty-two, had been drinking heavily for about fifteen years. When she was thirty-five, her husband divorced her after repeated pleading that she do something about her drinking problem. He also obtained custody of their two children. Emma was sufficiently shocked by this turn of events to give up drinking. She joined AA, remarried at age thirty-seven, and had another child at age thirty-eight. She had hurried into her second marriage, the chief motive being that she wanted another child.

A year later, Emma began drinking again and was threatened with divorce by her second husband. Emma made superficial attempts to stop drinking and began substituting an antianxiety prescription drug when she felt anxious or depressed. Her second husband divorced her six months later. This time, Emma retained custody of her child, though it was a close fight.

Emma took a job, was fired, went on welfare assistance, and began spending a lot of time in bars. On the urging of a friend, Emma finally decided to seek help for her alcohol and tranquilizer dependency. She gave up drinking but continued a heavy use of the antianxiety drug, sometimes taking as many as six a day. Emma was inconsistent in carrying out plans to reorganize her life to include less dependence on drugs and more constructive social outlets.

One day, a neighbor reported to the child protection agency that she believed Emma was neglecting her child and should be investigated. The child protection worker learned that Emma indeed had few social contacts outside the bars and occasionally left her two-year-old child unattended. Emma was allowed to maintain temporary custody of her child with regular home visits by a caseworker to supervise her parenting activity. The threat of loss of her third child was apparently a sufficient crisis to act as a turning point for Emma. The caseworker urged Emma to seek continued help with her problems from her counselor. Emma finally gave up her dependency on drugs, developed a more satisfying social life, and returned to work. She also made plans for another marriage, this time being more selective in her choice of a partner and less desperately dependent on a man for security.

The crisis of losing her children as a result of chronic dependence on alcohol and drugs led Emma to give up her self-destructive lifestyle. Two divorces resulting from her drug dependency were not enough to make her change. In fact, Emma did not seek available counseling on either of these occasions. She said she was ashamed to ask for help and in any case did not think she could afford it. Other people abusing drugs and alcohol seek help and make changes after serious financial or job failures, threats of imprisonment, or brushes with death, such as delirium tremens (DTs)—a sign of advanced alcoholism—bleeding ulcers, liver damage, or near fatal suicide attempts.

Emma's case illustrates the damaging effects of alcoholism on children. According to the National Institute on Alcoholism and Alcohol Abuse, an estimated 26 million American minors living at home have at least one alcoholic parent. Besides the daily stresses and crises experienced by these children, many become alcohol dependent themselves. College students in the United States engage in binge drinking at alarming rates. The increasing availability of crisis services and follow-up treatment programs should result in earlier choices toward growth rather than self-destruction for substance-dependent people. There are also increasing numbers of self-help groups for adult children of alcoholics that can be contacted through local AA branches.

Influence of Societal Attitudes and the Crisis in Psychiatry

The values of a given society naturally affect the use of drugs in that society. In the United States, many attitudes toward drug use are contradictory. For example, a drug such as marijuana is often regarded as dangerous, whereas some consider the excessive use of alcohol to be acceptable. A stable, law-abiding citizen can be censored or convicted for the use of marijuana, but if the same person chose to use alcohol, there would be no legal restrictions.

If alcohol is consumed privately with no damage to others, there are no sanctions against its use, even if excessive. Yet those who use alcohol chronically often suffer eventual liver or brain damage. A legal crisis can occur only for the user of alcohol who excessively indulges in public and then damages other people or their property, as in the case of reckless driving. For the drunken person's innocent victims, however, it is different. U.S. society's implicit support of alcohol abuse is illustrated by the looseness of laws punishing drunken drivers. For the most part, alcoholism has been decriminalized, and the concept of alcoholism as a disease is now widely accepted. However, whether or not alcoholism is a disease, the combination of drinking and driving takes an enormous social toll. The loss and crises of drunk-driving victims and their families are the focus of a concerted effort to stop what has been called a national slaughter on U.S. highways resulting from the abuse of alcohol.

The user of other drugs can experience a crisis simply by the purchase or possession of a substance such as marijuana. In the United States, a few states have changed the drug possession laws in this regard, but the use of drugs other than alcohol is still predominantly a political issue. Little effort is made to distinguish between the *user* and the *abuser* of drugs. Many crises, such as arrest and imprisonment of people using illegal drugs, occur by design of the social system. The most egregious U.S. examples of reactionary, punitive, and racially biased approaches to the problem of illegal drug use are the mandatory minimum sentencing and "three strikes and you're out" laws. With good reason, the majority of federal and state judges and others want to end the counterproductive policy of minimum drug sentencing, in that such sentencing is 7.5 times less effective than drug treatment in reducing cocaine consumption (Donnelly & Chacon, 2000; Dowdy, 1997; Jackson, 1997).

A public health perspective would focus first on prevention through early education, support of families, and collaborative parent-teacher efforts.[2] Unfortunately, the most serious drug abuse problems receive the least attention. The most widespread and dangerous abuse problems today are alcoholism and the overuse or misuse of prescribed drugs, both of which are legal. As physician Nahill (2000, p. C2) states, although drugs may possess lifesaving properties, the duality of nearly all drugs in use today means that "each pill we swallow carries with it certain risks that we downplay or ignore altogether."

[2]The U.S. Department of Health and Human Services, the National PTA, and the Center for Substance Abuse Prevention publish an informative and highly practical resource for parents, grandparents, and other caregivers, *Keeping Youth Drug Free*. Contact state departments of public health, or write the National Clearinghouse for Alcohol and Drug Information, P.O. Box 2345, Rockville, Maryland 20847-2345.

Among the most dramatic examples of adverse consequences are the results of some debatable experimental studies of psychoactive drugs, which prompted the appointment of a presidential commission to study the issue nationally. The questionable research tactics included giving a drug to induce a psychotic episode, withdrawing medications, and obtaining debatable forms of consent. These practices were reported in a four-part investigative journalism piece, "Doing Harm: Research on the Mentally Ill" (Whitaker & Kong, 1998). The report cites the "lure of riches," in that the studies are heavily funded by the pharmaceutical industry. This factor, however, is situated in the larger crisis in American psychiatry, compounded by managed-care preference for psychotropic drug treatment over talking therapies (Luhrmann, 2000).

The story of Ruth illustrates further the complex interplay between chronic problems and acute crises: beatings as a child, feelings of rejection, a troubled marriage, suicide attempts, depression, death of a husband by suicide, and alcohol dependence (see "Stress, Crisis, and Illness" in Chapter Two). It also highlights how crisis intervention (in contrast to something like electric shock "treatment") can be the occasion for a turning point in a chronically troubled life.

CASE EXAMPLE: RUTH

I called the crisis center because I was afraid I'd attempt to take my life again. All my suicide attempts stemmed from feeling rejected, especially by my father. He picked on me and favored my older sister. I couldn't do anything right. Once I stole some money from my mother's purse, so I could buy a gift for my friend (now I think I was trying to buy friendship). My father beat me so that my hands were bleeding; then he made me show my hands to my mother. My mother cried when he beat me, but I guess she was afraid to stop him. When my father was dying, he asked me to forgive him.

I dropped out of school after tenth grade and got a job in a stockroom and later worked as a bookkeeper. I got married when I was nineteen. Our first five years were beautiful. We had three boys. I loved my husband very much and waited on him hand and foot. We bought a home, and he helped finish it. During the second five years, he started changing and got involved with another woman. My family and everyone knew, but I kept denying it.

Then he left for about four months. I made a suicide attempt by turning on all the gas. I didn't really want to die; I just wanted him to stop seeing the other woman and come back to me. He came to pick me up at the hospital, and two weeks later I went over to his girlfriend's house and beat her up. I could have gotten in trouble with the law for that, but she didn't press charges.

After that, we tried to patch things up for about four months, but it didn't work. Then I started seeing other men. We had lots of arguments. I threatened divorce and he threatened to kill himself, but I didn't believe him.

One night, he sat in his car and wouldn't come in to go to bed when I asked him. At 7:00 A.M., my oldest son reported finding dad dead in his car. I thought it was my fault. Even today, I still tend to blame myself. His parents also blamed me. My father was still alive then, and he and my mother stood by me. After my husband's death, I made another suicide attempt. I was in and out of the hospital several times and received a lot of shock treatment. Nothing seemed to help in those days.

Three years after my first husband's death, I remarried. We argued and fought, and again I felt rejected. When I was afraid of taking an overdose of aspirin, I called the crisis center and was referred to the local crisis and counseling center near my home. I can't say enough good things about how my counselor, Jim, helped me. After all those years of being in and out of hospitals, having shock treatments, and

making several suicide attempts, I'm so glad I finally found the help I needed long ago.

I don't think I'd ever attempt suicide again. I still struggle with the problem of feeling rejected, which I think is the worst thing in the world to go through. Even though I feel I'm on the horizon of something much better, I still have my down days and have to watch that I don't drink too much. But I don't think I'd ever let myself get as down and out as I've been in the past. I've seen that real help is available when I need it.

Rescue Workers, Nurses, Physicians, and Social Workers in Acute-Care Settings

Crisis situations demanding response are as diverse as the people experiencing them. Health practitioners have numerous opportunities to assist people in crisis because of threats to health, life, and self-image from illness, accidents, and related problems. All human service workers have a responsibility to assist people in crisis, but health care personnel in emergency and acute-care settings are in a particularly strategic position to influence the outcome of high-risk crisis situations. The nature of emergency and acute-care settings, with a focus on lifesaving procedures, precludes the opportunity to assist a person to complete resolution of an emotional crisis originating from threats to health and life. If life is at stake, no one would place the expression of feelings, however intense these may be, before lifesaving measures.

Yet because of the tense atmosphere of emergency medical scenes, it is important to remember that emotional needs do not disappear when physical needs take on life-and-death importance. Both physical and emotional needs must be met. An appropriate attitude and a sensitivity to the emotional needs of victims and survivors must accompany necessary lifesaving procedures, and a team approach accomplishes this best; the strain on nurses, physicians, and emergency medical technicians would be enormous without teamwork. Staff burnout in these settings is often very high in any case, and the lack of teamwork and staff support, the inappropriate placement of personnel in high-risk work, or the lack of training in crisis intervention frequently contribute to such burnout (Fullerton, McCarroll, Ursano, & Wright, 1992; Hoff & Adamowski, 1998; McCarroll, Ursano, Wright, & Fullerton, 1993). Not everyone is suited for crisis work, but those who are should not suffer burnout or develop callous attitudes toward people in life-threatening situations. Acute-care nurses, for example, need the time and opportunity to air their feelings about the person who is comatose for days from a drug overdose. When the patient comes through the critical stage and survival seems certain, many nurses find it difficult to communicate empathetically with such a person.

In cases of cardiac arrest at hospitals, teamwork combines emergency medical work with crisis intervention. Nurses have observed that the emergency code system is so effective that it often brings more staff to the scene than are needed; however, provision is not always made for attending to the emotional needs of anxious family members (Davidhizar & Kirk, 1993). In one hospital, the psychiatric nurses—"surplus" personnel—routinely designate themselves to attend to family members who may otherwise be ignored. Nurses and physicians can be routinely trained to assist in emotional crises as well as medical emergencies (Adamowski et al., 1993; Bertman, 1991).

In general, health care practitioners in primary care, emergency, and acute-care settings need to focus on five key aspects of the crisis care process (discussed in detail in Chapters Three, Six, Eight, and Nine):

1. Identification of persons at risk through routine inquiry on initial contact
2. Level I assessment for (a) physical and emotional trauma and (b) risk to life—self and other
3. Empathic, supportive response
4. Safety planning (if assessment reveals risk to life)
5. Linkage, effective referral for Level II assessment, and follow-up

These basics of crisis work in general medical settings are interrelated: the likelihood of a person accepting a referral for crisis counseling, physical refuge, AA, or other service following emergency medical treatment (such as after a suicide attempt, rape, battering, or crisis related to drinking) will often be influenced by the health care worker's attitude and recognition of the many facets of the situation. In short, health practitioners in these settings are not usually expected to assist people through *all* phases of crisis resolution. Effective crisis care, however, does require assessing the emotional aspects of events threatening health and life, offering support, and linking people to reliable sources for further assistance. In addition to such clinical skills, workers in emergency settings need an up-to-date resource file with procedures to ensure follow-up when referrals are made. Social workers usually coordinate such resources.

The challenge of combining emergency medical treatment and crisis intervention protocols is compounded by the misuse of emergency medical centers for routine prenatal care and common ailments that should be treated in physicians' offices or primary health care settings. On the assumption that health care is a right, not a privilege, and that primary care is less costly than treatment in tertiary settings, some services must be publicly supported (Feingold, 1994; Rachlis & Kushner, 1994).

Summary

Health and assistance to people whose health is threatened constitute a major domain of social life. The loss or threat of losing life, limb, or healthy self-image are occasions of crisis for many. Most often, people who are thus threatened come to the attention of general health providers (for example, nurses and physicians) and frontline workers such as rescue teams, caseworkers, and others close to people's daily struggles. AIDS brings into perspective the intersection between personal health, the family, community, and global issues. It typifies life crises as a whole as it touches major themes of the crisis experience: loss, grief, suicide danger, violence, and the need for social support. AIDS reveals starkly the relationship between situational, transitional, and sociocultural origins of crisis as depicted in this book's Crisis Paradigm. The potential of workers in entry points to health and social service systems is enormous, as is the cost saving in human and financial terms when crisis assessment and intervention are routine parts of practice in these settings.

References

Adamowski, K., Dickinson, G., Weitzman, B., Roessler, C., & Carter-Snell, C. (1993). Sudden unexpected death in the emergency department: Caring for the survivors. *Canadian Medical Association Journal, 149*(10), 1445–1451.

Aiken, L. H., Lake, E. T., Semaan, S., Lehman, H. P., Cole, C. S., Dunbar, D., & Frank, I. (1993). Nurse practitioner managed care for persons with HIV infection. *Image: Journal of Nursing Scholarship, 25*(3), 172–177.

Auerbach, J. D., & Coates, T. J. (2000). HIV prevention research: Accomplishments and challenges for the third decade of AIDS. *American Journal of Public Health, 90*(7), 1029–1936.

Barry, K. (1979). *Female sexual slavery.* New York: Avon Books.

Barth, R. B., Pietrzak, J., & Ramler, M. (Eds.). (1993). *Families living with drugs and HIV: Intervention and treatment strategies.* New York: Guilford Press.

Battin, M. P. (1980). Manipulated suicide. In M. P. Battin & D. J. Mayo (Eds.), *Suicide: The philosophical issues* (pp. 169–182). New York: St. Martin's Press.

Bayer, R. (1994). AIDS prevention and cultural sensitivity: Are they compatible? *American Journal of Public Health, 84*(6), 895–898.

Becktell, P. J. (1994). Endemic stress: Environmental determinants of women's health in India. *Health Care for Women International, 15*(2), 111–122.

Bertman, S. L. (1991). *Facing death: Images, insights, and interventions.* Bristol, PA: Hemisphere.

Bianco, M. (1992). How HIV/AIDS changes development priorities. *Women's Health Journal/Isis International, 4,* 58–62.

Blumenfeld, W. J. (Ed.). (1992). *Homophobia: How we all pay the price.* Boston: Beacon Press.

Borysenko, J. (1987). *Minding the body: Mending the mind.* Reading, MA: Addison-Wesley.

Bral, E. E. (1998). Caring for adults with chronic cancer pain. *American Journal of Nursing, 98*(4), 27–33.

Bredenberg, P. (1991). *Who cares? Social support and women with breast cancer.* Unpublished doctoral dissertation, Syracuse University, Syracuse, NY.

Brody, H. (1988). *Stories of sickness.* New Haven, CT: Yale University Press.

Caplan, G. (1964). *Principles of preventive psychiatry.* New York: Basic Books.

Caudill, M. (1994). *Managing pain before it manages you.* New York: Guilford Press.

Chernin, K. (1985). *The hungry self: Women, eating, and identity.* New York: HarperCollins.

Childs, R. E. (1985). Maternal psychological conflicts associated with the birth of a retarded child. *Maternal Child Health Nursing, 14*(3), 175–182.

Congressional Joint Commission on Mental Health and Illness. (1961). *Action for mental health.* New York: Basic Books.

Conrad, P., & Kern, R. (Eds.). (1990). *The sociology of health and illness: Critical perspectives* (3rd ed.). New York: St. Martin's Press.

Dally, A. (1992). *Women under the knife: A history of surgery.* New York: Routledge.

Davidhizar, R., & Kirk, B. (1993). Emergency room nurses: Helping families cope with sudden death. *Journal of Practical Nursing, 43*(2), 14–19.

Des Jarlais, D. C. (2000). Prospects for a public health perspective on psychoactive drug use. *American Journal of Public Health, 90*(3), 335–337.

Donnelly, J., & Chacon, R. (2000, February 21). The endless war: A deadly grip. *Boston Globe,* pp. A1, A8–A10.

Dowdy, Z. R. (1997, November 25). Study queries mandatory sentences. *Boston Globe,* p. B2.

Durham, J. D., & Lashley, F. R. (2000). *The person with HIV/AIDS: Nursing perspectives* (3rd ed.). New York: Springer.

Edmands, M. S., Hoff, L. A., Kaylor, L., Mower, L., & Sorrell, S. (1999). Bridging gaps between mind, body and spirit: Healing the whole person. *Journal of Psychosocial Nursing, 37*(10), 1–7.

Ehrenreich, B., & English, D. (1979). *For her own good: 150 years of the experts' advice to women.* New York: Anchor Books.

Farberow, N. L. (1981). Suicide prevention in the hospital. *Hospital and Community Psychiatry, 32*(2), 99–104.

Farmer, P. (1999). Pathologies of power: Rethinking health and human rights. *American Journal of Public Health, 89*(10), 1486–1496.

Feingold, E. (1994). Health care reform—more than cost containment and universal access. *American Journal of Public Health, 84*(5), 727–728.

Fiedler, J. L., & Wight, J. B. (1989). *The medical offset effect and public health policy: Mental health industry in transition.* New York: Praeger.

Fishbain, D. A. (1996). Current research on chronic pain and suicide. *American Journal of Public Health, 86*(9), 1320–1321.

Fleming, P. L., Wortley, P. M., Karon, J. M., DeCock, K. M., & Janssen, R. S. (2000). Tracking the HIV epidemic: Current issues, future challenges. *American Journal of Public Health, 90*(7), 1037–1038.

Fuller, J. (1996). AIDS prevention: A challenge to the Catholic moral tradition. *America, 175*(7), 13–20.

Fullerton, C. S., McCarroll, J. E., Ursano, R. J., & Wright, K. M. (1992). Psychological responses of rescue workers: Fire fighters and trauma. *American Journal of Orthopsychiatry, 32*(3), 371–378.

Galea, R. P., Lewis, B. F., & Baker, L. A. (1988). Voluntary testing for HIV antibodies among clients in long-term substance-abuse treatment. *Social Work, 33*(3), 265–268.

Garrison, J. (1974). Network techniques: Case studies in the screening-linking-planning conference method. *Family Process, 13,* 337–353.

Goffman, E. (1963). *Stigma.* Englewood Cliffs, NJ: Prentice Hall.

Gollub, E. L. (1999). Human rights is a U.S. problem, too: The case of women and HIV. *American Journal of Public Health, 89*(10), 1479–1482.

Halldorsdottir, S., & Hamrin, E. (1997). Caring and uncaring encounters within nursing and health care: From the cancer patient's perspective. *Cancer Nursing, 20*(2), 120–128.

Hamilton, J. A., Jensvold, M. F., Rothblum, E. D., & Cole, E. (Eds.). (1995). *Psychopharmacology from a feminist perspective.* New York: Harrington Park Press.

Hansell, N. (1976). *The person in distress.* New York: Human Sciences Press.

Haygood, W. (1999, October 13). AIDS and the African. *Boston Globe,* pp. A1, A17.

Hoff, L. A. (1993). Review essay: Health policy and the plight of the mentally ill. *Psychiatry, 56*(4), 400–419.

Hoff, L. A. (2000). Crisis care. In B. Everett & R. Gallop *Linking childhood trauma and mental illness: Theory and practice for direct service practitioners* (pp. 227–251). Thousand Oaks: CA: Sage.

Hoff, L. A., & Adamowski, K. (1998). *Creating excellence in crisis care: A guide to effective training and program designs.* San Francisco: Jossey-Bass.

Hoff, L. A., & Rosenbaum, L. (1994). A victimization assessment tool: Instrument development and clinical implications. *Journal of Advanced Nursing, 20*(4), 627–634.

Hollibaugh, A. (1994, June). Transmission, transmission, where's the transmission? *Sojourner: The Women's Forum,* 5p., 7p.

Hoskins, C. N., & Haber, J. (2000). Adjusting to breast cancer. *American Journal of Nursing, 100*(4), 26–32.

Hughes, A., Martin, J. P., & Franks, P. (1987). *AIDS home care and hospice manual.* San Francisco: AIDS Home Care and Hospice Program, Visiting Nurse Association of San Francisco.

Jackson, D. Z. (1997, May 14). Study strikes a blow against mandatory sentencing for drug crimes. *Boston Globe,* p. A15.

Johnson, A. B. (1990). *Out of bedlam: The truth about deinstitutionalization.* New York: Basic Books.

Kavanagh, K. J. (1988). The cost of caring: Nursing on a psychiatric intensive care unit. *Human Organization, 47*(3), 242–251.

Kleeman, K. M. (1989). Families in crisis due to multiple trauma. *Critical Care Nursing Clinics of North America, 1*(1), 23–31.

Krieger, I. (1988). An approach to coping with anxiety about AIDS. *Social Work, 33*(3), 263–264.

Kruger, S. (1992). Parents in crisis: Helping them cope with a seriously ill child. *Journal of Pediatric Nursing, 7*(2), 133–140.

Link, B. G., Struening, E. L., Rahav, M., Phelan, J. C., & Nuttbrock, L. (1997). On stigma and its consequences: Evidence from a longitudinal study of men with dual diagnoses of mental illness and substance abuse. *Journal of Health and Social Behavior, 38,* 177–190.

Lloyd, M. (2000, March 7). United Nations campaign against AIDS focuses on men's attitudes. *Boston Globe,* p. A2.

Loustaunau, M. O., & Sobo, E. J. (1997). *The cultural context of health, illness, and medicine.* New York: Bergin & Garvey.

Luchterhand, C., & Murphy, N. E. (1998). *Helping adults with mental retardation grieve a death loss.* Philadelphia: Brunner/Mazel.

Lugina, H. I. (1994). Factors that influence women's health in Tanzania. *Health Care for Women International, 15*(1), 61–68.

Luhrmann, T. M. (2000). *Of two minds: The growing disorder in American psychiatry.* New York: Knopf.

Lynn, J., & Childress, J. F. (1991). Must patients always be given food and water? In C. Levine (Ed.), *Taking sides: Clashing views on controversial bioethical issues* (4th ed., pp. 118–126). Guilford, CT: Dushkin.

Mann, J. M. (1993). We are all Berliners: Notes from the ninth international conference on AIDS. *American Journal of Public Health, 83*(10), 1378–1379.

Maxwell, M. B. (1982). The use of social networks to help cancer patients maximize support. *Cancer Nursing, 5,* 275–281.

McCarroll, J. E., Ursano, R. J., Wright, K. M., & Fullerton, C. S. (1993). Handling bodies after violent death: Strategies for coping. *American Journal of Orthopsychiatry, 63*(2), 209–214.

Meisenhelder, J. B. (1994). Contributing factors to fear of HIV contagion in registered nurses. *Image: Journal of Nursing Scholarship, 26*(1), 65–69.

Millman, M. (1978). Medical mortality review: A cordial affair. In H. D. Schwartz & C. S. Kart (Eds.), *Dominant issues in medical sociology* (pp. 288–244). Reading, MA: Addison-Wesley.

Moore, K. W., & Schwartz, K. S. (1993). Psychosocial support of trauma patients in the emergency department by nurses, as indicated by communication. *Journal of Emergency Nursing, 19*(4), 297–302.

Murphy, B. (1994). *The politics of AIDS.* Unpublished manuscript.

Nahill, A. (2000, January 3). A doctor's lesson on duality of drugs: Second opinion. *Boston Globe,* p. C2.

Navarro, V. (1994). The future of public health in health care reform. *American Journal of Public Health, 84*(5), 729–730.

Neufeld, S. (1999, August 23). Black groups turn focus on AIDS fight. *Boston Globe,* pp. A1, A7.

Oakley, L. D., & Potter, L. (1997). *Psychiatric primary care.* St. Louis: Mosby-Year Book.

O'Rourke, M. E. (1999). Narrowing the options: The process of deciding on prostate cancer treatment. *Cancer Investigation, 17,* 349–359.

Pappano, L. (1998, July 26). Alone together. *Boston Globe Magazine,* pp. 14–22, 26–31.

Parkes, C. M. (1975). *Bereavement: Studies of grief in adult life.* Harmondsworth, England: Penguin Books.

Polak, P. (1971). Social systems intervention. *Archives of General Psychiatry, 25,* 10–17.

Polak, P. (1976). A model to replace psychiatric hospitalization. *Journal of Nervous and Mental Disease, 162,* 13–22.

Pruchno, R. A., & Potashnik, S. L. (1989). Caregiving spouses: Physical and mental health in perspective. *Journal of the American Geriatrics Society, 37,* 697–705.

Ptacek, L. J. (1982). Respite care for families of children with severe handicaps: An evaluation study of parent satisfaction. *Journal of Community Psychology, 10,* 222–227.

Rachlis, M., & Kushner, C. (1994). *Strong medicine: How to save Canada's health care system.* Toronto: HarperCollins.

Richardson, B. K. (1987, July/August). Psychiatric inpatients' perception of seclusion room experience. *Nursing Research, 36,* 234–238.

Root-Berstein, R. S. (1993). *Rethinking AIDS: The tragic cost of premature consensus.* New York: Free Press-Maxwell Macmillan International.

Sande, M. A., & Volberding, P. (Eds.). (1995). *The medical management of AIDS* (4th ed.). Philadelphia: Saunders.

Seeman, M., & Seeman, A. Z. (1992). Life strains, alienation, and drinking behavior. *Alcoholism, 16*(2), 199–205.

Shalev, A. Y., Schreiber, S., Galai, T., & Melmed, R. N. (1993). Post-traumatic stress disorder following medical events. *British Journal of Clinical Psychology, 32*(Part 2), 247–253.

Shilts, R. (1987). *And the band played on.* New York: St. Martin's Press.

Shipes, E., & Lehr, S. (1982). Sexuality and the male cancer patient. *Cancer Nursing, 5,* 375–381.

Singer, M. (1992). AIDS and U.S. ethnic minorities: The crisis and alternative anthropological responses. *Human Organization, 51*(1), 89–95.

Smith, D. R. (1994). Porches, politics, and public health. *American Journal of Public Health, 84*(5), 725–726.

Solomon, M. Z., O'Donnell, L., Jennings, B., Guilfoy, V., Wolf, S. M., Nolan, K., Jackson, B. A., Koch-Weser, D., & Donnelley, S. (1993). Decisions near the end of life: Professional views on life-sustaining treatments. *American Journal of Public Health, 83*(1), 14–23.

Sontag, S. (1978). *Illness as metaphor.* New York: Farrar, Straus & Giroux.

Stein, Z. A. (1995). Editorial: More on women and the prevention of HIV infection [Editorial]. *American Journal of Public Health, 85*(11), 1485–1487.

Sugg, N. K., & Inui, T. (1992). Primary care physicians' response to domestic violence: Opening Pandora's box. *Journal of the American Medical Association, 267*(23), 3157–3160.

Thea, D. M., Rosen, S., & Simon, J. (1999, September 14). AIDS is devastating whole societies. *Boston Globe,* p. A23.

U.S. Department of Health and Human Services. (1986). *Surgeon General's workshop on violence and public health: Report.* Washington, DC: Author.

Watson, J. E. (2000, January 27). Deadly denial: Doctor confronts scourge of AIDS in Latino men. *Boston Globe,* pp. B1, B5.

Whitaker, R., & Kong, D. (1998, November 15–18). Doing Harm: Research on the mentally ill [A four-part series], *Boston Globe.* Testing takes human toll [First of four parts], pp. A1, A32–A33. Lure of riches fuels testing [Third of four parts], pp. A1, A34–A35.

Zborowski, M. (1952). Cultural components in responses to pain. *Journal of Social Issues, 8,* 16–30.

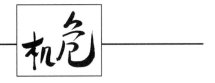

CHAPTER TWELVE

THREATS TO OCCUPATIONAL AND RESIDENTIAL SECURITY

Basic human needs include success in one's ascribed and achieved social roles and a secure, stable dwelling place. Meeting these needs implies

- The ability and opportunity to be creative and productive in a way that is meaningful to us and accepted by others
- Membership in a supportive community that values our presence and contribution
- Enough material supplies to maintain self-sufficiency and protection from the elements

As discussed in the last chapter, a serious change in health status threatens a person's self-image as well as the ability to be self-supportive. Underscoring the interacting relationship between health, occupational, and general social security, many people—especially in the United States where there is no comprehensive health care system—remain in unfulfilling jobs that can literally make them sick (Illich, 1976) to keep from losing insurance coverage. If they lose their jobs, the loss of insurance as well adds to their stress, fear, and insecurity about the future. In turn, these additional stressors affect one's health status and ability to function at precisely the time of greatest need. When occupation-based stress intersects with domestic issues, depression is not uncommon (Phelan et al., 1991). This includes stress from overwork by people who cannot afford to build regular leisure time into their lives (Schor, 1993). A study by Barnett and Rivers (1998) reveals that people who occupy multiple roles are more resilient than workaholics, who feel most disillusioned and more easily plunge into depression if something goes wrong on the job, having placed all their eggs in one basket, so to speak. Generally, job security is the fundamental means of maintaining residential security, since housing constitutes most people's major financial liability. The most extreme response to job loss is violence by the dismissed employee against the employer and others, a phenomenon more common in the United States than elsewhere.

These intertwined hazards around health, occupational, and residential security are compounded for those with a prior history of mental illness and for victims of violence, especially women and children. Most people look forward to the comfort and security of returning to a secure dwelling after a day's work or to welcoming coworkers after a vacation or business trip. When occupational and residential status are threatened, however, a person's status may be dramatically changed from

- Home to streets
- Having a job to the unemployment lines or poverty
- A sense of self-sufficiency to unexpected dependency
- A sense of security to uncertainty about where the next meal is coming from or where the next night will be spent: On someone's couch? In a welfare hotel? A shelter? The mean streets?

In the following pages, the principles and techniques of crisis intervention that frontline workers can apply on behalf of people in crisis around housing and occupational loss are discussed. People need to mourn the losses that characterize these unanticipated transitions, some of which are life threatening. And they need the hope that comes from advocacy and social change to alleviate the conditions that deprive people of jobs and home and perpetuate the widening gap between the world's rich and poor.

Occupational Changes

This section discusses the complex issues that pertain to working, earning money, and maintaining oneself and one's family economically.

Promotion, Success, and Economic Security

Promotion and success are not hazardous events or occasions of crisis for most. But suicide studies reveal that promotion can be the last straw that leads some people to commit suicide. The person who is promoted to a prestigious position may feel incapable of performing as expected in the new role. An anticipated promotion can also be a crisis point, as a new position brings increased responsibility, higher rank and status, and a change in role relationships among peers. If the move is from ordinary staff worker to a management position, the person may fear loss of acceptance by the peer group he or she leaves (Kanter, 1977).

The combination of loss of familiar supportive relationships at work and the challenge of unfamiliar work becomes too much to handle. A person's vulnerability to crisis in these circumstances is affected by several factors:

1. The general openness of communication in the company or agency
2. The person's ability to openly discuss questions and fears with a trusted confidant, because expressing worries about self-confidence, for example, might jeopardize the promotion
3. The person's perception of self and how one should perform in a given role—especially difficult for perfectionists

The Success Neurosis and Sex Roles. A crisis stemming from promotion has also been called the *success neurosis,* which is sometimes seen in women who view themselves as occupying second-rate or second-best positions. If they have worked primarily in the role of housewife and mother, they may suddenly become immobilized when other opportunities arise. This can happen even when they have openly expressed a desire for new opportunities.

Crises associated with promotion and success are usually quiet crises. People in this kind of crisis are not acutely upset but feel generally anxious and depressed and express bewilderment about being depressed. They feel disappointed that they cannot measure up to their own expectations; they know they have every reason to be happy. They cannot relate their feelings of depression to their lack of self-confidence and rigid expectations of themselves. A deep fear of failure may lead to the idea of suicide in the event that the person really does fail.

Anxiety, depression, and suicidal thoughts may move a person in this kind of crisis to seek help. Usually, such a person will go to a local crisis clinic or a private therapist. Several crisis counseling sessions are often sufficient for the person to

- Express underlying fears, insecurity, and disappointment with self
- Gain a realistic perspective on his or her abilities
- Grow in self-confidence and self-acceptance
- Use family and friends to discuss feelings and concerns openly rather than viewing such expressions as another failure

CASE EXAMPLE: ANGIE

Angie, age thirty-seven, had been doing volunteer work with the mental health association in her community. One of her special projects was helping handicapped people run a confection stand for local Parks and Recreation Department events. Because of the high quality of her work—which she could only acknowledge self-consciously—her friends urged her to open and manage her own coffeehouse.

She finally did so, and the project was a glowing success. Angie suddenly found herself in the limelight, a situation she had not anticipated. She could not believe it would last. After a few months, she began feeling tense and depressed and thought vaguely about suicide. She talked with her physician about her problem and was referred to a psychotherapist for help.

Short-term crisis counseling may reveal deeper problems of low self-esteem, rigid role expectations, inflexible behavior patterns, and habitual reluctance to communicate feelings of distress to significant people. Psychotherapy should be offered and encouraged, as these people are high risks for suicide if other crisis situations arise. But in addition to offering individual assistance, as crisis workers and as a society, we need to examine the structures and differential expectations and rewards that place women at greater risk of failing in their career aspirations. For example, executive women (unlike executive men) who want to avoid being derailed from the career ladder typically must jump through two hoops: traditional masculine behavior and traditional feminine behavior (Morrison, White, & Van Velsor, 1987). This is a new version of the old adage "Women must be twice as good to get half as far." One consequence of such stress might be an obsession with work, to the detriment of a healthy balance between work and other activities. Although women have made progress in traditionally male-dominated professions—for example, law, medicine, and engineering—they are vulnerable to the same gender-based harassment and abuse as women in traditionally female-dominated professions such as nursing (Phillips & Schneider, 1993). Finally, despite their high professional status, they shoulder the same dual burden that most women carry: they still do the bulk of unpaid domestic work such as child care.

The origins of work-related crises can be traced to cultural values and the tradition that men do public work and are paid well for it, whereas women do private work and are not paid at all (Waring, 1990). When women do work outside the home, the majority do so in traditionally female, nurturant or supportive jobs, such as nursing, child care, and clerical work (Foner, 1994; Kavanagh, 1988; Reverby, 1987). Because most women today work outside the home for economic, psychological, and social survival, the points of stress and potential crises are numerous as long as traditional values prevail. The internationally publicized murder trial of au pair Louise Woodward in 1997 underscored the persistence of these values: of the parents, both physicians with active careers, only the mother worked part-time in order to be available more for parenting; yet it was only the *mother* who was publicly vilified for not setting her career aside so she could be at home full-time and eliminate the need for an au pair. This response is more dramatic in the context of statistics from the U.S. Advisory Board on Child Abuse and Neglect: of those charged with shaking a baby into injury and death, 60 percent are fathers or boyfriends, 17 percent are female baby-sitters, and 12 percent are mothers (Jackson, 1997). For many women, the cost of caring is very high (Facione, 1994; Sommers & Shields, 1987) and will get higher as the number of seniors and people with AIDS increases, unless men assume more equal responsibility for the caring work of society. Crisis counseling or therapy is indicated for individual men and women struggling with these issues. The long-term results, however, will be limited without simultaneous attention directed to the social change strategies relevant to these crises of sociocultural origin (see Chapter Two).

Institutional Barriers to Promotion and Economic Security. Aside from regressive cultural values about men, women, and work, there are institutional barriers to promotion for millions of workers, especially ethnic minorities and poor women (Dujon & Withorn, 1996; Sidel, 1996). Globalization has led to ever widening gaps between the rich and traditionally disadvantaged groups. These social problems can lead to homelessness, child neglect, marital discord, bitterness, withdrawal from the mainstream of social life, substance abuse, suicide, and violence.

Numerous studies (see Chapter Two) underscore the work of Caplan (1964), Hansell (1976), and others documenting the need for intactness of one's social, cultural, and material supplies in order to avoid personal crisis (Perese, 1997; Schmidt, Weisner, & Wiley, 1998). Pearce and McAdoo (1982), writing for the National Advisory Council on Economic Opportunity regarding the "feminization of poverty," point out the differing results of divorce for women and men: the postdivorce poverty of most women is associated with the burden of single parenting and minimal financial support from the children's father, a situation exacerbated in cases of domestic violence.

Despite some exceptions to this pattern and some divorce settlements unfair to men, this situation is dramatized by the fact that within a year of divorce, the standard of living for most women decreases significantly and for men it increases. The largest percentage of poor women and children are members of racial minorities, which underscores the combination of race, gender, and class bias. Labor statistics show that women with children in the United States still earn only 70 percent of wages earned by men, despite the Equal Pay Act passed in 1965 (Crittenden, 2001). To offer psychotherapy or crisis counseling alone, without job training, day care, and advocacy for adequate housing for disadvantaged workers, represents a misunderstanding of the problem, its origins, and its solutions. Rather than recycling these old problems, a fresh look upstream to their source holds the most promise for reducing crisis proneness and long-term negative outcomes for victims of discrimination. Even many in the business community are recognizing that continued wage disparities hurt not only the individuals affected but also business as a whole (Lewis, 2000).

Paid and Unpaid Work

Worldwide, in labor statistics jargon, *work* is defined as paid work. In Africa, for example, 60 to 80 percent of agricultural work is done by women, though it is not included in official labor force counts. In Canada, according to 1992 data, household work, two-thirds of which is done by women, accounts for 41.4 percent of national output. As Mollison (1993, p. 15A) states, "The economy would shudder if homemakers stopped doing unpaid work. Families would have to choose between recruiting other unpaid volunteers, hiring replacements, or settling for a life in which unfed, ignorant children and grouchy, unkempt adults struggled for survival under burned-out light bulbs and amid mountains of stinky socks."

In sum, women probably will not achieve equality in the paid workforce until men do an equal share of society's unpaid—but nevertheless very necessary—work. Statistics compiled for the 1985 United Nations Decade for Women Conference in Nairobi, Kenya, reveal that women do two-thirds of the world's work (not counting unpaid child care), earn one-tenth of the world's income, and own less than one-hundredth of the world's property (Seager & Olson, 1986). As Waring (1990) notes, if women's work "counted," official labor statistics and potentially the entire social landscape could be transformed. In the United States, a national debate is in progress about "reforming welfare as we know it."

Few would contest the negative—even damaging—outcomes of intergenerational welfare dependency for some recipients (see Schmidt et al., 1998). Results of reform thus far throw into sharp relief the public denigration of women's work in rearing children alone, often following abuse and because some divorced fathers do not pay child support. Success in welfare reform would also link the worldwide correlation of teenage motherhood and general birthrates with equity in women's economic and educational status. Contrary to popular perception, adolescent pregnancy is not just a racial minority issue; rather, it reflects poverty and the increasing unwillingness of teens to defer sexual activity, factors that cross racial boundaries (Desmond, 1994).

Welfare reform acts in the mid-1990s by many states reveal very mixed results. Among states that enacted a "work-first" policy, in 1999 only 25 percent of those who had gone from welfare to work were employed at wages above $250 per week for a full year (Albelda, 1999). A $250 weekly income translates to $13,000 per year, $36,687 *below* the median annual income for a family of four, which in 1998 was $49,687 (U.S. Census Bureau, 2000). The $13,000 annual income level is $4,050 below the official U.S. poverty level for a family of four, which is $17,050 (*Economic Report of the President Transmitted to the Congress*, 2000). According to a study by the Educational Testing Service, most welfare recipients lack the education and training needed to escape poverty, but work-first overhaul programs do not provide such training (Meckler, 1999). Another reason for "reform" outcomes like this is the lack of affordable child care for poor mothers, while the role of fathers in parenting is virtually unchanged from traditional patterns. As Kuttner (2000) asks, "When was the last time you read an article about the stresses of being a working father?" (p. C7). But when fathers do share equitably in caring for their children, they often suffer more negative repercussions than women do in the workplace, thereby reinforcing the traditional value that child care is really just "women's work."

There is a perverse irony or double standard in expressed values and policy regarding women's work and welfare reform: in the Louise Woodward case, the mother with a comfortable income from her own and her husband's professional work is expected to stay home full-time to ensure proper child care; whereas poor mothers—many on welfare because of abuse—are expected to work outside the home whether or not child care is available. The hazards of these policies to the education and healthy development of children are great. This neglect of the nation's greatest resource—its children—means that future generations will pay the ultimate price (see Kozol, 1988, 2000). A similar double standard is evident in the fact that there is little organized effort by government to reform policies of tax credits to corporations that expand to cheap labor markets, subsidies to wealthy agribusiness originally intended for small farmers, tax-supported outlays to sports clubs and their wealthy players, tax rebates on mortgages for those lucky enough to own a home, and so forth.

Despite these grim results of regressive U.S. social policy affecting children and the society's communal health, the state of Wyoming has implemented a very effective, nonpunitive welfare reform effort in the United States, although Wyoming's economy lags the rest of the nation. Its 65 percent reduction in its welfare caseload is attributed to several policy decisions: in a people-to-people small-town approach, caseworkers offer support instead of threat. Their caseloads were reduced, and guidelines replaced rigid rules. Recipients are assured of continued benefits so long as they actively pursue a job, classes in preparing for a job, and opportunities for job training. Overall, the program is "work eventually" instead of "work first" (Grunwald, 1998).

This issue of welfare and *workfare* is especially urgent because it is connected to the hopelessness and apathy of chronically poor people, especially in inner cities and on Indian reservations. The heralded booming U.S. economy leaves these groups untouched, while their education in many substandard schools has not prepared them to command a living-wage job in the era of high technology and a globalized economy. In such a climate, despair and violence flourish. Perhaps in no instance is the link between personal crisis and socioeconomic and cultural factors more dramatically illustrated. The tandem approach discussed in Chapter Nine most aptly applies here: assist individuals through traumatic life events like joblessness and unemployment (often based on race and class status), hold them accountable for violence and child supervision, and *simultaneously* engage them and others to address the roots of their plight (see Crisis Paradigm, Box 3).

Following the 1992 Los Angeles riots, Bondi Gabrel, an ethnic minority owner of an apartment complex in that riot-torn community, could have abandoned his damaged building. Instead he *employed* gang members and provided leadership options and a vision of another lifestyle. Gang members now, instead of vandalizing property, are paid to guard it. When chosen as *person of the week* by a national television network, Mr. Gabrel said, "This is what happens when you invest in people. . . . We haven't asked for enough." As this example and Medoff and Sklar's account (1994) of the death and life of an urban neighborhood demonstrate, models for such multifaceted approaches are there and need to be widely replicated.

Work Disruption

Just as promotion, success, or disadvantaged status can be a source of crisis or threat to health, so can disruption or change in work role, especially for a person accustomed to a lifetime of job security. The depression of inner-city neighborhoods is connected to global economic changes and the widespread loss of manufacturing jobs, which had been the mainstay of security for many who are now desperate. Although median household incomes rose by 3.5 percent in 1998, inequality between wage earners has steadily widened since 1980, according to U.S. census data. Ethnic minority and immigrant groups are the most affected by the loss of manufacturing jobs, many of which have been transferred to countries with cheaper labor and looser laws protecting both workers and the environment. Many of these workers have little choice but low-paying service jobs with few benefits and few chances for advancement.

Western society's attitude toward work, especially in the United States, is highlighted by a tendency to value people in proportion to how much money they earn and to respect them in proportion to the socioeconomic status they derive from their earnings. In other words, many have absorbed the deeply embedded cultural value, "You're worth what you earn." This value system helps fuel the welfare reform debate and the suspicion on the part of the haves that the have-nots are ultimately responsible for their own misfortune and could remedy that misfortune if they simply tried harder. Such judgments fail to account for the complex relationship between most unemployment situations and either global economics or discrimination based on race, gender, age, disability, or ill health. Usually, the unemployed or underemployed in a changing economy are deeply regretful of their position and struggle continually to correct it. These complexities and troubles are compounded for recent immigrants, who have few rights and legal protections and often live in fear of deportation if they make their plight known. Unemployment, then—or the threat of same—whether by firing, layoff, or because of a personal problem like illness, is frequently the occasion of emotional crisis, including violent responses like suicide or murder. While unemployed people must act on their misfortune, they will be much more empowered to do so if they are not inappropriately blamed for their plight.

Regardless of the reasons, the person in crisis because of unemployment is usually in need of a great deal of support. If unemployment originates from personal sources, social support and individual crisis intervention are indicated. However, people who are unemployed because of economic recession or discrimination are less likely to feel hopeless and powerless if they are also put into contact with groups devoted to removing the underlying sources of their stress through social change strategies. This includes policy changes that would prevent corporations from simply closing U.S. plants, laying off hundreds of employees, and moving to a country where labor is cheaper without any collaboration with or consideration of the workers who have built their lives around the company. The primary origin of crisis for a worker thus laid off is the profit motive. The appropriate response, therefore, should include linking such a person to groups advocating labor-management policy change (see Crisis Paradigm). In Germany, for example, workers in an automobile manufacturing plant decided on a four-day workweek so that *none* lost their jobs. Recent protests during meetings of the World Trade Organization, the World Bank, the International Monetary Fund, and the Organization of American States suggest a new era of social change as activists clash with police to demonstrate for fairness to workers and for environmental protection in the face of global trade policies and agreements.

Standards of personal success for most of us hinge on involvement in work that is personally satisfying and of value to the external community. For example, a fifty-five-year-old man in a middle-management position who is prematurely retired may begin to drink or may attempt suicide as a way of dealing with the crisis of job disruption. These and other work-related crises are within the common province of personnel directors, occupational physicians and nurses, or anyone the person turns to in distress.

CASE EXAMPLE: RUSSELL AND JENNY OWENS

Russell Owens, age fifty-two, was a civil engineer employed for twenty years as a research consultant in a large industrial corporation. When he lost his job because of a surplus of engineers with his qualifications, he tried without success to find other employment, even at lower pay. Family financial needs forced his wife, Jenny, age forty-seven, to seek full-time employment as a biology instructor; she had worked only part-time before. Jenny was grateful for this opportunity to advance herself professionally. She always regretted the fact that she had never tried to excel at a job, partly because Russell did not want her to work full-time. Gradually, however, Jenny became resentful of having to support herself, her husband, and their sixteen-year-old daughter, Gwen, in addition to assuming all responsibility for household tasks. She urged Russell to do at least some of the housework. Because

Russell had never helped in this way, except for occasional errands and emergencies, Jenny's expectations struck a blow to his masculine self-image beyond the sense of failure and inadequacy he already felt from his job loss.

Russell also found it difficult to follow Jenny's advice that he seek help with his depression and increasing dependence on alcohol. The strain in their marital relationship increased. Jenny eventually divorced Russell, and he committed suicide. This case illustrates the importance of preventive intervention. Russell's drinking problem and eventual suicide might have been avoided if immediate help had been available to him at the crisis points of job loss and threat of divorce. Such help might also have resulted in a constructive resolution of Jenny's resentment of Russell concerning the housework.

Rural and Urban Occupational Transitions

Similar dynamics are apparent in the farm crisis. Farmers not only face a threat to their source of livelihood but also to their way of life. Although some farm foreclosures can be traced to individual mismanagement, the problem originates in policies that favor unbridled corporate accumulations of agricultural resources and profits at the expense of individual farm families. For example, federal price supports for farm products are cut back because of a "surplus." Yet in New England, where hundreds of Vermont dairy families have been driven off their farms, there is no milk surplus. Rather, the large amounts of milk at issue are from huge corporate farms in California. It is ironic that in a country of immigrants who fled Europe and prized the opportunity to earn an honest living on the land, people are now in crisis because public policy favors corporate monopoly over the nation's breadbasket. No doubt the suicides, alcoholism, violence, and family conflicts arising from the farm crisis will continue unless grassroots efforts and public policy (such as that proposed by the Vermont legislature) reverse the conditions causing so much pain and despair among the nation's rural citizens. One such grassroots organization is Farm Aid Rural Management in Bismarck, North Dakota. A similar program, the Kitchen Table Alliance, was organized as a countywide community development project in Ontario for farm families in financial, legal, or emotional difficulty or crisis to regain their health and productivity. These groups offer support, advocacy, crisis prevention, and referral for these distressed workers and their families.

Although the farm crisis in North America has abated, similar disruption of a way of life is now occurring in fishing communities worldwide. In poor countries, millions of rural dwellers flock to shantytowns near water, only to continue their grim struggle for survival, often with additional threats of violence in crowded slums or death from tidal waves. The threat in fishing communities is not only to a way of life taken for granted for generations but also to marine life, because overfishing depletes the fish supply. Support and crisis intervention groups like the Kitchen Table Alliance for farmers are crucial to the health and social welfare of affected fishing community members, in order to prevent suicide, violence, and substance abuse as governments and international agencies address the long-term facets of this issue.

Retirement

Some people look forward to retirement. Others dread it. For many people, retirement signifies loss of status, a reduced standard of living, and a feeling of being discarded by society. The experience is more pronounced when one is forced to retire at an early age due to illness or other disability. It is a time of stress not only for the retired person but also for family members, especially wives who do not work outside the home. Suddenly, a homemaker has to adjust to having at home all day a husband who may feel worthless and who may have developed few outside interests or hobbies apart from work. Fortunately, these patterns are changing as the population ages, and more older persons realize and take advantage of the fact that for many, formal retirement means the continuation, not the end, of a fulfilling life.

The attitude people hold toward retirement depends on the situation they retire to; whether retirement is pleasant or not is also influenced by lifestyle. Key areas of concern in evaluating a person's retirement situation include the following:

1. Does the person have any satisfying interests or hobbies outside of work? For many, work has been their main focus all of their adult lives, and most of their

pleasures are work related. For many overworked Americans, this may be a key issue requiring focused preretirement planning.

2. Does the person have a specifically planned retirement project? For example, some people plan to study literature, carpentry, or cooking when they retire. For people of means, Elderhostel offers many such programs.

3. Does the person have a comfortable place to live? This factor is highly influenced by the job issues already discussed.

4. Does the person have enough retirement income to manage without excessive dependence?

5. Is the person in reasonably good health and free to manage without hardship?

6. Has the person been well-adjusted socially and emotionally before retirement?

Even if the retired person's circumstances are favorable in all or most of these areas, retirement can still be stressful. We live in a youth-oriented society, and retirement signals that one is nearing or has already reached old age; after that, death approaches.

For some people, retirement is not an issue or occasion for crisis. They may be self-employed and simply keep working at a pace compatible with their needs and inclinations. Such people usually prepare for a reduced pace and have a healthy attitude toward life in each development phase, including old age. A new view of the life cycle suggests three phases: learning, earning, and returning. Thus, instead of retiring, people have an opportunity to return wisdom and other values to society and to have something returned to them after their years of learning, earning, and caring for others (P. Schoonover, personal communication, 1987).

Those who are crisis prone as a result of retirement should have the assistance accorded anyone experiencing a loss. They need the opportunity to grieve the loss of their former status, explore new ways of feeling useful, and eventually accept their changed roles.

Residential Changes

Moves across country or to a different continent require leaving familiar surroundings and friends for a place with many unknowns. Even though the person moving may have many problems at home, at least he or she knows what the problems are. Pulling up stakes and starting over can be an exciting venture, an occasion for joy and for gaining a new lease on life, or a source of deep distress and an occasion for crisis.

Consider the young woman who grew up in the country and moves to the city for the first time. She asks herself, Will I find a job? Will I be able to make friends? Will I be unbearably lonely? Will I be safe? Or the career person looking for opportunities wonders, Will things be any better there? How will I manage not seeing my family and friends very often? And last, consider the war refugee or immigrant, who worries, How will those foreigners accept me? Will I be able to learn the language so I can get along? Who will help me if things go wrong? What if I want to come back and don't have the money?

Anticipated Moves

These are a few of the many questions and potential problems faced by people who plan a move in hopes of improving their situation. Even in these instances, moving is a source of considerable stress. It takes courage to leave familiar territory, even when the move would free one from many negative situations. No matter what the motive for the move, and despite the anticipation of better things to come, people in this transition state often experience a sense of loss.

To prevent a crisis at this time, the person planning and looking forward to a move should avoid denying feelings of loss. Even when a person is moving to much better circumstances, there is usually the loss of close associations with friends or relatives. As in the case of promotion or success, the would-be mover often does not understand the sense of depression, which is probably related to the denial of feelings and guilt about leaving friends and relatives. Understanding and expressing these feelings helps the person keep an open relationship with friends left behind and frees the person to use and enjoy new opportunities more fully, unburdened of misplaced guilt or depression.

People who plan and look forward to a move are vulnerable to other crises. Once they reach their destination, the situation may not work out as anticipated: the new job may be less enjoyable than the old one; the escape from a violent city to a farm may seem less secure than expected; new friends may be hard to find; envisioned job opportunities may not exist.

Social isolation and the inability to establish and maintain satisfying social attachments make a person vulnerable to crises and even suicide. People who have satisfying supports can help prevent crises among those who have recently moved and have not yet established a reliable social support system. Elderly people, for example, who are moved to a group residential setting have a much improved chance of adjusting well to the change and perceiving it as a challenge if (1) they had a choice in relocation, (2) relocation was predictable and understandable within their meaning system, and (3) they received necessary social support (Armer, 1993). In the Cohousing movement discussed in Chapter Five, diversity by age is one of the goals, with some groups reserving a certain number of units (for example, five households out of twenty-five) for persons fifty-five and older. A planned move of this sort for people who dread living in housing complexes only for old people could do much to avoid a crisis during this major life transition.

Unanticipated Moves

The potential for crisis is even greater for those who do not want to move but are forced to—for example,

- The family uprooted to an unknown place because of a job transfer

- Inner-city dwellers—especially older people—dislocated because of urban renewal and priced out of the housing market
- Victims of disaster moving from a destroyed community
- People evicted because of unpaid rent
- Mental patients who have been discharged to the community without adequate shelter and social support
- Abused women and their children who are forced to leave their homes to avoid beatings or death
- Political or war refugees who must leave their homelands
- Migrant farmworkers who must move each year in the hope of earning a marginal subsistence

Many Afghan refugee women, for example, not only have lost family members and property but also face dramatic cultural differences, tripled social burdens, and lack of appropriate mates where they have now settled, in northern California (Lipson & Miller, 1994).

Thousands of teenagers and young people either run away from home, or they are simply "on the move." Many young people who run away do so because they are physically or sexually abused, or because they have come out as gay, lesbian, bisexual, or transgendered and are wholly rejected by their families. Often they lack housing, food, and money; many are further exploited sexually or feel forced into prostitution for survival; still others succumb to substance abuse (Greene, Ennett, & Ringwalt, 1997); in extreme cases they are killed by police for petty stealing and vagrancy.

War refugees who are crowded into camps in neighboring countries face similar hazards—unsanitary conditions, indifference, brutality, and even rape by soldiers and officials. As if these prices of civil and ethnic strife were not enough, some refugees face grim prospects for immigration, depending on race and political considerations of a prospective host country (Radin, 2000, p. A24). In the United States, for example, because of immigration quotas negotiated between Congress and the Immigration and Naturalization Service, far fewer African refugees are admitted than are admitted from Asia, Latin America, and Europe. There is congressional action pending to protect refugees who are the most vulnerable and are fleeing from persecution (Amnesty International, 2000, p. 21).

There are also groups of people who have been relocated by governments. Some of the most dramatic examples of such forced relocation and its long-term damaging effects are the destruction of Boston's West End in the 1950s to build Government Center (Gans, 1962); the 1953 dispatching of eighty-five Inuit people from northern Quebec to the High Arctic, where their families were wrenched apart and they endured extreme hardship and deprivation (Aubry, 1994); and the creation of racially segregated communities in South Africa (Sparks, 1990). As a result of these government actions, Boston's former West Enders are still mourning the loss of their homes, and the Inuit and South African majority are still seeking justice. Finally, there is the ordinary traveler who is en route from one place to another and loses money or belongings or is attacked.

In spite of the crisis potential of moves for many, moving can also be an occasion for growth through success in facing new challenges. Although highly mobile families may have fewer deep friendships, the family unit may feel closer and have a stronger self-concept as a result of successful coping in diverse circumstances. When counseling people with emotional problems related to relocation, psychologists identify four phases in coping with a move: (1) decision making—the less a person contributes to the decision, the more potential there is for trouble, (2) preparation—mastering the many details preceding a move, (3) separation from the old community—including acceptance of the sadness and loss involved, and (4) reinvestment—through involvement in one's new community (Singular, 1983, p. 46). These phases are akin to grief work and the rites of passage discussed in Chapters Four and Thirteen.

Helping the Migrant

Where is help available for the people in crisis related to migration? Crisis centers and mental health agencies are appropriate for people who are under great stress before a move as well as those who are anxious and upset afterward. Special programs for stranded youth and for refugees are on the rise. Social service agencies and services for aging persons should also provide anticipatory guidance and crisis counseling to all groups forced to move because of a planned project such as urban renewal. Unfortunately, such support and counseling are either not available or are not offered regularly.

CASE EXAMPLE: NOREEN ANDERSON

Noreen Anderson, age sixty-one, was confined to her apartment with a serious muscle disease. She was forced to retire at age fifty-eight and had felt lonely and isolated since then. She did not have family in the area but did have many friends. However, they gradually stopped visiting her after she had been confined for a year. Now her apartment building was being converted to condominiums that she could not afford. Everyone in the building had moved out except Noreen, who was unable to move without help. Fortunately, Noreen's phone was not disconnected. She called various social service agencies for help and was finally referred to a local crisis center.

An outreach crisis counselor went to Noreen's apartment. She expedited an application through a federal housing agency for a place for Noreen in a senior citizen's housing project. The counselor also engaged an interfaith volunteer agency to help Noreen pack and processed a request for immediate physical supplies through Catholic Charities. Noreen was grateful for the help she received after her several desperate telephone calls, but by this time she was depressed and suicidal. The crisis counselor saw her in her new apartment in the senior citizen's housing project for several counseling sessions. She helped Noreen get

in touch with old friends again and
encouraged the friends to visit on a
regular basis. A number of Retired Senior
Citizen Volunteers also visited Noreen,

which helped relieve her isolation and
loneliness. Noreen was no longer suicidal
at the termination of the counseling
sessions.

Travelers Aid Society. The Travelers Aid Society has been doing crisis intervention work with people in transit for years. Caseworkers of this agency see travelers
at the peak of their distress. The traveler who calls the society is often without
money or resources and is fearful in a strange city. In extreme cases, the person
may have been beaten, robbed, or raped. The Travelers Aid Society caseworker
gets in touch with relatives; ensures emergency medical services, food, and
emergency housing; provides travel money; and ensures the traveler a safe trip
home. Unfortunately, the Travelers Aid Society is poorly linked to other crisis
services in most communities. It has low visibility as a social service agency, is often
poorly funded, and does not operate on a twenty-four-hour basis in most places.
A close working relationship with a twenty-four-hour crisis service could remedy
this situation. The relative isolation of this agency often results in the Travelers
Aid staff handling suicidal or emotionally upset travelers by themselves, without
the support of crisis specialists who should be available.

International Institute and Other Support. The International Institute and
special refugee groups also help people in crisis related to immigration. The
institute's unique contribution is crisis work with refugees and immigrants who do
not know the local language. Inability to speak a country's language can be the
source of acute crises related to housing, employment, health, welfare, and legal
matters. Institute workers, all of whom speak several languages, assist refugees and
immigrants in these essential life areas.

There is an International Institute in nearly all major metropolitan areas,
where most refugees and immigrants first settle. Health and social service personnel can refer immigrants who are unaware of this service on arrival. The
language crisis is so acute for some immigrants that they may be mistakenly judged
psychotic and taken to a mental hospital, or they may have to rely inappropriately
on their own children for translation. Intervention by a multilingual person is a
critical part of care in such cases.

As is the case with the Travelers Aid Society, this important social service
agency has low visibility in the community and often is not linked adequately with
twenty-four-hour crisis services. Needed linkages may become routine as health
and crisis services become more comprehensive and cosmopolitan (Hoff &
Adamowski, 1998; Rachlis & Kushner, 1994).

The actual and potential crises of immigrants and refugees have become more
visible as ethnic conflict and international tensions have grown. People persecuted
or sought out for protest seek refuge and political asylum in friendly countries with
greater frequency. Cooperation between private and public agencies on behalf of
these people is paramount to avoid unnecessary distress and crisis. In addition to

legal, housing, language, and immediate survival issues, refugees experience the psychological pain of losing their homeland. No matter how we may have been treated, most of us have a strong attachment to our country of birth. Whether this bond is broken voluntarily or by threat to life, we need an opportunity to mourn the loss and find substitutes for what was left behind.

One way that refugees and immigrants cope with their loss is to preserve their customs, art, language, ritual celebrations, and food habits. These practices provide immigrants with the security that comes from association with their familiar cultural heritage. Sensitivity of neighbors and agency personnel to immigrants' cultural values, along with control of their own ethnocentrism, can go a long way in helping refugees feel at home. In contrast, members of host countries need particular sensitivity regarding a practice like female genital mutilation, which some immigrants wish to continue. See Chapter Thirteen regarding this cultural issue and what many groups define as a human rights violation.

Homelessness and Vulnerability to Violence

Some people live in cardboard boxes, ride the subway all night long, or stay in doorways of public buildings until they are asked or ordered by the police to move. Some sleep on steel grates to catch steam heat from below. Some abused women and their children move from shelter to shelter, staying the limit at each because battering does not fit the city's criteria of eligibility for emergency housing; one mother of three finally bought a tent and camped in a city park.

In the early 1990s, there were an estimated three million homeless people in the United States, an increase of 246 percent from 1983, and three or four times that many stay with family and friends (National Coalition for the Homeless, 1998, p. 12). Unless drastic action is taken, this figure will increase to nineteen million by the end of the century. The majority of these people are women and children. Besides having no secure place to stay, homeless people are frequent victims of rape or robbery of their few possessions; homeless youth are often victims of child prostitution; among the elderly homeless, some are disabled, some are deaf or blind, and some have symptoms of Alzheimer's disease. Contrary to popular perception, a good percentage of the homeless hold low-paying jobs that do not provide enough income to pay inflated rental prices. Many are victims of eviction when apartments are converted to condominiums for upwardly mobile, mostly white professionals. At no time since the Great Depression have homeless people represented such a cross-section of a wealthy Western society.

Among industrialized nations, the most visible and the highest numbers of homeless people are in the United States. In fact, as the problem continues unabated, many worry that homelessness will become institutionalized as a permanent feature of social life. Several factors that help explain the apparent intractability of this problem are (1) the growing disparity between rich and poor, (2) the lack of a national health program that includes sufficient coverage for crisis and mental health services, and (3) the continuing bias against the mentally ill and the resulting inadequate transitional housing and support services to prevent homelessness (Hoff, Briar, Knighton, & Van Ry, 1992; Jencks, 1994; Shinn et al., 1998; Weitzman, Knickman, & Shinn, 1992). But the problem is by no means limited to the United States. Worldwide recession and similar bias against the mentally ill occur cross-culturally and in any society where community values are sacrificed in favor of an individualistic paradigm such as the one that dominates in the United States (Bellah, 1986; Luhrmann, 2000). Perhaps most alarming of all is the fact that families with children in the United States now constitute the largest segment of homeless people (Davidhizar & Frank, 1992). For these families, getting to work or school is a maze of buses and subway rides, taking as long as two hours one way, while they await their turn for transfer from temporary housing in a motel to placement in affordable housing that is all too scarce.

Homelessness strips people of their self-respect, denies them their elementary rights as citizens, and blights the future of a nation's greatest resource—children. The crisis of homelessness is dramatized by happenings that took place in San Francisco under the rubric of the Matrix Program. For a number of years, San Francisco law allowed a team of city workers from the police, sanitation, and mental health departments to search out the homeless on the streets. When a homeless person was encountered, he or she was questioned and very likely either arrested or committed involuntarily to a psychiatric facility. If the person was sleeping, the police officer would gently tap the individual, who typically reacted in a startled or frightened manner. It was described as follows: the mental health professional steps in with a "rapid diagnosis of paranoia, or somehow makes the determination that the person may be a danger to him/herself or others and commits said person to a determined observation period in the hospital. As the hapless individual is taken away, all his belongings are trashed by the . . . Sanitation Engineers" (Dean, 1994, p. 3). Under the Matrix Program, a person could be charged with "sleeping in a park at night for lodging." For the sixty-two thousand citations issued in 1994, each carried a fine of $79. Dean (p. 3) compares the Matrix Program with scenarios from World War II:

> Right now, the government of San Francisco is doing things that you think only fascist countries are doing.
>
> Right now, someone who is homeless in San Francisco is being stripped of his/her meager belongings.
>
> Right now, a human being in San Francisco is being caged like a criminal because she/he is homeless.
>
> Right now, Keith McHenry is awaiting trial, which begins on Halloween day, because he chooses to feed the homeless in San Francisco. [McHenry was cited for serving food to the homeless at the United Nations Plaza under auspices of the Food Not Bombs program.]
>
> Right now, there is someone locked in a psych ward in San Francisco because he/she has been "diagnosed as homeless."

Right now, a child in San Francisco is selling his/her body for a meal or shelter.

Right now, in San Francisco, the Matrix program is in effect.

Right now, San Francisco is getting cold.

The victim-blaming practice of attributing homelessness to personal deficits is not supported by research that corrects the methodological flaws of earlier prevalence studies (Link et al., 1994). This study also suggests that the problem is of greater magnitude than has commonly been assumed. The crisis of homelessness is due primarily to the severe cuts in federal funds to build or rehabilitate low-income housing and to the overpriced real estate market that is generally free of obligation to include low-income and moderate-income housing in their speculative ventures. Haphazard policies and bureaucratic ineptness are also responsible. As Jonathan Kozol (1988) relates from his months with homeless people in one of New York's welfare hotels, the city spends $1,900 per month for a family of four, thus supporting enormous profits for a modernized poorhouse. But Kozol's informants wondered why so much money was spent on such hotels rather than designated for rent support in regular housing.

These problems are all exacerbated in the case of the homeless mentally ill, some of whom also have prison records. These homeless people are victims of failed deinstitutionalization programs and inadequate community planning (Cella, Besancon, & Zipple, 1997; Farrell & Deeds, 1997; Johnson, 1990; Kaplan, 2000; Scheper-Hughes & Lovell, 1986; Walker, 1998).

It would seem a foregone conclusion that what homeless people need is a home—a hallmark of the American dream. Yet despite numerous references to the crisis of affordable housing in major U.S. cities, the response to this crisis is essentially reactionary, individualistic, and biomedically focused, rather than being recognized as primarily a social problem demanding a policy response in accord with its social character. Lyon-Callo's (1998) ethnographic exploration of funding concerns dramatically illustrates this point. From his ten years of work and field study in homeless shelters, Lyon-Callo uncovered a funding focus on tertiary-level sheltering, case management, and "treatment" (that is, changing or reforming) of the "disordered" homeless harbored there. This funding emphasis suppressed efforts to change the dynamics of inequality around jobs and housing that fuels homelessness. Despite rhetoric from public officials regarding the homelessness problem, coalitions of shelter workers and homeless persons themselves who focused on obtaining stable homes were thwarted by governmental and nongovernmental funders who threatened to withdraw financial support if staff failed to focus on treatment as opposed to activity addressing the roots of the problem. Progress on this issue demands a both-and, not an either-or, approach, particularly since some psychiatric facilities discharge mental patients to these shelters for lack of other appropriate resources for persons needing continuing mental health service.

What do we do for people who have no place to sleep or who are at risk of dying from exposure to the elements in spite of affluence all around them in the richest country in the world? People often react with embarrassment and discomfort to a homeless person who appears on a doorstep or begs for spare change. But regardless of how charitably people respond to individual appeals for help, the crisis of homelessness in a humane, democratic society entails more than goodwill or charity. Although there is still a tendency to blame the victim, as Ryan's classic book (1971) expounds, people do not choose to be poor or homeless.

One of the most tragic examples of the failure to address the systemic problems fueling homelessness is the 1999 deaths of six firefighters in Worcester, Massachusetts, resulting from their attempt to rescue a homeless couple in an abandoned warehouse; firefighters from across the nation and abroad attended the funerals of these fallen heroes. The homeless young couple, expecting a child, were charged with manslaughter and prosecuted because they failed to report the fire that started from their tipped-over candle during a domestic fight. As emphasized throughout this book, a crisis of social origin demands a social response. In this tragic case, once again, the focus was on individual rather than on the social dimensions of the crisis. In sum, the interrelated social, cultural, and economic factors—along with discrimination based on race, sex, and age—that precipitate crises of homelessness (and in this case, the death of six firefighters in the prime of life) must be addressed in a comprehensive proactive manner.

A hopeful and empowering example of moving beyond shelter and stopgap measures is the first federally funded farm (in Cape Cod, Massachusetts) to be staffed by residents who have histories of chronic homelessness. Each will have a private room with shared dining and bathroom facilities—reminiscent of the single room occupancy (SROs) living quarters that were plentiful in most cities before gentrification and the reduction of government housing assistance. Residents must work thirty-five hours per week at the farm or in neighboring businesses, pay about 25 percent of their income to rent, commit to teaching newly acquired skills to at least one new arrival, try to get a high school diploma if they do not have one, and abide by the strict rules of no alcohol or drugs (Gaines, 2000).

We should support individual and communal efforts like this and those of Moshe Dean and others who write for and sell *Spare Change*. In Boston and New England, this newspaper is published by and for homeless people. Individuals who sell the paper for $1 are provided a means for some meager income. There is an international association of "street" newspapers, dedicated to advocacy and social change around this global problem. Such efforts, however, will never be sufficient to avoid further crises of homelessness without a change in public policies affecting housing (see Crisis Paradigm, Box 3, right circle).

Summary

To be happy, we need some meaningful work to support ourselves and a secure place to live. Many people are threatened with the loss of these basic necessities—and for refugees, even their homeland. Opportunities to assist people in crisis because of occupational or housing loss cross the social service and health care landscape. Helping people at these initial crisis points can make an enormous difference in the final outcomes of these transition states. Removing the socioeconomic roots of crises like unemployment and homelessness is urgent public business.

References

Albelda, R. (1999, May 24). Now we know: "Work first" hasn't worked. *Boston Globe,* p. A13.

Amnesty International. (2000, Summer). Pass the refugee protection act. *Amnesty International,* p. 21.

Armer, J. M. (1993). Elderly relocation to a congregate setting: Factors influencing adjustment. *Issues in Mental Health Nursing, 14*(2), 157–172.

Aubry, J. (1994, March 5). Exiled to a forsaken place. *Ottawa Citizen,* pp. 1, B1–B6.

Barnett, R. C., & Rivers, C. (1998). *She works/he works: How two-income families are happy, healthy, and thriving.* Cambridge, MA: Harvard University Press.

Bellah, R. (1986). *Habits of the heart: Individualism and commitment in American life.* New York: HarperCollins.

Caplan, G. (1964). *Principles of preventive psychiatry.* New York: Basic Books.

Cella, E. P., Besancon, V., & Zipple, A. M. (1997). Expanding the role of clubhouses: Guidelines for establishing a system of integrated day services. *Psychiatric Rehabilitation Journal, 21*(1), 10–15.

Crittenden, A. (2001). *The price of motherhood: Why the most important job in the world is still the least valued.* New York: Metropolitan Books.

Davidhizar, R. & Frank, B. (1992). Understanding the physical and psychosocial stressors of the child who is homeless. *Pediatric Nursing, 18*(6), 559–562.

Dean, M. (1994). The beginnings of genocide, or San Francisco's homeless living under the yoke of the Matrix Program. *Spare Change, 3*(7), 3.

Desmond, A. M. (1994). Adolescent pregnancy in the United States: Not a minority issue. *Health Care for Women International, 15*(4), 325–332.

Dujon, D., & Withorn, A. (Eds.). (1996). *For crying out loud: Women's poverty in the United States.* Boston: South End Press.

Economic Report of the President Transmitted to the Congress. (2000, February 1). Washington, DC: U.S. Government Printing Office.

Facione, N. C. (1994). Role overload and health: The married mother in the waged labor force. *Health Care for Women International, 15*(2), 157–167.

Farrell, S. P., & Deeds, E. S. (1997). The clubhouse model as exemplar. *Journal of Psychosocial Nursing, 35*(1), 27–34.

Foner, N. (1994). *The caregiving dilemma: Work in an American nursing home.* Berkeley: University of California Press.

Gaines, J. (2000, January 3). Home grown: Farm for homeless planned on Cape. *Boston Globe,* pp. A1, B5.

Gans, H. J. (1962). *The urban villagers.* New York: Free Press.

Greene, J. M., Ennett, S. T., & Ringwalt, C. L. (1997). Substance use among runaway and homeless youth in three national samples. *American Journal of Public Health, 87*(2), 229–235.

Grunwald, M. (1998, February 27). Wyoming cuts rolls by putting some heart into welfare reform. *Boston Globe,* pp. A1, A12.

Hansell, N. (1976). *The person in distress.* New York: Human Sciences Press.

Hoff, L. A., & Adamowski, K. (1998). *Creating excellence in crisis care: A guide to effective training and program designs.* San Francisco: Jossey-Bass.

Hoff, M. D., Briar, K. H., Knighton, K., & Van Ry, A. (1992). To survive and to thrive: Integrating services for the homeless mentally ill. *Journal of Sociology and Social Welfare, 29*(4), 235–252.

Illich, I. (1976). *Limits to medicine.* Harmondsworth, England: Penguin Books.

Jackson, D. Z. (1997, February 26). The wrong message on au pairs. *Boston Globe,* p. A19.

Jencks, C. (1994). *The homeless.* Cambridge, MA: Harvard University Press.

Johnson, A. B. (1990). *Out of bedlam: The truth about deinstitutionalization.* New York: Basic Books.

Kanter, R. M. (1977). *Men and women of the corporation.* New York: Basis Books.

Kaplan, F. (2000, August 23). For mentally ill, jail means care. *Boston Globe,* pp. A1, A8.

Kavanagh, K. J. (1988). The cost of caring: Nursing on a psychiatric intensive care unit. *Human Organization, 47*(3), 242–251.

Kozol, J. (1988), *Rachel and her children: Homeless families in America.* New York: Crown.

Kozol, J. (2000). *Ordinary resurrections: Children in the years of hope.* New York: Crown.

Kuttner, R. (2000, February 2). The hidden failure of welfare reform. *Boston Sunday Globe,* p. C7.

Lewis, D. E. (2000, May 9). Drive launched to ensure equal pay. *Boston Globe,* p. D5.

Link, B. G., Susser, E., Stueve, A., Phelan, J., Moore, R. E., & Struening, E. (1994). Lifetime and five-year prevalence of homelessness in the United States. *American Journal of Public Health, 84*(12), 1907–1912.

Lipson, J., & Miller, S. (1994). Changing roles of Afghan refugee women in the United States. *Health Care for Women International, 15*(3), 171–180.

Luhrmann, T. M. (2000). *Of two minds: The growing disorder in American psychiatry.* New York: Knopf.

Lyon-Callo, V. (1998). Constraining responses to homelessness: An ethnographic exploration of the impact of funding concerns on resistance. *Human Organization, 57*(1), 1–20.

Meckler, L. (1999, March 11). Train welfare mothers, study urges. *Boston Globe,* p. A20.

Medoff, P., & Sklar, H. (1994). *Streets of hope: The fall and rise of an urban neighborhood.* Boston: South End Press.

Mollison, A. (1993, June 27). Unpaid work by homemakers under scrutiny. *St. Paul Pioneer Press,* p. 15A.

Morrison, A. M., White, R. P., & Van Velsor, E. (1987). Executive women: Substance plus style. *Psychology Today, 21*(8), 18–27.

National Coalition for the Homeless. (1998). Report documents dramatic rise in homelessness. *Spare Change,* p. 12.

Pearce, D., & McAdoo, H. (1982). *Women and children: Alone and in poverty.* Washington, DC: National Advisory Council on Economic Opportunity.

Perese, E. F. (1997). Unmet needs of persons with chronic mental illnesses: Relationship to their adaptation to community living. *Issues in Mental Health Nursing, 18*(1), 19–34.

Phelan, J., Schwartz, J. E., Bromet, E. J., Dew, M. A., Parkinson, D. K., Schulberg, H. C., Duran, L. O., Blane, H., & Curtis, E. C. (1991). Work stress, family stress, and depression in professional and managerial employees. *Psychological Medicine, 21*(4), 999–1012.

Phillips, S. P., & Schneider, M. S. (1993). Sexual harassment of female doctors by patients. *New England Journal of Medicine, 329*(26), 1936–1939.

Rachlis, M., & Kushner, C. (1994). *Strong medicine: How to save Canada's health care system.* Toronto: HarperCollins.

Radin, C. A. (2000, August 20). Foreign policy plays a top role in U.S. decisions on refugees. *Boston Globe,* p. A24.

Reverby, S. (1987). *Ordered to care.* Cambridge: Cambridge University Press.

Ryan, W. (1971). *Blaming the victim.* New York: Vintage Books.

Scheper-Hughes, N., & Lovell, A. M. (1986). Breaking the circuit of social control: Lessons in public psychiatry from Italy and Franco Basaglia. *Social Science and Medicine, 23*(2), 159–178.

Schmidt, L., Weisner, C., & Wiley, J. (1998). Substance abuse and the course of welfare dependency. *American Journal of Public Health, 88*(11), 1616–1622.

Schor, J. B. (1993). *The overworked American: The unexpected decline of leisure.* New York: Basic Books.

Seager, J., & Olson, A. (1986). *Women in the world: An international atlas.* New York: Simon & Schuster.

Shinn, M., Weitzman, B. D., Stojanovic, D., Knickman, J. R., Jimenez, L., Duchon, L., James, S., & Drantz, D. H. (1998). Predictors of homelessness among families in New York City: From shelter request to housing stability. *American Journal of Public Health, 88*(11), 1651–1657.

Sidel, R. (1996). *Women and children last: The plight of poor women in affluent America.* New York: Penguin Books.

Singular, S. (1983). Moving on. *Psychology Today, 17,* 40–47.

Sommers, T., & Shields, L. (1987). *Women take care: The consequences of caregiving in today's society.* Gainesville, FL: Triad.

Sparks, A. (1990). *The mind of South Africa: The story of the rise and fall of apartheid.* London: Mandarin.

U.S. Bureau of the Census. (2000, December 29). Available at: http://www.census.gov/hhes/income/4person.html.

Walker, C. (1998). Homeless people and mental health: A nursing concern. *American Journal of Nursing, 98*(11), 26–32.

Waring, M. (1990). *If women counted: A new feminist economics.* San Francisco: Harper San Francisco.

Weitzman, B. C., Knickman, J. R., & Shinn, M. (1992). Predictors of shelter use among low-income families: Psychiatric history, substance abuse, and victimization. *American Journal of Public Health, 82*(11), 1547–1550.

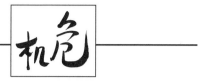

CHAPTER THIRTEEN

STRESS AND CHANGE
DURING LIFE PASSAGES

How are the terms *transition* or *passage* and *status* and *role change* related? What do they mean for people in crisis? Transition refers to passage or change from one place or stage of development to another. Status designates the place of individuals and groups with respect to their prestige, rights, obligations, power, and authority within a society. People are evaluated socially by their contribution to the common good and by other criteria such as birth, marital alliance, sex, race, age, sexual identity, wealth, and power. One's status is related to but different from one's *role:* status refers to *who* a person is, whereas role refers to *what* a person is expected to *do* within a given sociocultural milieu (Gil & Gil, 1987; Zelditch, 1968, p. 251).

What do these social concepts have to do with people in crisis in the clinical sense? It is, after all, a normal part of human life to grow and develop through childhood, adolescence, middle age, and old age to death. It is also common to marry, give birth, and lose one's spouse. Anthropologists and psychoanalysts for years have referred to these transition states as *life crises* (Erikson, 1963; Freud, 1950; Kimball, 1909/1960). There is a difference, however, in the anthropological concept of life crisis and its common usage by crisis intervention clinicians, even though, as Golan (1981, p. 7) states, there is something in common between the two conceptions of high-stress situations. In anthropology, life crisis refers to a highly significant, expectable event or phase in the life cycle that marks one's passage to a new social status, with accompanying changes in rights and duties. Traditionally, such status changes are accompanied by rituals (such as puberty and marriage rites) designed to assist the individual in fulfilling new role expectations and to buffer the stress associated with these critical, though normal, life events. In traditional societies, families and the entire community, led by "ritual experts," are intensely involved in the life passages of individual community members. This *anthropological* concept of life crisis corresponds roughly to the anticipated crises discussed in the clinical literature on crisis (see "The Origins of Crisis" in Chapter Two).

Crisis in its *clinical* meaning flows from the tradition of Caplan (1964) and others, who emphasize the sudden onset and brief duration of acute emotional upsets in response to identifiable traumatic events. In this sense, adolescence, marriage, giving birth, and entering middle age are *not* crises except in extraordinary circumstances, such as when the bridegroom fails to show up or the expected infant is stillborn—unanticipated traumatic events that accompany the transition. Transition states are critical life phases, not necessarily traumatic, but with the *potential* for activating an *acute emotional upset* in the clinical sense. They are *turning points*, social and psychological processes involving the challenge of successfully completing social, developmental, and instrumental tasks—for example,

- Changing social role, such as single to married
- Changing image of self, such as young to middle aged, healthy to sick
- Gathering material resources to support a new family member

As turning points in the developmental process, these life crises fit the classic definition of crisis as a period of both danger and opportunity. They also highlight the importance of the social, cultural, and material resources necessary for individuals to avoid acute emotional upset. Another connection between the anthropological and clinical definitions of crisis is the fact that individuals in acute emotional upset do not exist in a social vacuum; they are members of cultural communities. People in crisis are therefore influenced by social expectations of how to behave and by values guiding their interpretation of expected and unexpected life events, factors that figure strongly in the way one resolves a particular emotional crisis.

Thus, if it is unclear *who* a person is, *what* the person is expected to do, or *how* the person fits into familiar social arrangements based on cultural values, status or role ambiguity is activated. Status and role ambiguity can create so much stress that a person with conflicting or changed roles may withdraw from social interaction or may try to change the social structure to redefine the anxiety-provoking statuses (Douglas, 1966; Weiss, 1976). For example,

- If pregnant teenage girls sense that they are expected to drop out of high school, they are more likely to be poorly educated, unemployed, and dependent on welfare and to marry early, which enhances their potential for future crises.
- If widowed people sense that they are a threat to social groups of married people, they may feel cut off from social support and thereby increase their risk of emotional crisis around traumatic events.

- If children of parents feuding about divorce are not allowed to see their grand-parents, they may ask, Who is my family? The deprived grandparent may ask, What have I done wrong?

Rites of Passage: Traditional and Contemporary

An important means of reducing the stress and minimizing the chaos associated with such role ambiguity is the constructive use of ritual. One of the most dramatic differences between traditional and urban or industrialized societies is the relative importance of ritual and the separation between the sacred and the profane. With an increase in industrialization comes a corresponding increase in secularization and a decrease in sacred ceremonialism. In his classic work, *Rites of Passage,* van Gennep (1909/1960, p. 11) distinguished three phases in the ceremonies associated with an individual's life crises: rites of separation (prominent in funeral ceremonies), rites of transition (important in initiation and pregnancy), and rites of incorporation (prominent in marriage). A complete schema of rites of passage theoretically includes all three phases. For example, a widow is *separated* from her husband by death; she occupies a *liminal* (transitional) status for a time, and finally is *reincorporated* into a new marriage relationship (Goody, 1962).

These rites protect the individual during the hazardous process of life passages, times considered potentially dangerous to the person if not supported by the community. Ritual thus makes public what is private, makes social what is personal, and gives the individual new knowledge and strength (LaFontaine, 1977; Turner, 1967, p. 50). For example,

- A person who loses a loved one needs a public occasion to mourn.
- A couple who are intimate and cohabiting desire social approval (often through marriage).
- A dying person who is anointed has new knowledge of the imminence of death and greater strength to accept death.
- A divorced person needs community support following a failed marriage—in short, a ritual for public recognition and acceptance of a new role.

Rites of passage are not developed to the same extent by all societies (Fried & Fried, 1980). Until recently, it was generally assumed that rites of passage are relatively unimportant in modern societies: public and private spheres of activity and various social roles (such as worker, parent, or political leader) are more clearly separated than in traditional societies and hence in less need of ritual specification. However, there is no evidence that people in a secular urban world have less need for ritualized expression during transition states (Kimball, 1909/1960, pp. xvi–xvii). The modern discarding of ritual can be understood in part as a move toward greater freedom of the individual. Ritual can be a powerful mechanism for maintaining the status quo in traditional and contemporary societies (Durkheim, 1915); less ritual implies more personal freedom. Thus, while some rituals protect the individual during stressful transitions, they have a social purpose as well. For example, the traditional Samburu of Kenya, a polygynous gerontocracy (society ruled by elders) kept young men in a marginal position relative to the total society and forbade them to marry until around age thirty, an institution known as *moranhood*. This ritual preserved the concentration of power and wives among the older men (Hoff, 1978; Spencer, 1973). A contemporary negative ritual is the heavy drinking—hazing—associated with admission to college campus clubs.

The practice of hazing has come under increasing scrutiny over past decades. Many states have passed antihazing legislation. In Massachusetts, for example, the law forbids any dangerous initiation activities, requires pledges to be informed of the law, and specifies punishment of violators or those who fail to report hazing. These laws were based on a premise similar to one in child abuse dynamics: if one is abused, one learns to abuse others. It appears that this negative rite of passage has moved from fraternity houses to the football field and hockey arenas, where demonstrating team spirit often involves violence. And despite U.S. college campus efforts to control the purchase and use of alcohol, binge drinking is indulged in by thousands of young people. A 1997 survey of 113 colleges and universities revealed that 52.3 percent of students say they drink to get drunk (Daley, 1998; Kelly, 1999). In a contemporary twist on traditional rites of passage, these young people (not unlike their Samburu brothers or Somali sisters) feel pressured to drink in order to "belong" in a new environment without the usual supports of family and neighborhood. Wherever these destructive rituals occur, students have poorer grades, reduced career motivation, and increased dropout rates—all challenges for school and parents' groups to create positive rituals for students under stress, who have a powerful need to belong.

Another ritual under scrutiny is female genital mutilation, affecting an estimated 100 to 136 million women and girls, most in African, Far Eastern, and Middle Eastern countries. Sometimes referred to as female circumcision, unlike male circumcision, the operation (categorized in four types) damages or destroys a woman's normal sexual response and can cause life-threatening physical complications. The World Health Organization has declared the ritual a harmful practice and a human rights violation and urges abolishing it (World Health Organization, 1994). Novelist Alice Walker's fictionalized account (1992), *Possessing the Secret of Joy*, has made the practice and its context of gender-based oppression widely visible in the Western world. Canada and the United States have declared the practice illegal (Affara, 2000). The Nigerian Nurses and Midwives Association, Somali immigrant physicians, and other groups worldwide advocate for elimination of the practice and the education of health professionals in how to deal sensitively with women presenting their daughters for the ritual in Western medical settings. However, as with teen pregnancy and similar issues, this culturally embedded practice is complex, controversial, and intricately tied to socioeconomic and educational equity for women worldwide (Boddy, 1998; Ngugi, 1965).

CASE EXAMPLE: MARRIAGE AMONG THE SAMBURU

The social value imbuing everything in Samburu society is called *nkanyit*. This keystone of Samburu morality includes notions of respect, honor, shame, duty, politeness, avoidance, and decency, with the overriding emphasis on respect. A woman is taught to respect, fear, and avoid the elders from an early age. Her training induces her to accept the difficulties of marriage to an elder two to three times older than she, a situation that makes the marital strains more understandable. As in most societies, girls and women are valued less than boys and men; all girls are brought up with the idea of being good wives, an investment for their kin and husbands.

After marriage, a woman rarely goes home again, as this would endanger the tenuous stability of the marriage even more. Samburu women learn very early their inevitable lot of subordination and that the reputation of the clan hinges on their good behavior, not unlike the sexual double standard elsewhere. These notions are reinforced through the marriage ritual. Spencer characterizes the marriage ritual as a form of "brainwashing" and marriage for the average woman as *the* crisis of her life (Hoff, 1978; Spencer, 1973).

CASE EXAMPLE: MARRIAGE FOR CONTEMPORARY NORTH AMERICAN WOMEN

Unlike their Samburu sisters, many contemporary women view marriage and especially the ritual of the wedding day as high points in their lives. Like their Samburu sisters, however, many girls and women today still view themselves as failures if they cannot marry and retain a husband. Caught up in the emotional high of the wedding ritual, with dreams of "living happily ever after," the average bride is unconscious of the social significance of the ritual of being "given away" by her father and relinquishing her own name to assume that of her husband (Chapman & Gates, 1977). Many women willingly interrupt or delay careers to support their families through unpaid and devalued household work. Many are happy and secure in their role and testify that their dreams have come true. Millions, however, are battered, as the marriage license seems to have been transformed for some into a "hitting license" (Straus, Gelles, & Steinmetz, 1980); they feel trapped and become convenient objects of violence (Dobash & Dobash, 1979; Hoff, 1990). Or they become "displaced homemakers" (Jacobs, 1979). Many women are left behind for younger women, especially during middle age, when women are considered "over the hill" whereas men become more "distinguished." Often this occurs after women have sacrificed education and career opportunities in order to fulfill the social expectation of building a stable home (see Hyman & Rome, 1996). Among women heading households alone, a large percentage are poor.

These examples suggest that ritual serves to maintain society or various subgroups in a state of traditional equilibrium, with each person behaving according to accepted roles. As discussed in earlier chapters, however, maintaining traditional social roles, often reinforced through the negative use of ritual, can exact a considerable price from certain individuals—for example, more heart disease and suicides for men, social isolation or death for adolescents by suicide or manslaughter, and battering or poverty for women. The case examples also illustrate a continuum between traditional and contemporary rites of passage and suggest that people in all times and places need ritual. But what kinds of rituals are needed, and under what circumstances should they take place? How can ritual be helpful for the individual in transition as well as for society?

Ritual holds a paradoxical place in a secularized society. On the one hand, it is viewed as a sign of an earlier stage of social evolution (Moore, 1992). On the other hand, certain rituals are retained without critical examination of their expression in contemporary life. In modern life, three approaches to ritual are observed: (1) ritual is often denied any relevance; (2) some of its most oppressive and destructive aspects for individuals remain from ancient tradition or are recycled to include the abuse of alcohol, guns, or cars and medical technology to prolong life; (3) when ritual is observed, it is highly individualized, as in the rite of psychotherapy, in which the fifty-minute session and other practices are observed. Such rituals are complemented by medicalization and its focus on individuals rather than groups in modern urban societies.

These interpretations of ritual, however, are in the process of change. Meaningless and destructive rituals are being dropped entirely or are being questioned. For example, many women today retain their last names after marriage, and *both* parents of the bride *and* groom (rather than only the father of the bride) participate in the marriage ceremony. Similarly, with cultural awareness, barbaric rituals, oppression, and violence are no longer seen as the province of any one society, traditional or modern.

Our task as crisis workers is to consider the place of ritual during challenging turning points of life, particularly as it relates to crisis prevention. Whether critical life passages also become occasions of emotional crisis will depend on

1. What the individual does to prepare for anticipated transitions
2. The nature and extent of social support available to the individual during turning points
3. The occurrence of unanticipated hazardous events (such as fire, accident, illness, or loss of job) during transitional phases of life, when vulnerability is often greater
4. Our creativity as crisis workers in helping individuals and families develop positive contemporary rites of passage where there are few or none

Traditional and contemporary rites of passage are compared and the continuity between them illustrated in Table 13.1. The successful passage of individuals through critical stages in the developmental process depends on a combination of personal and social factors (Panchuck, 1994). Transition states highlight the dynamic relationship between the individual, family, and society (see "Privacy, Intimacy, Community" in Chapter Five). For example, adolescents who choose marriage or parenthood even though they are not ready for those responsibilities may become liabilities to society and may face more complex problems during

TABLE 13.1. RITES OF PASSAGE IN COMPARATIVE PERSPECTIVE.

Life Passage	Traditional Rites*	Contemporary North American Rites	
		Unexamined or Questionable	Newly Emerging or Suggested
Birth	Attended by family and/or midwife, birth occurs in natural squatting position Death risk is high if there are complications	Medicalized birth: pubic shaving, ultrasound, drugs, episiotomy or forceps, horizontal position Absence of family and friends unless specially arranged Death risk in the U.S. is high among developed countries	Natural childbirth aided by husband's or friends' coaching in home or birthing center, attended by midwife with backup medical care for complications Death risk is low when attended by properly trained midwife, and medical backup is available for special cases
Adolescence	Puberty rites	Hazing and binge drinking on college campuses Religious rites of confirmation and Bar and Bat Mitzvah[†] Obtaining driver's licenses[†]	Supervised college initiation Support and education groups in high schools, churches, and colleges, such as those concerning menstruation, sexuality, driving responsibly without drinking, and parenthood Relating traditional religious rites to modern life, for example, Mikvah in Judaism
Intimate relationships: beginnings and endings	Betrothal and marriage rites; required remarriage of widow; or remarriage may be forbidden	Bridal showers; stag parties[†] Traditional marriage rites	Egalitarian marriage ceremony and contract Consciousness-raising groups for men and women regarding traditional versus egalitarian male and female roles Divorce ceremonies Support groups for the divorced or for parents without partners
Middle age	Not generally ritualized; general increase in social value and respect by community; postmenopausal women may be regarded as asexual	Labeling of menopause as "illness"; individual psychotherapy and drugs for depression; estrogen replacement therapy for women Men past youth become more "distinguished"; women are often devalued further	Education and peer support groups for menopausal women Support groups for couples to redefine marriage (or other committed) relationship to avoid "empty nest" and other midlife crises

TABLE 13.1. RITES OF PASSAGE IN COMPARATIVE PERSPECTIVE. (*continued*)

Life Passage	Traditional Rites*	Contemporary North American Rites	
		Unexamined or Questionable	Newly Emerging or Suggested
Old age	Not generally ritualized; general increase in social value and respect by family and community Infirm elderly are cared for by family	Forced retirement Institutional placement for care	Economic and social policies to support care of elderly at home; respite services for caretakers Senior citizen programs such as part-time or shared jobs Volunteer work
Death	Usually elaborate, extended rituals involving family and entire community	80 percent die in institutions with restricted family involvement Mortician has become the main "ritual expert" Children often barred from death and burial rituals Prescription of tranquilizers to survivors after death of a loved one	Social support to aid in grief work Hospice care for the dying; support for family to care for dying member at home Support groups for cancer patients Inclusion of children in death and burial rituals Enhancement of funeral director's role to assist with grief work Widow to Widow and other self-help groups for survivors

*These rites vary widely among societies. No attempt is made to summarize them here; they are cited to illustrate continuity with modern practice. For an introduction to traditional transition rituals and further references, see Fried and Fried (1980).

†These rites are not always used to their greatest positive potential.

later stages of development. But the reason they are personally unfit might be traced to inadequate support from adults and to the complex social, economic, and cultural factors that affect adolescents and their families (Leach, 1994). Some legislators and schools favor requiring psychoeducation courses as a condition for a marriage license. Many church groups have required such courses for decades; clergy say that marriage is religion's turf, not the government's (Russo, 1997). These contemporary rituals are an attempt to increase marital happiness and prevent the often negative results of divorce, especially for children.

The role of individuals and families during transition states demands the successful completion of several tasks. For instance, among the traditional LoDagaa in Ghana (Goody, 1962), widows are metaphorically buried by being dressed in premarital *fibers* to signify that they are again adolescents without husbands. They are also fed, as a symbolic last supper of husband and wife and as a test of the widow's possible complicity in her husband's death. The widow's acceptance of food is equivalent to an oath to the ancestors of her innocence. The widow cooks porridge and flicks some on her husband's shrine to show that she has not committed adultery. These rituals are dramatic in that they involve not only the individual and the family but also the entire community.

In contrast, in contemporary society there is the stereotype of the widow who ritually sets the table every night for her dead husband. A possible reason for this behavior may be that the widow had no social, public occasion to cook her "last supper." She lacks the necessary community support to separate from her previous role, abandon her private illusion that her husband is still alive, and proceed to a new role without her husband. This example illustrates the tremendous importance of moving beyond the individual and the family to such social creations as Widow to Widow clubs, a contemporary substitute for the elaborate death rituals of traditional societies (see Lopata, 1995).

Golan (1981, pp. 21–22) outlines the specific tasks to be accomplished by individuals and families during transition states. Her division of "material-arrangemental" tasks (such as exploring resources and choices in the new role) and "psychosocial" or "affective tasks" (such as dealing with feelings of loss and longing for the past) corresponds to the emotional, cognitive, and behavioral steps in effective crisis coping discussed in Chapter Four. However, the effectiveness of these individual and family coping strategies greatly depends on the social and cultural setting. If a society is poor in constructive ritual, if familiar and secure routines and supports in an old role are not replaced, and if there is little awareness of the need for social support, even the strongest individuals may be unnecessarily scarred during passage through life's developmental stages. The challenge of moving on to a new stage of development or role becomes a threat: "Will I succeed or fail?" "What will people think if I fail?" "No, I don't think I can face having this baby—not without the help of its father." "Life just isn't worth living if I can't keep on working. I'm worth more dead than alive."

Keeping in mind the traditional and contemporary rites of passage and their relationship to stress and crisis in modern society, we can discuss the hazards and opportunities of these normal passages from birth to death. During these passages, crisis counselors and health and mental health professionals can be thought of as contemporary "ritual experts" (see Crisis Paradigm, Box 3, lower circle).

Birth and Parenthood

Parenthood places continual demands on a person from the time of conception until at least the child's eighteenth birthday. Parents must adjust to include an additional member in their family group. Such adjustment is especially difficult for first-time parents, even when they assume the role of parenthood willingly and regard their children as a welcome responsibility. The unique pleasure and challenge of bearing and nurturing a child through childhood into adult life usually outweighs the ordinary problems of parenthood.

Some parents fall into their role unwillingly or use it to escape less tolerable roles. Consider, for example, the adolescent who seeks relief from a disturbed family home and uses pregnancy as an avenue of escape or the woman who may have more children than she can properly care for emotionally and physically. Some women still view themselves as having no other significant role than that of mother and wife. Others do not limit their pregnancies because of religious beliefs forbidding artificial contraception. Still others lack the knowledge and means to limit their pregnancies. Unwanted children and their parents are more crisis prone than others. Emotional, social, and material poverty are important contributors to their crisis vulnerability (see McKenry & Price, 2000).

All parents, whether or not their children were wanted, are under stress and strain in their parental role. Parenthood requires a constant giving of self. Except for the joy of self-fulfillment and watching a child grow and develop, the parent-child relationship is essentially nonreciprocal. Infants, toddlers, and young children need continuous care and supervision. In their natural state of dependency, they give only the needy love of a child who says, in effect, "I am helpless without you, take care of me, protect me."

Some children, in fact, not only are dependent and needy but also for various reasons are a source of great distress and grief to their parents. Their difficult behaviors, for example, trouble at school or drug abuse, often signal trouble in the parents' marriage or in the entire family system. Sometimes parents try to deal with these troubles by themselves, struggling for a long time with whatever resources they have. Often they are ashamed to acknowledge that there is a problem with the child. They view any problem as a reflection of their own failure. Still other parents may not have access to child and family resources for help, either because the resources do not exist or because they cannot afford them. Religion professor Cornell West and economist Sylvia Ann Hewlett (1999) have produced a manifesto, *The War Against Parents*, to bridge the race, class, and gender divide in the "family values–government handout" debate.

Chronic problems of parenthood often persist until a crisis occurs and finally forces parents to seek outside help. Common examples of ongoing problems are a child's getting into trouble with the law, running away from home, becoming pregnant during adolescence, truancy, being expelled from school, or making a suicide attempt.

Parents usually seem surprised when these problems occur, but evaluation of the whole family often reveals signs of trouble that were formerly unobserved or ignored. Teachers, recreation directors, pastors, truant officers, and guidance counselors who are sensitive to the needs of children and adolescents can help prevent some of these crises. They should urge parents to participate in a family counseling program *early*, at the first sign of a problem. It is important for counselors and parents to keep in mind that even if preventive programs are lacking, it is never too late to act. An acute crisis situation provides, once again, the opportunity for parents and child to move in the direction of growth and development and for the parents to fulfill their needs for generativity.

Common Crisis Points for Parents

There are several common points of crisis for parents.

Death of a Child. Crisis often occurs after the death of a child, not only because of the parents' acute loss but also because the death requires parents to reorder their expectations about the normal progression of life to death—that parents usually precede their children in death. Thus, the loss of a child (including an adult child) is like no other death experience. Some claim it is felt more acutely than loss of a spouse. It is also keenly painful to accept the fact that death has cut off the child's passage through life. Besides being a profound loss, death of a child threatens the parents' perception of parenthood and the normal life cycle (Cacace & Williamson. 1996; Covington & Theut, 1993; Walsh & McGoldrick, 1991).

The sudden death of infants is known as *crib death*. The exact cause of these deaths is still unknown, hence the medical designation—sudden infant death syndrome (SIDS). With no warning signs, parents or a baby-sitter will find the infant dead in its crib. They bring the infant to the hospital emergency department in a desperate, futile hope of reviving it. The parents or caregiver have fears and guilt that they may somehow have caused the death. The fact that emergency service staff may seem suspicious or appear to blame the parents complicates this crisis. Indeed, the emergency staff must rule out the possibility of child battering, which they cannot do without examination.

Whether or not the child was battered, emergency personnel should withhold judgment. Parents in either case are in crisis and need understanding and support. Those in crisis over SIDS should be offered the opportunity to express their grief in private and with the support of a nurse. Hospital chaplains can often assist during this time and should be called in accordance with the parents' wishes. Parents should also be given information about sleeping position and self-help groups of other parents whose infants died suddenly in their cribs.

Until the fifty-year rate increase in SIDS was closely examined, it had been widely assumed that the exact cause of these deaths was unknown. Now Hogberg & Bergstrom's epidemiological and historical research (2000) in Sweden and other Western countries has uncovered the *prone* (lying on the stomach) sleeping position as the missing risk factor in all previous research aimed at finding a cause. It turns out that the fifty-year rise in SIDS rates corresponded with the widespread medical advice against the *supine* position (infant lying face up) to prevent swallowing vomitus or the turned-from-side-to-side position—advice popularized by Dr. Spock's and other baby books in the 1960s, 1970s, and 1980s. With the drop in SIDS rates in the mid-1990s, after a gradual shift from prone to supine positions, the study authors refer to SIDS as an "iatrogenic" tragedy, in showing that the misdirected infant care advice was targeted to and accepted by whole populations.

The most widely known and used group for parents whose infants have died is the Sudden Infant Death Syndrome Foundation. This is a national organization with chapters in all states and major cities. The program includes support from other parents, counseling from maternal-child nurse specialists, education through films, and a speakers' bureau with medical and lay experts on the topic. Education should include information about sleeping position, preferably supine.

The following case example illustrates the crisis of SIDS for parents and shows how negative outcomes of this crisis might have been avoided through crisis intervention by the pediatrician and others.

CASE EXAMPLE: LORRAINE

I can't begin to tell you what my life was like before Doris at our counseling center helped me. Six months ago, my second child died from crib death. She was two months old. When Deborah stopped breathing at home, I called the rescue squad. They resuscitated her and took her to the hospital. Deborah was kept in the intensive care unit for two months. Finally, the hospital and doctor insisted that we take her home. When we did, she died the very same day. I was completely grief stricken, especially since I am forty-one years old and had waited so long to have a second child. Our other child, David, is seven. I just couldn't accept the fact that Deborah was dead. My husband and the doctors kept telling me to face reality, but I kept insisting on an answer from the pediatrician as to why Deborah had died. I began having chest pains and problems breathing. Several times, my husband called the ambulance and had me taken to the hospital for elaborate heart tests. My doctor told me there was nothing physically wrong with me.

I went home and things got worse. My husband became impatient and annoyed. I worried day and night about doing something wrong with David and eventually causing his death. The school principal finally called me to say that David was having problems at school. I realized

I was being overprotective, but I couldn't help myself. The school recommended that we go to a child guidance clinic with David. I resisted and went back instead to my pediatrician and insisted once again on knowing the cause of Deborah's death. The pediatrician was apparently tired of my demands and recommended that I see a psychiatrist. I felt he was probably right but also felt we couldn't afford a psychiatrist; we had spent so much money on medical and hospital bills during the past year. I became so depressed that suicide began to seem like my only way out. One night, after an attack of chest pain and a crying spell, I was so desperate that I called the suicide prevention center. The counselor referred me to the local counseling center, where I saw Doris.

With Doris's help, I discovered that I was suffering from a delayed grief reaction. Through several counseling sessions, I was able to truly mourn the loss of my child, which I had not really done through all those months of trying to be brave, as my doctor and husband wanted me to be. Doris and I included my husband in some of the sessions. On her recommendation, I finally joined a group of other parents whose infants had died of crib death. I began to understand my fear of causing David's probable death and could finally let go of my overprotectiveness of him.

Although crib death has special features, the death of children in other ways is also traumatic and requires similar support and opportunities for grief work. In their study of mothers' and fathers' grief resolution, Kachoyeanos and Selder (1993) identified three processes: "presencing" the child through memory, reactivating the trauma of loss, and identifying missed options.

Compassionate Friends is a self-help group offering friendship and understanding to bereaved parents after the death of a child, whether by illness, murder, accident, or suicide. This international organization was founded by a pastor in England and now has over two hundred chapters around the United States.

Miscarried or Stillborn Child. The response of a mother at this crisis point is similar to that of a mother giving birth to a handicapped child: anger, loss, guilt, and questioning (see Chapter Eleven). Mothers ask, Why did this have to happen to me? What did I do wrong? What did I do to deserve this? Parents' need for grief work and the critical role of medical and hospital personnel are highlighted in the case of Gerry.

CASE EXAMPLE: GERRY HENDERSON

Gerry Henderson, age twenty-nine, gave birth to a stillborn child. Immediately after delivery, the child was taken out of the delivery room. Gerry never saw the baby; she was asleep from the anesthetic given her. Together with hospital authorities, Gerry's husband, Tom, who was numb and frightened, made arrangements to cremate the baby without consulting Gerry. The baby was not given a name. No one from the family attended the burial service. Tom was convinced that this was the best way to spare his wife and family any unnecessary grief.

When Gerry woke up and these facts were announced to her, she was beside herself with shock and grief, but Tom thought it best not to talk about the matter. Gerry was essentially alone with her grief. The nurses had a hard time handling their own grief and so were unable to offer Gerry support.

When Gerry returned home, her cousin invited her for a visit. The cousin had just had a new baby herself. Gerry felt she could not possibly face seeing another woman's live and healthy baby without breaking down. She was urged, however, to make the visit by her mother-in-law and husband, who said, "After all, you have to face reality sometime." Gerry refused to go to her cousin's house, though this caused further strain between her and her husband. Gerry's grief and tension reached the point that she began hearing the sound of a baby crying at various times during the day and during her sleepless nights. Because she knew there was no baby, Gerry was afraid she was going crazy. She was barely able to complete simple household chores.

After a week of lonely agony, Gerry walked into a nearby crisis clinic, where she cried inconsolably and poured out her story to a counselor. Gerry's husband, Tom, was asked to come in as well. Through several crisis counseling sessions, it became apparent that Tom was as shocked and grief stricken as his wife but believed that the only way to handle the infant's death was to "act like a man," not talk about his grief, and try to keep going. The cremation and not naming the baby were Tom's symbolic way of trying to wash away the problem. Gerry's mother-in-law and cousin joined in one of the counseling sessions. They were helped to understand the importance of not forcing Gerry to relate

to another child while she was actively grieving the loss of her own.

After Gerry and Tom did their grief work with the counselor's help, Gerry was able to resume a normal life without the child she had anticipated, Eventually, she was also able to relate to her cousin and her cousin's child without hostility.

The discomfort that some health professionals still feel with death and loss is compounded by ethical issues in cases of miscarriage—that is, some hospitals consider a miscarried fetus as just tissue, not a baby. By state law in Massachusetts, for example, hospitals must inform parents of their option of private arrangements for burial or other disposition or entrusting this to the hospital. The grief counseling that should always be offered does not occur routinely (Pfeiffer, 1999). The lack of contemporary rites of passage for mourning and dealing with death in hospitals is highlighted by another example.

CASE EXAMPLE: INFANT DEATH

A woman gave birth to twins, who both died about ten minutes after birth. The parents were not religious and struggled alone with their decision about how to mark the short life and death of their children. Their grief work was not

helped by the fact that people kept referring to the infants as stillborn. To the mother especially, it was very important for people to realize and acknowledge that she had given birth to live, not dead, infants.

Miscarriage is another common source of misunderstanding. Because many women miscarry without knowing it, some regard all miscarriages as the simple passing of body fluids. An insensitive remark such as, "You can always try again," fails to consider the mother's bonding with the unborn life or that she may not want to try again. A mother needs to mourn this loss within the framework of the meaning the pregnancy had for her and her family, in spite of others' possible dismissals of the event as relatively unimportant.

Similarly, women who have an abortion need to grieve the loss, regardless of the moral and religious conflicts that may accompany the event (Teichman, Shenhar, & Segal, 1993). Despite continued public controversy over abortion, for most women faced with an unwanted pregnancy, abortion is rarely a matter of good versus evil, but rather the lesser of two evils in the face of daunting odds.

The Medicalization of Birth. The potential crises surrounding birth and parenthood are colored further by controversy about cesarean births. Traditionally, cesarean birth was selected when life was at risk for the child or mother (less than 10 percent of births, though the rate of cesareans still exceeds this figure in some U.S. hospitals). There is perhaps no event arising from birth and parenthood that shows more sharply the difference between traditional societies and Western societies. Birth in North America has come to be identified as an elaborate medical event in which mothers turn over the unique birthing process to physicians, drugs, and surgery. The hazards of medicalizing the natural event of birth are increasingly challenged (Jordan, 1993; Mitford, 1993). The development of birthing centers and the increasing use of midwives is an outgrowth of public debate over birth as a natural event (Boston Women's Health Book Collective, 1998; Inch, 1984). Ideally, the management of birth should be in natural settings with trained midwives, with obstetrical consultation available for medical complications during birth to avoid the possible crisis of unnecessary death. Such medical intervention is required in only a small percentage of total births. For most births, medicalization is itself a hazard to be avoided (Jordan, 1993).

Illness or Behavior Problems of a Child. Similar intervention is indicated for parents whose children are seriously ill, have had a serious accident, or are dying. The modern, relaxed visiting regulations in most hospital wards for children have reduced the crisis possibility at this time for both parents and child. Parents are encouraged to participate in their child's care, so that the child feels less isolated and anxious about separation from parents, and the parents feel less threatened about their child's welfare. When behavioral problems are the issue, parents, teachers, and health providers should note the cautions and dangers of using psychoactive drugs as a first-level response, as discussed in Chapter Five (see also Leach, 1997, and Child Screening Checklist, Chapter Three).

Divorce and Single Parenthood

The high rate of divorce in North America has stabilized. The parent who gains custody of the children has the responsibility of rearing them alone, at least until remarriage; the other parent experiences a loss of the children. The loss is more acute if the divorced parents live in different cities or different parts of the country. If the loss is accompanied by a sense of relief, guilt usually follows. To assuage guilt, the relieved parent may shower the children inappropriately with material gifts or accuse the other parent of being too strict, inattentive, or uncaring. This crisis point of parenthood can be anticipated whenever the divorce itself is a crisis for either parent. Divorce counseling can help avoid future crisis.

The increase of no-fault divorce laws and attention to the needs of children in divorce settlements will also help prevent crises for parents, children, and grandparents. Although divorce affects children of all ages, preschoolers are at greatest risk following divorce. However, as already discussed, it is not so much the divorce itself as it is the manner in which parents conduct themselves and the poverty (especially for women) that cause the greatest stress on children of divorced parents (Sidel, 1996). Existing laws do not adequately address the crisis of divorce, as attested by the incidence of child snatching by the parent denied custody. Another problem faced by many mothers is the awarding of custody to fathers on the basis of their greater financial security and attendant access to legal services (which many women cannot afford), even when these fathers have not been the primary caretakers of the children (Chesler, 1986). Although the increasing interest of fathers in parenting their children is to be applauded, to award them custody primarily on a class basis is a cruel punishment of mothers, who have assumed the major burden of child care throughout history. This growing practice highlights the need for social change to address women's economic inequality.

Single Fathers. U.S. census figures show that rates of single fatherhood increased by 25 percent between 1995 and 1998. Fathers who do assume full-time parenting responsibility face stereotypes about that role, struggle with the same issues as single mothers, and have fewer support groups available to them (Wong, 1999). A new group of professionals, certified divorce planners, are available to divorcing parents, who must always remember that they are divorcing each other, not their children. During custody conflicts, these new professionals can help prevent such abuses as (1) awarding visitation rights to a father who abused his partner and children and (2) charging a nonabusive father with child molestation as a means of denying him visitation or joint custody rights (see Arendell, 1995; Irving & Benjamin, 1995).

Teenage Parenthood. The problems and hazards of single parenthood are increased for a teenager with no job and an unfinished education. The infants of teen mothers are also at increased risk of death, battering, and other problems exacerbated by the poverty of most adolescent parents. Increasingly, teenage mothers do not automatically drop out of high school because of pregnancy, do not marry only because they are pregnant, and do not give up their babies. Hospitals and social service agencies are now establishing collaborative programs with high schools, which include an emphasis on health, sex education, parenthood, and career planning. There is also growing recognition that the prevalence, problems, and hazards of teenage pregnancy will not subside until values and opportunities for women in society change. Counselors and others working with young mothers, many of whom are from low-income or troubled homes, repeatedly note that these girls see mothering as their only chance for fulfillment. Life seems to offer them no prospect of happiness through career or an education. Indeed, there is still widespread social, cultural, and economic reinforcement of the notion that a woman's major value to society is her capacity for motherhood, a view bolstered by Freudian psychoanalytic theory (see Chodorow, 1978). A young woman may sense that she has little chance to contribute anything else to society and says in effect, "But I can produce a baby." In fact, some young women request pregnancy tests not because they fear they are pregnant but because they wish to gain assurance of their fertility. So even if a girl does not plan to conceive, once pregnant she finally finds meaning in her life; she now will be important and necessary—at least to a helpless infant. Current efforts to reform welfare will probably fail if they do not consider these issues and emphasize the joint responsibility of mothers and fathers for the children they produce (Eyre & Eyre, 1993).

Stepfamilies and Adoption

In addition to the high rate of divorce and teen pregnancy in North America is the high rate of remarriage and the increasing presence of blended families. As with any major transition, families in these situations face many challenges and need support through crises in order to reap the potential riches of new family structures while avoiding the pitfalls, especially for children. There is now a growing body of literature on this topic, including the need for communitywide approaches to helping such families (for example, O'Callaghan, 1993; Papernow, 1993).

Adoption is another parenting issue ripe with opportunity and danger for the child, parents, and entire groups. One married woman who could not bear a child and wanted to adopt sacrificed her marriage because her husband wanted no children. A single person desiring parenthood usually faces many more challenges during the approval process than a heterosexual couple with the same desire. Anyone, married or single, who attempts interracial adoption in the United States must navigate not only the usual hurdles but also the national debate on the topic. While acknowledging the importance of racial identity, emphasis should be on the common humanity and needs of all children for nurturance and love in a stable family, needs that are rarely met in institutional settings or with frequent shifts between foster families (Bartholet, 1993; Bates, 1993).

Lesbian and Gay Parenthood

The contemporary stresses of parenthood include those of gay, lesbian, bisexual, and transgendered parents. There is probably no group of parents more misunderstood than gay parents. The myth and fear is that gay parents will bring up their children to be gay. Another myth is that gay men are much more likely than straight men to abuse children. As a result, lesbian and gay parents may lose custody of their children for no other reason than their sexual identity. Gay people of both sexes may be denied adoption if their sexual identity is known. For example, community protest in Massachusetts resulted in the removal of a foster child from the home of two gay foster parents, only to have the child abused six months later in a "normal" foster home. Crises around gay parenthood might decline with reflection on the following facts: the vast majority of parents are heterosexual; yet these straight parents have reared millions of gay people. The necessary role models of either sex and sexual identity exist for all children in many social contexts besides the home. Also, the majority of child sexual abusers are heterosexual male relatives (see Blumenfeld & Raymond, 1993; Raymond, 1992; Williams, 1992).

Surrogate Parenthood

In a landmark decision, the New Jersey supreme court declared that paying a woman to have a baby constitutes illegal baby selling and perhaps is criminal and potentially degrading to women. Legal, ethical, and emotional controversy over this technological response to the desire of childless couples for children will probably continue nevertheless, with proponents citing the Bible in support of their position and opponents noting that the last time human beings were bred for transfer of ownership was during slavery (Arditti, Klein, & Minden, 1984; Corea, 1985). The parenting issues of infertility and the right of procreation are cited as rationales justifying surrogacy. However, infertility rates are highest among low-income racial minority groups, due in part to greater exposure to various hazards, whereas lower rates among affluent women are traced largely to later age at attempting pregnancy. Surrogate babies, therefore, are usually born to poor women and paid for by affluent white couples. In the United States, the price of a surrogate arrangement is usually many thousands of dollars, while women in poor countries are paid much less or nothing at all. And although procreation is a right, this right cannot be exercised at the expense of the primordial right of a woman to the child she has nurtured and birthed.

The *preventive* approach to the infertility that has spawned surrogacy includes removal of environmental and workplace hazards affecting fertility and child care provisions that would allow career women to have children at earlier ages without compromising their jobs. The continuing controversy in wealthy countries surrounding this issue is illustrated in the 1993 report of the Royal Commission on New Reproductive Technology in Canada. Although the commission was mired in controversy for years, it did reach consensus on some issues, such as tighter licensing standards and the banning of surrogate motherhood and sex-selection techniques (Mickleburgh, 1993; Krishnan, 1994). In the United States, there is a move toward such federal regulation of birth technology, especially for protecting the rights of children.

The complexity of this issue is compounded by a resurgence of nineteenth-century *natalism*, which emphasizes the biological reproduction role of women. Natalism's seductive power is dramatized in the stories of two Montreal couples who began in vitro technology; one couple followed through for years at enormous financial and personal cost, whereas the other dropped out in favor of adoption and a more global (versus individualistic) approach to their desire to care for children (see *The Technological Stork*, Canadian Film Board). But among those parents who in good faith choose adoption, after weathering the crisis of infertility, some are confronted with the loss of their adopted child to biological parents, whose rights are almost always favored by courts, sometimes apparently irrespective of the child's best interests. One couple who faced this crisis made meaning out of their loss by successfully advocating for a change in laws that more fairly protects the rights of all concerned in such cases.

Fatherhood in Transition

A discussion of parenthood is incomplete without considering the changing notion of fatherhood, especially in regard to prevention of parent-child crises. The changing role of fathers is related to several factors: (1) the necessity for most mothers to work outside the home, (2) financial and other risks of single parenting to all concerned, (3) increasing realization of the benefits to children of being reared by two parents rather than one, (4) growing awareness by fathers of what they miss emotionally through marginal involvement in parenting. However, there are strains in this transitional process. Several factors work against contemporary fathers' assuming a more active role in child rearing: (1) continued sex-role socialization at home and in school (Sadker & Sadker, 1994), (2) continued gender-based inequality in the paid labor force, (3) the tenacious notion that it is more appropriate for a mother than a father to take time from a job on behalf of family needs (Thurer, 1994), (4) lack of role models for male participation in child care, (5) gender-based stereotypes in such professions as nursing and child development, (6) some women's continued ambivalence about men's active participation.

Because child care is the only arena in which women routinely have exercised control, it is unlikely that they will readily give it up so long as their limited access to other areas of power continues. Language is a barometer of our success here; for example, we still hear that mothers "take care of their children," whereas fathers "baby-sit" or "watch" them. In North America and worldwide, the poverty of children usually mirrors the poverty of their mothers. A 1993 United Nations Human Development Report on thirty-three countries that keep gender-based statistics reveals that no country (including rich nations like Canada, Germany, Switzerland, and the United States) treats women as well as it treats men. And a social health index measuring, among other items, child poverty and teen suicide reveals that the United States lags behind Western European countries in policies and practices that address the needs of working parents. For example, Western European countries grant paid work leave for attending to family issues, whereas in the United States many cannot afford to take the unpaid family leave available— and this, only to workers in companies of fifty or more employees (Crittenden, 2001; Dvorchak, 1992). Poverty and inadequate child care services are not just issues for welfare mothers; they adversely affect increasing numbers of intact families and struggling parents. Some corporations are also realizing greater business returns, more employee satisfaction, and reduced absenteeism as a result of providing child care benefits. As Ruddick (1989) suggests, children, women, men, and the whole social order would benefit by balancing domestic and public work between women and men.

Adolescence and Young Adulthood

Opinion regarding the age span of adolescence varies in different cultures and according to different theorists. The Joint Commission on Mental Health of Children in the United States considered youth up to age twenty-five in the program it recommended for youth in the 1970s. The extent of adolescence is influenced by such factors as (1) length of time spent in school, (2) age at first marriage, (3) parenthood or the lack of it, (4) age at first self-supporting job, and (5) residence (with or apart from parents). In general, adolescence can be considered in two stages—early and late. Late adolescence overlaps with young adulthood, particularly for those who prolong vocational and educational preparation into their early and middle twenties.

Developmental Challenges and Stress

During early adolescence, the major developmental task is achievement of "ego identity" (Erikson, 1963). Adolescents and young adults must give up the security of dependence on parents and accept new roles in society, including assuming responsibility in the work world and achieving a capacity for intimacy. The adolescent struggles with the issue of independence and freedom from family. On the one hand, the young person is very much in need of the family's material and emotional support. On the other hand, the young person may resent the continued necessity of dependence on parents. Interdependence—a balance between excessive dependence and independence—is a mark of growth during this stage.

Developmental tasks during late adolescence include finding and adjusting to a place in the world apart from immediate family and developing a capacity for intimacy in one's chosen sex role. These tasks may involve finding and holding a satisfying job; succeeding in college, technical training, or graduate school; and choosing and adjusting to a lifestyle such as marriage or communal living.

Success with the developmental tasks of adolescence depends on what happened during one's infancy and childhood, including transitions such as toilet training, weaning, and starting school. An unhappy childhood is the usual precursor to unhappiness for an adolescent or young adult. Successful completion of the tasks of adolescence or young adulthood can be accomplished only if parents know when to let go and do not prevent the young person from making decisions she or he is capable of making independently. Young people today simultaneously face new opportunities and terrifying threats, often with insufficient support in either instance.

U.S. society has been described as youth oriented. This does not mean that Americans particularly value younger people; instead, it shows a devaluation of older people. In fact, the necessary services for both normal and troubled young people are grossly lacking in many communities. For example, many schools do not have guidance counselors or school social workers. The youthful population in every community should have access to emergency hostels, where young people abused by their parents or seeking refuge from conflict can go. There should be housing for youthful offenders in special facilities with a strong community focus, not with hardened criminals. And all schools should provide suicide prevention programs. The lack of specialized services for disturbed children and adolescents needing psychiatric hospitalization has reached crisis proportions in many places, a problem exacerbated by managed care policies and the misuse of psychotropic drugs on young children (see Chapters Four, Six, and Seven).

Sexual-Identity Crisis

As already noted in the chapters on suicide and violence, many adolescents today are at increased risk of destructive behaviors toward self and others, and gay, lesbian, bisexual, and transgendered youth are at even greater risk, especially of suicide. Though complex factors intersect during all adolescent crises, homophobia in mainstream North America is commonly assumed to underpin the crises and chronic problems faced by gay youth. Williams (1992, 1986), an anthropologist who has studied among Native people of North American, Pacific, and Southeast Asian cultures, points out how these people revere androgynous members of the community as "higher" because the spirit from which all life (human, animal, plant) emanates has blessed the person with *two* spirits; hence the person is respected as a "double person," with particular roles and contributions to make in religion, the family, the workplace, and the community at large. Thus "difference is transformed—from *deviant* to *exceptional*— becoming a basis for respect rather than stigma" (Williams, 1992, p. 267). From his fieldwork with the Lakota, for example, Williams notes that the *berdache* (androgynous men) are the first choice to become adoptive parents when there is a homeless child—a marked contrast to nearly universal policy in most North American jurisdictions, which forbid such adoption, allegedly to prevent sexual molestation.

Blumenfeld (1992) shows the enormous costs of homophobia to *all*—those who are stigmatized, victimized, and deprived of an opportunity to live peaceful and fruitful lives, as well as those who have accepted the notion that these "different" people are also evil. But the highest price is paid by adolescents during the vulnerable developmental stage of discovering their sexual identity in a homophobic mainstream society and coming to terms with who they are without engaging in self-destructive behaviors. Figure 13.1 illustrates the sexual-identity crisis that many lesbian, gay, bisexual, and transgendered youth experience. It depicts the Crisis Paradigm applied to this at-risk group of adolescents, highlighting both the danger and the opportunity to move beyond homophobia toward a more egalitarian value system, as espoused by many pre-Columbian Native communities (see also Blumenfeld & Lindop, 1994).

FIGURE 13.1. SEXUAL-IDENTITY CRISIS.

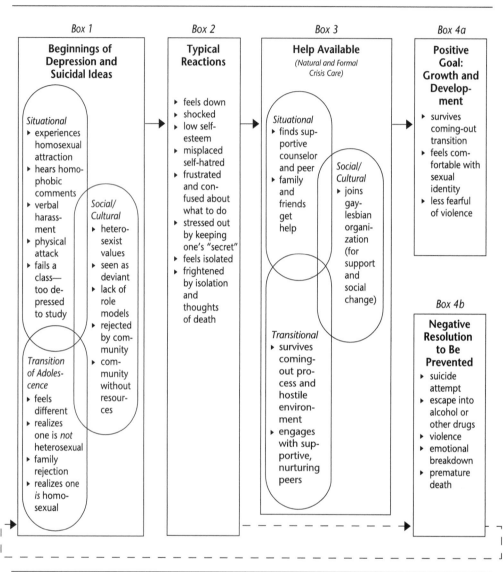

Crisis origins, manifestations, and outcomes and the respective functions of crisis care have an interactional relationship. The intertwined circles represent the distinct yet interrelated origins of crisis and aids to positive resolution, even though personal manifestations are often similar. The arrows pointing from origins to positive resolution illustrate the *opportunity for growth and development* through crisis; the broken line at bottom depicts the potential *danger of crisis* in the absence of appropriate aids. The loop between Box 4b and Box 1 denotes the *vulnerability* to future crisis episodes following negative resolution.

Helping Young People

Parents, teachers, pastors, youth directors, guidance and residence counselors, primary care providers, and school nurses are in powerful positions to help or hinder young people in their quest for identity and a meaningful place in society (Novello, 1993; Van Ornum & Mordock, 1987). Help may mean simply being available and attentive when a young person is upset and wants to talk; offering information the young person needs in order to make decisions about career, education, or marriage; guiding young people in the use of counseling and other resources when they find themselves in a crisis; or acting as a youth advocate in instances of neglect, abuse, or other injustice.

The crisis intervention principle of doing things *with*, rather than *to* and *for*, troubled people is particularly important when trying to help the young (see Chapter Four). Because a major developmental task of adolescence is finding a unique place and achieving healthy interdependence, a counselor's inattention to this principle can defeat the purpose of the helping relationship. Certainly, a young person in trouble may need a caring adult to help make certain decisions. But the same principle applies here as in work with troubled adults: the troubled person should participate in any decision affecting him or her unless that is clearly impossible under certain circumstances. Then the counselor should be ready and available to act on the person's behalf. Some adults assume that young people are incapable of making decisions or of accepting responsibility. In contrast, others force adolescents to make decisions and assume responsibilities they may not be ready for. Either attitude causes trouble. Crises and ongoing problems such as drug abuse, delinquency, and violence can often be avoided when young people have the support they need to meet the demands of this phase of development.

CASE EXAMPLE: NORA STAPLES

Nora Staples, age seventeen, and her sister, Jennifer, age sixteen, moved to a large city three hundred miles from their home in order to get away from their abusive father. Their elderly grandparents invited Nora and Jennifer to stay with them, despite their cramped living quarters and financial straits. Nora and Jennifer's parents divorced when the children were eleven and ten. Their mother left the area after the divorce, and the girls had not seen her since. For four years, Nora and Jennifer stayed with an aunt and uncle who lived near their father's home.

When Nora was fifteen and Jennifer fourteen, their father insisted that they live with him. He expected them to cook and keep house, which they did without complaint; they were afraid of what he would do if they rebelled. On weekends, their father went on drinking binges. Every month or two after such a binge, he would put both girls out of the house and lock the door; they would then go back to their aunt and uncle's house for a few days until their father insisted they come home again. The aunt and uncle were finally threatened by the father if they ever took the girls in again. When they heard this, Nora and Jennifer hitchhiked to their grandparents' home.

Two weeks after arrival at her grandparents' home, Nora began talking about shooting herself. The grandmother called a local crisis service and persuaded Nora to talk with the counselor. Indeed, Nora had obtained a gun and was seriously considering suicide. She felt angry with her father, though she had never let him know that. She also felt guilty about leaving him, although she could not bear being with him any longer. Now she felt she was a burden to her grandparents and saw no point in going on. Nora agreed, however, to come to the crisis clinic for counseling to deal with her problem. She also agreed to a plan to dispose of the gun, with the help of her grandparents and the police. Nora's grandparents were helped to deal with their anger and disgust with their son for the way he had treated Nora and Jennifer.

In spite of her problems, Nora managed to graduate from high school with honors at age seventeen and was offered a scholarship by a nearby private college. She was undecided about whether to start college immediately or get a job to help support herself while living with her grandparents.

The service plan for Nora and her grandparents included the following:

1. Individual counseling sessions for Nora to deal with her anger and misplaced guilt regarding her father, to help her make a decision about college or work, and to explore alternatives other than suicide as a way out of her despair
2. Family counseling sessions for Nora, her grandparents, and her sister, Jennifer, to help them deal together with their feelings about the situation, to find ways of supporting one another, and to find a solution to the problem of crowded living quarters
3. Collateral conferences with the Department of Family Services to obtain financial support for Nora and Jennifer and to enable the grandparents to find a larger residence

Nora, Jennifer, and their grandparents were also advised of their rights and of the resources available to them to press charges of neglect against the father if he came to take the young women away with him, as they suspected he would do within weeks.

By the end of eight individual counseling sessions and six family sessions, Nora was no longer suicidal. She had learned that the scholarship would be available to her the following year if she chose to delay going to college. She therefore decided to stay with her grandparents for a year and get a job to help support herself. One factor in this decision was Nora's realization, through counseling, that she was very resentful of having had to assume so much responsibility for her father and his needs. She said she wanted the chance to live in peace and quiet with a family for a while. She also felt deprived, as a result of her disturbed home situation, of the opportunity to live the way most teenagers do.

Nora gained the strength and courage to file charges against her father when he came to demand that she and Jennifer return to his home. A restraining order was obtained, and he was directed by a family court to make regular support payments to Nora and Jennifer while they continued to live in their grandparents' home. Custody of Nora and Jennifer was vested with their grandparents.

A six-month follow-up contact revealed that Nora was much happier and had decided to go ahead with college plans. She was advised of college counseling services available to her should she become upset and suicidal again.

Young women like Nora and Jennifer need special support to avoid crisis during their passage through adolescence. If adolescents come from troubled families, we should pay particular attention to the social and family approaches discussed in Chapter Five. The role of grandparents in such situations is becoming more common as drug abuse, joblessness, poverty, incarceration, and death among parents leave many children—even infants—without the family support they need. Grandparents are not only essential in these cases but also need extra support themselves as they "weather the storm" of resumed parenting roles during a major transition state of their own (Minkler & Fuller-Thomson, 1999; Newby, 1993). Conversely, grandparents who feel useless and discarded may gain a new lease on life by tending to the needs of children within familial and community circles. A loosening of the dominant nuclear family structure, enhancement of extended family roles, and community developments such as Cohousing (see Chapter Five) can serve not only distressed children but also the community at large.

But even if family disturbance, rejection, and deprivation are not apparent, many young people complain that they do not feel listened to. Parent effectiveness training should begin in high school and include a focus on listening, loving, and giving, as well as discipline and nonviolent positive control approaches. Adult guidance from schools, churches, and recreation directors should supplement family support with creative approaches (Blau & Gullotta, 1995; Brendtro, Brokenleg, & Van Bockern, 1990). Hazing tragedies, teenage gangs, binge drinking, and similar negative group associations attest to the tremendous need of young people for peer belonging and acceptance along with adult guidance. Dangerous hazing activities are remarkable for their destructiveness and for their lack of any mature adult influence. Although rites of passage for adolescents are necessary, the challenge is to develop contemporary alternatives that reflect sensitivity to adolescents' simultaneous needs for support, guidance, independence, and group belonging. For example, when considering the threat of HIV-AIDS and of adolescents' continuing abuse of alcohol, groups such as Students Against Drunk Driving or discussion sessions on AIDS and responsible sexual behavior can function as contemporary rites of passage during this critical developmental phase (see Crisis Paradigm, Box 3, lower circle).

Helping a Family in Crisis

More consistent efforts are also needed within social service and mental health agencies for family approaches to the problems of adolescents. The interrelated stresses and crises of parents and their children, along with several intervention strategies, are illustrated in the following example of a family in crisis.

CASE EXAMPLE: THE PAGE FAMILY

Donald Page, forty-four, and Ann Page, thirty-nine, had been married for twenty years and had four children—Alice, age twenty; Michael, eighteen; Betsy, fourteen; and Gary, nine. Donald worked in a local automobile factory. After two years in military service, he returned home as a disabled veteran. Ann worked as a secretary prior to their marriage and returned to work when her husband joined the service. When Donald returned, the Pages moved to a small farm on the outskirts of a large city. They leased the farmland, and Donald stayed at home most of every day doing odd jobs around the farm. He did few routine household chores, even though Ann worked full-time outside the home. The Pages had a bleak social life, and in general their marriage and family life were strained.

The Page children felt isolated because it was difficult to see their friends except during school hours. Alice had a baby at age seventeen and dropped out of her junior year in high school. She and her mother quarreled constantly over responsibility for the baby, who lived in the family home. After two years of this fighting, Alice's parents asked her to find a place of her own, which she did. Ann, meanwhile, threatened to report Alice to child protection authorities if she did not start assuming more responsibility for her child. Ann really wanted to keep Alice's baby herself, for she had wanted another child. Alice also talked about giving her baby away to her mother.

Betsy, meanwhile, was reported to be having problems in school, and teachers suspected her of taking drugs. Betsy had been belligerent at home, refusing to do chores and staying out late. Finally, Betsy ran away from home and was returned by police after three days. Donald and Ann were advised by police and school authorities to seek help for Betsy. They did not follow through and continued alone in their struggle to control her behavior. Michael tried to help both Betsy and his parents, but he felt pulled between the two parties. Gary was the "spoiled" child and occasionally asked why everyone was fighting all the time.

When Betsy's school problems heightened, she was threatened with expulsion and a week later ran away again. This time when police found her, she threatened suicide if she was taken home. Police therefore took her to a community mental health emergency service, where she saw a crisis counselor; she begged to be placed in a detention center rather than go back home. After several hours with Betsy, the counselor was able to persuade her that she could help her and her family make things more tolerable at home and that a detention center was no place for a girl her age, at least not until other alternatives had been tried.

Betsy's parents, meanwhile, were called and asked to come to the crisis clinic. Betsy felt hopeless about anything changing at home, though she expressed the wish that somehow things could get better. She particularly hated two situations: (1) her father and mother fighting about what she could and could not do and whom she could and could not see and (2) her mother's and Alice's constant fighting about Alice's baby. If these situations at home did not change, she said she just wanted to die.

The Pages agreed to a contract for eight crisis counseling sessions that were to involve the entire family, including Alice. One of the sessions was with the parents, Alice, and Betsy only. Another session was with the parents, Betsy, the school guidance counselor, principal, and homeroom teacher. The following goals were established for the counseling sessions:

1. Improve communication among all members of the family and cut out the contradictory messages Betsy was receiving
2. Help family members detect signs of distress among themselves and learn to listen and support one another when troubled
3. Work out a mutually agreeable program of social outlets for Betsy
4. Work out a plan to divide the chores in a reasonable and consistent way among all family members
5. Arrive at an agreeable system of discipline that includes rewards and punishments appropriate to various behaviors
6. Help Alice make satisfying decisions regarding herself and her baby
7. Develop a plan to work cooperatively with Betsy's teachers and the guidance counselor to resolve Betsy's problems in school

Family members agreed on various tasks to achieve these goals. For example, Donald and Ann would set aside some private time each day to discuss their problems and disagreements about discipline—out of the children's range of hearing. Betsy agreed to follow through on certain chores around the house. If she failed to do so, Ann agreed not to pick up after her and to discuss disciplinary measures with Donald. Alice would seek individual counseling to assist her in making a decision about herself and her child.

Two of the counseling sessions were held in the home, which the counselor observed was quite crowded. One result of this meeting was that the family found ways of ensuring individual privacy in spite of cramped quarters.

The threats of Betsy's suicide attempt and school expulsion were crisis points that moved Donald and Ann to work on underlying problems in their marriage. These problems made parenthood more difficult than it might otherwise have been. After eight crisis counseling sessions, the Page family existence was much less disturbed but by no means tranquil. However, Betsy was no longer in danger of being expelled from school, and she at least preferred her home to a detention house. Donald and Ann Page agreed to marriage counseling for themselves after termination of the crisis counseling contract in an effort to make their future years as parents less burdensome. The attention directed to dealing with marriage and family problems may decrease the chance that Betsy will follow in her sister's footsteps and become pregnant out of wedlock (see Weingarten, 1994).

Intimate Relationships: Beginnings and Endings

Because intimacy is basic to the human condition, a break in intimate attachments can lead to crisis. In this section, the beginnings and endings of intimate relationships are discussed briefly as one of the major transition states.

Intimacy as a Basic Need

An intimate relationship refers to any close bond between two people in which there is affection, reciprocity, mutual trust, and a willingness to stand by each other in distress without expectation of reward. The emphasis in this definition is on psychological and social intimacy, although a sexual relationship may also exist. Whether one is married, single, or living with someone of the same or opposite sex, intimate relationships are essential to a happy, productive life. Sexual relationships alone do not necessarily imply intimacy as here defined (see the "Service Forms" section in Chapter Three).

Intimate relationships—the social and emotional bonds between people—constitute a significant portion of the fabric of society. Some of the more common of these relationships and intimacies are courtship, marriage, and deeply committed friendships outside marriage. Entering into such a relationship is a major event with important social and psychological ramifications. Common endings include divorce or widowhood. These endings are highly visible, but other, less official, disruptions of close bonds can be equally traumatic and often produce crisis.

At the beginning and ending of an intimate relationship, the people involved undergo a change in role and status: from single to married, from spouse to divorcé, from associate to friend, or from friend to forgotten one. When beginning a new intimate relationship, an old, secure role must be abandoned and replaced by a new and unfamiliar one. If the person changing roles is lacking in personal and social resources, taking on a new role may be the source of crisis. Often a role change results in feelings of loss, including mourning what one has given up. When the familiar role of lover, spouse, or trusted friend ends, a sense of insecurity may result. The person may experience crisis because a basic needed attachment is severed and may again face the challenge of role and status change. Transitions into and out of supportive intimate relationships are therefore among the more common occasions of crisis for many people, with adolescents being particularly vulnerable.

Besides couples who begin and end intimate relationships, couples who choose to remain childless also experience strain. Reasons for remaining childless include support for zero population growth, inability to cope with the responsibility of parenthood, or simply choosing a way other than child rearing to make a social contribution. Childless couples often meet with social disapproval from others who assume that the basic purpose of marriage is procreation. In effect, the message is this: you can have intimacy if you assume the social responsibility of producing and rearing children. The National Alliance for Optional Parenthood is working on gradually changing the public's attitude toward childless marriage.

Gay and lesbian couples face similar disapproval, despite the movement to ensure equal rights for gay people. Various municipal and other jurisdictions, for example, have recently guaranteed gay couples the same employment insurance benefits as other couples, and some jurisdictions recognize civil unions that provide benefits traditionally limited to heterosexual couples. Gay men in particular often face additional threats to intimate attachments related to HIV-AIDS.

Excessive Dependence on Intimate Attachments

Because intimacy with others is an integral part of our lives, deep emotion and importance are attached to intimate relationships. Our feelings about these attachments affect our thoughts and behavior. For example, some people have unrealistic expectations of those they love and may behave in unusual ways when the bond is threatened or severed (Fehr, 1995). In contrast, some people have such deep fear of possible rejection that they repeatedly resist offers of friendship, love, and intimacy. Crisis can occur at the beginning of attachments or when the intimate relationship is disrupted, as in divorce, death of a spouse, or betrayal by a friend.

Halpern (1982) discusses "addictions" to people—the excessive need to be attached to someone special—as well as the dynamics of ending such an addiction, which involve breaking away and appreciating the beauty and positive aspects of solitude. Remembering Halpern's maxims and those described in other self-help books can help buffer the crisis potential when breaking out of addictive or destructive relationships; for example,

1. You can live—and possibly live better—without the person to whom you are attached.
2. A mutual love relationship should help one feel better, not worse, about oneself.
3. Guilt is not reason enough to stay in a relationship.
4. Some people die of destructive relationships. Do you want to be one of them?
5. If someone says, "I'm not ready for a relationship," or "I'm not going to leave my spouse," or "I don't want to be tied down," believe it.
6. The pain of ending a relationship, like other crises, will not last forever. In fact, it will not last as long as the pain of sustaining it.
7. We are whole and valuable as individuals apart from particular relationships.
8. When we end a destructive relationship, we open our lives to new possibilities.

Singles, Isolation, and Divorce

Considered within the privacy, intimacy, and community dynamic (see Chapter Five), an excessive dependency on intimacy usually results in a neglect of basic needs for privacy and community. Conversely, attachments to people who are not good for us can be fostered by the threat of social isolation.

Social opportunities, especially for the single person who has moved recently to a new community, are often lacking. In many communities, social events are organized around couple relationships. Consequently, a single person may find it extremely difficult or impossible to feel comfortable in a tightly knit society that demands that people participate as couples. Many communities now have singles organizations, where single people of any age can make friends and enjoy a wide range of social activities. However, despite the existence of these clubs, it is still difficult for a single person to establish satisfying social relationships after changing location. Fortunately, the single state is now being accepted by many as a fulfilling lifestyle, making it easier for the single person to establish social contacts in a new community.

A person who is not single by choice and is unable to make friends easily is likely to be crisis prone. Psychotherapy may be indicated if the person is chronically unhappy or depressed about being single; if living alone, that person is also a greater risk for suicide. In general, the risks of isolation and crisis responses like suicide are greater when the person is single because of divorce, separation, or widowhood (see Buehlman, Gottman, & Katz, 1992).

Divorce is particularly hazardous when the burden of care and support of young children falls entirely on one parent and when older people divorce and their value system has no place for divorce. Until very recently, divorce in the latter category was rare. It is now increasing rapidly and is overwhelmingly initiated by men. The crisis potential of these nonmutual divorce actions is high because of

- Lack of expectation
- Contradiction of deeply held values
- Widespread absence of social support structures for these special groups

Consider the following example of what divorce can mean to an older person.

CASE EXAMPLE: HELEN

Helen, age sixty-four, was not allowed to continue working in the same government agency as her husband, Tom, when they married thirty-five years ago. It was understood and accepted then that a husband should have the advantage of career development, and the wife should tend the home and children. Giving up her fledgling career as a civil servant was not a problem for Helen, as it was also understood and expected that marriage was for a lifetime and that her future economic support was secure. When Helen was sixty, Tom, then age sixty-four, left her for a woman twenty-five years his junior. Helen felt devastated and suicidal, saying over and over to her friends and two adult children that somehow it must have been her fault. She said repeatedly that Tom's death would have been preferable to a divorce.

Helen had a hard time acknowledging to anyone but her family and closest friends that she was divorced. She felt ashamed and frequently referred to herself as a widow. Helen could not understand how her daughter Caroline, also divorced, could be so apparently unruffled by the event. (Caroline had no children, worked as a writer, and preferred her single life.) At age sixty, Helen's only marketable job skill was baby-sitting. She was also a good gardener and cook but had no paid work experience in these fields. Besides being mateless at age sixty, Helen barely escaped homelessness. By a stroke of luck, she obtained the marital home and was able to rent one room so she could pay taxes and utilities. There was no legal provision, however, for her to receive benefits from her husband's pension.

In spite of these hardships, Helen scraped by and came out of her depression after two years. She now takes advantage of senior citizen travel packages and attends adult education classes. She is attractive, charming, and dearly loved by her friends and family, and she acknowledges at times that she may be better off without Tom in spite of occasional loneliness. Two years ago, Helen turned down the marriage proposal of a courtly but sickly man, age eighty. Although she was fond of this man, she resisted tying herself down to what she anticipated would eventually turn into a nursing role, especially after she had adjusted to her new freedom.

The harsh realities of the single life are contradicted by the stereotypes of swinging singles with a carefree existence. The single state without children does provide greater freedom to pursue one's career or engage in other activities, but the hazards of single parenthood speak for themselves. Every lifestyle has its advantages and trade-offs; for example, greater freedom and less responsibility may be balanced against greater insecurity in old age. Social research in the last century, beginning with Durkheim (1915), consistently reveals that marriage is in fact more advantageous and ego protective for men than it is for women (Martikainen & Valkonen, 1996). But women and men who have never married are better adjusted and are less at risk for suicide than those who have lost a spouse by any means. The hazards to individuals in these transition states would be modified by contemporary rites of passage, such as divorce ceremonies and acceptance into widows' clubs. Lacking such social supports can leave single people in a permanent liminal (transitional) state (van Gennep, 1909/1960), as they are never quite reincorporated into the community in their new role.

Middle Age

The term *middlescence* has been applied to those past adolescence but not yet in senescence. Stevenson (1977, p. 1) identifies two stages in this period of adult life: *middlescence I*, the core of the middle years between thirty and fifty, and *middlescence II*, the new middle years, extending from fifty to seventy or seventy-five. This division contrasts with the U.S. Census Bureau and popular opinion, which define middle age as the time between the ages of forty-five and sixty-four. Until very recently, little attention has been paid to the middle years except in the negative sense of stereotypes about being over the hill, sexually unattractive, unhappy, and depressed (Anderson & Stewart, 1994; Golan, 1981; Levinson, Darrow, Klein, Levinson, & McKee, 1978; Panchuck, 1994). People in midlife are literally caught in the middle: they have major responsibilities for the young and the old. They are the primary figures in society's major institutions: family, business, education, health and social service, religion, and politics. Besides doing most of the regular work of society, they are also its major researchers, with the understandable result that they have focused their research primarily on groups other than themselves.

Because of the relative lack of attention given to the midlife period, it is not surprising that many popular notions about midlife are the result of myth and folklore. Considering also the influence of medicalization, this major life passage is often recast as a "disease" to be "treated." The reality is that most people in midlife

- Are happier than they were when younger
- Lead highly productive and satisfying lives
- Have stable jobs and have met the major challenges of education and parenthood
- Are securely settled in a community in purchased rather than rented housing
- Enjoy a network of satisfying social relationships
- Have more disposable income and financial security than either the young or the old
- Enjoy good health and feel physically and mentally vigorous

In general, middle-agers today have more options than in earlier times because they are healthier. Census data reveal that North American and Western European women who are age forty-five can expect to live thirty-five more years and men, twenty-nine more years. Popular beliefs about middle age lag behind these statistical predictions.

Many, however, experience midlife as a threat. If a person at midlife is married and has children, familiar parenting roles may no longer fill one's day; spousal roles may need redefining (Maltas, 1992). If not single by choice, a middle-ager may see the chances for marriage as decreasing. Men may be threatened by a diminished sex drive and leveling off of career advancement opportunities. Women in careers face the same threat; women without careers must meet the challenge of returning to school or resuming an interrupted career. The onset of menopause may threaten a woman's sense of feminine identity and attractiveness. Both men and women may perceive their lives at middle age as quickly slipping away before they achieve what they want for themselves and others.

The success of men and women in dealing with these midlife changes depends on

- Psychological health and general outlook on life
- Lifelong preparation for this stage of human development
- Social support and economic security

Some people are trapped into the false security of living as though life were an unending fountain of youth. Such people may avoid healthy preparation for the developmental tasks of midlife. Or if they are socially isolated and lack the financial assets necessary to pursue education and leisure activities, midlife can increase their crisis proneness. In spite of the advantages middle-aged people have, this developmental passage is as hazardous as other transitions, though it is not as hazardous as popular stereotypes would have us believe.

Among all the myths associated with middle age, none is more widespread than that of female menopause as a disease. Significant efforts to undo this stereotype include publications such as *The New Our Bodies, Ourselves for the New Century* by the Boston Women's Health Book Collective (1998), which has been translated into many foreign languages. It is now widely accepted that menopause is a natural transition state, not a disease, in spite of bodily and mental changes such as hot flashes and a changing view of self past child-bearing age. Not only does menopause not require medical intervention for distress in the majority of cases, but estrogen replacement therapy, so popular in the past, is linked with various complications and remains controversial (MacPherson, 1992). Menopause support groups now sometimes take the place of estrogen replacement therapy during this important transition state. In such groups, women receive factual information (which is often rare and imprecise from the mainstream gynecology profession) and support in coping with the physical, social, and psychological changes accompanying the cessation of menstruation.

Men undergoing the climacteric could benefit from similar support groups. Coming to terms with middle age could influence the behavior of men who cope with changes in themselves by establishing liaisons with younger women.

Old Age

It has been said that we are as old as we feel. Many of the issues discussed regarding middle age apply to old age: psychological outlook, social support, and economic security are critical factors affecting the crisis proneness of old people. The issues concerning retirement, noted in Chapter Twelve, also apply to many elderly people, and many are at special risk for crisis. For example, minority elders have lower incomes than white elders; three-fourths of elderly people below poverty level are female; older women earn much less than older men; low-income elders are much more likely to have limiting chronic conditions than high-income elders (Estes, 1986). With the federal cutbacks in domestic programs since 1981, greater burdens of caring for increasing numbers of elders fall on women (Doress & Siegal, 1987; Pillemer, Moen, Wetherington, & Glasgow, 2000; Sommers & Shields, 1987). Typically, those caring for impoverished and chronically ill women are underpaid, overworked, and overwhelmed.

The needs of elders are being addressed through the work of advocates such as senior legislators, the Gray Panthers, the Older Women's League, the American Association of Retired Persons, and increasing numbers of individuals. A recent emphasis on gerontological research and graduate training programs in universities also can contribute to the long-range welfare of the elderly. Many of the myths about old age are an extension of those about middle age: old age is a disease, and old people are uniformly needy, dependent, and asexual.

Attitudes Toward Seniors

Despite increased political advocacy and advances in gerontological research, ageism and stereotypes about old people persist. Cultural values and the policies and practices flowing from them do not change rapidly. Old people are not as highly valued in mainstream North American society as they are, for example, in some Native communities and most non-Western societies. Recent social emphasis on the small nuclear family has virtually displaced the extended family arrangement in most Western societies. Grandparents, aunts, and uncles are rarely integrated into a family home. Most children, therefore, routinely have only two adults (their parents) as role models and supporters. In cases of death, desertion, or divorce, children are even more deprived of adult models. Fortunately, this is changing with attempts to get children and old people together—for example, through nursing home visits by groups of children and other intergenerational volunteer programs in schools.

Older people experience even greater hardship than children do by their exclusion from the nuclear family. They feel—and often are—unwanted. Often they are treated as guests and have no significant role in matters of consequence in their children's families. When older people, because of health or other problems, do live with their grown children, additional tensions arise. The older person may become impatient and irritable with the normal behavior of the grandchildren. Space is sometimes insufficient to give everyone some privacy, or the old person may seem demanding and unreasonable (Killeen, 1990).

Services for Elderly People

Stress can be relieved and crisis situations prevented when special public health and social services are available to families caring for an older person. As a parallel to child care needs, many workers and advocacy groups for elders are demanding inclusion of elder care in benefit packages. A first-of-its-kind public housing venture in Boston was designed to meet the physical and social needs of elderly residents and young children. The twenty-six subsidized units for grandparents who are raising their grandchildren were developed from an abandoned nursing home and are called Grand Families House (Davis, 2000). In some areas of North America, outreach workers from the public office for aging make regular contacts with older people in their homes. Names of needy people are obtained from pastors, welfare, and mental health workers.

Outreach service such as this is very helpful in preventing crises and avoiding institutionalization. Contrary to public perception, only 5 percent of old people in the United States live in nursing homes, and even people a hundred years old and older are often highly engaged in living (Clayton, Martin, Poon, Lawhorn, & Avery, 1993). Where public services are lacking, the lives of many older people can take on a truly desperate character (see "Abuse of Older Persons" in Chapter Eight). The situation is particularly acute for the older person living alone who (for physical or psychological reasons) is unable to get out. Senior citizen centers now exist in nearly every community. Every effort should be made to encourage older people to use the services of these centers. This may be the only real source for keeping active physically and for establishing and maintaining social contacts. Such physical and social involvement is essential to prevent emotional, mental, and physical deterioration. Some people will need help in order to use these services—money and transportation to get there or counseling to convince them to use the service.

Other services for seniors in the United States and Canada include

- Retired Senior Citizen Volunteers Program, a group available for various kinds of volunteer tasks
- Phone Line, which maintains a roster of names of shut-in people (elderly or disabled) and calls to ensure their safety and contact with a helping agency
- Meals on Wheels, an organization that makes and delivers hot meals to the incapacitated
- Help Your Neighbor and similar public and private organizations available to the isolated and distressed

Visiting nurses are another key resource. Often a nurse can detect stress or suicidal tendencies. A fast-growing service in the United States, Program for All-Inclusive Care for the Elderly, aims to keep frail elderly people in their homes while providing medical and housekeeping support. In addition to the services for older people cited here, all agencies for the aging should maintain active contact with the local crisis center for consultation and direct assistance in acute crisis situations. The tragic deaths discussed in the following case example might not have occurred had there been preventive intervention.

CASE EXAMPLE: MARJORIE JONES AND DAUGHTER ROSE

After the death of her elderly husband, Marjorie Jones was overwhelmed caring alone for Rose, her mentally retarded adult daughter. She had resisted neighbors' offers of assistance. After a postal worker became concerned and alerted authorities, she and her daughter were found dead in their trash-filled home in a middle-class neighborhood. The neighbors anguished about what they might have done to avoid this tragedy.

This case suggests the need for more proactive social services following loss, as well as for people caring for any disabled person. It also illustrates the need for community education about how to offer neighborly help or make early referrals without invading the privacy of people who may feel too proud to ask for or receive assistance.

CASE EXAMPLE: ANTONE CARLTON

Antone Carlton, age seventy-seven, lived with his wife, Marion, in a run-down section of a city. Antone was nearly blind and had had both legs amputated, due to complications of diabetes. Antone and Marion survived on a poverty-level income. Marion, age sixty-eight, was able to take care of Antone. Then she was hospitalized and died of complications following abdominal surgery. Antone was grief stricken. After Marion's death, a visiting nurse came regularly to give Antone his insulin injections and arrange for help with meals.

One day, Antone's house was broken into, and he was beaten and robbed of the few dollars he had. The nurse found Antone with minor physical injuries, but he was also depressed and suicidal. The local crisis center was called and an outreach visit made. The crisis outreach team assessed Antone as a very high risk for suicide. Antone, however, insisted on remaining in his own home. The services of Help Your Neighbor were enlisted for Antone, especially to provide for an occasional visitor. Homemaker services were also arranged. A week later, Antone was beaten and robbed again, but he still refused to move out of his home. The nurse inquired about a senior citizen housing project for Antone. They refused to accept anyone as handicapped as Antone, although he did consider leaving if he could move to such a place. After a third robbery and beating a few weeks later, Antone agreed to move to a nursing home.

Institutional Placement of Elders

In Antone's case, a nursing home placement was a means of resolving a crisis with housing, health care, and physical safety. However, admission to a nursing home is itself an occasion for crisis for nearly every resident. Also, while some people do well in a nursing home, for many, institutionalization marks the beginning of a rapid decline in physical and emotional health. A new nursing home resident will invariably mourn the loss of his or her own home or apartment and whatever privacy it afforded, no matter how difficult the prior circumstances were. New residents resent their dependence on others, regardless of how serious their physical condition may be. These problems are less acute for those who need intermediate-level care; their health status does not require such complete dependence. In domiciliary-level care, residents remain independent and are much less subject to crisis.

A person who has been placed in a nursing home by family members may feel unloved and abandoned. Some families do abandon an old parent, often not by choice but because they cannot handle their own guilt feelings about placing the parent in a nursing home, no matter how necessary that placement might be.

The most stressful time for a nursing home resident is the first few weeks after admission. The new resident's problems are similar to those of people admitted to other institutions: hospitals, detention facilities, or group homes for adolescents. Crisis intervention at this time will prevent many more serious problems later, such as depression, suicidal tendencies, withdrawal, refusal to participate in activities, and an increase in physical complaints. Studies reveal that a significant number of elderly people simply give up after retirement or admission to a nursing home and die very soon thereafter (Richman, 1993). Hopelessness in these cases is the forerunner to death. Elderly people admitted to nursing homes should be routinely assessed for suicide risk.

Besides having to deal with feelings of loss, resentment, and rejection, some people placed in nursing homes do not get a clear, honest statement from their family about the need for and nature of the placement. This contributes further to the person's denial of the need to be in the nursing home.

Nursing staff who are sensitive to this crisis of admission to a nursing care facility are in a key position to prevent some negative outcomes. The newly admitted resident, along with the family, should be provided ample opportunity to express feelings associated with the event. Family members persuaded to be honest with the resident about the situation and not deny reality will feel less guilty and more able to maintain the social contact needed by the resident. Staff should actively reach out to family members, inviting them to participate in planning for their parent's or relative's needs in the nursing care facility. This will greatly relieve the stress experienced by an older person during the crisis of admission and adjustment. It will also reduce staff crises. When families are not included in the planning and have no opportunity to express their own feelings about the placement, they often handle their stress by blaming the nursing staff for poor care. This is a desperate means of managing their own guilt as well as the older person's complaints about the placement.

Besides the crisis of admission, other crises can be prevented when nursing care facilities have (1) activity programs in keeping with the age and sociocultural values of the residents, (2) programs involving the residents in outside community events, and (3) special family programs. Unfortunately, the quality of nursing care facilities frequently reflects a society's devaluation of older people. Funding is often inadequate, which prevents employment of sufficient professional staff.

Retirement and the realization of old age are times of stress but need not lead to crisis. Societal attitudes toward old age are changing, so that this stage of life is now anticipated by more and more people as another opportunity for human growth. In some societies, retired people are called on regularly to work several weeks a year when full-time workers go on vacation. There are many other opportunities in progressive societies for older people to remain active and involved. Many crises in the lives of elderly citizens can be avoided if they are accorded more honor and some postretirement responsibilities.

How we treat our elderly citizens can account for the marked difference in death rituals in traditional and modern urban societies: in modern societies, many

people are dead *socially* (by forced retirement or familial rejection) long before physical death occurs. Society need therefore only dispose of the body; no rituals are
needed to transfer social functions (Bloch, 1971; Goody, 1962). This cross-cultural
observation invites further consideration of death, the final passage.

Death

Death is the final stage of growth (Kübler-Ross, 1975). It marks the end of life and
is the most powerful reminder we have that we have only one life to live and that
to waste it would be folly.

Death has been a favorite topic of philosophers, poets, psychologists, physicians, and anthropologists for centuries. Volumes have been written by authors
such as Aries (1974), Bertman (1991), Feifel (1977), Fulton, Markusen, Owen, &
Scheiber (1978), Glaser and Strauss (1965), Mitford (1963), Kastenbaum (2000),
and Kübler-Ross (1969, 1975). There is even a science of *thanatology* (study of
death and dying). Yet death is still a taboo topic for many people, which is unfortunate because it means the loss of death as a "friendly companion" to remind us
that our lives are finite. Such denial is the root of the crisis situation that death
becomes for many. Vast and important as the subject of death is, consideration of
it here is limited to its crisis aspect for health and human service workers.

Attitudes Toward Death

Death is not a crisis in itself but becomes one for the dying person and survivors
because of the widespread denial of death as the final stage of growth. As Tolstoy
(1886/1960) wrote so eloquently in *The Death of Ivan Ilyich*, the real agony of death
is the final realization that we have not really lived our life, the regret that we did
not do what we wanted to do, that we did not realize in and for ourselves what we
most dearly desired. This fact was borne out in research by Goodman (1981), who
compared top performing artists' and scientists' attitudes toward death with a
group who were not performing artists or scientists but were similar in other respects. She found significant evidence that the performing artists and scientists
were less fearful of death, more accepting of death, and much less inclined to want
to return to earth after their death if they had a chance. Having led full and satisfying lives, they were able to anticipate their deaths with peace and acceptance.
They had "won the race with death."

The denial of death, so common in U.S. society, is a far greater enemy than
death itself. It allows us to live our lives less fully than we might with an awareness
and acceptance of death's inevitability. Through the works of Elisabeth Kübler-
Ross (1969, 1975) and many others, we have made progress in dealing with death
openly. However, some health professionals and families still are reluctant to discuss the subject openly with a dying person (see Christakis & Asch, 1995; Ross,
Fisher, & MacLean, 2000).

This is changing through the promotion of living wills, advance directives regarding the use of extraordinary treatment, and the public debate about physician-assisted suicide. For many, the assisted-suicide issue is primarily one of maintaining control over one's last days and not suffering unnecessary pain. More and more physicians and nurses are concerned about the influence of technology on the care of the dying and the undertreatment of pain (Solomon et al., 1993), and they avail themselves of courses on death and dying (see Bertman, 1991). Increased public awareness, a more realistic approach to death, and a loosening of denial's grip are now evident as people consider (especially through media attention) the prospect of dying in an institution attached to tubes and with no control over or conscious awareness of the process. As Dubler (1993) notes, the culture of medical institutions must change to accommodate the notion of negotiated death. The Patient Self-Determination Act passed by Congress in 1990 facilitates such change by requiring health care institutions to inform patients of their rights to make advance medical directives. The act encourages people to think about what treatment they wish if terminally ill. It also ensures compliance with their wishes for the kind of death they envision. The AIDS crisis makes the need to come to terms with death more urgent than ever (see Chapter Eleven). See Haynor (1998) for detailed information on how health professionals can empower patients and assist them in decision making around advance directive requirements.

Many problems and crises associated with death, dying people, their families, and those who attend them in their last days might be avoided if death were faced more directly. As noted by Kübler-Ross (1969, 1975), Fagerhaugh and Strauss (1977), and others, nurses, physicians, ministers, and family need to become open, communicative companions to those who are dying. However, nurses and physicians often avoid talking openly with dying people about their condition. Dying patients pay a high emotional price when this happens. The numerous examples of avoidance that are cited in Kübler-Ross's classic book, *On Death and Dying* (1969), still apply in many situations unless the staff has had extensive sensitization to the practices she recommends. *How We Die* (Nuland, 1994), written by a physician, is another attempt to break through denial by his blunt account of the physiological process of ending life.

The inability or refusal to come to terms with death is a critical issue for crisis workers in general, not just on behalf of the dying. Why? Because death, as suggested in earlier chapters, is a kind of prototype for *all* crisis experiences—that is, many crises arise directly from the death of a loved one, but all crises and life passages are like a "minideath" in the *loss experience* common to them all. The successful resolution of crisis, then, is crucially connected to the process of coming to terms with loss. Helping others through their losses and helping them find new roles, new relationships, and emotional healing depends heavily on whether we are comfortable with the topic of death and our own mortality. A healthy attitude toward our own death is our most powerful asset in assisting the dying through this final life passage and comforting their survivors.

In a culture without strong ritual and social support around dying, the major burden of positively dealing with death falls on individuals. Crisis workers and health professionals associated with death in their professions can make their work easier by attending courses on death and dying, which are widely offered on college campuses. Sensitization to death and its denial in modern society and to ethical issues such as assisted dying (Schwarz, 1999; de Vries, 1999) is also aided by reading literary and other works on the topic (Cutter, 1974; Fried & Fried, 1980; Goodman, 1981; Goody, 1962; Rosenthal, 1973; Tolstoy, 1886/1960). Intensive workshops focusing on our own denial of death through sensitizing exercises are another means of forming death awareness. Such workshops have provided the stimulus for some to become aware of the preciousness of every moment (Bertman, 1991). Coming to terms with our own death not only can change our life and eventual death but also lays the foundation for assisting others through death.

Helping a Dying Person

In U.S. and Canadian society, many people whose deaths are anticipated die in institutions such as hospitals or nursing homes, not in their own homes. Proportionately more people with AIDS, however, die at home. Rosenthal, a young poet dying of leukemia, struck out against the coldness and technology that awaited him along with death in a hospital. He tells his remarkable story of facing death and living fully until that time in *How Could I Not Be Among You?* (1973). On learning of his imminent death from leukemia, Rosenthal checked out of the hospital, moved to the country, and did the things he wanted to do before dying.

Many others are not able to die in self-chosen circumstances; most will spend the last phase of their lives in hospitals or nursing homes. These dying people deserve to have the shock of their terminal illness tempered by those who attend them. Crisis intervention for a person who has learned of a diagnosis of fatal illness begins with awareness of one's own feelings about death. Next in the helping process is understanding what the dying person is going through. Wright (1985) refers to the acute, chronic-living, and terminal phases of a person's response to a life-threatening illness. Family members and everyone working with the dying will recognize the phases of dying as described by Kübler-Ross (1969) from her interviews with over two hundred dying patients.

Kübler-Ross identifies five stages of dying: denial, anger, bargaining, depression, and acceptance. All people do not necessarily experience all the stages, nor do these stages occur in a fixed, orderly sequence. Kübler-Ross's work is most useful for sensitizing health and hospice workers to some of the major issues and problems faced by the dying.

1. *Denial.* Typically, denial is expressed with, "No, not me," on becoming aware of a terminal illness. People deny even when they are told the facts explicitly. Denial is expressed by disbelief in X-ray or other reports, insistence on repeat

examinations, or getting additional opinions from other doctors. Denial is the basis for the persistence of quack remedies. But denial may be necessary as a delaying mechanism, so the person can absorb the reality of having a terminal illness. During this phase, the person is withdrawn and often refuses to talk. Nurses, physicians, clergy, and social workers must wait through this phase and let the person know that they will still be available when he or she is finally ready to talk. Pressing a person to acknowledge and accept a bitter reality before the person is psychologically ready may reinforce the need for defensive denial. Self-help groups (such as those sponsored by Omega and the AIDS Action Committee in the Boston area) are a contemporary substitute for traditional rites of passage through this important transition state.

2. *Anger.* When denial finally gives way, it is often replaced by anger: "Why me?" This is more difficult for hospital staff and family to deal with than denial, as the person often expresses the anger by accusations against the people who are trying to help. The person becomes very demanding. No one can do anything right. The person is angry at those who can go on living. Nurses are frequently the targets of anger. It is important for them to understand that the anger is really at the person's unchosen fate, not at the nurses. They must support the patient, not retaliate or withdraw, recognizing that the anger must be expressed and will eventually pass.

3. *Bargaining.* Faced with evidence that the illness is still there in spite of angry protests, the person in effect says, "Maybe if I ask nicely, I'll be heard." This is the stage of bargaining, which goes on mostly with God, even among those who do not believe in God. Bargaining usually consists of private promises: "I'll live a good life," or "I'll donate my life and my money to a great cause." During this phase, it is important to note any underlying feelings of guilt the person may have or any regrets that life has not been lived as idealized. The dying person needs someone who can listen to those expressions of regret.

4. *Depression.* During this stage of dying, people mourn the losses they have borne: losses of body image, income, people they loved, joy, or the role of wife, husband, lover, or parent. Finally, they begin the grief of separation from life itself. This is the time when another person's presence or touch of the hand means much more than words. Again, acceptance of one's own eventual death and the ability to be with a person in silence are the chief sources of helpfulness at this time.

5. *Acceptance.* This follows when anger and depression have been worked through. The dying person becomes weaker and may want to be left alone more. It is the final acceptance of the end, awaited quietly with a certain expectation. Again, quiet presence and communication of caring by a touch or a look are important at this time. The person needs to have the assurance that he or she will not be alone when dying and that any wishes made, such as in advance directives, will be respected. Messages of caring will give such assurance.

Awareness and understanding of our own and of the dying person's feelings are the foundation of care during the crisis of terminal illness and death. Crisis intervention with the families of dying people will also be aided by such awareness and understanding. Because dying alone is a dying person's greatest fear, communication with families is essential. Families should not be excluded from this final phase of life by machines and procedures that unnecessarily prolong physical life beyond conscious life. Family members who help by their presence will very likely become more accepting of their own future deaths. Denial of death and death in isolation do nothing to foster growth.

The Hospice Movement

One of the most significant recent developments aiding the dying person is the hospice movement, founded by a physician, Cecily Saunders (1978), in London in 1967. Sylvia Lack (Lack & Buckingham, 1978), also a physician, extended the hospice concept to the United States (McCabe, 1982). The hospice movement, now taking root worldwide (Saunders & Kastenbaum, 1997), grew out of awareness of the needs of the dying and concern that these needs could not be met adequately in hospitals engaged primarily with curing and acute-care procedures. A main focus of the hospice concept is the control of pain and the provision of surroundings that will enhance the possibility of dying as naturally as possible (Carson & Eisner, 1999). The growing emphasis on palliative-care research and service extends this concept. A groundbreaking work in Canada (Fisher, Ross, & MacLean, 2000) provides guidelines for comprehensive care at the end of life, which, if widely implemented, would go far in alleviating unnecessary pain and preventing emotional crisis during this final life stage (see also Field & Cassel, 1997).

Lack has identified ten components of hospice care (McCabe, 1982, p. 104):

1. Coordinated home care with inpatient beds under a central, autonomous hospice administration
2. Control of symptoms (physical, social, psychological, and spiritual)
3. Physician-directed services (due to the medical nature of symptoms)
4. Provision of care by an interdisciplinary team
5. Services available twenty-four hours a day, seven days a week, with emphasis on availability of medical and nursing skills
6. Patient and family regarded as the unit of care
7. Provision for bereavement follow-up
8. Use of volunteers as an integral part of the interdisciplinary team
9. Structured personnel support and communication systems
10. Patients accepted into the program on the basis of health care needs rather than ability to pay

The hospice movement is a promising example of a new awareness of death in modern society and the importance of supporting the rights of the dying. The pivotal place of this service for the dying is underscored by the AIDS crisis and by increasing numbers of other people who may prefer to die at home. As more people select hospice care, however, the need for respite for families and more hospital-based hospices will also increase (Wegman, 1987). Assistance for the dying person is supported by the "Dying Person's Bill of Rights," adopted by the General Assembly of the United Nations (1975, p. 99):

> I have the right to be treated as a living human being until I die.
>
> I have the right to maintain a sense of hopefulness however changing its focus may be.
>
> I have the right to be cared for by those who can maintain a sense of hopefulness, however changing this might be.
>
> I have the right to express my feelings and emotions about my approaching death in my own way.
>
> I have the right to participate in decisions concerning my care.
>
> I have the right to expect continuing medical and nursing attention even though "cure" goals must be changed to "comfort" goals.
>
> I have the right not to die alone.
>
> I have the right to be free from pain. I have the right to have my questions answered honestly.
>
> I have the right not to be deceived.
>
> I have the right to have help from and for my family in accepting my death.
>
> I have the right to die in peace and dignity.
>
> I have the right to retain my individuality and not be judged for my decision, which may be contrary to beliefs of others.
>
> I have the right to discuss and enlarge my religious and/or spiritual experiences, whatever these may mean to others.
>
> I have the right to expect that the sanctity of the human body will be respected after death.
>
> I have the right to be cared for by caring, sensitive, knowledgeable people who will attempt to understand my needs and will be able to gain some satisfaction in helping me face my death.

Throughout our lives, hazardous events and transitions can be occasions of crisis, growth, or deterioration. So in death, our last passage, we may experience our most acute agony or the final stage of growth. Whether or not we "win the race with death" depends on

- How we have lived
- What we believe about life and death
- The support of those close to us during our final life crisis

Summary

Life passages are minideaths. In each of these transition states, we leave something cherished and familiar for something unknown and threatening. We must mourn what is lost in order to move without terror to whatever awaits us. Preparation for transitions—whether from one role to another, one stage of life to another, or from life to death—is helpful in averting acute emotional crisis during passage. To assist us in this all-important life task, we need contemporary ritual experts—that is, mature, caring people who are willing to support and protect us from tumultuous waves that might block our successful passage. These modern-day ritual experts are crisis counselors, members of self-help groups, pastors, health professionals, family, neighbors, and friends—people who care about people in crisis.

References

Affara, F. A. (2000). When tradition maims. *American Journal of Nursing, 100*(8), 52–70.

Anderson, C. M., & Stewart, S. (1994). *Flying solo: Single women at midlife.* New York: Norton.

Arditti, R., Klein, R. D., & Minden, S. (Eds.). (1984). *Test-tube women.* London: Pandora Press.

Arendell, T. (1995). *Fathers and divorce.* Thousand Oaks, CA: Sage.

Aries, P. (1974). *Western attitudes toward death from the middle ages to the present.* Baltimore: Johns Hopkins University Press.

Bartholet, E. (1993). *Family bonds: Adoption and the politics of parenting.* Boston: Houghton Mifflin.

Bates, J. D. (1993). *Gift children: A story of race, family, and adoption.* New York: Ticknor & Fields.

Bertman, S. L. (1991). *Facing death: Images, insights, and interventions.* Bristol, PA: Hemisphere.

Blau, G. M., & Gullotta, T. P. (1995). *Adolescent dysfunctional behavior: Causes, interventions, and prevention.* Thousand Oaks, CA: Sage.

Bloch, M. (1971). *Placing the dead.* London: Seminar Press.

Blumenfeld, W. J. (Ed.). (1992). *Homophobia: How we all pay the price.* Boston: Beacon Press.

Blumenfeld, W. J., & Lindop, L. (1994). *Family, schools, and students' resource guide.* Boston: Safe Schools Program for Gay and Lesbian Students, Massachusetts Department of Education.

Blumenfeld, W. J., & Raymond, D. (1993). *Looking at gay and lesbian life* (2nd ed.). Boston: Beacon Press.

Boddy, J. (1998). Violence embodied? Circumcision, gender politics, and cultural aesthetics. In R. E. Dobash & R. P. Dobash (Eds.), *Rethinking violence against women* (pp. 77–110). Thousand Oaks, CA: Sage.

Boston Women's Health Book Collective. (1998). *The new our bodies, ourselves for the new century.* New York: Simon & Schuster.

Brendtro, L. K., Brokenleg, M., & Van Bockern, S. (1990). *Reclaiming youth at risk: Our hope for the future.* Bloomington, IN: National Educational Service.

Buehlman, K. T., Gottman, J. M., & Katz, L. F. (1992). How a couple views their past predicts their future: Predicting divorce from an oral history interview. *Journal of Family Psychology, 5*(3/4), 295–318.

Cacace, M., & Williamson, E. (1996). Grieving the death of an adult child. *Journal of Gerontological Nursing, 22*(2), 16–22.

Caplan, G. (1964). *Principles of preventive psychiatry.* New York: Basic Books.

Carson, M., & Eisner, M. (1999). *Caregiving guide for seniors.* Ottawa: Algonquin.

Chapman, J. R., & Gates, M. (1977). *Women into wives: The legal and economic impact of marriage.* Thousand Oaks, CA: Sage.

Chesler, P. (1986). *Mothers on trial: The battle for children and custody.* Seattle: Seal Press.

Chodorow, N. (1978). *The reproduction of mothering.* Berkeley: University of California Press.

Christakis, N. A., & Asch, D. A. (1995). Physician characteristics associated with decisions to withdraw life support. *American Journal of Public Health, 85*(3), 367–372.

Clayton, G. M., Martin, P., Poon, L. W., Lawhorn, L. A., & Avery, K. L. (1993). Survivors of the century. *Nursing and Health Care, 14*(5), 256–260.

Corea, G. (1985). *The mother machine.* New York: HarperCollins.

Covington, S. N., & Theut, S. K. (1993). Reactions to perinatal loss: A qualitative analysis of the National Maternal and Infant Health Survey. *American Journal of Orthopsychiatry, 63*(2), 215–222.

Crittenden, A. (2001). *The price of motherhood: Why the most important job in the world is still the least valued.* New York: Metropolitan Books.

Cutter, F. (1974). *Coming to terms with death.* Chicago: Nelson-Hall.

Daley, B. (1998, December 7). Colleges declare war on drinking. *Boston Globe,* pp. B1, B8.

Davis, W. A. (2000, April 6). Grand central. *Boston Globe,* pp. F1, F8.

de Vries, B. (Ed.). (1999). *End of life issues: Interdisciplinary and multidimensional perspectives.* New York: Springer.

Dobash, R. P., & Dobash, R. E. (1979). *Violence against wives: A case against the patriarchy.* New York: Free Press.

Doress, P. B., & Siegal, D. L. (1987). *Ourselves, growing older.* New York: Simon & Schuster.

Douglas, M. (1966). *Purity and danger.* London: Routledge.

Dubler, N. N. (1993). Commentary: Balancing life and death—proceed with caution. *American Journal of Public Health, 83*(1), 23–25.

Durkheim, E. (1915). *Elementary forms of the religious life.* London: Hollen St. Press.

Dvorchak, R. (1992, October 5). Social health "index" puts U.S. at 21-year low. *Boston Globe,* p. 3.

Erikson, E. (1963). *Childhood and society* (2nd ed.). New York: Norton.

Estes, C. L. (1986, June 30). *Older women and health policy.* Paper presented at the Women, Health, and Healing Summer Institute, University of California, Berkeley.

Eyre, J., & Eyre, R. (1993). *Teaching your children values.* New York: Simon & Schuster.

Fagerhaugh, S. Y., & Strauss, A. (1977). *Politics of pain management.* Menlo Park, CA: Addison-Wesley.

Fehr, B. (1995). *Friendship process.* Thousand Oaks, CA: Sage.

Feifel, H. (Ed.). (1977). *New meanings of death.* New York: McGraw-Hill.

Field, M. J., & Cassel, C. K. (Eds.). (1997). *Approaching death: Improving care at the end of life.* Washington, DC: National Academy Press.

Fisher, R., Ross, M. M., & MacLean, M. J. (2000). *A guide to end-of-life care for seniors.* Toronto and Ottawa: University of Toronto and University of Ottawa.

Freud, S. (1950). *Totem and taboo.* London: Routledge.

Fried, N. N., & Fried, M. H. (1980). *Transitions: Four rituals in eight cultures.* New York: Norton.

Fulton, R., Markusen, R., Owen, G., & Scheiber, J. J. (Eds.). (1978). *Death and dying.* Reading, MA: Addison-Wesley.

General Assembly of the United Nations. (1975). Dying person's bill of rights. *American Journal of Nursing, 75,* 99.

Gil, D., & Gil, E. (1987). *The future of work.* Rochester, VT: Schenkman.

Glaser, B. G., & Strauss, A. (1965). *Awareness of dying.* Hawthorne, NY: Aldine de Gruyter.

Golan, N. (1981). *Passing through transitions.* New York: Free Press.

Goodman, L. M. (1981). *Death and the creative life.* New York: Springer.

Goody, J. (1962). *Death, property, and the ancestors.* London: Tavistock.

Halpern, H. (1982). *How to break your addiction to a person.* New York: McGraw-Hill.

Haynor, P. M. (1998). Meeting the challenge of advance directives. *American Journal of Nursing, 98*(3), 26–32.

Hoff, L. A. (1978). *The status of widows: Analysis of selected examples from Africa and India.* Unpublished master's dissertation, London School of Economics.

Hoff, L. A. (1990). *Battered women as survivors.* London: Routledge.

Hogberg, U., & Bergstrom, E. (2000). Suffocated prone: The iatrogenic tragedy of SIDS. *American Journal of Public Health, 90*(4), 527–531.

Hyman, J. W., & Rome, E. R. (1996). *Sacrificing our selves for love.* Freedom, CA: Crossing Press.

Inch, S. (1984). *Birth rights.* New York: Pantheon Books.

Irving, H. H., & Benjamin, M. (1995). *Family mediation: Contemporary issues.* Thousand Oaks, CA: Sage.

Jacobs, R. H. (1979). *Life after youth.* Boston: Beacon Press.

Jordan, B. (1993). *Birth in four cultures* (4th ed.). Prospect Heights, IL: Waveland Press.

Kachoyeanos, M. K., & Selder, F. E. (1993). Life transitions of parents at the unexpected death of a school-age and older child. *Journal of Pediatric Nursing, 8*(1), 41–49.

Kastenbaum, R. (2000). *The psychology of death.* (3rd ed.). New York: Springer.

Kelly, K. (1999, January 3). Legislators, colleges move to curb students' binge drinking. *Boston Sunday Globe,* p. N7.

Killeen, M. (1990). The influence of stress and coping on family caregivers' perceptions of health. *International Journal of Aging and Human Development, 30*(3), 197–211.

Kimball, S. T. (1960). *Introduction: Rites of passage* (A. van Gennep, Trans.). Chicago: University of Chicago Press. (Original French edition published 1909)

Krishnan, V. (1994). Attitudes toward surrogate motherhood in Canada. *Health Care for Women International, 15*(4), 333–358.

Kübler-Ross, E. (1969). *On death and dying.* New York: Macmillan.

Kübler-Ross, E. (1975). *Death, the final stage of growth.* Englewood Cliffs, NJ: Prentice Hall.

Lack, S., & Buckingham, R. W. (1978). *First American hospice.* New Haven, CT: Hospice.

LaFontaine, J. (1977). The power of rights. *Man, 12,* 421–437.

Leach, P. (1994). *What our society must do—and is not doing—for our children today.* New York: Knopf.

Leach, P. (1997). *Your baby and child: New visions for the '90s.* New York: Knopf.

Levinson, D. J., Darrow, C. N., Klein, E. N., Levinson, M. H., & McKee, B. (1978). *The seasons of a man's life.* New York: Knopf.

Lopata, H. Z. (1995). *Current widowhood: Myths and realities.* Thousand Oaks, CA: Sage.

Maltas, C. (1992). Trouble in paradise: Marital crises of midlife. *Psychiatry, 55*(2), 122–131.

MacPherson, K. (1992). Cardiovascular disease prevention in women and noncontraceptive use of hormones: A feminist analysis. *Advances in Nursing Science, 14*(4), 34–49.

Martikainen, P., & Valkonen, T. (1996). Mortality after the death of a spouse: Rates and causes of death in a large Finnish cohort. *American Journal of Public Health, 86*(8), 1087–1093.

McCabe, S. V. (1982). An overview of hospice care. *Cancer Nursing, 5,* 103–108.

McKenry, P. C., & Price, S. J. (Eds.). (2000). *Families and change: Coping with stressful events and transitions* (2nd ed.). Thousand Oaks, CA: Sage.

Mickleburgh, R. (1993, November 30). Prohibit surrogate mothers, report says—controls urged for technology. *Globe and Mail,* pp. 1, A6–A7.

Minkler, M., & Fuller-Thomson, E. (1999). The health of grandparents raising grandchildren: Results of a national study. *American Journal of Public Health, 89*(9), 1384–1389.

Mitford, J. (1963). *The American way of death.* New York: Simon & Schuster.

Mitford, J. (1993). *The American way of birth.* New York: NAL/Dutton.

Moore, T. (1992). *Care of the soul: A guide for cultivating depth and sacredness in everyday life.* New York: Walker.

Newby, D. (1993). *Intergenerational caregiving: Transition from grandparent to parent.* Unpublished doctoral dissertation, Boston College.

Ngugi, W. (1965). *The river between.* London: Heinemann.

Novello, J. (1993). *What to do until the grown-up arrives.* Kirkland, WA: Hogrefe & Huber.

Nuland, S. B. (1994). *How we die: Reflections on life's final chapter.* New York: Random House.

O'Callaghan, J. B. (1993). *School-based collaboration with families.* San Francisco: Jossey-Bass.

Panchuck, P. (1994). *The midlife experience of contemporary women: Views along the midway.* Unpublished doctoral dissertation, Leslie College, Boston.

Papernow, P. L. (1993). *Becoming a stepfamily: Patterns of development in remarried families.* San Francisco: Jossey-Bass.

Pfeiffer, S. (1999, December 5). Parental grief of loss compounded. *Boston Sunday Globe,* pp. B1, B6.

Pillemer, K., Moen, P., Wethington, E., & Glasgow, N. (Eds.). (2000). *Social integration in the second half of life.* Baltimore: Johns Hopkins University Press.

Raymond, D. (1992). "In the best interests of the child": Thoughts on homophobia and parenting. In W. J. Blumenfeld (Ed.), *Homophobia: How we all pay the price* (pp. 114–130). Boston: Beacon Press.

Richman, J. (1993). *Preventing elderly suicide: Overcoming personal despair, professional indifference and social bias.* New York: Springer.

Rosenthal, T. (1973). *How could I not be among you?* New York: Braziller.

Ross, M. M., Fisher, R., & MacLean, M. J. (2000, June–August). Toward optimal care for seniors who are dying: An approach to care. *Mature Medicine Canada,* 127–130.

Ruddick, S. (1989). *Maternal thinking: Toward a politics of peace.* Boston: Beacon Press.

Russo, F. (1997, October). Can the government prevent divorce? *Atlantic Monthly,* 28–42.

Sadker, M., & Sadker, D. (1994). *Failing at fairness: How America's schools cheat girls.* New York: Scribner.

Saunders, C. (1978). Hospice care. *American Journal of Medicine, 65,* 726–728.

Saunders, C., & Kastenbaum, R. (Eds.). (1997). *Hospice care on the international scene.* New York: Springer.

Schwarz, J. K. (1999). Assisted dying and nursing practice. *Image: Journal of Nursing Scholarship, 31*(4), 367–373

Sidel, R. (1996). *Women and children last: The plight of poor women in affluent America.* New York: Penguin Books.

Solomon, M. Z., O'Donnell, L., Jennings, B., Guilfoy, V., Wolf, S. M., Nolan, K., Jackson, B. A., Koch-Weser, D., & Donnelley, S. (1993). Decisions near the end of life: Professional views on life-sustaining treatments. *American Journal of Public Health, 83*(1), 14–23.

Sommers, T., & Shields, L. (1987). *Women take care: The consequences of caregiving in today's society.* Gainesville, Fl: Triad.

Spencer, P. (1973). *Nomads in alliance.* Oxford: Oxford University Press.

Stevenson, J. S. (1977). *Issues and crises during middlescence.* Englewood Cliffs, NJ: Appleton-Century-Crofts.

Straus, M. A., Gelles, R. J., & Steinmetz, S. K. (1980). *Behind closed doors: Violence in the American family.* New York: Anchor Books.

Teichman, Y., Shenhar, S., & Segal, S. (1993). Emotional distress in Israeli women before and after abortion. *American Journal of Orthopsychiatry, 63*(2), 277–288.

Thurer, S. L. (1994). *The myths of motherhood: How culture reinvents the good mother.* Boston: Houghton Mifflin.

Tolstoy, L. (1960). *The death of Ivan Ilyich.* New York: New American Library. (Original work published 1886)

Turner, V. (1967). *The forest of souls.* Ithaca, NY: Cornell University Press.

van Gennep, A. (1960). *Rites of passage.* Chicago: University of Chicago Press. (Original French edition published 1909)

Van Ornum, W., & Mordock, J. B. (1987). *Crisis counseling with children and adolescents.* New York: Continuum.

Walker, A. (1992). *Possessing the secret of joy.* Orlando: Harcourt Brace.

Walsh, F., & McGoldrick, M. (Eds.). (1991). *Living beyond loss: Death in the family.* New York: Norton.

Wegman, J. A. (1987). Hospice home death, hospital death, and coping abilities of widows. *Cancer Nursing, 10*(3), 148–155.

Weingarten, K. (1994). *The mother's voice: Strengthening intimacies in families.* Orlando: Harcourt Brace.

Weiss, R. S. (1976). Transition states and other stressful situations: Their nature and programs for their management. In G. Caplan & M. Killilea (Eds.), *Support systems and mutual help: A multi-disciplinary exploration* (pp. 213–232). Philadelphia: Grune & Stratton.

West, C., & Hewlett, S. A. (1999). *The war against parents.* Boston: Houghton Mifflin

Williams, W. L. (1986). *The spirit and the flesh: Sexual diversity in American Indian culture.* Boston: Beacon Press.

Williams, W. L. (1992). Benefits for nonhomophobic societies: An anthropological perspective. In W. J. Blumenfeld (Ed.), *Homophobia: How we all pay the price* (pp. 258–274). Boston: Beacon Press.

Wong, D. S. (1999, July 5). Single fathers embrace role, fight stereotype. *Boston Globe,* pp. A1, A16.

World Health Organization. (1994). *Maternal and child health and family planning: Traditional practices harmful to the health of women and children* (Resolution WHA 47). Geneva: World Health Assembly, 47th.

Wright, L. K. (1985). Life-threatening illness. *Journal of Psychosocial Nursing, 23*(9), 7–11.

Zelditch, M. (1968). Status, social. In D. L. Sills (Ed.), *International encyclopedia of the social sciences.* New York: Macmillan and Free Press.

NAME INDEX

A

Adamek, M. E., 220
Adamowski, K., 4, 14, 15, 19, 23, 66, 71, 72, 89, 105, 124, 156, 215, 216, 229, 296, 297, 352, 353, 356, 391
Advocacy Centre for the Elderly and Community Legal Education Ontario, 274
Affara, F. A., 422
Aguilera, D. C., 8, 10
Ahmed, F. A., 324–325
Aiken, L. H., 378
Akhter, M. N., 10, 112
Albelda, R., 402
Allen, K. R., 140
Alvarez, A., 190
American Association of Colleges of Nursing, 237, 312
Amnesty International, 409
Anderson, C. M., 449
Andrews, B., 331
Antonovsky, A., 17, 25, 42, 133, 340
Apfel, R. J., 338, 342
Arditti, R., 436
Arendell, T., 434
Aries, P., 456
Armer, J. M., 408
Arnetz, B. B., 299
Arnetz, J. E., 299

Arnold, E., 108
Asch, D. A., 456
Atkinson, J. M., 169
Attneave, C., 133
Aubry, J., 409
Auerbach, J. D., 365
Austin, J. B., 305
Avery, K. L., 453
Avison, W. R., 34, 41

B

Babcock, J., 305
Baber, K. M., 140
Badger, T. A., 169
Baechler, J., 184
Bagley, C., 245
Baker, L. A., 377
Balach, L., 193
Baldessarini, R. J., 217
Baracos, H. A., 295
Bard, M., 292
Barnett, R. C., 397
Barney, K., 22, 72, 127
Barry, K., 375
Barter, J. T., 204, 301
Barth, R. B., 366
Bartholet, E., 435
Bates, J. D., 435
Bateson, G., 108
Battin, M. P., 175, 177, 180, 231
Baugher, M., 193

Baum, A., 39, 320, 339
Baum, M., 79
Bayer, R., 368–369
Beardslee, W. R., 167
Bebbington, P., 42
Beck, A. T., 196
Beck, J. S., 196
Becker, H., 66, 173
Becktell, P. J., 355
Begun, J. W., 11
Bell, C. C., 58, 204, 241, 301, 303
Bellah, R., 413
Bengtson, V. L., 42
Benjamin, M., 434
Benne, K. D., 57, 58
Bennett, L., 290, 305, 306
Bennett, R. T., 247
Bentovim, A., 236
Bergstrom, E., 35, 429
Berk, R. A., 304, 312
Berkman, L. F., 133
Berlin, I. N., 205
Berman, A. L., 179, 193, 204, 214, 215, 216, 218, 222, 226, 228–229
Bernardi, P. J., 177
Bertalanffy, L. von, 11
Bertman, S. L., 391, 456, 457, 458
Besancon, V., 19, 91, 414
Besharov, D., 239
Bianco, M., 375, 379
Bishop, E. E., 137

SUBJECT INDEX

A

AA. *See* Alcoholics
    Anonymous (AA)
AAC. *See* AIDS Action Committee
    (AAC)
AACN. *See* American Association
    of Colleges of Nurses (AACN)
AARP. *See* American Association of
    Retired Persons (AARP)
AAS. *See* American Association of
    Suicidology (AAS)
Abortion, 382–383, 432
Abuse: communication in cases of,
    277–278; and crisis assessment,
    73–74; and victim blaming,
    44–45, 45f. *See also* Victims;
    Violence; Woman battering
Acquaintance rape, 236, 252
Acquired immune deficiency
    syndrome (AIDS): and
    adolescents, 443; and anger,
    369–371; and anxiety, 371; and
    blame, 375, 376; caretakers of
    people with, 377–380; children
    with, 375–376, 443; and
    churches, 379; community
    responses to, 379–380; coping
    with, 371–374, 372t, 378–379;
    counseling in cases of, 370, 376,
    377; crisis manifestations of,
    369–371; as crisis origin,

364–365, 368–369; and Crisis
    Paradigm, 368, 370f; crisis
    resolution for people with,
    371–374; and crisis workers,
    378; and dementia, 371; and
    discrimination, 364, 365–366,
    376, 379; and families, 372t,
    377–380; feelings of patients
    with, 359; and guilt, 369–371;
    and HIV testing, 377; and
    lesbians, 375–376; mothers of
    people with, 377–378; and
    poverty, 365; and pregnancy,
    374, 375; prevalence of, 365;
    preventive intervention for, 376;
    and rape, 375–396; resources
    for people with, 371, 373; risk
    factors for, 365; social network
    and, 374; society's response to,
    365–366; sociocultural factors
    affecting people with, 365–366,
    369, 371, 375; and stress, 371,
    378–379; and suicide, 374;
    support groups for people with,
    378–379; women with,
    374–376
Action for Mental Health, 12–13, 352
Acute care, 390–391
Addiction, 447. *See also* Alcohol
    abuse; Drug abuse
Adolescents: and AIDS, 443; and
    alcohol abuse, 443; counseling

for, 160, 216, 441–442, 445;
    crisis intervention for, 438–439,
    440f, 441–443, 445; crisis
    management for, 440f; crisis
    services for, 438–439; and
    culture, 204–205; dependence
    of, 223–224, 438; and depres-
    sion, 196; development of, 224,
    438; homosexual, 439, 440f;
    listening to, 443; as parents,
    248, 434–435; rituals of,
    424–426, 425t; self-destructive
    behavior of, 439; and suicide,
    167, 168–169, 178, 193, 194,
    196, 216; and suicide attempts,
    192; suicide prevention for,
    223–224; and suicide risk
    assessment, 204–205; transition
    states of, 438–439.*See also*
    Children
Adoption, 435, 436
Advertising, 253
Africa, 236, 275, 303, 365, 375, 409
Ageism, 275
Agent Orange, 338
Aid to Incarcerated Mothers, 310
AIDS. *See* Acquired immune
    deficiency syndrome (AIDS)
AIDS Action Committee (AAC),
    366, 367, 373, 377, 378, 379
AIDS Dementia Complex, 371
Al-Anon, 161

Wilbert O. Galitz

Humanizing Office Automation

The Impact of Ergonomics on Productivity

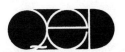

QED Information Sciences, Inc.
Wellesley, Massachusetts

To Sharon, and the growing family:
Kevin, Lisa, Mitchell, and Barry;
Karin and Mark; and Kim

Acknowledgments

The following material is reproduced with the kind permission of the copyright owners listed: Tables 4.2, 4.3, and 4.4 are from J. D. Hodges and B. W. Angalet, "The prime technical information source—the local work environment," *Human Factors*, Vol. 10, No. 4, copyright 1968, and Figure 7.1 from J. P. Duncanson and A. D. Williams, "Video conferencing; reactions of users," *Human Factors*, Vol. 15, No. 5, copyright 1973. Table 9.1 is from "The Steelcase National Study of Office Environments," *Contract*, January 1979, Gralla Publications, Inc., and is reproduced courtesy Gralla Publications, Inc., and Steelcase, Inc. Figure 9.1 is from *Modern Office Procedures*, March 1978, copyright 1978 by Penton/IPC, subsidiary of Pittway Corporation. Figure 9.2 is from *The Office*, March 1978, courtesy Office Publications, Inc. Table 10.1 is from *On Language*, by William Safire, copyright 1980, TIMES BOOKS /The New York Times Book Co., Inc.

Contents

Foreword

The retail distribution of computer technology was inconceivable to the data processing professionals five years ago. Most veterans of the computer revolution still find it disquieting to hear the media extol the virtues of hardware and software products. It seems, too, as if every commercial promises that the product is "user friendly."

Certainly, designers of microcomputer equipment and programs have made tremendous strides in advancing the "friendliness" of these products. In fact, one might argue that it was the "ease of use" phenomenon that fanned the acceptance and sales of these products, instead of the pricing, even though the latter reflects magnificent advances in engineering and manufacturing.

But are these products really "user friendly"? No doubt, they are much friendlier than their predecessors, which intimidated users for decades. Remember, however, that the intelligent application of knowledge about human factors and behavioral science in the architecture and construction of computer-based systems is still in the earliest stages of evolution. It is likely that today's "friendlier" products will be ridiculed as naive, awkward, and ineffective five years from now. While the value of the art of incorporating human factors in computer technology is recognized, the body of knowledge and experience required to refine the art is still sparse.

The signs of substantive progress will be conspicuous when college catalogs offer courses in "Human Factors in Systems Design," along with programming and technical courses. Or when MIS departments routinely employ full-time behavioral scientists. Or when software allows users to design their own system.

In the meantime, the more enlightened designers and managers will recognize the need for orientation to this new discipline, and will at least familiarize themselves with current methods, techniques, and concepts. This book should assist them in that process.

GERALD MASKOVSKY

Managing Director
Marsh & McLennan

Preface

In this book I have attempted to bring into as clear a focus as possible a constantly shifting and moving target—the human being in the automated office. My objectives have been

- to define the discipline of human factors/ergonomics as it relates to office automation, in order to provide a coherent viewpoint;
- to classify behavioral considerations in office automation so that principles and findings can be cataloged;
- to describe the relevant principles and research results (both applied and laboratory).

Gaps will inevitably appear in any body of knowledge; by its nature, knowledge can never be complete. This book is an extension of and improvement upon its predecessor, *Human Factors in Office Automation* (Life Office Management Association, Inc., 1980); undoubtedly, we will be able to say the same of any successor. Nevertheless, I believe this volume describes the state of the art for human factors/ergonomics.

I would like to thank the many researchers and practitioners actively involved in this complex and challenging field for their contribution to this body of knowledge. Without each and every one, this book could not exist.

This work also reflects the past and continuing support of a number of people and organizations, some of which associations predate this effort by a great number of years. The individuals, for all of whom I at one time worked, are Ralph Notto, Gerry Maskovsky, and Jack Endicott. The organizations are QED Information Sciences, Inc. (Wellesley, Massachusetts), Business Forms Management Association (Portland, Oregon), and Administrative Management Society (Willow Grove, Pennsylvania). To them all I give my thanks.

Last, this effort could not have been completed without the unstinting support of my wife, Sharon. To her I give special thanks.

1

Planning for Office Automation

The office, an indistinct arena of human interactions, ambiguous communications, poorly understood actions, and rigid habit patterns, is being besieged by a force that promises to free it from the drudgery and inefficiencies that have plagued it for decades. This force is composed of a variety of entities like word processing, personal computers, electronic mail, and video conferencing, and is known collectively as office automation. Those who are seduced by its technological promise have predicted a speedy solution to office woes through its implementation. Some feel that automation offers a far greater promise than meets the most perceptive eye—greater perhaps than any previous technological application, including data processing (Bair 1979). It is also felt that automation may bring about an organizational revolution among white-collar workers comparable to that caused by the advent of the assembly line among blue-collar workers (Carlisle 1976).

But a funny thing has happened along this path to the pot of gold at the end of the rainbow. Few technologists took the time to ascertain whether the office worker needed, wanted, or could cope with the onslaught of technology. Common worker reactions have included outright rejection of technology, feelings of job erosion, and work alienation brought about by more specialized tasks and dehumanized communications, concerns for health and safety, and increasing resistance to all new technology. For the implementors of technology the result was often shattered dreams and spectacular failures.

Past results, current trends, and future fears have for many years led automation experts to conclude that, in the long run, behavioral considerations are the key factor in introducing new office technologies (Bair 1979; Connell 1979; Drageset 1979; Kirkley 1980; and Maskovsky 1979). Indeed, the past decade is littered with the corpses of systems that failed because people were forgotten in the design process (Bryce 1979; Diran 1978; Igersheim 1976; Johnson et al. 1978; and Lucas 1976). Today, behavioral considerations are a paramount concern whenever office automation issues are addressed. Office

1

automation can no longer be viewed as a technological end in itself. It must reflect the needs and goals of the office worker as well as the organization if greater human efficiency, effectiveness, and productivity are to be achieved. Only when both organizational and personal goals are harmonious will greater productivity ultimately result. Technology must remain a tool of people, not the reverse.

Before beginning a survey of the office and its human factors, a look at the office of yesterday and today is appropriate. Such a survey will provide a context for the remainder of this book.

Yesterday's Office

The office of the 1800s was very different from that which exists today (Markus and Yates 1982). Most organizations were small and occupied a single location. The few employees located outside the office were usually agents marketing the company's products elsewhere. The bulk of written communication occurred between the company and the outside world. Internal communications were generally face-to-face, and internal written documents were infrequent. Storage for written communications usually consisted of pigeonholes in rolltop desks and boxes or drawers in which paper was stored flat. Outgoing correspondence was copied by pressing it between the dampened tissue leaves of a bound *press book*. Searching for correspondence required knowing the approximate dates of creation, the frequent moving of storage boxes, and shuffling of papers. Since incoming and outgoing correspondence was stored in a different manner, it was impossible to retrieve all on the same subject at a single try. Technological support to yesterday's office first occurred with the invention and mass production of the typewriter in the 1870s and the telephone at about the same time.

In the late 1800s companies began to grow larger and more complex. The volume of external correspondence ballooned, and the need for internal correspondence became obvious. Two more technological innovations were needed to cope with changing needs. The first was a way of vertically storing information to make it more accessible. In 1876 vertical card files were created for libraries, and in 1893 vertical office files were introduced by a library supply company. Drawers eliminated the need to unstack boxes, and vertical positioning of their contents enabled them to be searched without removing the contents. The second innovation was a way of producing loose, rather than bound, copies of documents. This need was satisfied by Edison's invention of the mimeograph machine about 1870, and the creation of carbon paper, which achieved widespread use shortly after 1900. Combined with vertical filing, these reproduction methods enabled incoming and outgoing correspondence to be easily stored and retrieved together. It created an *organization memory* independent of the people who stored the information.

Vertical filing created a revolution in offices. In the first two decades of this century a dramatic increase in the number of internal memoranda occurred. Standard formats were devised, and various indexing schemes developed. Filing areas sprang up in all organizations and in many company departments.

The elements of this office, the desks, chairs, files, lights, floor plans, kinds of job, and so forth, were created to expedite the flow of paper through the system. Since paper was handled manually, control over the form and pace of the information flow and job performance rested primarily with the worker. The design of the office components were standardized, reflecting primarily engineering and manufacturing considerations. The modern office had arrived—or so it seemed.

Today's Office

The seeds for today's office were sown in the late 1930s and '40s with the invention of the photocopier and computer. In the 1960s xerography began to unleash tons of paper into the office at the push of a button. In the 1960s and '70s the computer began providing a viable alternative means of information storage by permitting it to be done electronically. It also made possible the creation and transmission of information electronically, and reduced the time in which tasks could be performed from hours to microseconds. The computer's invasion into the office has been meteoric. Various estimates indicate that one in every seven to ten white-collar workers today interact with a computer in one way or another. Some occupations, such as banking and insurance, will find 90 percent of their tasks done electronically before the decade is over.

The office in which automation is firmly trying to entrench itself, however, has solid roots. Since the revolutionary changes around the turn of this century, the office has been geared to stability and slow change. It is a nebulous environment of human interactions, communications, and rigid habits, and its pulse is difficult to grasp. Its costs are increasing at a rate of 12–15 percent a year while the typical person working within it utilizes only 40 percent of his or her potential. Many of its occupants, especially the managers and professionals, have traditionally been told only what to do and not how to do it. They have tended to develop highly personalized ways of working. The office elements, its desks, chairs, and so on, are primarily a carryover from the earlier era when manufacturing considerations prevailed.

The work ethic of the modern office worker is also changing. The desire for material things is being expanded to include psychological incentives. Workers are much more concerned today with the quality of the work life and the humanization of the work environment. Interesting and meaningful work is a sought-after goal. Variety is preferred to routine, and informality to structured settings. The authority of management is being questioned, and participation in decisions affecting a person's work is valued (McKendrick 1982).

It is into this complex cauldron that automation moves. Managing the changes automation requires is difficult because few meaningful precedents exist, and there are many uncertainties. Coping with change no longer means simply adapting to a new status quo. It means adapting to continuous change in an environment that is dynamic, not static. Managing such change is complicated by the fact that it is doubtful that management and office personnel are absorbing and utilizing those changes that have already occurred. Toffler (1971) points out that there is a limited pace at which humans can respond to change. The increasing lag between this human response and rapid change is the basis for his *future shock*.

The Changing Medium of Information

As the information in today's office moves from a paper-based to an electronic-based medium, the characteristics of the information are changing in both substance and style. The most common electronic-based medium—the visual display terminal, or VDT—possesses many characteristics that are almost the opposite of paper. Table 1-1, derived from Springer (1982), compares these two visual display media.

Display characteristics. Information displayed on paper is legible and readable, based upon years of research toward developing a quality product. The matte surface of the paper diffuses reflected light, scarcely affecting the quality of the material presented. Paper-based information may be read under a variety of lighting conditions, with the upper limit of illumination seldom a concern. By contrast, VDT characters are luminous and often of a dot-matrix construction. The character image may be blurred by dust on the VDT screen or by reflections from overhead lights or windows. In general, reading information on a display screen imposes greater visual demands on a person than does reading information on a piece of paper.

Viewing plane. Papers are normally read horizontally, such as resting on a desk top. They may be read vertically, however, by physically raising the paper to a position perpendicular to the eye. VDTs are normally read in a

Table 1-1.   Characteristics of Two Visual Display Media

Paper/Hard Copy	*Electronic/VDT*
Dark characters on a light background	Light characters on a dark background
Continuous-line characters	Dot-matrix characters
Matte surface	Reflective surface
Horizontal plane	Vertical plane
Manual input	Keyboard input
Easy to handle	Difficult to manipulate
Perceptually permanent	Perceptually transient
Date stored physically	Data stored electronically
Information presented simultaneously	Information presented serially

vertical plane since internal mechanics and concerns with light reflections permit little flexibility.

Kind of input. Papers are normally completed by hand, VDTs through use of a keyboard. Writing skills are far more common than keying skills. When writing, a person's eyes follow the hands, providing immediate feedback. When keying, the hands operate in a different visual plane than that of the information display. Therefore, keying is a more complex visual motor task.

Handling characteristics. Paper can be easily manipulated to get it into a comfortable viewing position. It can be held forward, backward, tilted, placed on the desk, placed or held at arm's length. VDTs, on the other hand, are difficult to move. Viewing angles and distances can usually be changed only by posture changes of the viewer, such as leaning forward, backward, or to the side.

Information permanence. A hard copy is relatively permanent. Information seldom disappears from paper. Visual confirmation of presence is seldom required. Paper can, however, be misplaced or misfiled. Information on a VDT screen can disappear as a result of a burp by the machine or the inadvertent pressing of a wrong key. The perceptual and physical permanence of information can affect the way people think and feel about it. Physical permanence and control is usually preferred to transience and lack of control.

Information presentation. Display of information on a VDT is limited by the boundaries or size of the display area. Often information must be presented serially, such as a string of snapshots viewed in sequence. Comparisons of information displayed on different screens is difficult. To do so requires an exceptional memory or, more often, paper-and-pencil notes. The breadth of display of paper information is only restricted by the physical size of the work area.

The new nature of the display medium is a fundamental change accompanying the introduction of computer-based technology. This seemingly simple change from paper to electronics has had profound consequences in the demands imposed on the office's personnel and the environment.

Automation's Users

Office automation is being presented to two kinds of users. The first includes the fairly young and well educated who have been exposed to automation as part of their education. These people know what technology offers and demand its application. The second group—those educated before technology began infiltrating educational institutions—have been exposed to technology only from a distance. These people are busy, untrained, and nontechnical. The sole criteria by which they judge technology will be its ability to help them perform jobs faster and easier than traditional methods. These are the users to whom technology must be sold. Martin (1973) has described them as follows:

- *Highly intelligent.* They demand system speeds that match their information-absorption speed. Typewriter-like terminals, for example, are frustratingly slow.
- *Not amenable to training.* The extent and pressures of their daily activities leave time for only rudimentary training.
- *Not code- or mnemonic-oriented.* The system's language must be the same as that used in the users' daily activities.
- *Highly impatient.* They have a low tolerance level for delays in learning to use new systems or tools.
- *Requiring a high information bandwidth.* They must absorb or communicate a maximum amount of information and make decisions in a minimum amount of time.
- *Nonrugged.* They will reject a system if confused by unintelligible messages or unclear procedures.
- *Having a low panic threshold.* If they perceive themselves as looking foolish to others (especially to subordinates), they will rapidly reject a system. This is common in people approaching a system for the first time.
- *Demanding a worthwhile payoff.* They must perceive that the gains they can achieve from a system exceed the energies they must expend to use it.

The Road to the Future

The objective of any advanced office system should be to support people who have jobs to do. The road to be followed should lead to improved productivity and worker satisfaction through harmonization of the workers, the organization, and technology. A behavioral-technical system must be created where jobs, computer systems, the work environment, and people's motivations and psychological needs are properly woven into the entire office fabric.

Human needs, considerations, and goals in office automation—the human factors or ergonomic aspects—are the topic of this book. It begins with a review of what *human factors* and its sibling *ergonomics* really are. It then focuses on the behavioral problems and concerns that office automation has unleashed. This is followed by a look at the tasks that comprise the office worker's job. Finally, a series of behavioral design guidelines are presented for the aspects of the office that influence the well-being of the workers and the organization. Included are the design of systems, jobs, equipment, the environment, documentaion, and training. Special chapters are devoted to electronic meetings and other new communication technologies as well as to managing the change process. The objective is to give the reader a well-rounded look at all the considerations. Office automation, if it is to be successful, cannot afford to ignore these issues, for they are all interrelated.

References

Bair, J. H. "Planning for Office Automation." *The Automated Office*, pp. 449–462. American Inst. of Industrial Engr., 1979.

Bryce, M. "In Perspective," edited by R. B. Frost. *Infosystems*, July 1979.

Carlisle, J. H. "Evaluating the Impact of Office Automation on Top Management Communication." *AFIPS Conference Proceedings*. 45 (1976): 611–616.

Connell, J. J. "Opening Remarks." *Summary of Proceedings*, Fall 1979. Pasadena, Calif.: Office Technology Research Group, 1979.

Diran, K. M. "Management Information Systems: The Human Factor." *Journal of Higher Education* 49, No. 3 (May/June 1978): 273–282.

Drageset, D. J. "Remarks." *Summary of Proceedings (Fall 1979)*. Pasadena, Calif.: Office Technology Research Group, 1979.

Igersheim, R. H. "Managerial Response to an Information System," edited by Stanley Winkler. *AFIPS National Computer Conference Proceedings* 1976. Montvale, N. J.: AFIPS Press, 1976, pp. 877–882.

Johnson, J. H.; Williams, T. A.; Giannetti, R. A.; Klinger, D. E.; and Nakashima, S. R. "Organizational Preparedness for Change: Staff Acceptance of an On-Line Computer–Assisted Assessment System." *Behavioral Research Methods and Instrumentation* 10, No. 2 (April 1978): 186–190.

Kirkley, J. L. "The Office Merry-Go-Round." *Datamation* 26, No. 2 (February 1980): 43.

Lucas, H. C. *Why Information Systems Fail*. New York: Columbia University Press, 1976.

Martin, J. *Design of Man-Computer Dialogues*. Englewood Cliffs, N.J.: Prentice-Hall, 1973.

Maskovsky, G.S. "Planning for the Office of the Future." *Summary of Proceedings,* Fall 1979. Pasadena, Calif.: Office Technology Research Group, 1979.

Markus, M. L., and Yates, J. "Historical Lessons for the Automated Office." *Computer Decisions,* June 1982, pp. 116–121.

McKendrick, J. "The Office of 1990–Human Resources." *Management World*, 1982.

Springer, T. J. "Automation, Ergonomics and Offices: Evolution or Revolution?" *Journal of Information Management* 4, No. 1 (Fall 1982).

Toffler, A. *Future Shock.* New York: Bantam Books, 1971.

2

Human Factors/Ergonomics

What are the human factors and behavioral considerations that we hear so much about? What is *ergonomics*? Scattered through popular literature is little of substance to assist those who try to apply exploding technologies. The definitions given for *human factors* and *ergonomics* are sometimes misleading. Many practitioners still associate human factors with vague concerns for the needs of people, with specifics seldom pinned down.

We shall begin by defining the science of human factors and its sister science of ergonomics. We shall then examine their history, both pre- and post-computer. This will be followed by examples of how they are applied and how their effectiveness is measured. Finally, we shall summarize some human characteristics of crucial importance in the design and implementation of technology.

Human Factors and Ergonomics Defined

Human factors has assumed a number of meanings in recent years. It has been used to refer to the characteristics of people, a design philosophy, the name for a profession, and the name for a branch of science.

As a science, human factors is the scientific study of people at work. It involves systematically applying knowledge of people's sensory, physical, intellectual, and motivational attributes to the design of the equipment, software and systems, tasks, documentation, and environment of the office. Its ultimate objective is to achieve maximum human efficiency and effectiveness in system development, operation, and maintenance. At its core is systematic analysis of human/machine problems through research. As a design philosophy, it simply means that people should get top priority in the way things are designed.

The term *human factors* is historically of North American derivation. For years practitioners in the United States and Canada have used this and similar terms (such as *human engineering* or *human factors engineering* which will be described more fully in the history to follow).

In recent years in North America another term has come into popular use to describe what human factors is and does. It is essentially the European term for the same thing and was imported because of its catchy name. The word is *ergonomics.*

Ergonomics is a word derived from the Greek term "ergo," meaning *work,* and "nomos," meaning *natural laws.* Specifically, it was used to connote a worker's relationship to the physical things around him or her, including the equipment, workplace layout, and the environmental conditions. Its original intent was narrower than human factors, implying more of an engineering thrust. The design of human/computer interactions and software were not addressed in the traditional setting of ergonomics.

This is changing, however. The term *software ergonomics* was recently coined, which completely closed the definition gap between ergonomics and human factors. Soon, the words will be interchangeable, ergonomics encompassing everything that human factors does. Whether ergonomics will assume ascendency as the word to fully describe the scientific study of people at work remains to be seen.

A Brief History

The objectives of human factors are old. Mankind's history has been characterized by efforts to do things more efficiently and to economize both time and effort. The primitive person who lived more than 600,000 years ago fashioned stones into crude choppers to aid in cutting. The same motivation was evident in the ingenuity of the person who first used sails instead of paddles to propel a boat. It is evident today in the person who buys push-button appliances to do housework. But while the objectives of human factors are as ancient as people themselves, the crystallization of these concepts into a specific field of endeavor is a recent development.

Historically, much of the progress in designing tasks or implements for human use has been the result of experience. Many devices used in the home and factory evolved this way, such as kitchen utensils, doorknobs, and hand tools. Experience is a good test of such devices and procedures, at least to the extent that it identifies those that are inadequate for human use.

Twentieth-century developments of more complex equipment and procedures, however, necessitated more than just human experience to determine the adequacy of designs. By the late 1930s two new approaches to solving modern design problems had developed. One concerned work methods and involved the use of time-and-motion studies to further simplify repetitive tasks. The other was selection and training of people to match whatever tasks existed.

World War II, however, brought complex weapons systems that required more complicated human/machine interaction. The selection-and-training approach could no longer provide enough personnel to meet operational needs. The focus shifted to developing devices that large numbers of people could use. Equipment and devices became *human engineered*, as it was called in America.

In Europe, *ergonomics* was born. After the war, human engineering continued to thrive in the military environment.

By 1960 military system design was becoming more complex. It became evident that fulfilling a system's design requirements would require the simultaneous design and development of its hardware, software, and human elements. Human factors expanded to include software and job design and became known as personnel subsystem development. By the mid-1960s, human factors engineering, as it was then popularly called, had moved into the commercial world (Belt and Galitz 1967), where it has steadily made inroads.

Today no single professional group is responsible for research in human factors or the application of its principles to system design. Anthropologists, physicians, physiologists, industrial designers, data-processing specialists, and especially engineers and psychologists all participate. In a broad sense, anyone who is concerned with trying to improve the devices and systems people use or the ways of using them is practicing human factors.

Human Factors in Computer Systems

During its first twenty years, the data-processing industry paid little attention to the human/computer interface in system design. The focus instead was on efficient use of central processing units and storage media. The high cost of technology and the fact that computers were used by a relatively few specialists sublimated the interface between humans and computers. Systems were, in effect, designed from the inside out.

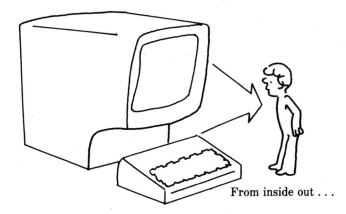

From inside out . . .

As computing power increased and computing costs decreased, computers touched more work lives. As computer usage by several users became usage by several hundred users, personnel costs became a dominant factor in total systems costs.

The kind of system user was also changing. The traditional non-discretionary user, a programmer or clerk, was being joined by one who possessed job discretion, the executive or manager. The programmer or clerk is non-discretionary in that a choice whether or not to use a computer in one's job does not exist. Tasks demand that computers be the vehicle by which they are performed. To avoid the computer requires changing jobs or vocations. The non-discretionary manager or executive, however, is able to view the computer as simply a tool akin to a pencil or stapler. If this tool results in something better than the old manual ways of doing things, it will be used. If not, it is ignored.

Economics and the greatly ascending importance of the discretionary user has forced a refocusing of system design emphasis on the user. It became more widely recognized that the ease and effectiveness of human interactions with computers would depend on how well the interface reflected people's needs. Thus, the system design emphasis shifted to outside in. A new buzzword was coined—*user-friendly*.

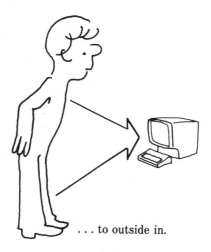

. . . to outside in.

The new outside-in orientation is illustrated by some examples. Yesterday, a request for a specific piece of information resulted in a lengthy, almost indigestible printout. Today, the same request yields the specific item on a visual display unit. Requests for computer service once had to be made in rigidly structured machine languages, but now they can be made in languages that are natural to people.

The late 1970s and early 1980s were characterized by a great deal of progress in developing a true outside-in orientation. Much still remains to be accomplished, however. We are still developing too many systems that do not adequately reflect user requirements and are paying only sporadic attention to human factors. The fault lies partly with the designers of such systems and partly with the users themselves. From a design standpoint, human-oriented design solutions have frequently been too complex for user environments, too full of inconsistencies, and overreliant on training to compensate for design holes. Often, the result is a user who is bewildered and overtaxed by learning requirements. The problem from a user standpoint is one of human nature. Because people are flexible, intuitive, and capable of making decisions and handling unforeseen situations, they accept design inadequacies and inconsistencies and they develop and implement strategies to handle them. This does work, but only until a system failure results from the interference of the compensating strategies with system objectives.

The late 1970s has also been characterized by the emergence of another problem with computer systems. Reported visual and postural problems and work stress associated with the use of visual display terminals has sparked much interest in the design of the hardware, the workstation, the office environment, and jobs. These concerns, described in Chapter 3, have underscored the depth of human factors issues in computer systems. These concerns have also resulted in legislation concerning terminal use in a number of European countries and legislation interest in several American states. Legislation issues will be addressed in Chapter 13.

The promise of the 1980s for office automation is that the outside-in design orientation will continue to accelerate, flourish, and mature and that all aspects of office system design will achieve the full human factors attention they deserve.

Human Factors Applied

Human factors addresses a variety of office system elements that affect human performance. Among them are system design, the human/machine interface, information transfer, documentation, training, the environment, and personal factors (Fox 1974).

System design refers to overall design conditions that reduce human effectiveness, such as:

- definitions of activities to be performed by people and machines;
- human interface with computer software;
- manual subsystem design logic and compatibility with existing procedures;
- effective use of human skills and knowledge; and
- development of effective feedback loops.

Faulty design decisions made during system development will lead to faulty and far-from-optimum systems. Such decisions include those that:

- prevent people from completing manual activities in the shortest possible time and with the fewest errors;
- require that people communicate on a system's terms, instead of in language natural to humans; and
- result in people not continually knowing their status and the system's status.

The human/machine interface refers to the interaction of people with the physical design of display screens, keyboards, controls, and other hardware. It involves the factors addressed by the human engineering of the 1940s and 1950s and today falls largely under the jurisdiction of equipment manufacturers.

Information transfer refers to methods of collecting and transmitting data and the characteristics of information itself. Important variables include information content, structure, and amount. Each can significantly affect human understanding, handling and keying of information, as well as error rates.

Documentation includes all printed materials needed to install, operate, and maintain an office system. Obviously, the goal of documentation design is completeness, clarity, and accuracy of procedures, training manuals, reference materials, and job aids. If these objectives are not met, human efficiency will decline, and the probability of data errors contaminating a system will increase.

Training includes both formal training programs and informal on-the-job learning. An office system may be well designed and adequately documented, but if people are not taught what to do and how to do it, their performance will suffer, and errors will increase. Training is often de-emphasized. Also, some designers feel that the training responsibility is fulfilled simply by preparing training materials. The objective of effecting a behavior change through use of the training materials is sometimes forgotten.

Environment refers to the conditions existing in a person's life space or work world, such as noise, lighting, temperature, the workstation and work area. Improper design of these factors can distract people from their tasks and thus have a negative impact on their performance.

Personal factors include the traits, characteristics, or conditions peculiar to the nature of humans that affect their performance. One significant personal factor in computer-based systems is the lack of necessary education, experience, or skills to benefit from systems training. Another critical personal factor is motivation—people's feelings toward their jobs. Those feelings can range from enthusiasm or simple satisfaction to total apathy, or any shade of gray in between. Other factors include people's reaction to and acceptance of change, physiological needs, fatigue, and age.

Human Factors, then, addresses all the elements described here, as its principles and methods apply to achieving optimum human performance, comfort, efficiency, and effectiveness in office systems design.

Measures of Effectiveness

A person's effectiveness is the most difficult project success criterion to measure. But ultimately, it is the only true measure of an office system's success. The following specific cost/benefit measures can be used to judge the effectiveness of Human Factors and thus justify its existence.

Improved efficiency or productivity is achieved by minimizing the time required to perform tasks, procedures, or operations and maximizing the accuracy of the final product.

Increased dependability or reliability refers to minimizing instances of human malfunctions or human-induced system malfunctions, permitting human dependability under stress or overload situations, and minimizing update or maintenance costs.

Minimum training and manpower costs refers to a system's ability to minimize requirements for unusual skills or unique abilities, reduce training time, and facilitate efficiency.

Improved safety and palatability involves minimizing occupational hazards and personnel injuries, and maintaining optimum user workloads and stress levels.

User acceptance refers to enhancing job satisfaction—both intrinsic and aesthetic—and morale. Achieving user acceptance requires that a system reflect individual differences in people.

Flexibility and adaptability to change means the system's adaptability to changing user requirements and technological advances, and its applicability to new environments. It should permit ease of reprogramming.

Human Functions Important to Design

A basic tenet of an office system is that its design be within the capabilities and limits of the people using it. What are these capabilities and limits? Even a small dissertation is well beyond the scope of this book since many textbooks, handbooks, and articles have been written on the subject (for example: Bailey 1982; McCormick 1976; Gagne 1966; Morgan et al. 1963). But a brief discussion of some human characteristics is necessary since they form the basis upon which many design and implementation decisions will be made. Human functions important to any design effort include input, processing, output, skill, learning, motivation, individual differences, and errors.

Input

The human input function has two components: *sensing* and *perception*.

Sensing. The sensing apparatus reports the presence or absence of differences in physical energy. From a systems standpoint, the most commonly used senses are vision and audition, while the less frequently used include taste, smell, and balance.

All senses have a limited spectrum in which they are useful. Vision is sensitive to brightness, color, and movement; it is directional in nature; and has limited powers of differentiation. Audition is nondirectional and especially prone to masking—the covering of one signal by another.

Normally, the human is not capable of absorbing all the stimuli present at one time. Consequently, people exercise selectivity in what they sense or pay attention to, maintaining selectivity rules in memory. Vision is used most effectively when:

- spatial orientations or search are required,
- simultaneous comparisons must be made,
- multidimensional material is presented, or
- high ambient noise levels exist.

Audition is preferable when:

- interruption of attention is required,
- small temporal relations are important, or
- poor ambient lighting exists.

Perception. Humans classify sensed stimuli based on models stored in their memories. Their perceptions have the following qualities:

- *Limited Channel Capacity.* One's capacity to perceive has a distinct and stable upper boundary. It is unknown whether this boundary results from the sensory apparatus itself or from central nervous system processes.
- *Inconsistency.* Perception is affected by one's general health, fatigue, environment, or previous perceptual activity. Low activity will cause a decrement in perceptual ability.
- *Interference.* Many stimuli, including irrelevant signals or noise, bombard the senses and can mask critical signals. The basic determining factor in interferences is the similarity between the critical signal and the noise signal.
- *Constancy.* Perception is synthetic rather than analytic. It tends to put things into wholes so that even though the physical signal may vary over a wide range, stimuli classifications are not disturbed.

The ability to perceive the world in terms of context often works against people because it causes them to ignore important signals. On the positive side, however, perception in context enables people to make order out of chaos and to extract a great deal of information from sketchy data. This ability to identify partial information, though, can cause perceptual errors—making identifications with inadequate facts.

Some important perceptual design considerations are:

- Do not overload or underuse perceptual capacity.
- Enhance the human ability to abstract signals from the noise components of stimuli, or minimize the noise itself.
- Provide enough signals so that proper classifications are made.

Processing

The processing function involves establishing meanings for what has been perceived—identifying and interpreting stimuli. The human tendency is to recreate stimuli into what has meaning to the observer. People recognize what they expect to recognize.

Interpretation is also influenced to some extent by motives. People recognize what they want or need to recognize. In the processing phase appropriate responses are determined, and both short- and long-term memory play an important role. Long-term memory is a permanent storage mechanism with undefined limits, while short-term memory is a temporary storage mechanism.

Short-term memory. Information enters the short-term memory by perception through the sense organs or through cognition from long-term memory. Short-term memory is highly susceptible to interference, and its contents are constantly in danger of being replaced by new information. Its capacity is about seven items. Remembering a telephone number long enough to complete the dialing operation taxes the memories of many people. Up to a point, the number of items that can be stored in short-term memory is independent of the information content of the items. It is just as easy to remember several informationally rich items as it is to remember the same number of informationally poor items. Short-term memory has great flexibility, and suitable instructions can easily change its programming. It can also store short-action sequences.

Long-term memory. This memory contains programs that consist of rules for selective sensing, classification models for perception, rules for establishing meanings, and sequences of actions for implementing motor activities. The programs are established and modified by learning. The greater the program's complexity, the longer it will take to develop and store. Programs may be retained for long periods.

An important memory consideration, with significant implications for system design, is the difference in ability to recognize or recall words. The human active vocabulary, words that can be recalled, typically ranges from 2,000–3,000 words. Passive vocabulary, words that can be recognized, typically numbers about 100,000.

Response determination. The final step in the processing function is reorganizing the input into meaningful output. The ease of determining a response depends on how well models, rules, and action sequences are ingrained (learned) in long-term memory.

Output

The human processing function frequently culminates in some action, either motor or verbal. Motor movements are limited in kind, direction, angle, speed, strength, and accuracy. Diverse movements, such as those involved in typing, have an upper limit of approximately ten per second, but when discrimination is required, the response rate is about five per second. Motor-movement limits appear to be caused by the central nervous system, not muscles. In any motor activity, people try to achieve economy of effort. This involves trying to substitute primary or ballistic movements for secondary or controlled movements.

Skill

The objective of human performance is to perform skillfully. Skill involves linking input and output into a sequence of action. The essence of skill is performance of actions in correct time sequence, with adequate precision.

Skillful performance is characterized by consistency and economy of effort. Humans seek consistency by compensating for their inherent variability, and they seek economy of effort by establishing a work pace that represents optimum efficiency. Skillful performance is subject to finite limits. In many perceptual-motor skills, motor limits are exceeded before perceptual limits.

Figure 2–1 illustrates the limits of the human capacity to perform skillfully. Increased input results in increased output only until a physical performance limit is reached, at which point a plateau occurs. Individuals can still handle the increasing load by finding more efficient ways to perform tasks, by time sharing between tasks, or by omitting operations or actions. Eventually, however, they reach an overload condition, which causes them to omit critical actions, make errors, and produce less. Ultimately a breakdown results.

Performance can also suffer when required human activities are few. Through inactivity, the individual becomes bored, misses cues, and makes errors.

Skills are hierarchical in nature, and many basic skills may be integrated to form increasingly complex ones. Lower-order skills tend to become routine and drop out of consciousness, while higher-level skills are flexible, adaptable, and more under the momentary control of the human purpose.

Learning

The human ability to learn is important—it clearly differentiates people from machines. A design developed with the intent of minimizing learning time can accelerate human performance. Given enough time, of course, humans can improve their performance in almost any task. Most could be taught to

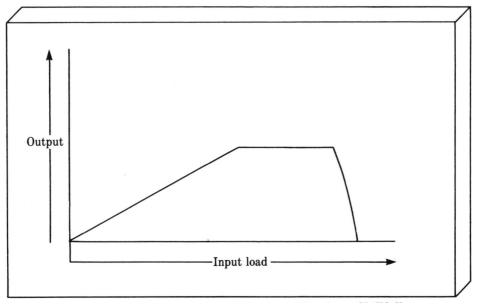

Figure 2-1.   The Human Capacity to Perform Skillfully

walk a tightrope. But a designer shouldn't call for using a tightrope if a walkway is feasible.

Most learning is a combination of trial-and-error and insight. Learning can be enhanced if it:

- allows skills acquired in one situation to be used in another somewhat like it (design standards can accomplish this);
- provides complete and prompt feedback; and
- is phased, that is, it requires that people know only the information needed at that point in the learning process.

Motivation

Motivation and stress levels can greatly influence human capacities to work. Factors both within and outside the job can affect a person's motivational state. High motivation results in higher productivity and more consistent, accurate performance. Low motivation makes performance inconsistent and error prone.

Motivational influences outside the job cannot be controlled in an office system design, but they must be understood and considered.

Individual Differences

A complicating but also advantageous characteristic of people is that they all differ—in looks, feelings, motor abilities, strengths, intellectual abilities, and so on. In a keyboard data entry task, for example, the best operators will probably be twice as fast as the poorest and make ten times fewer errors.

Individual differences complicate design because design must permit individuals with widely varying characteristics to satisfactorily and comfortably perform the same task. This adjustable range normally must encompass 90 percent (fifth to ninety-fifth percentile) of a system's users. In the past this has usually resulted in bringing designs down to the level of lowest abilities or selecting of people with the minimum skills necessary to perform a job. But office technology now offers new possibilities of tailoring jobs to the specific needs of users with varying learning or skill levels.

Errors

The ultimate objective of system design is to allow humans to perform required activities in the correct pattern and time sequence, with adequate precision. The inhibiting factor in achieving this objective is error. The capacity of humans to make errors is, in fact, the most significant deterrent to successful system operation.

Most human errors are not random. People have a tendency to make certain kinds of errors. For example, they tend to:

- abbreviate or simplify by omitting details and elements, or to condense by combining elements;
- lose the middle parts of an element, or drop elements from the middle of a series;
- close or fill in gaps, by giving a value to a missing element;
- create symmetry by completing one item to match the pattern of a preceding one;
- show bias toward the center by bringing extreme values closer to the norm; and
- assimilate an element into a prior or an expected input.

Nothing inherent in manual activities will produce errors. Errors only occur when one or more factors impair performance. Theoretically, all factors that cause people to make errors could be identified and controlled, but from a practical standpoint, the time and energy to do this are not usually available. Errors can be reduced to an acceptable level simply by understanding what causes them and by developing a design that minimizes the opportunities for them to occur.

Looking Ahead

Human Factors in office automation, then, has many facets and covers a wide, ever-changing landscape. No office system can succeed without true commitment to and conscious application of human factors techniques and principles.

The next chapter begins a survey of the state of the art of human factors in office automation. It begins with a review of the behavioral problems and concerns being widely discussed today. Attention is then directed to the various components over which the system designer or implementor has some control, such as system design, equipment design, the office environment, documentation, and training. Because of the importance of job design, the change process and the burgeoning electronic meetings, chapters are devoted to these topics as well.

Because human factors is such an immense field, there is no attempt to restate detailed principles and findings covered in other readily available documents. Relevant references are provided as needed.

References

Bailey, R. W., *Human Performance Engineering: A Guide for System Designers.* Englewood Cliffs, N. J.: Prentice-Hall, 1982.

Belt, S. L., and Galitz, W. O. "Upgrading the Man–Computer Relationship." *Sperry Rand Engineering Review*, Summer 1967.

Fox, F. W. Paper presented at the Seventh International Symposium on Human Factors in Telecommunications, Montreal, Canada, 1974.

Gagne, R. M., ed. *Psychological Principles in System Development.* New York: Holt, Reinhart and Winston, 1966.

McCormick, E. J. *Human Factors in Engineering and Design.* 4th ed. New York: McGraw-Hill, 1976.

Morgan, C. T.; Cook, J. S.; Chapanis, A.; and Lund, M. W. *Human Engineering Guide to Equipment Design.* New York: McGraw-Hill, 1963.

3

Automation Concerns

The introduction of computer technology into the office, while producing many benefits, has unleashed a wave of growing concern over potential negative side effects for some of its users. These concerns over such issues as increased visual and postural problems, increased work stress, reduction in the quality of working life, lost jobs, and health hazards, have created a storm of rhetoric and a growing number of studies around the world. The realities are increasingly difficult to pin down owing to the enormity and complexity of the considerations. The issues are also being clouded by those whose interests may be more political than humanitarian. The safest and most practical approach is to take one step backward in order to obtain a global view. The more significant considerations should then emerge and the risk of bogging down in detail should lessen.

Visual Problems

Numerous field studies in recent years have uncovered a variety of complaints about eye troubles associated with using visual display terminals. (For example, Crane 1979; Meyer et al. 1979; Hultgreen and Knave 1974; Elias et al. 1980; Smith et al. 1981; and Laubli et al. 1980.) The most commonly reported visual discomforts are eye strain, burning eyes, irritated eyes, and blurred or double vision. Dainoff et al. (1981) found a moderate but significant correlation with time spent using the VDT.

Buttressing these field studies are a number of experimental studies addressing the eye mechanism itself. Haider et al. (1975, 1980) found a reduction in the eye's visual acuity after three to four hours of continuous work on a VDT. Gunnersson and Soderberg (1980) have found that the near point of accommodation and convergence moves away during the workday, and it is greater for VDT than non-VDT work. Mourant et al. (1979) found that the time to visually focus on a far point increased as a function of time using a VDT. The former studies also reported a tendency for subjective symptoms of

23

visual fatigue to be correlated with the psychological changes measured. Other studies, however, have reported no problems, or at least no differences in reported eye discomforts, between VDT and non-VDT users. Falling into this category are De Groot (1981) and Starr et al. (1982). Many of the studies reporting problems have also been criticized for methodological deficiencies (Starr et al. 1982 and Schurick et al. 1982). Described methodological problems include failure to use control groups, improper subject selection, failure to control for other influences such as those of the task or workstation, and failure to control emotional issues touching on sensitive concerns, such as health and job security, which could bias the results.

All researchers agree that the visual discomforts are transient, not permanent. What then can we conclude? Before venturing an opinion, let us examine the source of concern: the human eye.

Human Vision

The eye is much like a camera. Entering light passes through an opening in the iris called the pupil and is focused by the lens onto an area of the retina called the fovea. There it is translated into electrical impulses and transmitted by the optic nerve to the brain. The visual system is controlled by a series of muscles that work in opposition to one another.

One set of muscles controls the shapes of the lens which brings images at varying distances into sharp focus (accommodation and convergence). A second set of muscles in the iris controls the amount of light entering the eye (adaptation). With light stimulation the retina gradually loses its sensitivity, while in the absence of light it gradually recovers it. While normal viewing occurs in the center of the retina, incidental light is absorbed throughout it. Excessive light in the periphery of the field of vision, then, can cause some light adaptation throughout the retina and subsequent degradation of visual ability.

The eye perceives differences by detecting differences in brightness or color within the visual field. With little or no contrast, no edge is perceived, but as contrast increases, edge perception improves until finally additional contrast no longer helps. At a certain point, extreme brightness contrast begins to impair visual performance by creating a contrast glare. Luminance brightness relationships, must therefore be kept within narrow limits.

Another series of muscles gives the brain a more reliable picture by providing slightly different views through quick small movements of the eye. These movements, called rapid saccadic movements, compensate for the tendency of the retina's cells to tire.

Problems with the human optic system may be either physiological or induced by the environment. Environmental conditions that force extensive use of eye muscles can cause fatigue. The muscles' function will be impaired until they have had time to rest and recover. Excessive muscle fatigue lowers a person's visual skills, and tasks then become more difficult, requiring more effort and concentration.

Physiologically, the lens may have an improper shape, which results in an out-of-focus image being projected onto the retina. This is commonly called nearsightedness or farsightedness. With age the lens loses its elasticity, thereby reducing the range of eye focus that can be achieved. With age the lens also loses its transparency, thereby reducing visual acuity. These physiological problems are commonly corrected through use of eyeglasses or contact lenses.

Discomfort can have a major impact on reading performance. If a display is irritating or difficult to read, reading performance will probably suffer (Snyder and Taylor 1979 and Vartebedian 1971).

Many attempts have been made to find objective criteria to measure visual fatigue. That is, is there some objective measure such as blink rate, pupil diameter, or eye fixations that correlates with a measurable discomfort symptom? So far, efforts have been unsuccessful. Human feelings remain the primary descriptive source of information.

A Conclusion

Examination of the results of the research, knowledge of the haphazard ways in which VDTs have been installed in offices around the world, and comparison of the physical attributes of displays with the functioning of the human eye, leads to the inescapable conclusion that something is wrong. The evidence is too strong to suggest otherwise. But it would be as unreasonable to conclude that VDTs cause eye discomfort as it would be to conclude that they do not cause eye discomfort. To reach one or the other conclusion would be like saying that reading a magazine does or does not cause eye discomfort. A magazine with clear legible characters being viewed under the proper amount of light normally yields little if any eye discomfort. The same magazine read under the harsh glare of a desk lamp, or on a moving train with a bad roadbed and poor springs, or in an automobile being driven down a road through flickering tree shadows on a bright sunny day would probably result in considerable discomfort. Whether the magazine was the first or last in the press run and has dark or 'washed-out' print, will also influence reading comfort.

No two VDTs are exactly alike. Design characteristics vary, the environments in which they are used vary, and the tasks being performed vary. No wonder the results are confusing. Like magazines, VDTs can be made more difficult to work with, or easier to work with. Problems may exist, or they may not. If a fault exists, it is that we have not understood the breadth and complexity of the issues, and we have placed too much faith in the inherent adaptability of people to technology. In some cases we have made bad judgments.

Potential Causes of Visual Discomfort

Based on the physiology of the eye, what are some of the characteristics of VDTs and the environment that contribute toward eye discomfort? Table 3–1 summarizes the factors that are described below.

Table 3–1. Potential Causes of Visual Discomforts Associated with Using Visual Display Terminals

Equipment/Environment

- Excessive luminance contrast in the visual field
- Variable focus distance in the visual field
- Screen reflections
- Oscillating display character brightness (flicker)

Equipment

- Low contrast between display characters and background
- Excessive display character brightness
- Low display character stability
- Poor display character sharpness
- Poor display character legibility
- Divergent light wavelengths (color)

Human

- Uncorrected eye defects
- Eyeglasses

Excessive luminance contrast in the visual field. Large brightness contrast between display screen, source documents, windows, and lights may strain the eye's adaptive mechanism. A bright light source close to the line of sight can cause the iris muscle to open and close repeatedly. So can frequent eye movements between a dark display screen and a brightly lit source document. Research performed by TUV Reinland found 8,000 to 25,000 movements between a display screen and source documents over an eight-hour day (*Mini-Micro Systems* 1981).

Large brightness contrast in the field of vision can cause eye adaptation to the brightest source. If the bright source is in the background, the eyes may adjust to the background and make reading the display difficult. Several studies reporting visual discomfort found excessive luminance contrast ratios on the visual field (Hultgreen and Knave 1974; Luabli et al. 1982; Stammerjohn et al. 1981; and Coe et al. 1980).

Variable focus distance in the visual field. Muscles may tire if the eyes have to converge and diverge repeatedly in looking rapidly between objects at different distances. This is a special problem for older people whose refocusing distance and time has degraded. Rapid changes in visual focal points may occur thousands of times daily if information sources are positioned at different viewing distances.

Screen reflections. Display screens frequently have highly reflective glass surfaces that reflect light from such environmental sources as windows, lights, and other bright surfaces. When these reflections diminish the contrast between characters and background, visual acuity drops and reading difficulties occur. In some cases the reflected light is bright enough to cause glare. Almost all studies reporting visual discomfort found screen reflections to be serious problems.

Oscillating display character brightness (flicker). To maintain a constant display image, a VDTs phosphor must be continually refreshed. If it falls below a certain level, the oscillation is perceived as a flickering light. Flicker has adverse effects because it overloads the adaptation mechanism of the eye. Little is known about the effects of non-visible flicker, or nonperceived oscillation, of VDTs. But it is known that nonperceived oscillation of fluorescent lights may cause complaints of irritated eyes from some people working under them. There are reasons to assume that nonvisible oscillation in VDTs may also have adverse effects on the retina of very sensitive persons (Grandjean, undated).

The degree of perceived flicker depends upon some physical characteristics of the VDT itself as well as some environmental conditions. Generally, flicker is more noticeable with:

- lower phosphor refresh rates,
- shorter phosphor persistence rates,
- higher display character brightness,
- lower display background brightness, and
- lower room illumination levels.

Low contrast between display characters and background. The characters displayed on some VDTs are not very bright. In this case visual acuity drops and reading difficulties occur.

Excessive display character brightness. High levels of character brightness can create contrast or direct glare. Bright images can cause the characters to be indistinct and also cause reading problems.

Low display character stability, sharpness, and legibility. Characters that "swim," are fuzzy, or are poorly designed, also stress the eye's accommodating power.

Divergent light wavelengths (color). The eye refracts light of different wavelengths (color) in different ways. Light simultaneously entering the eye from sources with widely divergent color compositions (dual source light) cannot be brought into simultaneous sharp focus. The eye must adapt individually to each light source to clarify each image. Eye irritation may result when frequent adaptations are necessary. Colors close to the end of the visual spectrum create the worst problems.

Uncorrected eye defects. People generally do not take care of their eyes as they should. It is variously estimated that from one-third to one-half of all people have an uncorrected eye defect of one kind or another. Above the age of forty, eye defects become the rule rather than the exception. Wearing glasses or contact lenses is not always the solution. One study of clerical and administrative workers found that 37 percent of the eyeglass wearers were in need of a new prescription (Cakir, Hart, and Stewart 1979). For those with uncorrected eye defects, working at what may be a visually demanding task will certainly not make the job any easier. The result will be only to make existing poor conditions worse.

Eyeglasses. As the eye lens gradually begins to stiffen around the age of forty, and refocusing becomes more difficult, eyeglasses are often needed for normal reading. Reading glasses are set for a normal reading distance of about 12–15 inches. VDTs are often read at distances of 18 inches or more, thereby lowering visual acuity. Continued stiffening of the eye lens with advancing years often results in the need for an additional set of glasses for long-distance viewing. The common solution is a pair of double-lens glasses (bifocals), the lower portion used for near viewing and the upper for distance. Again, these are not set for normal VDT viewing distances, resulting in the same problem.

Where to from Here?

Current evidence indicates that visual discomfort associated with working with VDTs may be attributed to a combination of three factors: improperly designed display units, unsuitable lighting conditions, or the task itself.

Improperly designed display units take their toll on the accommodation and adaptation mechanisms of the eye. Laubli et al. (1982) found significant differences in eye discomfort when comparing terminals possessing good character sharpness, high character stability, and low degree of oscillation with those lacking these qualities. The better-designed terminals gave fewer problems. However, many characteristics of the display screen cannot be considered independently of the environment in which they are used. Perception of flicker and luminance contrast ratios both depend somewhat on one another. Some environmental factors may act independently of the equipment, of course. A severe direct glare source maybe almost totally debilitating. Here the toll is on the accommodation and adaptation mechanisms of the eye.

Finally, the task being performed may cause reported visual discomfort. Thousands of eye movements a day between a display screen and surrounding source materials are likely to be the result of a poorly designed task or series of tasks. Such a situation can only magnify any equipment/environmental problems that may exist. The relationship of visual discomfort to one's job has further critical implications that will be discussed later.

It is evident that we still have much to learn. The depth and complexity of the considerations yield no easy answers. Needed is a more comprehensive and dynamic model in which the specific attributes of the visual environment are linked to the specific aspects of the visual function. It is also evident that individual differences play a significant role in the perception of discomfort. Some people find a situation uncomfortable that others can tolerate. Ultimate answers must satisfy a range of people. Until this is achieved—if it ever is achieved—we must use the knowledge available today to create as fine a viewing environment as possible.

What we do know, if consciously applied, can eliminate, or alleviate, much of the reported discomfort. Later chapters will address these solutions. The benefits, in addition to the obvious physical one for VDT users, can also be measured in performance. Wodka (1982) has derived a formula for determining reading rate of VDT displays based upon calculations that the Illuminating Engineering Society Research Institute has derived for calculating changes in industrial and paper-oriented office tasks. Using this formula, Ryburg (1981) has estimated that VDT reading speeds and task accuracy at a large office studied can be improved 3–7 percent by establishing proper lighting for VDT use.

Postural Problems

Like visual discomfort, innumerable studies have uncovered reports of postural problems associated with using VDTs. In addition to those previously referenced in the preceding discussion, further problems have been uncovered by Ferguson (1971); Hunting (1980); and Maeda (1977) in using other office equipment. As in the case of vision, not all studies have yielded problems (Starr et al. 1982) and many of the studies have been criticized for methodological deficiencies. The most common reported problems are pains in the neck, shoulder, back, arms, and hands.

While eyestrain may be a more sensitive issue, postural problems can be more serious in the long term. The body muscles are sensitive tissues. Underused they will atrophy, overloaded or improperly used they may fatigue, suffer temporary damage, or even suffer permanent damage. Fatigued muscles will impair performance; damaged muscles may prevent a task from being performed.

Atrophy is prevented by building variety into manual tasks. Astronauts in the confines of a space capsule are forced to reach for some controls and materials to provide needed muscle exercise. Muscle fatigue is reduced by letting a person assume relaxing and comfortable positions, and not forcing a set of muscles to undergo continuous activity.

Again, the depth and breadth of complaints must lead one to the conclusion that something is amiss. To understand more fully, let us look at the office worker's desk.

The Changing Office Desk

Before the use of visual display terminals, the office desk was characterized by a collection of working materials (forms, files, books, manuals, etc.) tools (pencils, ruler, stapler, etc.), and storage facilities (drawers, shelves, etc.). Commonly shared items (file cabinets, photocopy machines, etc.) were a short walk away. Most items on the desk were movable and portable by the desk's occupant. To create a comfortable working position simply involved arranging the items in a manner deemed most appropriate by the worker. Changes in position could easily be accomplished. A manual, for example, could be read flat on the desk surface, on one's lap, or even lying on the floor if desired. In essence the worker controlled the working environment, easily modifying it to achieve maximum comfort. Periodic movements throughout the work area were often required and changes in seated posture easily accomplished.

Gradually, however, working materials, tools, and storage facilities have been replaced by VDTs. The VDT is large, bulky, and difficult to move. It is placed on desks intended to support the manual materials that it replaces. Location of the display screen and keyboard is generally fixed, often in a location far less than optimum for human comfort. VDT users have been forced to adapt their posture to the rigid requirements imposed by the machine. As more and more tasks are internalized within the system, the diversity of movements to accomplish a job are diminished. A variety of muscular movements are replaced by one—the keystroke.

Possible Causes of Postural Problems

Muscle fatigue and injuries associated with the use of VDTs can be ascribed to several factors: awkward posture, constrained posture, and repetitive movements. Those who wear bifocal eyeglasses may have to assume an awkward posture in order to read a display screen. They must tilt their heads backward and incline their torso forward to bring the image into focus through the reading lens.

A person is linked to the VDT through both the keyboard and the screen. Both head and hands must be kept in practically a fixed position, with the remainder of the body, neck, shoulders, trunk, and arms, following suit. The keying and viewing tasks constrain both posture and movement. If the position assumed is not comfortable, the problems are magnified.

Repetitive movement injuries are caused by repeated rapid movements, not necessarily involving heavy loads or long duration. Such injuries often take the form of tenosynovitis and tendonitis. Teniswood (1982), in a study of the data entry department of a large Australian bank, found twenty cases of compensable tenosynovitis over a four-year period. These injuries occurred in a staff of about ninety people who performed predominantly right-handed keying tasks at rates of 16,000 keystrokes per hour.

Discomfort and injuries of this type cannot be attributed solely to VDTs in the workplace, however. Back trouble has been a hazard facing typists and machine operators for years. Patkin (1983) reports treating an office worker for a hand injury caused by improper use of a pencil. The problem was pressing the pencil too firmly on the paper. The cure was not to press so hard!

Unlike vision, the components of comfortable posture are more fully understood. Factors which contribute to postural discomfort include the following:

High or low keyboards. More often the problem is with keyboards that are too high, the result of placing VDT's on desks traditionally designed for manual activities. This places more strain on the forearm or wrist. The ability to rest one's arms or hands on the desk or keyboard can alleviate this problem somewhat (Hunting et al. 1980).

Improper viewing angles. Display screens are often set too high with the result that the normal downward inclination of the head is not achieved. This increases the strain on neck muscles. Screen viewing problems created by display and environmental deficiencies often force people to assume awkward body positions in order to read the display. This can lead to postural problems.

Poor chairs. Proper chair height and back support is a necessity for sedentary activities. Without it, the muscles surrounding the spinal cord may be strained and the delicate ligaments and tissues around the vertebrae may be pinched.

High rates of input. High input rates force the maintenance of constrained positions for extended periods of time. They can also lead to repetitive movement injuries.

What Are Some Solutions?

There is reasonable agreement on the desired posture of a seated person using a VDT. Guidelines will be presented in Chapter 9. The problem of high input rates is not an environmental problem. It is a function of the design of the job and the equipment used. These will be addressed in Chapters 5 and 8.

Psychosocial Problems

A third area of concern centers around a person's psychological reactions to automation. Limited research evidence now available indicates that some users of VDTs are more likely to show higher stress symptoms than their colleagues who do not use VDTs. Factors measured include anxiety, depression, irritability, boredom, inner security, anger, confusion, and general fatigue. Complementing the research data are a growing number of voices expressing fears about the direction automation is steering the quality of work life, and the effect this is having on the psychological well-being of the worker. Factors suggested as potential causes of work stress are summarized in Table 3–2 and described below.

Potential Causes of Work Stress

Rigid work procedures. Rigid work procedures do not permit any flexibility in how a task is accomplished. Cohen et al. (1982) found rigid work procedures were one of the distinguishing features when comparing two kinds of VDT jobs for level of stress. A job with rigid work procedures was found to yield higher stress levels for its performers.

Oversimplified, repetitive, and routine jobs. Oversimplification, repetitiveness, and routineness create boredom and monotony. Boredom and monotony were cited in the studies by Smith et al. (1981) and Stammerjohn et al. (1981), as among the most important factors in job stress. Oversimplified and repetitive jobs do not permit office personnel to utilize their education and experience, so they lack challenge. It is interesting to compare the activities of office VDT users and video-game players. Both activities require simultaneous viewing of a display screen and performance of complex manual dexterity tasks. The challenge of winning makes the video game interesting and fun, however, while the lack of challenge in the office job often leads to boredom.

Lost sense of job meaning. There is little sense of accomplishment if the fruit of one's labors does not yield a tangible product—a product shaped by human craftmanship. Many automated jobs are but a small part of a larger process in which the final product is rarely visible. Consequently there can be little identification with, or pride in, the end product. Cohen et al. (1982) also found lack of job meaning to be a distinguishing feature of more highly stressful jobs.

Table 3–2. Potential Causes of Work Stress

• Rigid work procedures	• Monitored performance
• Oversimplified, repetitive, and routine jobs	• Disrupted social relationships
• Lost sense of job meaning	• Reduced status and self-esteem
• Lack of control	• Reduced mobility
• Heavy workloads	• Concern for safety
• Pressures for performance	• Concern for career and job future

Lack of control. Automated systems often do not permit people to exercise control over the manner, order, and pace of their work. Tasks must be performed in the prescribed way, in the prescribed order, and at a pace dictated by the system's response time. The psychological need for autonomy is severely threatened. Cohen et al. (1982) found lack of autonomy to be another distinguishing feature of highly stressful jobs. A number of researchers have found that being able to exercise control over the work situation can relieve many work-stress situations (Gardell 1979; Johansson et al. 1978; Karasek 1979; Karasek et al. 1981; and Frankenhaeuser 1979). People cannot perform at a steady stream of excellence.

A recent report by the Opinion Research Corporation indicates that job dissatisfaction caused by lack of control is creeping into the ranks of middle management as well. Many managers are finding themselves to be simple passers of information up and down through the corporate hierarchy (*Training and Development Journal* 1981).

Heavy workloads. Automation frequently brings with it calls for high production standards. A person is often asked to perform at maximum rates for long periods of time with the peaks and valleys of normal human performance rarely achievable. When valleys do occur, they usually are imposed by the system (slow response times or down systems), not a reflection of human needs.

Pressures for performance. Constant pressures to achieve high performance, to achieve a machine-like efficiency, may be both outwardly imposed (by management) or inwardly imposed (by the worker). Pressures for performance were another distinguishing feature of stressful jobs in the study by Cohen et al. (1982).

Monitored performance. Automated systems can easily be monitored, be it by keystrokes, pages created, or transactions processed. Monitoring conjures up grim images of "Big Brother" for many. A Canadian government-appointed task forced regarded " . . . close monitoring of work as an employment practice based on mistrust and lack of respect for basic human dignity. It is an infringement of the rights of the individual . . . ." (Labour Canada Task Force 1982). Others argue, however, that the power of monitoring can work for the individual. It provides an objective measure of performance that is hard to dispute. It appears that monitoring itself is not the danger but whether the worker is informed, and how the results are interpreted and used, that are the key issues.

Disrupted social relationships. Automation can seriously impair or destroy the social relationships that exist in the office. People need to encounter and interact with others. Social reinforcement of the peer group is important to many people.

Reduced status and self-esteem. The negative qualities of automation, taken in total, can impair a person's conception of worth and self-esteem. It is important that one have some pride in oneself, and a sense of contribution to an ultimate goal.

Reduced mobility. Being tied to a VDT reduces one's mobility. Calmer, more positive feelings are associated with mobility (Johansson 1980).

Concern for safety. A critical concern for safety is being threatened by fears of health hazards associated with using VDTs. This issue will be addressed later.

Concern for career and job future. As computers perform more of the tasks accomplished by clerical personnel, employment opportunities will diminish. European studies indicate a 15–20 percent clerical job loss in the next ten to twenty years. Some experts feel that since many clerical positions are filled by women, and few women are promoted to professional ranks because of a lack of technical knowledge and prevailing management attitudes, job opportunities for women will thereby diminish. Being replaced by a machine is a valid fear expressed by many. Job future concerns may not only be restricted to the clerical workforce, however. Widespread use of computer-aided design may eliminate future drafters, a potential loss of some 300,000 skilled positions (*Computerworld* 1983).

Some Implications

Psychosocial problems and the physical ailments associated with posture and vision cannot really be neatly divided into separate categories. Nor can the effects of the hardware, the system, the environment, and an organization's management. The worker, too, must be looked upon not just as one but as many with a variety of needs, interests, attitudes, and susceptibilities. In the past we have tended to look upon the VDT as a collection of steel, plastic, glass, silicon chips, and electrons—a physical entity to blame for many of today's perceived ills. It is something one can feel and touch. We have also looked at the worker as a kind of robot, a standard collection of muscles, bones, and fluids, adaptable to most anything. This entity is somehow immune from feeling and emotions, and damage of the body or psyche. We have looked at the work environment as a placid lake, not as a raging sea serving as a battleground between management and worker—between management and unions. We have looked at the worker as an unnecessary expense, something that can be replaced by a machine with far less cost, both financially and emotionally. Our vision has tended to be safe and rather narrow. To broaden it is frightening. But broaden it we must. The questions are difficult and the answers even more so, but they must be addressed. What, then, are the implications of what we know today and what should be the future directions?

The VDT, and the VDT workstation, play a role in reported discomforts. A large portion of the reported problems appear to be real. The physiology of the human eye and body is not always compatible with the way VDTs are manufactured and installed. VDTs have been manufactured with display characteristics that can fatigue the human eye, and with components arranged to force their users to assume uncomfortable, constrained, and fatiguing postures. VDTs have also often been installed in offices in a haphazard way with little thought to good viewing and operating conditions.

Use of VDTs need not be physically fatiguing, however, as evidenced by the people and studies that report no problems. A properly designed VDT and good work environment, while probably not totally devoid of discomforts in today's state of the art, can be made much more comfortable to work with than is commonly the case. Solutions to problems, however, cannot be accomplished by independently addressing the equipment and environment. One problem, for example, the large luminance contrast between a dark display screen and the brighter work environment, can be resolved by brightening the display screen or darkening the room. It might even be resolved by redesigning the task so as not to require so many eye movements between the display screen and the surrounding materials.

Job content also plays a significant role in reported discomforts. Reports of physical ailments can be influenced by the content of the job being performed. Some studies (Smith et al. 1981 and Coe et al. 1980) have found higher incidences of physical complaints among clerical users than among professional users of VDTs. The job content of professional users included flexibility in accomplishing goals, control over tasks, utilization of experience and education, and satisfaction and pride in an end product—the kinds of qualities missing from many clerical tasks. The impact of the job, and the design of the system, has a much larger impact on satisfaction and work stress than many early researchers suspected. The psychosocial needs can overshadow physical needs in a variety of human experiences. Imagine the strains and discomforts imposed on the body of the marathon runner or the driver of a racing car in Indianapolis in late May. The gratification one receives for these kinds of endeavors is certainly not physical.

Length of working time plays a role in reported discomforts. Johansson and Aronsson (1980) found that as the amount of working time at various VDT jobs increased, so did the percentage of workers expressing psychosocial problems. This study corroborates what has long been assumed. Shorter time periods at VDTs provide opportunities to rest muscles and permit a greater variety in movements and tasks. Studies have yet to be made on optimum time periods but observation indicates that two hours or less a day at the VDT relieves many of the physical problems.

Individual differences play a role in susceptibility to discomfort. No two people are alike. Human physiques, traits, and sensitivities are distributed along the normal distribution curve. The viewing angle of a VDT located in a standardized position may be proper for one person but not for another. One person may perceive display flicker while a second does not in an identical viewing condition. Even the effect of job-related frustrations on people varies. When confronted with on-the-job obstacles, high-ability persons tend to suffer more (Peters 1983). Solutions must consider individual differences; variable opinions and responses are the norm.

Political issues often muddy the water. Issues of discomfort and stress often become intertwined with difficult labor negotiations or attempts at unionization. Facts are submerged under emotions and political strategies. To admit that a problem does or does not exist may strengthen or weaken one's position, depending upon one's viewpoint. Adversarial relationships seldom yield true and meaningful solutions.

A displaced workforce is a problem that cannot be ignored. The justification for technology in the workplace is, in corporate lingo, the *bottom line*. That technology replaces people, whether it is spoken or unspoken, cannot be denied. The savings have to come from somewhere and that somewhere is a shrinking labor force. In many cases the survival of an organization is at stake, and automation is all that stands between survival and an obituary in the *Wall Street Journal*. An individual organization cannot be faulted for the measures forced upon it by today's competitive marketplace.

For years applied technology in manufacturing yielded increased productivity in wide-open markets. The result was the creation of more jobs in service areas where displaced workers had a place to go. Today, technology is being applied everywhere in a shrinking world with limited market shares. Places for the displaced worker to be absorbed are rapidly disappearing or have already disappeared. The worker's buying power is diminishing accordingly. Carried to its logical extreme we could end up with totally automated offices and few individuals possessing the financial ability to purchase their products or services.

The questions that must be asked are: Is this a desirable direction for business and, more importantly, mankind? Do the costs of progress outweigh the negative impacts, or not? This issue cannot be addressed in many individual boardrooms because of the pressures at work in each organization. It must be attacked nationally and internationally. Is the worker a human being or a resource? Are people the tool of automation or is automation a tool of the people? The questions, and answers, have profound implications in the generations ahead.

Health Hazards

The proliferation of VDTs in the office has given rise to many concerns over possible adverse health effects associated with their use. Reports of unusually high numbers of miscarriages, birth defects, and eye cataracts have created feelings of uneasiness among many VDT users. Among commonly cited examples are children with deformities born to four out of seven VDT operators at a Canadian newspaper and seven miscarriages in twelve pregnancies at a mail-order computer center in Texas (*Health and Safety Bulletin* 1982). Instances such as these have spurred calls for protective measures in VDT use and even legislation to enforce compliance. While most VDT critics agree that the numbers do not prove anything, they do feel the evidence must warrant concern, and to err should be on the side of safety. Others maintain that these high percentages are simply statistical quirks.

In reaction to these concerns, a number of studies of the radiation emission qualities of VDTs have been performed by a variety of governmental and nongovernmental organizations around the world. Among these are Moss et al. (1977); Weiss and Petersen (1979); Wolbarsht et al. (1980); Vetter (1979); Cox (1980); Terrana et al. (1980); Murray et al. (1981); United States Bureau of Radiological Health (1981); and the *Environmental Health Directorate* (1983).

Potential Kinds of Radiation in VDTs

The kinds of radiation that are thought to be generated by cathode ray tubes (CRTs) and the electronic components of VDTs are x-rays, microwave, radiofrequency, extremely low frequency, ultraviolet, infrared, and visible radiations.

X-rays. Whenever fast-moving electrons are slowed down or stopped suddenly by a material, x-rays are produced. When electrons from the cathode strike the fluorescent material on the viewing face of a CRT, visible light is emitted. Ideally, all electrons should be converted to visible light. In practice, however, some electrons are converted to x-rays instead. These x-rays are perceived as a potential source of danger to humans.

Measurements of x-ray emissions over a wide variety of models repeatedly show that none are detectable above the natural background levels. The Bureau of Radiological Health has examined 250 VDTs consisting of 150 different models. Emission levels 500,000 times lower than the mandatory standard for VDTs have failed to be detected. X-rays produced by a CRT are of low energy and not very penetrating. Those x-rays produced are absorbed by the glass face and never reach the outside of the device itself. In fact, the thick glass face on the CRT is actually capable of absorbing x-rays of energies considerably higher than those now produced in the VDT.

Microwave. VDTs have no components that can generate microwave radiation. No microwave radiation has been detected in any of the studies.

Radiofrequency (RF). Radiofrequency radiation in a VDT is caused by the rapid pulsing on and off of the voltage as the image is created on the CRT. In some instances radiofrequency radiation has been found near the surface of the VDT. The level, however, decreases very rapidly with distance from the surface and at distances of about 8–12 inches radiofrequency is either not detectable or well below harmful levels, including the most stringent exposure standards in the world. The level of the radiofrequency radiation that has been detected is of the low frequency kind (up to 150 kiloHertz), and the human body is highly reflective of frequencies below 200 kiloHertz. Therefore only a minimal amount of that which is present is actually absorbed by the body.

Extremely low frequency (ELF). Extremely low frequency emissions, or magnetic field intensities, have been found to be of very low intensity. They are comparable to, or even exceeded by, other common electrical and electronic devices found in the home.

Ultraviolet (UV) and infrared (IR). Ultraviolet and infrared radiation may also be produced at the fluorescent screen by the bombarding electrons. While most of it is also absorbed by the glass surface on the screen, some ultraviolet radiation has been detected at the viewing screen. Where it has been detected, however, the measured levels have been thousands of times lower than those permitted for continuous occupational exposure.

Visible light. The purpose of a CRT is to produce visible light. The amount produced, however, is really quite low. It is about 200 times lower than the outdoor light level on a cloudy day and about 100 times lower than occupational exposure limits.

Conclusion

Based on the results of other studies, and the findings of their own study, the authors of the Environmental Health Directorate report (1983) conclude: "There is no reason for any person, male or female, young or old, pregnant or not, to be concerned about radiation health effects from VDTs." Statements like this, however, will probably not end the controversy. With tragedies from asbestos, thalidomide, dioxin, and the medical use of x-rays earlier this century still in our minds, the feeling that science does not know all the answers may very well persist. What if our standards are too high? What if our measuring instruments are not sensitive enough? What if we are measuring the wrong thing? These are representative questions that might still be asked. We must continue to search for answers that assure everyone that the accelerating use of VDTs is a safe path to follow. At the same time we cannot turn away from a tool with so much promise.

The proper course would seem to be to continue the research needed to establish causes and effects while at the same time assuring that VDTs are used properly within the limits of today's knowledge.

References

Cakir, A.; Hart, D. J.; and Stewart, D. F. M. *The VDT manual.* Darmstadt, Federal Republic of Germany: IFRA, 1979.

Coe, J. B.; Cuttle, K.; McClellan, W. C.; Warden, N. J.; and Turner, P. J. *Visual Display Units.* Wellington: New Zealand Department of Health, Report W/1/80, 1980.

Cohen, G. F.; Smith, M. J.; and Stammerjohn, L. W., Jr. "Psychosocial Factors Contributing to Job Stress of Clerical VDT Operators." *Office Automation Conference Digest.* San Francisco, April 5–7, 1982.

Computerworld, 1983.

Cox, E. A. "Radiation Emissions from Visual Display Units" and "Health Hazards of VDUs?" *Papers presented at a One Day Conference, the HUSAT Research Group, Loughborough University of Technology* 11 (December 1980): 25–38.

Crane, P. M. "Effects of Work at Video Display Computer Terminals on Vision, Mood, and Fatigue Symptoms." Unpublished technical report, 1979.

Dainoff, M. J.; Happ, A.; and Crane, P. "Visual Fatigue and Occupational Stress in VDT Operators." *Human Factors* 23 (1981): 421–438.

DeGroot, J. P. "Eyestrain in Video Terminal Users." *Paper presented at the European Conference of Postal and Telecommunications Administrations Symposium on Ergonomics in PTT-Administrations.* The Hague, September 1981.

"Discontent Is Growing among Middle Managers." *Training and Development Journal,* April 1981, p. 8.

Elias, R.; Cail, F.; Christmann, H.; Tisserand, M.; and Horvat, F. *"Conditions de Travail Devant Les Ecrans Cathodiques. Organisation Des Taches et Astreintes de L'organisme." Cahiers et notes documentaires (INRS) 101* (1980): 499.

Environmental Health Directorate. *"Investigation of Radiation Emissions from Video Display Terminals."* Canada, 83-EHD-91. 1983.

Ferguson, D. "An Australian Study of Telegraphists' Cramp." *British Journal of Industrial Medicine* 28 (1971): 280–285.

Frankenhaeuser, M. "Psychoneuroendocrine Approaches to the Study of Emotion as Related to Stress and Coping." In *Nebraska Symposium on Motivation (1978),* edited by H. E. Howe and R. A. Dienstabier, pp 123-161. Lincoln: University of Nebraska Press, 1979.

Gardell, B. *"Tjanstemannens Arbetsmiljoer* (Work Environment of White-collar workers)." Preliminary report. The research group for social psychology of work. Department of Psychology, University of Stockholm, Report No. 24, 1979.

Grandjean, E. *"Ergonomics Related to the VDT Workstation,"* Zurich, Switzerland: Swiss Federal Institute of Technology, Department of Hygiene and Ergonomics.

Gunnarsson, E., and Söderberg, I. "Eyestrain Resulting from VDT Work at the Swedish Telecommunications Administration." *National Board of Occupational Safety and Health, Staff Conference Summary.* Stockholm, 1980.

Haider, M., and Slezak, H. "Stresses and Strains on the Eyes Produced by Work with Video Display Screens. *Committee on Automation of the Trade Union of Employees in the Private Sector*. Vienna, 1975.

Haider, M.; Kundi, M.; and Weisenbock, "Strain of the Worker Related to VDU with Differently Colored Characters." Paper presented at Ergonomic Aspects of Visual Display Units Workshop. Milan, Italy, March 1980.

Health and Safety Bulletin, edited by John Mathews and Nick Calabrese. ACTU-VTHC Occupational Health and Safety Unit. ISSN 0727-3304. Carlton South, Victoria, Australia, 1982.

Hultgreen, G. V., and Knave, B. "Discomfort Glare and Disturbances from Light Reflections in an Office Landscape with CRT Display Terminals." *Applied Ergonomics* 5(1) (1974): 2–8.

Hunting, W.; Grandjean, E.; and Maeda, K. "Constrained Postures in Accounting Machine Operators." *Applied Ergonomics*. 11 (3) (1980): 143–149.

Johansson, G. "Individual Control in Monotonous Task: Effects on Performance, Effort, and Physiological Arousal." *Reports from the Department of Psychology*. Stockholm: University of Stockholm, 1980.

Johansson, G., and Aronsson, G. *Stress Reactions in Computerized Administrative Work*. Stockholm, 1980.

Johansson, G.; Aronsson, G.; and Lindstrom, B. "Social, Psychological and Neuroendocrine Stress Reactions in Highly Mechanized Work." *Ergonomics*. 21 (1978): 583–599.

Karasek, R. A. "Job Demands, Decision Latitude, and Mental Strain: Implications for Job Redesign". *Administrative Science Quarterly* 24 (1979): 285–311.

Karasek. R. A.; Baker, D.; Marxer, F.; Ahlbom, A.; and Theorell, T. "Job Design Latitude, Job Demands, and Cardiovascular Disease: A Prospective Study of Swedish Men." *American Journal of Public Health* 71 (1981): 694–705.

Labour Canada Task Force. "In the Chips: Opportunities People Partnerships." *Report of the Labour Canada Task Force on Micro-Electronics and Employment*. (Members: E. Margaret Fulton; Zavis Zeman; Jeannine David McNeil; Murray S. Hardie; Harish C. Jain; Ratna Ray). Cat. No. L35-1982/E. 1982.

Laubli, T.; Hunting W.; and Grandjean, E. "Postural and Visual Loads at VDT Workplaces. Part 2: Lighting Conditions and Visual Impairments." Ergonomics, 1982.

Maeda, K. "Occupational Cervicobrachial Disorder and Its Causative Factors." *Journal Human Ergology* 6 (1977): 193–202.

Meyer, J. J.; Gramoni, R.; Korol, S.; and Rey, P. "Quelques Aspects de la Charge Visuelle aux Postes de Travail Impliquant un Ecran de Visualisation." *Le Travail Humain* 42 (1979): 275–301.

Mini-Micro Systems, August 1981.

Moss, C.E.; Murray, W. E.; Parr, W. H.; Messite, J.; and Karches, G. J. "A Report on Electromagnetic Radiation Surveys of Video Display Terminals." *National Institute of Occupational Safety and Health*. Report DHEW (NIOSH) No. 78-129. NIOSH. Cincinnati, 1977.

Mourant, R. R.; Lakshmanan, R.; and Herman, M. "Hard Copy and Cathode Ray Tube Visual Performance—Are There Differences?" *Proceedings of the Human Factors Society—23rd Annual Meeting*, 1979, pp. 367–68. Santa Monica, Calif., 1979.

Murray, W. E., et al. "Potential Health Hazards of Video Display Terminals." *NIOSH Research Report*. DHHs (NIOSH) Publication No. 81-129. Cincinnati: 1981.

Patkin, M. Personal conversation. Whyalla, Australia. 14 June 1983.

Peters, L. "Battling the Office Blues." *Office Administration and Administration*, 1983.

Ryburg, J. Personal conversation. Ann Arbor, MI, November 1981.

Schurick, J. M.; Helander, M. G.; and Billingsley, P. A. "Critique of Methods Employed in Human Factors Research on VDTs." *Proceedings of the Human Factors Society— 26th Annual Meeting (1982)*. Santa Monica, Calif., 1982.

Smith, M. J.; Cohen, B. G. F.; Stammerjohn, L. W., Jr; and Happ, A. "An Investigation of Health Complaints and Job Stress in Video Display Operations." *Human Factors* 23 (4) (1981): 387–400.

Snyder, H. L.; and Taylor, G. B. "The Sensitivity of Response Measures of Alphanumeric Legibility to Variations in Dot Matrix Display Parameters." *Human Factors*. 21 (1979): 457–471.

Stammerjohn, L. W., Jr.; Smith, M. J; and Cohen, B. G. F. "Evaluation of Workstation Design Factors in VDT Operations." *Human Factors* 23 (4) (1981): 401–412.

Starr, S. J.; Thompson, C. R.; and Shute, S. "Effects of Video Display Terminals on Telephone Operators." *Human Factors* 24 (6) (1982): 699–711.

Teniswood, C. F. In *Health and Safety Bulletin # 12*. Victoria, Australia; ACTU-VTHC Occupational Health and Safety Unit, May 1982.

Terrana, T.; Merluzzi, F.; and Giudici, E. "Electromagnetic Radiations Emitted by Visual Display Units." In *Ergonomic Aspects of Visual Display Terminals* edited by E. Grandjean and E. Vigliani, London: pp. 13–21 Taylor and Francis Ltd., 1980.

United States Bureau of Radiological Health. "An Evaluation of Radiation Emission from Video Display Terminals." HHS Publication FDA 81-8153. 1981.

Vartebedian, A. C. "Legibility of Symbols on CRT Displays." *Applied Ergonomics* (1971): 130–132.

Vetter, H. "Health Hazards Associated with the Use of Visual Display Units." *IAEA Report*, 1979.

Weiss, M. M., and Petersen, R. C. "Electromagnetic Radiation Emitted from Video Computer Terminals." *American Industrial Hygiene Association Journal* 40 (1979): 300–309.

Wodka, M. A. "Which Light to See." *Course: Office Automation: The Facility Management Perspective*. Ann Arbor, Mich.: Facility Management Institute, 1982.

Wolbarsht, M. L.; O'Foghludha, F. A.; Sliney, D. H.; Guy, A. W.; Smith, A. A., Jr.; and Johnson, G. A. "Electromagnetic Emission from Visual Display Units: A Non-hazard." In *Occular Effects of Non-Ionizing Radiation, Proceedings, Society of Photo-Optical Instrumentation Engineers*, Volume 229, 1980.

4

Office Tasks

Classifying Office Activities

As the modern office evolved with its various processes, tasks, and inter-relationships poorly defined, practitioners realized that the effective implementation of automation would require a much better understanding of each worker's office role. This has led in recent years to a number of studies attempting to define exactly what office workers do, and how much time they spend doing it. An IBM office study, for example, identified about twenty-five general human functions (Engel et al. 1979), while XEROX, in a branch office study, defined more than six hundred unique clerical and administrative tasks (Wenig and Pardoe 1979). Other representative studies include those of Booz Allen Hamilton (Poppel 1983) and Arthur Andersen & Co. (Baxter 1982).

The general conclusion that can be drawn from these studies is that a classification of activities is difficult to derive, and that a great diversity exists among business organizations, and among individuals within each organization. The studies also reveal that today's office worker may spend 30 percent or more of his or her time performing nonproductive tasks. Typical time-wasters include:

- unnecessary travel or time away;
- nonproductive meetings or telephone calls;
- trying to find and digest the right information;
- expediting previously assigned tasks;
- generating and disseminating documents;
- doing nonprofessional tasks such as setting up meetings, filing, and making photocopies.

In order to provide a meaningful discussion, however, a classification scheme must be formulated. One such scheme is given in Table 4–1. The major

Table 4–1. Human Office Activities

Cognitive	Communicating	Physical
Information gathering	Conferring/meeting	Travel
Data analysis/calculating	Telephoning	Typing/keying
Planning/scheduling	Writing	Filing/retrieval
Reading/proofreading	Dictating	Mail handling
Decision making		Copying/reproducing
Information storage/	*Procedural*	Collating/sorting
retrieval	Completing forms	Pickup/delivery
	Checking documents	Using equipment

groupings—cognitive, communicating, procedural, and physical—are derived from Bennett (1971), while specific office tasks are built on those described by Engel et al. The importance of these activities to job performance varies, as does their amenability to technological assistance. Much can be said of some, and little or nothing of others right now. This classification scheme does, however, provide a meaningful organization and starting point for discussion.

Whether twenty-five human functions are sufficient for complete understanding of office functions is doubtful, but whether six hundred are manageable is also questionable. What is known, however, is that the ability of office systems to replicate familiar and comfortable activities and to employ familiar thinking processes will be the most important factor in how office workers accept automation.

Cognitive Activities

Cognitive activities are mental—the act or process of knowing through awareness or judgment. They range from straightforward tasks, such as reading, to relatively complex activities, such as decision making. This discussion focuses on gathering, storing, and retrieving information; planning; data analysis; and decision making.

Information Development and Gathering

Gathering information is often required to accomplish another function, such as calculating or decision making. But occasionally the gathering may be an end in itself.

This activity was studied by Hodges and Angalet (1968), and although their subject matter was technical, they did uncover some interesting results. The basic questions they addressed were when information is first needed, where it is obtained, how much of it is received, and in what form. Tables 4-2, 4-3, and 4-4 summarize their results. The subjects satisfied nearly one-third of their information needs without search, and sought about half the information they needed within the local work environment. They found part or all of

Table 4-2.   First Source of Information

	Source	Frequency (percent)
No search required	Recall	19.0
	Received with task	10.5
Local work environment	Asked a colleague	14.5
	Searched own collection	13.0
	Internal company consultant	9.5
	Department files	5.5
	Assigned to subordinate	4.5
	Respondent's own action	2.5
	Asked supervisor	1.0
External to work environment	Library or librarian	10.0
	Manufacturer or supplier	6.0
	Customer	2.0
	External consultant	1.0
	DOD information systems	1.0

Table 4-3.   Acquisition from First Source

Acquisition	Frequency (percent)
All the information needed	46.9
Part of the information	46.9
Reference to another source	4.4
Nothing	1.1
Irrelevant or inappropriate information	0.7

Table 4-4.   Types of Information Media

Medium	Frequency (percent)
Recall	13.5
Oral	27.1
Informal documentation	20.2
Semiformal documentation (company or government publication)	29.2
Formal documentation (publishing house, etc.)	9.3

the needed information at the first source. The study also showed that these individuals received about one-quarter of their information orally and one-fifth through informal documentation. Formal documentation was rarely used. Information sought in the local work environment had a greater probability of acquisition success than that sought from distant sources.

The first-used source depended primarily on the characteristics of the information itself, not on the people, tasks, or jobs. Generally, the subjects used remote sources when they knew the sources had the desired information, when the information acquisition time permitted it, or when they perceived the information to be of a formal type.

The implications of this research for office systems are:

- Dominant initial information sources are informal and personal and must be defined and incorporated into system design.
- Formal information sources must be brought closer to people so they may use them more productively.
- The ultimate objective of a system should be to become a supplier of information, not simply a storer of documents.

Data Analysis and Calculating

Pure analytical time—the time spent contemplating, problem solving, or conceptualizing—is a valuable and rewarding professional activity. Participants in the Booz Allen Hamilton study, however, spent only 8 percent of their time in this way (Poppel 1983). Professionals with tenure, though, spent 30 percent more time analyzing than those with little tenure. Most workers overestimated the time they actually spent on analysis, and many felt even more time was needed than their overinflated estimate of what time actually was spent.

Planning and Scheduling

Bolt Beranek and Newman (1980) found that activity management accounted for 5–10 percent of a worker's time. Carlisle (1976) concluded that most managers, unable to escape a daily avalanche of instruction communications, do not have a clear model of their communication environment. Therefore, they cannot use their time effectively by scheduling and monitoring high-priority communications.

It was felt that a *personal assistant* tool attracts less computer-oriented people to using a system. Its short-term payoff and appeal is quite high (Morgan 1976). Engel et al. (1979) found that in the case of principals, the most frequently used functions were individual. Functions such as mail queue, schedule calendar, hold queue, retrieval, and calendar update helped organize and control work efficiently.

Information Storage and Retrieval

Files are the backbone of the paper office. Records of the past, present, and occasionally the future, find their way into more file drawers than wastebaskets. One individual may have access to thousands of files that may be indexed mentally or with simple filing schemes.

Cole (1982) studied thirty office filing schemes. Those studied interacted with three kinds of filed information: action information, personal work files, and archive storage. *Action information* is that being dealt with now or in the immediate future. It is immediately accessible, being found in in-trays, on desks, and even on chairs or the floor. It is only used efficiently if the quantity is manageable, permitting remembering items and their location. Large quantities often require painstaking searches. *Personal work files* are information filed according to some strategy in the immediate workstation environment. It is relevant to a person's ongoing work schedules. It may be located in the desk, in workstation storage drawers, or in filing cabinets. *Archive storage* includes long-term structured storage systems, often at some distance from the office. This information has no direct relevance to predicted work schedules.

The organization of action information is the most important of the three. Action information items relating to a particular function have to be kept together and be easily accessible. If not, fragmentation of information will create inefficiencies in use. Information stored is categorized as simply as possible. Elaborate mechanisms (such as color coding) are often developed, but frequently fall into disuse. There is a general lack of motivation among people in maintaining filing systems.

The most important factor in enabling people to relate to stored information is spatial memory. Stored materials are viewed as assuming a position in three-dimensional space. Interaction with information has to be frequent, however, to prevent spatial awareness from becoming indistinct. As spatial awareness fails, categorical relations and structure become more important in accessing information. Ultimately, information retrieval becomes entirely dependent on one's knowledge of formal organization and structure. People also use temporal and physical cues in accessing information. Date, color, size, and shape, for example, enable one to relate to information in many different ways. In general, action information is accessed spatially and archive storage categorically, with personal work files utilizing both. Table 4-5 summarizes the characteristics of the kinds of filed information.

Many computer filing schemes have not been successful because of their inability to replicate spatial searches. Complex operational procedures, rigid command languages, keywords, and keyboard entry are often incompatible with one's concept of how information is stored.

Cole concludes that an information storage and retrieval system must reflect the following:

- An understanding of the system user's information needs, including type, form, volume, complexity, functions, and levels of storage.
- The realization that people prefer to spend as little time as possible actually filing.
- Spatial awareness is a naturally dominant concept in humans.
- Color coding, symbols, images, and formatting should be used to enrich the cues available, provide ponts of reference in information, and aid conceptual understanding.

Decision Making

One of the greatest potentials of office automation is its ability to aid the decision-making process. That potential is so immense that experts say it will undoubtedly change the way organizations do business (Keen and Wagner 1979). Behavioral studies of manager and organization decision making are consequently becoming more important. Such studies are clearly mandatory if computer support of managerial decision making is to be effective.

There are few empirical or theoretical analyses of how people manipulate data to solve problems. Most office decisions are semistructured and irregular

Table 4-5. Summary of Information Kinds and Related Design Considerations

Action Information	*Archive Storage*
Detailed knowledge of information and its whereabouts	Contextual knowledge of information less sure of its whereabouts
Of direct relevance to present work	Possibly indirectly relevant to present work
Short-term memory and recent long-term memory considerations	Long-term memory considerations
Predominant spatial awareness of information	Predominant awareness is of information categories
Limit to the amount of information that can be related to in direct spatial terms	A very large amount of information can be related to with the correct strategy
Requires minimum organization	Requires extensive organization
Requires little retrieval aid (e.g., indexes or other user support)	Retrieval is most efficient using retrieval aids

Personal work files should be considered a hybrid of the two extreme levels.

Adapted from Cole (1982).

rather than routine or repetitive, and many are tactical rather than strategic (Morgan 1976). Habit, rules of thumb, and muddling through are very important in the decision-making process (Keen 1981).

Wright (1974) conducted a study of decision making, focusing on the harassed decision maker—one who must make a decision in an environment that discourages leisurely action. This individual characteristically accentuates negative evidence, uses few attributes in the decision-making process, and is quite likely to discredit evidence on a few salient dimensions.

Managers strongly favor concrete and verbal data over formal analysis. Reluctance to use computerized information sources is based on the belief, often justifiable, that the information is untimely, irrelevant, inaccurate, or incomplete (Eason 1974; Morgan 1980). Managers also often have difficulty in identifying their own needs (Nickerson 1981). Keen and Wagner, describing the results of an IBM study, claim that decision makers themselves don't really know how they make decisions; further, they don't want to reveal the details of the decision making they are aware of.

Based on the sketchy evidence available, Keen and Wagner provide some tentative general design criteria for systems used by decision makers:

- Systems applications must permit rapid creation, alteration, and extension of a system.
- Dialogue between the decision maker and the computer should be based on the decision maker's concepts, vocabulary, and problem definitions—not the machine's.
- Communication aspects of the decision-making process are important. The design must provide socially acceptable ways of presenting a decision or solution and consider the feedback of those affected by it.
- An interactive, menu-driven system is necessary.

In short, key system features are flexibility, ease of use, and adaptability.

Communicating Activities

The impact of new technology on office communication will be pervasive. Telecommunications will become the glue that ties new office systems together. But the promise of electronic communication is being tempered by an increasing awareness of the importance of social aspects of office system design. A solution that solves technical and administrative problems but fails to address social needs is doomed to failure.

Communication among people in organizations has been studied from many angles. The simplest distinction is between formal and informal communication. Formal communication reflects the organization's needs and goals and tends to be written and hierarchical. Informal communication is ad hoc, usually verbal, and lateral. It may or may not relate to the job. Such communication satisfies the individual's need for social satisfaction in the work environment.

Conrath (1973), in a study of an organization's communication structure, found the following relationships:

- Written communication tends to be vertical, following the organization's authority structure.
- Telephone communication is the most closely aligned with the organization's task structure.
- Face-to-face interactions are most influenced by the organization's physical structure and are fostered by close proximity, regardless of task or authority relationships.

New technologies, such as word processing, are addressing formal communication rather well. But the vital role that informal communication fulfills in the office must also be realized. Such communication must be encouraged and incorporated into system design because organizations of people need social support to maintain commitment to their jobs.

Conferring and Meeting

Conferring and meeting are simultaneous interactions between two or more people. Their purpose may range from simple information dissemination to complex problem solving and may involve superior/subordinate or peer relationships. Historically, business meetings have consisted of face-to-face encounters involving total sensory awareness, including tactile, gustatory, and olfactory dimensions. They permit easy perusal of documents and other materials and such peripheral niceties of hospitality as shaking hands, coffee breaks, or lunch.

The behavior of meeting participants has begun to come under the research microscope. Brecht (1978), in a study of academic, business, and government meetings, concluded that meetings do differ from one another, but the way they differ is not as obvious as it appears. Salient characteristics of a meeting, such as its purpose or the group conducting it, appear to have little or at the most an ambiguous effect on meeting communication processes. The more subtle characteristics of meetings, such as their size and complexity, do influence the nature of the communication. Implications of these differences are unclear, however.

In a 1973 office communications survey on meeting content, Hough and Panko (1977) found the most common meeting activities involve information give-and-take and problem solving. Meeting contents were directed as follows:

Table 4-6. Distribution of Meeting Content

Rank	Type of Information	Percent of Meetings
1	Information seeking	49
2	Information giving to keep people in the picture	48
3	Problem solving	48
4	Discussion of ideas	26
5	Delegation of work	12
6	Negotiation	11
7	Forming impression of others	9
8	Policy making	8
9	Presentation of a report	8
10	Inspection of fixed objects	7
11	Conflict	4
12	Disciplinary interview	1

Studies of how executives and managers spend their time (for example, Poppel 1983) reveal that meetings and conferences occupy a significant portion of the workday. Reports in a range of 30–70 percent of one's time are commonly found. Preferences for verbal communication over nonverbal communication (such as memos) appear to be reinforced by fact.

Increasingly, groups rather than individuals are accomplishing professional and managerial work. Group behavior has the following characteristics (Driscoll 1979):

- New groups do not work well together.
- The advantages of groups over individuals emerge only as groups mature.
- Groups experience an initial nonproductive period during which they must answer questions like, *Who is in charge? What's in it for me? What's expected of me?* But once these matters are resolved, the group can make rapid progress.

If face-to-face meetings have one disadvantage, it is that they are easily dominated by one or two powerful orators (Johansen et al. 1979).

Telephoning

The telephone is the primary electronic medium of informal communication in today's business office. Its advantages are: speed and range (anyone in the world with another telephone is almost immediately available), ease of use (simple key entry or dialing a short combination of numbers), accessibility (it fits on a desk), and acceptability (holding a telephone handset to one's ear during conversation is an established behavior pattern).

But, as Reid (1973) describes, the telephone has disadvantages as well. The first is its storage characteristics. The printed word can be scanned quickly without the aid of special equipment, but extracting information from an audio recording is, by comparison, quite tedious. Incorporation of a storage mechanism into a person-to-person telecommunication facility is an unsatisfactory method of establishing a permanent record of conversations.

A second disadvantage is the coordination necessary to complete a call. Deciding when to call is left to the individual, who has imperfect knowledge of the accessibility of the telecommunication network. All the phone lines may be busy, preventing the call from reaching its destination, or the called party may not be available. Studies show that only 30 percent of business calls reach their intended recipient on the first attempt (Saunders 1982).

Another disadvantage is that a telephone call can interrupt other work that is more important than the call itself. Executives report that this is true for about 60 percent of all calls (Saunders). An unannounced call may also catch a party at a bad moment, thus eliciting an unfavorable, irreversible response.

Nevertheless, office workers spend a significant portion of their day on the telephone (up to 15 percent or more) and a portion of all meetings are conducted over it (20 percent by one estimate). The impossibility of predicting with any confidence whether a phone call will reach a party at a good moment may be a poor incentive for substituting the telephone for a face-to-face meeting, however.

Dictation

Little is known of the behavioral aspects of composing documents. The normal methods include physical (writing and typing) and verbal (dictation to a machine or to another person). Using one's mouth instead of one's hand to compose a document would seem advantageous since people can speak memorized material about five times faster than they can write it (Gould 1978). It would also seem to allow them to function more effectively by speeding up the process of getting ideas out of the short-term working memory and onto a permanent record, before they are forgotten.

But dictation as a human communication function has had mixed success—some people like it, others do not. Lockwood (1979) argues that, in terms of real productivity, handwriting and typing are both faster than machine dictation, measured from the time dictating begins to when the document is signed off. Dictation time is longer because it requires more edit cycles. Lockwood does not present data to support this conclusion, however.

To date, Gould (1978) and Gould and Boies (1978) have performed the most thorough dictation studies. The former study tested the notion that dictating is hard to learn and requires practice before one dictates as well as one writes. This study concluded that adult subjects who had never dictated before, with a few hours practice, were able to dictate one-page letters of varying complexities as well as they wrote them. The composition time, quality, and gross linguistic characteristics of the dictated and written letters were similar. The Gould and Boies study tested the hypothesis that people who are learning to dictate believe their written documents are superior to their dictated documents. The study results confirmed this hypothesis. Immediately after composition, the subjects believed their written letters superior to their dictated letters, even though they and others later rated them equal. The study also notes that, depending on document complexity, an author's dictation speed is about 20 percent to 35 percent faster than writing after many years of dictation experience. These experimenters conclude that:

- Dictation yields faster performance.
- Performance, perception, and preference are all important in accepting dictation. Not only must the system lead to better performance, but the user must know it does.
- In writing, basic composition skills, not the composition method, are probably the limiting factor.

This final conclusion, however, is questioned by the study of Chapanis et al. (1977), which found that sentences generated in hard copy tend to be longer than those created orally.

Ultimately, the process of dictation involves speaking directly to the computer itself. What effect will the limitations imposed by the listening device have on the dictation rates of the document producer? This was studied by Gould et al. (1982), who compared unrestricted continuous speech dictation to a limited vocabulary dictation (1,000 and 5,000 words) and dictation necessitating speaking in isolated words. In all cases restrictions reduced performance. Compared to traditional dictation speeds with unlimited vocabularies of 25–30 words per minute, restricted vocabularies yielded connected speech dictation rates of 15 words per minute, and isolated speech dictation rates of 7.5–10 words per minute.

Procedural Activities

Procedural activities follow predefined rules or steps. They tend to be mechanical and are almost always performed simultaneously with other activities, such as reading and writing. Activities are placed in this category primarily because of intent, rather than task purity.

Completing Forms

A common procedural activity is completing forms. This is influenced by two form aspects: the language used and the spatial arrangement of the information. Traditionally, office forms are made of paper and may be completed outside the office system or within the system itself. As office technologies develop, the form medium will continue to evolve from a paper to an electronic base. Both electronic and paper form design will be considered in Chapter 6.

Physical Activities

Physical activities require the manual expenditure of human energy. As previously noted, the human objective in performing any manual task is economy of effort. Office automation—in the form of typewriters and dictating machines, for example—has already made some significant advances in achieving this. But further revolutionary gains are on the horizon. Still, while total elimination of some physical activities may be in the offing, an increased need for others, such as typing and keying and using equipment, will inevitably occur.

Typing and Keying

The basic communication mode between people and office systems has been, and will continue to be, keying, usually on a standard typewriter keyboard. Typewriter keying is a perceptual-motor skill familiar to almost everyone in the Western world. Most people have used a typewriter at some time. But typing skills vary enormously, ranging from a proficient 100 or more words per minute to the two-finger, hunt-and-peck variety. Does office systems effectiveness depend on typewriter proficiency? Preliminary evidence indicates not. The Weeks et al. (1974) and Chapanis et al. (1977) studies found that typing skill in itself does not represent an advantage in problem-solving tasks. The actual typing part of the process consumed only about a third of the problem-solving activity. Slight time advantages gained by proficient typing made little difference overall.

Growth of the proportion of office system tasks involving typing, however, will eventually create an advantage for skilled typists. The kind of typing required will also be a factor, with greater expert/novice differences occurring with text typing than with nontext keying. The crossover point will depend upon the task and cannot now be predicted with any accuracy.

A second factor in typewriter use is attitude. Skilled typing has traditionally been viewed as a clerical task. Will a widely divergent group of office users accept typing? Evidence is still sketchy, but a Rand Corporation study (Schindler 1982) found that resistance to typing cannot be predicted based on sex alone. Some women as well as men do not like typing. The best guess today is that some people will type and some won't, but the former should be in the majority.

Awareness of the benefits to be gained from keyboard use can probably overcome negative attitudes toward typing. Ease of keyboard (and system) use will be extremely important. And not making a lack of typing skill obvious to others will be important to some people.

Using Equipment

Equipment will soon pervade every office. Most jobs will require some interaction with devices that will gradually absorb more human activities. It is worth repeating that this equipment must be easy to use and designed in the image of human behavior patterns, and that technological complexity must not contaminate operations. One further point is also worth emphasizing: Human behavior patterns are often social. Designs (at least in their first generation of use) must not deviate from what is socially acceptable today. It is acceptable, for example, to hold a telephone to one's ear, but wearing headphones or a microphone in most business offices today would be deviating too far from the norm.

References

Baxter, R. I. "Study Sees Better Time Use with Voice, Electronic Mail." *Computerworld,* 25 October, 1982, p. 31.

Bennett, C. A. "Toward Empirical, Practicable, Comprehensive Task Taxonomy." *Human Factors* 13, No. 3 (1971): 229–235.

Brecht, M. "A Meeting Is Not a Meeting Is Not a Meeting: Implications for Teleconferencing." *Proceedings of the Human Factors Society—22nd Annual Meeting (1978).* Santa Monica, Calif., 1978.

Bolt, Beranek, and Newman, Inc. *Electronic Mail: The Messaging Systems Approach.* Cambridge, Mass., 1980.

Carlisle, J. H. "Evaluating the Impact of Office Automation on Top Management Communication." *AFIPS Conference Proceedings* 45 (1976): 611–616.

Chapanis, A.; Parrish, R. N.; Ochsman, R. B.; and Weeks, G. D. "Studies in Interactive Communication: II. The Effects of Four Communication Modes on the Linguistic Performance of Teams During Cooperative Problem Solving." *Human Factors* 19, No. 2 (1977): 101–126.

Cole, I. "Human Aspects of Office Filing: Implications for the Electronic Office." *Proceedings of the Human Factors Society—26th Annual Meeting (1982)*, pp. 59–63. Santa Monica, Calif., 1982.

Conrath, D. W. "Communication Patterns, Organizational Structure and Man: Some Relationships." *Human Factors* 15, No. 5 (1973): 459–470.

Driscoll, J. W. "People and the Automated Office." *Datamation*, November 1979, pp. 106–112.

Eason, K. D. "The Manager as a Computer User." *Applied Ergonomics* 5, No. 9 (1974): 9–14.

Engel, G. H.; Groppuso, J.; Lowenstein, R. A.; and Traub, W. G. "An Office Communications System." *IBM Systems Journal* 18, No. 3 (1979): 402–431.

Gould, J. D. "An Experimental Study of Writing, Dictating and Speaking." In *Attention and Performance VII*, edited by J. Pequin, pp. 299–319. Hillsdale, N. J.: Erlbaum Assoc., 1978.

Gould, J. D., and Boies, S. J. "How Authors Think About Their Writing, Dictating and Speaking." *Human Factors* 20, No. 4 (1978); 495–505.

Gould, J. D.; Conti, J.; and Bovanyecz, T. "Composing Letters with a Simulated Listening Typewriter." *Proceedings: Human Factors in Computer Systems*, pp. 367–370. Gaithersburg, Md. March 15–17, 1982.

Hodges, J. D. Jr., and Angalet, B. W. "The Prime Technical Information Source—The Local Work Environment." *Human Factors* 10, No. 4 (1968): 425–430.

Hough, R. W., and Panko, R. R. *Teleconferencing Systems: A State-of-the-Art Survey and Preliminary Analysis.* Stanford, CA: Stanford Research Inst., April 1977.

Keen, P. G. "Information Systems and Organizational Change." *Communications of the ACM* 24, No. 1 (1981): 24–33.

Keen, P. G., and Wagner, G. R. "DSS: An Executive Mind-Support System." *Datamation*, Nov. 1979, pp. 117–122.

Lockwood, D. "Forum: Implementing Advanced Office Systems." *Corporate Systems* 4, No. 5 (July/August 1979): 6–56.

Morgan, H. L. "Office Automation Project—A Research Prospective." *Proceedings of the National Computer Conference*, 1976, pp. 605–610.

Morgan, M. B. "Office of the Future—Is Management Ready?" *Journal of Systems Management* 31, No. 6 (1980): 28–32.

Nickerson, R. S. "Why Interactive Computer Systems Are Sometimes Not Used by People Who Might Benefit from Them." *International Journal of Man–Machine Studies* 15, No. 4 (1981): 469–483.

Poppel, H. L. "Study Reveals OA Expense and Effort Is Worth It." *Information System News*, 24 January 1983, p. 41.

Reid, A. A. L. "Channel Versus System Innovation Person/Person Telecommunications." *Human Factors* 15, No. 5 (1973): 449–457.

Saunders, S. "Voice Messaging: While You Were Out…A New System Called." *Today's Office*, October 1982, pp. 69–74.

Schindler, P. E. Jr. "New Rand Study Punctures Old Office Automation Myths." *Information Systems News*, 16 October 1982.

Weeks, G. D.; Kelly, M. J.; and Chapanis, A. "Studies in Interactive Communication: V. Cooperative Problem Solving by Skilled and Unskilled Typists in a Teletypewriter Mode." *Journal of Applied Psychology* 59, No. 6 (1974): 665–674.

Wenig, R. P., and Pardoe, T. D. *Office Automation Systems.* International Management Services, August 1979.

Wright, P. "The Harassed Decision Maker: Time Pressures, Distractions, and the Use of Evidence." *Journal of Applied Psychology* 59, No. 5 (1974): 555–561.

5

Designing Jobs
People Can and Will Do

The impact of office automation is most clearly felt in the jobs office workers are asked to perform. Research shows that the design of jobs, and related job-oriented considerations, have a significant effect on the acceptance and effective use of technology. Improper job design threatens the well-being and productivity of workers, whereas proper and thoughtful design creates the opportunity to make work-life more satisfying, and increases productivity as well.

Technically, a job is that portion of the employee's work role that consists of activities related to the transformation of objects or materials. For many years jobs were performed in the cottages and fields of peasants. These jobs tended to be holistic in nature. A plowed field culminated in a harvested and consumed crop. A shapeless piece of steel ended up attached to a horse's hoof. As technology became more complex, jobs moved into factories. Job fragmentation and division of labor promised greater productivity.

In the era of simple technology, jobs were made more efficient by applying time and motion studies. Workers were simply considered to be machines or extensions of machines—complicated, unreliable, and recalcitrant machines, but machines nevertheless. As technology became more sophisticated, the workers' role shifted from that of user or guider of tools to that of regulator, controller, or maintainer of systems. Blue shirts were replaced by white shirts. The design of jobs, however, did not change. Task and job rationalization was imported into the office environment with no regard for the consequences. Solutions developed for simple deterministic technology were imposed on quite different social systems. This has created a dilemma which began in the 1960s and continues today. How can the office technical and social system be effectively merged?

Continuing to treat people in ways they will not accept is not cost effective. System implementors must avoid a production-line mentality because they will be dealing with people who want to use their intelligence. Hird (1972) says that many new workers find it increasingly difficult to accept the idea that they have become measured units, robotized for the sake of production efficiency. If work offers them nothing more than burning up calories to meet production schedules, they will demand the highest possible pay for being kept in mental solitary confinement.

Swain (1973) and Kirkley (1980) feel that the biggest mistake employers can make is to automate functions without considering the tasks left for workers to perform. In their push for results, they might automate manual procedures and then measure the resulting efficiency simply by pointing to the number of people fired or not hired. If so, the fact that job dissatisfaction may have increased or that superfluous management systems or work environments have been perpetuated may be entirely overlooked. Thus, the office of the future could simply add to the country's growing malaise—its lack of pride in work and its products—and create a technological barrier between all workers and their work, whether they be clerks or executives.

Workers have reacted to today's offices in a variety of ways. The last two decades have seen greater resistance to managerial authority and job conditions, sagging productivity and commitment to the company, waning job satisfaction, and a rising sense of alienation. Absenteeism and turnover have increased as have non-wage-related strikes and sabotage. Traditional work ethic values are changing and there is a much greater emphasis on self-fulfillment. Sixty percent of the adults of the 1980s now consider this most important (Windsor 1982). Meaningful work and participation in decisions affecting work are now much sought after goals. If office systems are to achieve their true potential, we must reexamine and possibly restructure work itself, making it more palatable to those who perform it. Key elements include job enrichment, job redesign, and worker participation in the process. Before looking at these, however, let us review the potential causes of job stress and the criteria for a well-designed job.

Job Design and Work Stress

The potential causes of work stress were discussed in Chapter 3. We learned there that the tendency has been for computers to yield jobs that are more routine, fast-paced, and monitored, allowing less flexibility and social contact. The result has been heightened work stress caused by such factors as boredom, work overload, and the thwarting of psychological needs for autonomy, self-esteem, social regard, safety, and career development. A major deficiency is the perceived loss of control the user reports in the automated office. Automation tends to be accompanied by rigid work procedures, high production standards, constant pressure for performance, little control over tasks, and little identification or satisfaction with the end product. Research shows that lower job satisfaction occurs with tasks that are repetitive, oversimplified, and lacking in control, status, and participation.

It is interesting to note that studies have found higher stress levels in clerical users of VDTs and lower levels in professional VDT users. The jobs of clerical users are characterized by the qualities described above, while professional users' tasks are more flexible and controllable, utilize the workers' education, and provide more satisfaction and pride in the end product. Clerical users often perceive technology as taking the meaning out of work, raising their workload, and increasing anxiety about being replaced by a machine; professional users view it as a tool to enhance their productivity.

Research also indicates that the kind of job being performed correlates with reported physical ailments associated with VDT use. Professional users report fewer discomforts than do their clerical counterparts. Evidently one's job significantly colors one's attitudes about automation.

Technology and Restructured Jobs

Technology need not result in badly designed jobs. Its inherent flexibility can yield an array of configurations to satisfy the psychological needs of almost anyone. For example, technology can:

- Enlarge responsibilities through creating a need to understand the technology itself.
- Enlarge responsibility by providing access to a much greater range of capabilities and information. Performance may then be measured in more meaningful terms such as growth or business retention, not simply in error rates.
- Absorb routine clerical skills, permitting focusing on the nonroutine or nonautomatic.
- Absorb computational, scheduling, and routine decision-making tasks so as to permit focusing on goal setting, trend perception, and human contact.
- Increase responsibility and communication skills since one's work will affect others faster and more often.

The challenge will be to harness technology in a meaningful way.

Job Design Criteria

Variety	Control and self-regulation
Reasonably demanding	Feedback
Meaningfulness	A degree of social support
Closure	Participation in decisions affecting
Opportunity to learn, develop, and	work
grow	Connection to the future

The design of a job must balance the needs of the organization and its workers. Business needs include flexibility and adaptability in an environment that is growing turbulent. Human needs include the qualities listed that a job must possess before its holder will perceive it as satisfying. Without these qualities, productive performance can never be achieved, although this does not mean that their presence guarantees productiveness. Factors beyond the scope of this book, such as an organization's management style and how well it treats its employees, are influences as well. But without achieving the following job design criteria, productive performance is unlikely.

Variety. Variety is necessary to maintain alertness and responsiveness. Routineness and repetitiveness tend to extinguish one's interest. Adult human beings in a stimulus-free environment tend to hallucinate. For those tied to a piece of technology (such as a VDT) variety of physical activity is needed. Even a comfortable working position will become tiring after awhile. Desirable kinds of physical activity include walking to return materials to trays and interactions with other people, including coworkers and clients, either face-to-face or by telephone.

Reasonably demanding. A job must be demanding and challenging. The skills and capabilities the worker brings to the job must be used in the job. If not, the worker will become bored. On the other hand, if job requirements exceed one's capabilities, frustration will result. A good worker is one who performs the job skillfully, whereas the poor worker appears clumsy. For a task to demand skilled performance it must be of optimum difficulty—not too easy and not too hard.

Meaningfulness. The skills required to complete a job must be used in a meaningful context. The job must make sense. Something of consequence, relevance, or significance must be produced or accomplished.

Closure. A job must be complete in two ways. It must contain a series of tasks or responsibilities that the worker perceives as having an identifiable beginning and end. Secondly, the tasks or responsibilities must be performed for a specific, identifiable group of beneficiaries.

Opportunity to learn, develop, and grow. Workers must be able to do a job in many ways, some of which are better than others. The better ways should be achievable as the worker becomes more proficient. The ability to learn on the job implies performance standards and feedback. The enormous capacity of humans to learn is often overlooked.

Control and self-regulation. People should be able to plan, regulate, and control their own work worlds. Materials and processes should be regulated with a minimum of coercion. People must also have as much decision-making control as possible over how the job is carried out. They should not only have the responsibility to comply with routine procedures, but also have the authority to act in unusual situations. Control can mitigate many other undesirable factors.

Feedback. Feedback is essential. Workers must receive frequent, direct, and meaningful information on how they are performing. Information on performance is critical to reducing errors and to achieving self-confidence when accomplishments are recognized. To accelerate behavioral change in the desired direction, feedback must be frequent, and it must come directly and immediately from the receiver of the product or service.

A degree of social support. Work-related communication of employees must exist. Recognition for accomplishments must be provided.

Participation in decisions affecting work. Participation in work decisions aids learning and growth. It enables one to assess one's efforts when finished and gives a person a stake in the future.

Connection to the future. People must feel that the job leads to some sort of desirable future.

Whether these criteria have actually been achieved in job design is not as important as whether they are perceived by the worker to exist. Changing the objective state through meeting these criteria may not increase job satisfaction if the worker does not perceive their existence.

Job Redesign and Worker Participation in the Process

Job redesign will evolve as technology forces changes in task content, job responsibilities, and human interactions. This issue is important because it is entwined with worker acceptance of technological change. Naturally, any criteria for good job design must also be applied to job redesign. But a critical question is whether incumbents should be allowed to participate in the redesign process. Does this result in more acceptable job content? Does it help ensure the acceptance of change?

Those favoring worker involvement in redesign say that the person directly involved in a job is the most capable of innovating changes in it because no one else knows better what the operation is all about (Swain 1973). Incumbents who are more knowledgeable about the job will be more committed to and less threatened by changes (Glaser 1975; Hackman and Oldham 1976; Vroom 1964). The result will be increased motivation and job satisfaction (DeJong 1978; Swain 1973).

Those opposed to employee involvement argue that allowing people to participate in their own job redesign may raise their hopes unrealistically.

And if all their recommendations are not accepted, problems may be created (Ford 1969; Grote 1972).

Research supporting either view is scarce. A recent study by Seeborg (1978) does, however, provide some data. The study, in which managers, supervisors, and subordinates redesigned their own jobs, resulted in the following conclusions:

- Supervisors focused on vertically loading jobs—increasing task identity and the worker's area of responsibility.
- Workers were most concerned with the social aspects of their work.
- Neither supervisors nor workers made radical changes.
- Job satisfaction increased more when workers participated in the redesign.
- Identical changes were perceived to be better by workers who participated in the redesign than by those who did not participate.

A study by Hall et al. (1978) reached similar conclusions. It found that when organizational change is imposed, attitudes are less positive than when change is participative or representative. This was true even of changes that were favorable to the worker.

A Mumford and Banks (1967) study concluded that workers must want to participate and feel they have something to gain from doing so, and they must have low initial resistance to change. These experimenters also concluded that perceived participation is more important than active participation. Some people may not welcome participation and prefer to be told what to do. The results of this study and comments of others lead to the following general conclusions:

- The job redesign process should be participative.
- The workers involved should want their jobs and work situations redesigned.

Job Enrichment

The premise of advocates of job enrichment is that people have a need to find fulfillment in their work and that job enrichment provides the opportunity for that fulfillment. It is popularly thought to be a key to motivation and productivity.

Job enrichment comprises two forms—horizontal and vertical. Horizontal job enrichment consists of task diversification, or giving the worker a wider variety of similar tasks. Vertical enrichment involves expanding tasks to encompass some meaningful whole by permitting workers to do a job from beginning to end.

A review of job enrichment literature reveals an abundance of rhetoric, a lack of substance, and diverse opinions of its virtues. Its proponents continue to extol its benefits, while others caution that it is not the solution to all worker problems. Why such a wide divergence of conclusions?

First, over the last twenty years, innumerable studies have concluded that job enrichment (or job enlargement, its predecessor) is meant to increase motivation, decrease boredom and dissatisfaction, and improve attendance and productivity. The results of these studies are used to justify continued development and implementation of job enrichment programs in business.

While this has been occurring, but with much less publicity, a small body of findings has been accumulating which contradicts, questions, or qualifies the conclusions of job enrichment advocates. A study by Schoderbek and Reif (1969) revealed that out of more than 200 firms responding to a mailed questionnaire, only 19 percent (41 companies) were using a job enrichment program. Only 4 of those indicated their experience had been "very successful." Cummins and Salipante (1974), who reviewed 57 experimental job-redesign studies, found that almost every study showed severe methodological deficiencies that threatened the validity of their conclusions. The Hawthorne effect was a predominant factor.

Steers and Spencer (1977) found that increased job scope was associated with better job performance for high-need achievers, but not for low-need achievers. They concluded that since high performance is not motive-relevant for low-need achievers, enriched jobs should have little impact. Umstot et al. (1976) found that job enrichment had a substantial impact on job satisfaction, but little effect on productivity. But they concluded that increased satisfaction may result in other benefits, such as higher output quality and reduced turnover and absenteeism.

Another accumulating body of evidence indicates that the lower the worker's skill level, the less likely job enrichment will succeed. Schoderbek and Reif's study revealed that getting unskilled workers to accept job enrichment was more difficult than getting the skilled or semiskilled to accept it. This was because of the unskilled's preference for the status quo and highly specialized work, as well as their lack of interest in job improvements that require new skills or greater responsibility. Hulin and Blood (1968) and Fein (1970) conclude that many workers are alienated not necessarily from work, but from the middle-class norms and values inherent in job enrichment programs—positive regard for occupational achievement, belief in the intrinsic value of hard work, desire for attaining responsible positions, and the work-related aspects of the Protestant ethic. For these workers, job content is not necessarily related to job satisfaction nor is motivation necessarily a function of satisfaction. Such alienated workers find fulfillment outside the work environment. Any job satisfaction they do experience at work is largely the result of social interaction with other workers, not of job content or design.

Numerous other studies have pointed out that repetitive work can have motivating features or characteristics for some people (Smith 1955; Kilbridge 1960; and MacKinney et al. 1962).

Another argument of those not in full support of job enrichment focuses on failures that result from worker resistance to change. This argument has some merit if change is pursued for the sake of change alone. With new technology, however, change is inevitable, and problems associated with it must be directly confronted.

Job Enrichment: Some Conclusions

When the smoke clears, what can we conclude about job enrichment? Obviously, there are no simple answers since experts have been wrestling with solutions for years. Stepping back and looking at technological change and office systems from an overall perspective, however, one can see that human tasks, interactions, and skill requirements, as well as organizations themselves, will be changing. So natural human resistance to change can no longer be an argument against job enrichment.

For many workers, change will make tasks more routine, impose more rigor, and disrupt the traditional social aspects of the work environment. Job enrichment appears able to confront some of these problems. It has significant face validity (jobs can be made more interesting), and its implementation costs will be low as it rides the coattails of technological change. It can also be a psychological sales tool that can aid in getting workers to accept office automation. This should not be misconstrued as an end in itself but simply as a benefit of the mechanism used to get people to accept change. It can be concluded, then, that job enrichment appears to be a valuable tool in the arsenal of the agent of technological change.

Job enrichment, however, must not be indiscriminately applied. The evidence that some people's job performance or satisfaction is not affected by job content is compelling. Application of job enrichment to such workers may be more damaging than useful. Therefore, job enrichment should be used only for those who will benefit from it.

Making decisions about job enrichment requires thorough study of the needs and values of the workers affected by office automation. Unfortunately, job enrichment literature contains few specific design guidelines. But DeJong (1978) states that vertical job enrichment and increased autonomy of work groups should be given preference over horizontal job enrichment and job rotation. And Driscoll (1979) concludes that enriching jobs with discretionary tasks is the most effective method.

Sociotechnical Systems Approach

One approach to work design that deals with the human and social aspects as well as the technical aspects is that of sociotechnical systems. Whereas job enlargement and enrichment begin with individual jobs and proceed to redesign them from that viewpoint, the sociotechnical approach looks at the work system and creates jobs within a much broader perspective. Using structured analysis techniques to separate the technical and social aspects, tasks are combined in new ways that permit much greater worker control of the workload variances, greater decision-making, and more personal interaction. For more information on this approach see Taylor (1981).

Job Design and the Systems Analyst

Most jobs are no longer socially evolved. They are consciously created by someone who will probably never perform the job. In computer systems, this someone is quite often the computer systems analyst.

Two research studies by Hedberg and Mumford (1975) and Davis (1977) have attempted to uncover the principles adhered to by computer system designers in the development of such systems. This, they felt, would provide a better understanding of the manner in which the content of jobs was designed in industry. The results of both studies are similar. When designing systems the designers attempt to minimize total costs of production, minimize immediate costs by minimizing skills, and they deemphasize job satisfaction. Jobs are tightly defined with targets and controls set by supervisors, not by employees.

When asked to describe the person for whom they are designing jobs, however, designers have a somewhat different view. Workers are characterized as being capable of doing a variety of tasks, possessing considerable skill, and demanding interesting work. Worker satisfaction and motivation are acknowledged.

System designers appear to be caught in a dilemma. What they are producing in the way of systems does not totally agree with their views of the person who will use the system. Pressures to get the job going apparently prevent any serious attempt to satisfy the human needs of those for whom they are designing. Any program to address job design or redesign in the modern organization is going to have to confront system development methods that are often in direct conflict with the objectives sought.

Conclusion

If the office is to survive, it must come to grips with the continuing high rate of change of technology as well as the changing needs, aspirations, and expectations of those who populate it. Productivity improvements will never result from a population of mass production workers, those programmed to perform a small task and considered unreliable, obstinate, and not capable of innovation and dealing with variations. The only hope lies in the humanistic worker, a regulator and controller capable of innovating, learning, making judgments, and being flexible. Job restructuring may be wrenching for organizations and individuals but designing work around people, not machines, is a direction that we can no longer afford to ignore.

References

Cummins, T. G., and Salipante, P. F. "The Development of Research-Based Strategies for Improving the Quality of Work Life." *Paper presented at a NATO Conference on Personal Goals and Work Design.* York, England, 1974.

Davis, L. E. "Job Design Criteria 20 Years Later." In *Design of Jobs*, edited by L. E. Davis and J. C. Taylor. Glenview, Ill.: Scott Foresman, 1979.

DeJong, J. R. "The Method in Work Design: Some Recommendations Based Upon Experience Obtained in Job Redesign." *International Journal of Production Research* 16, No. 1 (January 1978): 39–49.

Driscoll, J. W. "People and the Automated Office." *Datamation*, November 1979, pp. 106–112.

Fein, M. *Approaches to Motivation.* Hillsdale, N. J., 1970.

Ford, R. N. *Motivation Through the Work Itself.* American Management Assn., 1969.

Glaser, E. M. *Improving the Quality of Work Life . . . And in the Process, Improving Productivity.* Los Angeles: Human Interaction Research Inst., 1975.

Grote, R. C. "Implementing Job Enrichment." *California Management Review* 15, No. 1 (1972): 16–21.

Hackman, J. R., and Oldham, G. R. "Motivation Through the Design of Work: Test of a Theory." *Organizational Behavioral and Human Performance* 16, No. 2 (1976): 250–279.

Hall, D. T.; Rabinowitz, S.; Goodale, J. G.; and Morgan, N. A. "Effects of Top–Down Departmental and Job Change Upon Perceived Employee Behavior and Attitudes: A Natural Field Experiment." *Journal of Applied Psychology* 63, No. 1 (1978): 62–72.

Hedberg, B., and Mumford, E. "The Design of Computer Systems: Man's Vision of Man as an Integral Part of the System Design Process." *Human Choices and Computers*, edited by E. Mumford and H. Sackman. New York: North Holland Publishing Company, 1975.

Hird, J. F. "What Makes Japan's Industry So Successful?" *Assembly Engineering* 15, No. 1 (1972): 20–24.

Hulin, C. L., and Blood, M. R. "Job Enrichment, Individual Differences and Worker Responses." *Psychological Bulletin* 69, No. 1 (1968).

Kilbridge, M. D. "Do Workers Prefer Larger Jobs?" *Personnel*, September/October 1960, pp. 45–48.

Kirkley, J. L. "The Office Merry-Go-Round." *Datamation* 26, No. 2 (February 1980): 43.

MacKinney, A. C.; Wernimont, P. F.; and Galitz, W. O. "Has Specialization Reduced Job Satisfaction?" *Personnel* 39, No. 1 (January/February 1962): 8–17.

Mumford, E., and Banks, O. *The Computer and the Clerk.* London: Routledge and Kegan Paul, 1967.

Schoderbek, P. P., and Reif, W. E. *Job Enlargement.* Ann Arbor, Mich.: Bureau of Industrial Relations; Graduate School of Business Administration, University of Michigan, 1969.

Seeborg, I. S. "The Influence of Employee Participation in Job Redesign." *The Journal of Applied Behavioral Science* 14, No. 1 (1978): 87–98.

Smith, P. C. "The Prediction of Individual Differences in Susceptibility to Industrial Monotony." *Journal of Applied Psychology* 39, No. 5 (1955): 322–329.

Steers, R. M., and Spencer, D. G. "The Role of Achievement Motivation in Job Design." *Journal of Applied Psychology* 62, No. 4 (1977): 472–479.

Swain, A. D. "Design of Industrial Jobs a Worker Can and Will Do." *Human Factors* 15, No. 2 (1973): 129–136.

Taylor, James. *Quality of Working Life and White-Collar Automation: A Socio-Technical Case.* Los Angeles, Calif.: Institute of Public Relations, UCLA, February 1981.

Umstot, D. D.; Bell, C. H.; and Mitchell, T. R. "Effects of Job Enrichment and Task Goals on Satisfaction and Productivity: Implications for Job Design." *Journal of Applied Psychology* 61, No. 4 (1976): 379–394.

Vroom, V. H. *Work and Motivation.* New York: John Wiley, 1964.

Windsor, R. K. "Management Opinion." *Administrative Management*, August 1982, p. 82.

6

System Design

A computer, the most powerful tool in the office worker's array of tools, must be an extension of the worker's own self. Consequently, the system and its software must reflect a person's capabilities and respond to his or her specific needs. As part of the overall person/computer interface, system design considerations focus upon these three considerations:

- the language by which people express their needs and desires to the computer;
- the display representations that show the state of the system to workers;
- the more abstract issues that affect a person's understanding of the system's behavior.

Ideally, a system's design should enable a person to develop a conceptual model of the system itself. The conceptual model is the concept a person gradually acquires to explain the computer's behavior. This model is developed in the mind and it enables a person to understand and interact with the system.

Why People Have Trouble with Computer Systems

System design and its behavioral implications are now coming under intense scrutiny by office automation practitioners. As we have seen, this has not always been the case. Historically, the design of computer systems has fallen within the realm of programmers, systems analysts, and system designers. Many of these people are technicians possessing extensive technical knowledge and little behavioral training. Design decisions have rested mostly upon the designers' intuition and wealth of specialized knowledge. Most designers do not realize the extent of their technical knowledge and have been unable to recognize poorly designed interfaces.

The intuition of designers or anyone else, no matter how good or bad they may be at what they do, is error-prone. It is too shallow a foundation for basing design decisions. Specialized knowledge lulls one into a false sense of security. It enables one to interpret and deal with complex or ambiguous situations on the basis of context cues not visible to users, as well as knowledge not possessed by naive users of the computer system. The result is a perfectly usable system to its designers—but one the office worker is unable or unwilling to face up to and master.

What makes a system complex in the eyes of its user? Listed below are five contributing factors.

Use of jargon. Included here is a proliferation of and reliance upon words alien to the office environment. Some examples are: *queue, background, paginate,* and *segment.*

Fine distinctions. These include actions that accomplish similar things but must only be used in specific situations; or the same action that culminates in a different result depending upon when it is performed. Often these distinctions are minute and difficult to keep track of.

Nonobvious design. By this we mean design elements that are not obvious or intuitive to the system user. Operations may have prerequisite conditions that must be satisfied before they can be accomplished; or outcomes may not always be immediate, obvious, or visible. The result is that workers cannot always relate results to the actions that accomplish them.

Disparity in problem-solving strategies. People learn best by doing. They have trouble following directions and do not always read instructions before taking an action. The human problem-solving strategy can be characterized as error correcting, whereby a tentative solution is formulated immediately based upon available evidence. This tentative solution often exhibits a low probability of success but is subject to revision in the light of further evidence. Most computers, however, enforce an *error-preventing* strategy. This strategy assumes that an action will be chosen and performed only if a high degree of confidence exists in its success. The result is that people often get into situations from which it is difficult to untangle themselves (Reed 1982).

Design inconsistency. The same action may have different names; for example, *save* and *keep, write* and *list.* Or the same result may be described differently; for example, *not legal* versus *not valid.* The result of all of this is that system learning becomes an exercise in rote memorization. Meaningful learning becomes difficult if not impossible.

Responses to Poor Design

Those unable to cope with poor design may exhibit a variety of responses ranging from the psychological to the physical. Psychological responses include the following (Foley and Wallace 1974).

Confusion. Detail overwhelms the perceived structure. Meaningful patterns are difficult to ascertain, and the conceptual model cannot be established.

Frustration. This results from an inability to easily convey one's intentions to the computer. It is heightened if an unexpected response cannot be undone or what really took place cannot be determined. Inflexible, and unforgiving systems are a primary cause of frustration.

Panic. Panic may be induced by unexpectedly long delays during times of unusual or severe pressure. Primary causes are unavailable systems and long response times.

Boredom. This results from improper computer pacing (slow response times) and overly simplistic jobs.

These psychological reactions diminish the effectiveness of people using the system because they are severe blocks to concentration. Thoughts irrelevant to the task at hand are forced to their attention and the necessary concentration is impossible. The result is often higher error rates and poor performance. They frequently lead to, or are accompanied by, the following physical reactions (Eason 1979; Stewart 1976).

Abandonment of the system. The system is rejected and other information sources are relied upon. Some other information source must be available, and the system user must have the discretion to perform the rejection. This is a common reaction of managerial and professional personnel.

Incomplete use of the system. Only a portion of the system's capabilities are used, usually those operations that are easiest to perform or provide the most benefits. Historically, this has been the most common reaction to most systems.

Indirect use of the system. An intermediary is placed between the would-be user and the computer. Again, this requires high status and discretion; it is another typical response of managers.

Modification of the task. The task is changed to match the capabilities of the system. This is a prevalent reaction when the tools are rigid and the problem is unstructured, such as in scientific problem solving.

Compensatory activity. Additional actions are performed to compensate for system inadequacies. A common example is the manual reformatting of information to match the structure required by the computer. This is a typical reaction by workers with low discretion, such as clerical personnel.

Misuse of the system. The rules are bent to shortcut operational difficulties. This requires significant knowledge of the system and may impact upon system integrity.

Direct programming. The system is reprogrammed by its user to meet specific needs. This is a typical response of the sophisticated worker.

Ease of Use

Ease of use is frequently mentioned as an ultimate design criterion for office systems. Although it is a simple expression, it has complicated implications. It may apply to a single operation, task, or procedure, or to an entire job. The following criteria, some of which were first described by Miller (1971), can measure a system's ease of use.

The training time required to achieve satisfactory performance is important because in office systems, brevity equals goodness. Most managerial and professional personnel are too busy to devote much time to training in new technologies. In light of this, and considering high turnover rates, satisfactory performance levels must be achieved as soon as possible. It is critical that workers be able to learn to operate a device within the time they are likely to commit to the learning process.

Number of errors deals with maintenance of a reasonable error rate by competent people measured in units of time or per number of operations.

Integration of automated and nonautomated tasks means that there must be a good fit between automated tasks and tasks the technology does not address. That fit must be achieved quickly and with few errors.

Exasperation responses are the "Oh damn!" reactions that express user annoyance or frustration. The frequency of these may foretell a strong rejection of a tool or technology. The absence of exasperation, however, may not represent attitudinal acceptance of a tool.

Habit formation rate refers to how quickly people learn to use a facility and how quickly that use becomes more or less automatic, so that they no longer have to think about what they are doing. This variable can be measured by observing a person's speed, lack of hesitation, and apparent ease in working with a device or system.

How many people want to use the system reflects the attitude of actual or potential users toward a device or system. There are, of course, many reasons for liking or disliking a system, and not all of them are necessarily connected with the device itself or the service it provides. However those attitudes result, they may be more powerful than any other factor in a given system's acceptance.

Irrelevant supporting actions required to perform a task are the incidental actions required for, but not directly related to, doing a job. They include such actions as translating computer code into English, performing frequent or extensive *log-on* procedures, or going through several operations to find the right page in an instruction manual.

Irrelevant display events include information items that must be disregarded but that use up part of the capacities an individual could devote to relevant tasks.

Time and frequency for user warm-up means how long it takes to relearn the necessary skills involved in using infrequently used tools or procedures. It also refers to the number of minutes required for warm-up each time a frequently used tool is used before satisfactory speed and accuracy are achieved.

Decision-making time is the amount of time required to decide what to do after receiving all the information necessary to analyze a problem and select a suitable action.

Shift or work time is the length of time a person can continue working without becoming fatigued.

Failure recovery time includes the amount of time, the number of operations, and the cost of resources required for the user to recover from failures caused by either operator or system errors.

Technology transition time means, where multiple systems are employed, the time necessary to achieve a satisfactory performance level after shifting from one tool to another.

Friendly Systems

Another descriptive term commonly used in today's systems literature is *friendly*—a quality that well-designed office systems are supposed to possess. The dictionary definition of friendly (relating to or befitting a friend; showing kindly interest or goodwill; not hostile; inclined to favor; comforting or cheerful) provides designers with little useful information for developing a system with this quality. Much is left to the imagination.

To put the term in a systems context, let us say that any design decision that allows a system to achieve a high score in ease-of-use criteria will get a high score in friendliness. But friendliness may mean something more—an effect achieved by the harmonious interaction of all the ease-of-use criteria. Achieving this will come slowly, as systems implementors gain a better understanding of the role of people in office systems, and as they test and then modify those systems.

The Desirable Qualities of a System

The computer, as the office worker's major tool, should be a pleasant companion. It should be seen as possessing a variety of desirable qualities. In recent years, a number of writers and researchers have begun to describe what these desired qualities are perceived to be. While too abstract to serve as design guidelines themselves, they provide useful criteria toward which design guidelines may be directed. These qualities, whose compilation was begun by Nemeth (1982), are discussed in the following paragraphs.

Adaptive. A system must be adaptable to the physical, emotional, intellectual, and knowledge traits of the people whom it serves. All office workers should be permitted to interact with a computer in a manner and style which best suits their needs. In essence, the system should be responsive to individual differences in interaction manner, depth, and style.

Transparent. A system must permit one's attention to be focused entirely on the task or job being performed, without concern for the mechanics of the interface. One's thoughts must be directed to the application, not the communication. Any operations which remind a worker of their presence are distracting.

Comprehendible. A system should be understandable. A person should know what to look at, what to do, when to do it, why to do it, and how to do it (Treu 1977). The flow of information, commands, responses, and visual presentations should be in a sensible order that is easy to recollect and place in context (Kaplow and Molnar 1976).

Natural. Operations should mimic the office worker's behavioral patterns. Dialogues should mimic the office worker's thought processes and vocabulary (Foley and Wallace 1974).

Predictable. System actions should be expected, within the context of other actions that are performed. All expectations should be fulfilled uniformly and completely (Martin 1973; Treu 1977).

Responsive. Every human request should be acknowledged, every system reaction clearly described. Feedback is the critical ingredient for shaping a person's performance.

Self-explanatory. Steps to complete a process should be obvious and, where not, supported and clarified by the system itself. Reading and digesting long explanations should never be necessary (Eason 1979).

Forgiving. A system should be tolerant of the human capacity to make errors, at least up to the point where the task or the integrity of the system are affected. Inflexible, unforgiving systems are critical causes of system dissatisfaction. The fear of making a mistake and not being able to recover from it is a primary contributor toward human fear of dealing with computers (Eason 1979; Hansen 1976).

Efficient. Eye and hand movements must not be wasted. Attention should be directed to relevant controls and displays of information. Visual and manual transitions between various system components should proceed easily and freely.

Flexible. People should be able to structure or change a system to meet their particular needs. Inexperienced people may wish to confront and utilize only a small portion of a system's capabilities in a specific manner. With experience, they may wish to utilize extended capabilities in some other manner. This extension and modification of interaction and control procedures should be permitted at the discretion of the workers (Kaplow and Molnar 1976; Schneiderman 1980).

Available. Like any tool, an office system must be available if it is to be effective. Any system unreliability, no matter how good normal system performance, will create dissatisfaction (Miller and Thomas, 1977).

Natural Language Dialogues

For an office system to be responsive to its users, a person and the system must have some means of communicating with one another. The most common and flexible means is an English-based language that includes the numbers, symbols, and punctuation found on a standard typewriter keyboard. The primary design criteria usually applied to languages is that they be natural to the user.

Natural languages are sometimes considered synonymous with English prose. Many argue that systems must accept English prose if they are to move smoothly into the office. Natural human communications, however, are characterized by an apparent unruliness. Gould et al. (1976) found that slight variations in instructions for achieving a goal led to large variations in the expressions people used to achieve the goal. There was no particularly strong natural tendency, but the adaptiveness of human linguistic and cognitive systems was apparent. Procedure manuals written by different analysts describing the same activity, or forms they design to collect the same data, are classic examples of this adaptiveness. Chapanis et al. (1977), in their study of communication modes, found numerous errors and irregularities and grammatical rules repeatedly violated or ignored.

If computers are ever to interact with people on human terms, the irregularities and inconsistencies that characterize natural human languages must be confronted. Although natural human communication appears to have no strict standards, it obviously follows some rules because information gets conveyed, and quite complex problems do get solved.

But perhaps a totally natural language is not necessary. Seeking economy of effort, people tend to be impatient with redundancies (Nickerson 1969), which English is full of. The whole objective of any communication is to transmit an idea quickly and accurately. The transmitter's degree of redundancy depends on the understanding characteristics of the recipient. If the communicator limits redundancies, will the message still be effectively conveyed?

The study by Kelly and Chapanis (1977) has a bearing on this question. They required subjects communicating by teletypewriter to use either 300-word, 500-word, or unlimited vocabularies. Subjects who worked with the restricted vocabularies interacted and solved problems as successfully as those who worked with no restrictions. Thus it appears possible, at least for the types of communications studied in this experiment, to develop limited vocabularies for use in human/machine interactions.

Another pertinent study is that of Gould et al. (1976). They found that subjects who showed a low preference for a restricted-syntax language would readily and sometimes spontaneously use such a language when called upon to communicate.

Schoonard and Boies (1975) tested the ability of typists to type abbreviated words (of one to three characters) in a text-entry process. The typists recognized and typed 93 percent of the to-be-abbreviated words, with an error rate no greater than when they were typing unabbreviated words. And the substitution process did not affect the keystroke rate.

The results of these studies and evidence from operating data-processing systems (Galitz 1979a) indicates that well-designed, restricted vocabularies can provide effective language interfaces between users and office systems. But the language must be natural from an application and job-related standpoint.

The search for the ideal language or languages must continue if people and machines are to work in total harmony. The ultimate solution is probably beyond today's technology and will require further refinement and the use of voice and touch. But for now, designs must develop within the limits of today's technology.

Current Directions and Guidelines

Design of the human/computer interface still remains more of an art than a science. The body of research needed to develop truly effective interfaces is small. Only now is this needed research effort showing signs of awakening. The issues also have great depth and subtlety. Even seemingly straightforward considerations such as minimizing the number of keystrokes may not make a system easier to use. Therefore, we cannot be optimistic that all the answers will be forthcoming in the months and years ahead.

The office and technology, however, will not wait. We must move forward with what is known today, making decisions as best we can. Toward that goal, what follows is a series of design guidelines addressing system design. The guidelines reflect not only what we know today but what we think we know today. Many are based upon research, others on the collective thinking of behaviorists working in the area of office automation. The guidelines address the behavioral considerations involved with office automation users in general, when nothing is known about individuals or their functions. Final system design will, of course, require understanding of specific user tasks and goals.

Consistency

A system should look, act, and feel the same throughout.

Design consistency is a common thread that runs throughout these guidelines. It is the first cardinal rule of all design activities. Consistency is important because it can reduce requirements for human learning by allowing skills learned in one situation to be transferred to another like it. While any new automated system must impose some learning requirements on its users, it should avoid encumbering productive learning with nonproductive activity.

In addition to increased learning requirements, variety in design has a number of other by-products, including:

- More specialization by system users;
- Greater demand for higher skills;
- More preparation time and less production time;
- More frequent changes in procedures;
- More error-tolerant systems (because errors are more likely);
- More kinds of documentation;
- More time to find information in documents;
- More unlearning and learning when systems are changed;
- More demands on supervisors and managers;
- More things to go wrong.

Inconsistencies in design are caused by differences in people. Several designers might each design the same system differently. Inconsistencies also occur when design activities are pressured by time constraints. All too often the solutions in those cases are exceptions that the user must learn to handle.

People, however, perceive a system as a single entity. To them it should look, act, and feel similarly throughout. Excess learning requirements become a burden to their achieving and maintaining high performance and can ultimately influence their acceptance of the system.

Design consistency is achieved primarily by applying design standards within a common framework. The designer creativity that this stifles (if indeed it does) would seem to be a small price to pay for an effective design.

Design Tradeoffs

Human requirements must always take precedence over machine processing requirements.

Design guidelines often cover a great deal of territory and will occasionally conflict with one another or with machine processing requirements. In such conflicts the designer must weigh alternatives and reach a decision based on accuracy, time, cost, and ease-of-use requirements. This leads to the second cardinal rule in office system development: *Human requirements always take precedence over machine processing requirements.* It might be easier for the designer to write a program or build a device at the expense of user ease, but this should not be tolerated.

Log-On

Only one simple action should be necessary to initiate a log-on.

Access to any office system must be easy. Difficult or cumbersome log-on procedures can discourage a system's use before its benefits have a chance to be demonstrated. This simple action should be nothing more than the depression of a log-on or start key. If more actions are required, the system must lead a person through the necessary steps.

Initiative

Initiative should be commensurate with the capabilities of the system users.
- For new and inexperienced people, provide a computer-initiated dialogue.
- For the experienced, permit a human-initiated dialogue.

Initiative is a system characteristic defining who leads the dialogue between an office worker and the computer. In a computer-initiated dialogue, the direction is placed in the hands of the system and a person responds to various kinds of prompts provided by the computer. These prompts may take the form of questions, directions, menus of alternatives, or forms to fill in. Computer-initiated dialogues are usually preferred by new users of systems. They rely on our powerful passive vocabulary (words that can be recognized and understood), and they are a learning vehicle, implicitly teaching a system model as one works.

Human-initiated dialogues place the responsibility of direction in the hands of the system's user. The computer becomes a blackboard waiting to be drawn upon. The user provides free form instructions from memory—either commands or information—and the system responds accordingly. Human-initiated dialogues are often preferred by experienced system users since they permit faster and more efficient interaction. A computer-initiated dialogue tends to slow down and disrupt the more experienced user.

Mixed-initiative dialogues have also been designed. An example of this are labeled function keys on display terminals. The label itself provides a prompt or memory aid but the user must remember when it can be used. Most of the earlier generation computer systems possessed human-initiated dialogues, since this has been the style their designers have been most comfortable with. As a result of the kinds of problems described earlier, and exposure of computer technology to more nonspecialists, there has been in recent years a shift in emphasis to computer-initiated methods. This new emphasis has brought into focus more clearly the problems of this approach for a person who becomes experienced with a system. The result is that today we are beginning to see systems that combine both initiative styles. The needs of both kinds of system users can then be simultaneously satisfied.

A question that has repeatedly been asked is at what point is a person ready to make the transition from a computer- to human-initiated dialogue? Some research has recently investigated this subject. Gilfoil (1982) provided novice system users with a choice of a menu-driven dialogue (computer-initiated) or a command-driven dialogue (human-initiated). The study participants chose the menu approach to start with and moved to the command approach after 16–20 hours of experience. At this point they were found to perform better and to be more satisfied with the command dialogue. A similar study (Chafin and Martin 1980) found the transition occurring at about 25–50 hours.

These numbers, of course, should not be interpreted literally. Many characteristics of the system, task, and using population would substantially influence the results. What is important is the direction these numbers take. They show that it does not take long for new users of a system to start moving from dependent to independent status. An office system, to be truly effective, must provide a dual-initiation capability.

Flexibility

A system must be sensitive to the differing needs of its users.

Flexibility is a measure of the system's capability to respond to individual differences in people. A truly flexible system will permit a person to interact with it in a manner commensurate with that person's knowledge, skills, and experience. One kind of flexibility has already been described in the discussion on initiation. A system that permits both human- and computer-initiated dialogues is flexible in that regard. Other areas of flexibility include the display or nondisplay of *prompts*, permitting defaults, or the creation of special vocabularies. Another example of flexibility can be found in an electronic mail system that permits its users to receive their messages in one of these ways:

- When a message is there, the system sends it (*assertive*).
- The system calls to indicate a message is there but the message must be asked for (*interrogative*).
- The system never calls, all messages must be asked for (*passive*).

Each person working with such a system can choose the method most comfortable to himself or herself.

Flexibility can have differing levels. At one extreme the user can choose the preferred method and the system will respond accordingly. At the other extreme the system constantly monitors a person's performance (errors, speeds, frequency of use of components, and so on) and modifies itself accordingly. The latter might more appropriately be called an *adaptive system*.

Other examples of flexibility are given in the pages that follow.

Complexity

Complexity should be commensurate with the capabilities of the system users. Four ways to *minimize complexity* are:

- Use progressive disclosure, hiding things until they are needed.
- Make common things simple at the expense of uncommon things made harder.
- Make things uniform and consistent.
- Minimize redundancy.

Complexity is a measure of the number of alternatives available to the office worker. It is the number of ways something can be done or the number of choices one has at any given point. A highly complex system is difficult to learn. For inexperienced users, complexity frequently degrades performance, especially by increasing error rates. Complex systems are often not fully used, or used ineffectively, because a person may follow known but more cumbersome methods instead of easier but unfamiliar methods. A system lacking complexity may have a different set of faults: it may be tedious to use or not accomplish much.

Complexity, then, is a two-edged sword. To effectively solve office problems it must exist. For the office tool to be effectively utilized by the office worker, it must not be apparent.

There are four specific ways to minimize complexity. First, provide progressive disclosure. That is, introduce new system parts only when workers see the need to do something they do not know how to do, or when they see they can do something in fewer steps. The inherent complexity is then less visible and learning made easier. Second, make the common things easier to do at the expense of the uncommon things that are made harder. Greater overall system effectiveness thereby results. Third, be consistent. Inconsistency is a foolish form of complexity. Fourth, minimize redundancy. Two or more ways to perform an operation increases complexity without increasing capability.

Power

Dialogue power should be commensurate with the capabilities of the system users.

Power is a measure of the amount of work accomplished by a given instruction to a system. A very powerful instruction can evoke a string of system operations doing many things. This same series of operations can also be evoked by a series of instructions, each directed toward one specific aspect. Each individual instruction would then be less powerful because it accomplishes less.

High power is usually associated with high dialogue complexity and reduced system generality. Therefore, while a powerful system can be effectively utilized in the hands of a well-trained person, the untrained may be unable or unwilling to cope. The result is often system rejection. Goodwin (1982) provides an interesting analysis of an electronic mail system whose utility was diminished because of the dialogue power it possessed.

Power, then, is another dialogue property whose effectiveness is directly related to the experience level of people working with a system and whose optimum level varies along a sliding scale that changes with user needs.

Information Load

Information load should be commensurate with the capabilities of the system user.

Six ways to reduce information load are:

- Provide graphic rather than alphanumeric displays.
- Format displays to correspond to users' immediate information requirements.
- Use languages that are natural.
- Move clerical operations into the system.
- Provide less powerful commands.
- Provide less complex dialogues.

Two ways to increase information load are:

- Permit more powerful commands.
- Permit more complex dialogues.

Information load is a measure of the degree to which a user's memory and/or processing resources are absorbed. It is a function of the task being performed, a person's familiarity with the task, and the design of the dialogue itself. Like other dialogue properties, the optimum level can change with a user's experience.

Information loads that are too high or too low can affect performance. High loads strain a person's capabilities and may cause an inability or unwillingness to cope. Low levels create boredom and inattentiveness, fostering errors.

Human memory is a weak link in the people/machine interface and should be supported whenever possible. Information load can be reduced by the actions listed above. As a user becomes more knowledgeable and the information load can be expanded, the direction should be toward greater dialogue power and complexity. These are positive steps toward greater system effectiveness.

Control

General

- The user must control the interaction.
- The context maintained must be that of the user.
- The means must be compatible with the user's skills and the desired end result.

Paths

- The capability to go from/to any point or step must exist.
- Input stacking must be possible.
- A home position must always be available.

Options

- Options or actions available at any time must be accessible either on a display or through a help function.
- Only relevant options should be available.

Control is the process of being responsible for determining and selecting what to do, entry of information into a display, transmission of that information to the system, processing of that information in conjunction with the system, and later retrieval of that information from the system. The design objective is user ease and efficiency in performing all these actions.

General. Control must always rest in the hands of the user. Actions must result from explicit human inputs and requests. No delays or paced delays beyond a person's expectancies should exist. The context maintained must always be from the perspective of the user. The knowledge carried forward by the system must be that which represents the user's level of understanding. To support human memory in ascertaining status or context, prior user entries should be available for review as needed. While processing modes are not desirable, if used, a facility should be available to remind the user of the one that is current.

Paths. A user should be able, at his or her option, to move from any one point or step in an interaction to any other step or point within the context of what is being done. In a series of menus, for example, the capability should exist for going from one menu to any other menu in the string. This kind of action is illustrative of a human-initiated dialogue overriding a computer-initiated dialogue.

Stacking of inputs or requests must be possible. Stacking is the process of stringing together a series of discrete requests or commands so that they comprise one input. The system will then perform each action consecutively while the user awaits the result. The order of stacked commands should be the same as if they were discrete commands. Command separators should be standard symbols with a slash (/) preferred. No concern with blanks should be required. If the system is unable to complete a series of stacked commands, it will stop and present the next appropriate step or menu. The user should be able to assign a single name to command strings that are frequently used together. This more powerful command should then be recognizable by the system and in the future elicit the discrete actions it refers to.

A home position, such as a primary or main system menu, should always be achievable by a simple user action.

Options. Options or actions available at any given time must be available on a display or through a help function. All relevant options should be displayed except those that are always available systemwide. Only relevant options should be displayed. Options not currently available to a person should not be provided. If options are designated by codes, these codes must also be provided.

Command languages must be logical, consistent, and flexible. A logical and consistent language will expedite the user's learning process and slow the forgetting that results from language disuse. Flexibility allows users to adapt the command language to themselves, instead of the other way around. The following guidelines highlight the more important features of a command language. Engel and Granda (1975) and Watson (1976) also provide detailed discussions.

Command Languages

Content. Command languages must be familiar, and reflect the user's viewpoint, not the system designer's. Users must be able to express their needs with command constructions similar to their own thought processes, natural problem-solving vocabularies, and language. Ledgard et al. (1980) found far better performance after redesigning a commercial text editor so that the commands more closely resembled English phrases. Black and Moran (1982) found words always better than nonwords in free recall.

All too often a system's command language has been that created by its designer. Jones (1978) pointed out the discrepancies between designers' assumptions and the realities of the users' language that have made many command languages difficult to use. He concludes that:

Content

- Use words that are familiar; highly suggestible; discriminating.

Structure

- Use words that are perceptually dissimilar and that can be abbreviated.

Organization

- Provide a structuring rule.
- Provide customized subsets.
- Permit naming flexibility.

Consistency

- Use a common command discipline throughout all applications.

Defaults

- Within a command, the system should supply missing arguments. Between commands, the system should supply missing commands if a predefined sequence is initiated; supply missing arguments based on previously supplied arguments; supply a missing command based on arguments.

Edits

- Only incorrectly entered command data should be reentered.

- Designers tend to assume a one-to-one correspondence between newly formed command statements and their meanings. Users see many of the commands as having the same meaning.
- Designers presume nothing is assumed by users except what is expressly stated about a command. Users possess innumerable unstated assumptions that are applied to the interpretation process.
- Designers assume that users' deductions are made from absolutely unvarying frames of reference. Users often establish meaning based upon immediate context.

Is the user the best creator of a command language for an office automation system? The evidence here is contradictory. Black and Moran (1982) conclude that computer naive people are not good command designers. They tend to create frequent and general words for commands whereas best performance is achieved with infrequent, discriminating words. Furnas et al. (1982) found great diversity in people's descriptions of even the most common objects. The average likelihood of any two people using the same main content word in their description of the same object ranged from 0.07 to 0.18. Therefore a common acceptable word to all is difficult to achieve. Similar conclusions have been reached by Barnard et al. (1981) and Carroll (1980).

Scapin (1982), however, found that people performed better with their own command language. Perhaps the best solution is a joint effort between users and designers with the final solution derived from testing and refinement.

Command names should be highly suggestible. A command name is good to the degree that it suggests directly what the command does (PRINT is better than LIST), and that it suggests directly the relationship (whether similar, opposite, or unrelated) of that command to other commands in the system (Rosenberg 1982). Hammond et al. (1980a) found that the pattern of errors in a dialogue correlates with the extent to which command names are ambiguous relative to their underlying operations.

Command names should be discriminating. Avoid small and subtle differences such as PRINT versus WRITE. Use specific instead of general words (SUBSTITUTE instead of CHANGE). As described above, both Barnard et al. (1982) and Black and Moran (1982) found specific words resulted in better performance than general words.

Structure. Choose command words that are perceptually dissimilar to avoid confusion errors. While command languages must be meaningful and not highly coded, permitting abbreviations and concise notation will support differing user proficiencies, from expert to novice. Advanced vocabularies and short, concise, control notations and conventions maximize the performance of expert users. Inability to truncate can contribute to user dissatisfaction with a system. Forcing people to enter long words increases keying time, error frequency, and associated time-consuming recovery procedures.

Organization. Provide a structuring rule for the population of commands. Scapin (1982) found that providing structure to a family of commands by breaking them into logical groupings was an important factor in aiding learning.

Customize the command language by providing subsets of the command language and features. This characteristic is particularly advantageous when the technology is first introduced, since it permits phased learning of system components.

Provide flexibility by permitting users to assign their own names to frequent command sequences. The result, as mentioned earlier, will be a more powerful dialogue.

Consistency. Consistency in command languages is mandatory if a collection of office systems with which a worker interacts is to be perceived as one system. Table 6-1 illustrates a variety of command words from current systems that are used to accomplish the same purpose. People must be able to learn additional functions by increasing their vocabulary, not by learning separate foreign languages.

Defaults. If a person fails to specify a command, the system may prompt the individual to supply the missing information by listing potential values. This approach is acceptable if the alternatives are limited; but when the list becomes complicated or time consuming, it is less desirable. A second alternative is to ask users to supply the missing information from memory, but this is not an optimal approach.

A third option is for the system to supply a default value for the missing information. A default is an agreement between the user and the system concerning the normal or usual working environment. Defaults are a powerful aid in achieving a user-oriented language, but they are not without problems. The user may not know or understand the default or may not have a convenient way of changing it. For these reasons, perhaps default usage should be optional.

Edits. A person should never have to reenter an entire command, especially if only one item on a line is incorrect. An appropriate mechanism, such as cursor positioning, should also exist to help the user by setting up the appropriate spot for reentry.

Command Language Arguments

Organization

- Few commands with many arguments is a better organization than many commands with a few arguments.

Format

- Key-word argument formats are superior to positional formats.

Table 6-1. Different Command Words Often Having the Same Meaning

To begin an interaction:	*To create a hard copy:*
LOGIN	WRITE
LOGON	OUTPUT
HELLO	PRINT
SIGNIN	LIST
SIGNON	DISPLAY

A command argument is an option that qualifies a general command. Figure 6–1 shows two command methods for obtaining a printout of two kinds of insurance transactions—incomplete and complete new business. The first method uses two separate commands, while the second has one command, each with two arguments.

Boies (1974) found that a majority of users in a large time-sharing system used only a few of the many system commands available and frequently employed commands in their simplest and least powerful form. He speculated that this could result from command structures that were difficult for users to recall when needed. Boies subsequently compared the use of a small number of commands and a large number of arguments with use of many specific commands and a few arguments. He found the former more useful (Miller and Thomas 1977). More study is needed, however, to find an optimal command language strategy.

Using a positional command language format, arguments are assigned a relative or absolute position in the argument string. With a key-word format, arguments may be in permutable strings, indicating the argument type and its value. The value of arguments must be remembered in both cases. Positional

Command:

    PRINT INCOMPLETE NEW BUSINESS

    (------------------------Command------------------------)

    PRINT COMPLETE NEW BUSINESS

    (------------------------Command------------------------)

Command and argument:

    PRINT   INCOMPLETE NEW BUSINESS

    (command)   (----------------Arguments----------------)

    PRINT   COMPLETE NEW BUSINESS

    (command)   (----------------Arguments----------------)

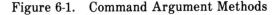

Figure 6-1. Command Argument Methods

formats appear to impose greater memory requirements on users since remembering positions is an additional burden. In an informal study, Weinberg (1971) found high error rates in using positional formats.

Assistance

A system should provide:

- user-selectable prompting;
- a HELP facility.

New users of an office system go through a learning process. This learning process is directed toward developing a conceptual model to explain the system's behavior and the task environment itself. HELP displays and prompting serve as cognitive development tools to aid this understanding.

Prompting is instructional, providing information or messages by the system as part of the dialogue to assist the user. It is the system's way of requesting additional or corrected information, or guiding users step by step through tasks in the proper order. Systems also use prompting to tell users what tools are available, which ones they can obtain from where they are, or anything else that can or must be done next. Inexperienced users will find prompting a valuable aid in learning to use a system. Experienced users, however, would probably not find prompting desirable as it may slow their interaction with the system. To those users, it should be available only as needed. Therefore, people should have the ability to selectively or completely turn prompting mechanisms on or off.

A HELP facility is instructional information that can be easily obtained as the need arises by a simple key action or command. When accessed, the HELP facility should be aware of the kind of difficulties a person is having and respond with relevant information. If the HELP facility is unsure of the source of trouble, it should work with the user through prompts and questions to resolve the problem.

In a study of menu-driven versus command-driven dialogues, Gilfoil (1982) found a dramatic upsurge in HELP referrals about the time users are making the transition to the command mode. He concludes that the highest frequency of HELP facility usage occurs when people are experiencing difficulties in creating structured mental representations of the task.

In another study, Barnard et al. (1982) found that a person's recall of command operations was related to frequency of HELP facility access. Fewer HELP requests were associated with better command recall. They speculate that the availability of HELP may become a crutch and lead to less effective retention. People may implement a passive cognitive strategy. A HELP facility may influence performance in systematic and subtle ways and must be investigated further.

Feedback

A system should acknowledge all actions by:

- immediate execution;
- in-progress message;
- correction message;
- confirmation message;
- change in state or value.

Knowledge of results, or feedback, is a necessary learning ingredient. It shapes human performance and instills confidence. All requests to the system must be acknowledged in some way. This acknowledgement is normally provided when the system completes the request, and normally takes the form of immediate execution, a confirmation message, a change in state or value, or an error message. If a request requires a long processing period (more than 10–15 seconds), the system should acknowledge its receipt and provide an interim *in-progress* message.

Recovery

A system should permit:

- commands or actions to be abolished or reversed;
- immediate return to a certain point if difficulties arise.

People should be able to retract an action by issuing what Miller and Thomas (1977) call an *undo* command. Knowing they could withdraw a command would reduce much of the distress of new users, who often worry about doing something wrong. The return point could be a recent mental closure point or the beginning of some predetermined period, such as back ten screens or some number of minutes.

Recovery should also allow users to return to a previous point in the interaction if difficulties arise. The goal is, as Martin (1973) says, stability—returning easily to the right track when a wrong track has been taken. Recovery should be obvious, automatic, and easy and natural to perform. In short, it should be hard to get into deep water or go too far astray.

If an action is not reversible, and its consequences are critical, it should be made difficult to accomplish.

Function Keys

Uses

- For frequent and basic control inputs.

Operation

- Require single action only.
- Disable keys when not applicable.

Labels

- Provide informative descriptions.
- If multifunctional, describe the current function.

Location

- Arrange in logical groupings
- Be compatible with importance.

Consistency

- Use a common meaning and location discipline across modes and applications.

Function keys are advantageous in that they reduce memory requirements, permit faster entry (fewer keystrokes), and reduce errors. Therefore, they are integral parts of almost all office system keyboards.

Uses. Function keys are ideal for inputs that are frequent and basic. The control functions described in the next section are ideal candidates for inclusion as function keys.

Operation. Require only single actions to activate. Shift key operations are especially prone to error. Hammond et al. (1980b) found that about one-third of the errors in a computer system were the result of mistyping, and half of these were due to using the correct key with the wrong shift. If a function key is not being used, it should be disabled.

Labels. Provide informative descriptions that clearly describe the key's purpose. If multifunctional, describe the current function through an overlay or on the display screen itself.

Location. Provide logical groupings of keys based upon an analysis of their sequence of use, frequency of use, function, and importance.

Consistency. Be consistent in labeling and usage between modes and across applications.

Control Functions

Desirable control functions include:

- Page forward;
- Page backward;
- Hold/store;
- Abort/cancel;
- End/stop;

- Retrieve;
- Help;
- Resume;
- Undo/back-up;
- Print.

Interacting with an office automation system requires that some basic control operations be available at all times. Logical candidates are these functions, which are ideal for incorporation into function keys.

Page forward and Page backward. These functions enable one to move rapidly through a series of display screens.

Hold/store. This stores something being worked on in a file facility whence it may later be retrieved.

Abort/cancel. This cancels or erases what one is working on.

End/stop. This stops processing immediately; it may be returned to at that point later.

Retrieve. This retrieves from a file facility that which has previously been stored.

Help. This accesses the HELP facility, as previously described.

Resume. This returns to the point where one is working after HELP or End/Stop.

Undo/back-up. This reverses the action just performed, as previously described.

Print. This provides hard-copy printout of the current display.

Any office system application may, of course, require additional control functions based upon its objectives.

Error Management

Prevention

- Handle common misspellings.
- Permit review of message about to be sent.
- Permit editing of message about to be sent.
- Provide common "send" mechanism.
- Advise of nonreversible changes.

Detection

- Immediately detect all errors.
- Visually identify the item in error.
- Never cause system to abort.

Correction

- Provide an explicit error message explaining how to make corrections.
- Initiate clarification dialogue.
- Require resending only erroneous information back to system.

Error management and control is really a cornerstone of this entire book in the sense that reducing the probability of human error is an objective of most design guidelines. The focus here is on the mechanics of error prevention, detection, and correction.

Prevention. Where possible, human misspellings of commands and requests should be accepted and handled by the system. Person-to-person communication does not require perfection. Person-to-computer communication should impose no more rigor. Inappropriate use of SHIFT keys should also be distinguished, where possible, since they are such a large cause of keying errors. Entries made into a system should be reviewable and editable by the person who has made them. Human memory is poor and keying errors will occur.

A common *send* mechanism should be provided to transmit an entry to the system. Two or more keys to accomplish the same purpose, especially if their use is mandated by different conditions, can be confusing and more prone to errors. If an action will cause a nonreversible change, and the change is critical, the user should be requested to confirm the change. A separate key should be used for this purpose, not the *send* key.

Detection. All errors should be immediately detected and visually identified to the user. Errors, of course, should never cause a system to abort.

Correction. An explicit error message explaining how to make corrections should be provided. If an explicit message is impossible, the system should initiate a clarification dialogue with the user. All ambiguities should be resolved by interrogation of the user by the system. Errors should be corrected with minimal typing. Only erroneous information should be sent back to the system.

Another important error control measure is to have the system identify and store errors. This will allow tracking of common errors, so that appropriate prevention programs can be implemented.

Response Time

- System responsiveness should match the speed and flow of human thought processes.

  - If continuity of thinking is required and information must be remembered throughout several responses, response time should be less than two seconds.
  - If human task closures exist, high levels of concentration are not necessary and moderate short-term memory requirements are imposed; response times of two to four seconds are acceptable.
  - If major task closures exist, minimal short-term memory requirements are imposed; responses within four to fifteen seconds are acceptable.
  - When the user is free to do other things and return when convenient, response time can be greater than fifteen seconds.

- Constant delays are preferable to variable delays.

Dissatisfaction with system response time is a function of both length and variability. The ideal situation is when a person perceives no delays. That perception, however, will vary with mental processes and activities. In general, response times should be geared to the short-term memory load to which an individual is subjected and to how that person has grouped the activities being performed. Intense short-term memory loads necessitate short response times. While completing chunks of work at task closures, users can withstand longer response delays.

The human *now*, or psychological present, is two to three seconds. This is why continuity of thinking requires a response time within this limit. Recent research indicates that for creative tasks, response times in the range of 0.4–0.9 seconds can yield dramatic increases in productivity, even greater in proportion to the increase in response time (Smith 1983). The probable reason is the elimination of restrictions caused by short-term memory limitations. There is, however, a point at which a person can be saturated by information presented more quickly than it can be comprehended. There is also some evidence indicating that when a system responds too quickly, there is subconscious pressure on users to also respond quickly, possibly threatening their overall comfort (Elam 1978).

As the response-time interval increases beyond 10–15 seconds, continuity of thought becomes increasingly difficult to maintain. Doherty (1979) suggests that this happens because the sequence of actions stored in short-term memory are badly disrupted and must be reloaded.

Carbonell et al. (1969) point out that it is the variability of delays, not their length, that most frequently distresses people. From a consistency standpoint, a good rule of thumb is that response-time deviations should never exceed half the mean response time. For example, if the mean response time is four seconds, a two-second deviation is permissible. Variations should range from three to five seconds.

The degree of frustration may also depend on such psychological factors as a person's uncertainty concerning how long the delay will be, the extent to which the actual delay contradicts those expectations, and what the person thinks is causing the delay. Such uncertainty concerning how long a wait there will be for a computer's response may in some cases be a greater source of aggravation than the delay itself (Nickerson 1969). A consistent, paced, and reasonable response time geared to the task at hand will alleviate many of the pressures that do exist.

Specific Response Times

- Log-on/initialization: up to 30 seconds, with immediate interim acknowledgment.
- Error messages: a brief pause after a closure.
- Inquiry: one to fifteen seconds.
- Browsing/scrolling: one second or less.
- Data entry: within a transaction, four to six seconds; after completing a transaction, up to fifteen seconds.

Acceptable response times for certain office system activities have been put forth. Delays in completing system log-on while the computer reorganizes resources and facilities are not as annoying as long delays during interactions. Therefore, delays of up to thirty seconds for log-on are acceptable, but a fairly quick acknowledgment that log-on is occurring should be given when the process begins.

Interruptions in concentration can be frustrating. People should be able to finish what they are doing before being told of an error. At task closures, the system should pause briefly to allow a person to change mental modes before having to attend to an error message.

Inquiry response times depend on urgency. They may range from one to fifteen seconds.

Browsing or scrolling usually involves rapid search for information. Additional information to be searched must maintain the visual searching pace established. A one-second response time should be expected.

Manual paper shuffling during data entry provides a good closure point. Longer response delays between screens can then be tolerated.

Messages

___

Words must be:

- short, meaningful, common, and spelled out;
- in a familiar language;
- interpretable in only one way;

Words should not consist of:

- contractions,
- short forms, or
- abbreviations (unless they are more meaningful than the full words).

Sentences must be:

- brief, simple, and clear;
- directly and immediately usable;
- affirmative;
- in an active voice;
- nonauthoritarian;
- nonthreatening;
- nonanthropomorphic;
- nonpatronizing;
- in the temporal sequence of events;
- structured so that the main topic is near the beginning;
- cautious in the use of humor;
- nonpunishing.

Other considerations are:

- The system must display abbreviated versions of the message when requested.
- Something that must be remembered must be at the beginning of the text.

___

A system communicates with people through many kinds of messages: prompts, diagnostic messages generated by errors, information messages, and status messages. A message must minimize ambiguity and confusion, allowing easy, correct, and fast interpretation. It must also be of the proper tone, evoking no negative reactions.

The following practices will lead to easy, correct, and fast message interpretation and acceptance.

Words:

Use short, meaningful, common, and familiar words. Because people can read short words faster than long ones and interpret them more easily, short words will improve performance and reduce errors. Words should be meaningful and common to the users, not the designers. Language perceived as *computerese* may confuse or intimidate some people (Loftus et al. 1970; Wason and Johnson-Laird 1972).

Interpretable in only one way. Avoid confusions between words that have different meanings. Invalid to many means not correct. An invalid in a hospital setting may be one suffering from illness or disease, however.

Do not use abbreviations. Use them only if the abbreviation is more meaningful than the full word or if the abbreviated form is absolutely necessary. If an abbreviation is used, it should be short, meaningful, and distinct from other abbreviations. If it is not significantly shorter than the full word, do not use it.

Do not use contractions or short forms. People are more likely to understand the sense of a message if it uses complete words. For example, say "not complete" rather than "incomplete," "not valid" rather than "invalid," and "do not" rather than "don't."

Sentences:

Use brief, simple sentences. Brief sentences are more readily understood than longer sentences containing multiple clauses. Break long sentences into two or more simple sentences if it can be done without changing the meaning. Roemer and Chapanis (1982) created messages at three levels of reading ability (fifth, tenth, and fifteenth grade) and tested them on people of varying verbal abilities. The fifth grade version was found to be best for all levels. People of high verbal ability did not perceive the fifth-grade version as insulting as some feared.

Provide directly and immediately usable sentences. Searching through reference material to translate a message is unacceptable, as are requirements for transposing, computing, interpolating, or mentally translating messages into other units.

Use affirmative statements. Affirmative statements are easier to understand than negative statements. For example, "Complete entry before returning to menu" is easier to grasp than, "Do not return to menu before completing entry." (Herriott 1970; Greene 1972.)

Use the active voice. It is usually easier to understand the active voice than the passive voice. For example, "Send the message by depressing TRANSMIT" is more understandable than, "The message is sent by depressing TRANSMIT." (Herriott 1970; Greene 1972; Barnard 1974.)

Be nonauthoritarian. Imply that the system is awaiting the user's direction, not that the system is directing the user. For example, phrase a message "Ready for next command," not "Enter next command."

Be nonthreatening. Avoid harsh and cold words; be factual instead. For example, say "Months are entered by name," not "Numbers are illegal."

Be nonanthropomorphic. Do not ascribe human personality to a machine, as many people are still threatened by it. Again, imply that the system is awaiting the user's direction, not vice versa. Say, for example, "What do you need?" not "How can I help you?"

Be nonpatronizing. The response, "Very good, you did it right" may thrill a fourth grader but would probably insult an adult. "Performed" would be a more agreeable response.

Order words chronologically. If a sentence describes a temporal sequence of events, the order of words should correspond to the sequence. A prompt should say "Enter address and page forward," rather than "Page forward after entering address."

Place the main topic near the beginning. As the more frequently occurring messages are learned, placing the main topic at the beginning will eliminate the need to always read the whole message.

Avoid humor and punishment. Until an optimal computer personality is designed, messages should remain factual and informative and should not attempt humor or punishment. Humor is a transitory and changeable thing. What is funny today may not be funny tomorrow. What is funny to some may not be to others. Punishment is not a desirable way to force a change in behavior, especially among adults.

Other considerations:

Display abbreviated versions of messages when requested. People are impatient with noninformative or redundant computer messages. A problem, however, is that the degree of computer-to-person message redundancy depends on the person's experience with the system. This may vary with different parts of a system. So the availability of abbreviated or detailed messages allows tailoring of the system to the needs of each person. During system training and early implementation stages, detailed versions can be used. Individuals can switch to abbreviated versions as their familiarity increases, but they should maintain the ability to receive detailed messages.

Place that which must be remembered at the beginning of text. One can remember something longer if it appears at the beginning of a message. Items in the middle of a message are harder to remember.

Text Editors

- Text should be represented as one continuous character string. Within the string, easy means must exist to add, move, assemble, and delete text.
- A facility should exist that permits easy identification of a specific target within a text string. Minimally, the target area specified should include characters, words, sentences, paragraphs, and pages.
- Automatic text processing features should include the capability to:

  - merge variable lists with standard formats;
  - locate a defined character string;
  - replace defined character strings with alternative strings.

- It should be easy to specify text formats, such as indentations, margins, tabs, spacing, and headings.
- Final format copy should be displayed exactly as it will be printed.
- Completed text should be easily stored, retrieved, and deleted.
- It should be easy to designate text printing specifications, such as number of copies, type style, and print priority.

Any text editor should fulfill the broad function requirements listed above. But even if these capabilities exist, the more important factor is how easily functions are then performed. Without the ability to easily use a capability, it becomes virtually useless.

Quite often, discussions of text editing merge the *what* (functions performed) into the *how* (methods of performance). When differences between the two become blurred, discussion becomes difficult. This review will focus on *what* with an occasional illustration of a possible *how*. But derermination of the most effective methods of performing these functions must ultimately be accomplished in light of all the guidelines described throughout this book.

An entity (such as a document) must be created or rearranged without concern for page breaks. The picture presented to the user must be a whole. Thus the ability to scroll through the file continuously and stop whenever wanted is important. Manipulating building blocks (pages) is not desirable.

Users must specify to the text processor where the text is to be placed. In generating initial text on display-oriented text processors, text position on the screen is usually defined by the location of a cursor, generally on a character-by-character basis. Characters are entered in positions designated by the cursor. Target location, then, implies a capability to move the cursor around the display surface as targets change.

Cursor movement may be of two kinds, contextual or screen-oriented. A contextual cursor's movements are limited to where characters (including spaces) have been placed. This movement may be by the character, word, line, or paragraph. A screen-oriented cursor can be moved anywhere on the screen without regard to whether text has been entered. It is controlled by keys such as *up*, *left*, and so on. Hicks and Keller (1982) recommend a screen-oriented cursor as being the better choice. People using this alternative performed faster, required fewer assistance calls, and made fewer errors.

As text is created it should be automatically formatted as entered. The editor should break lines at proper positions (word wrapping) and reformat it continuously if characters are deleted in the process. Neal and Emmons (1982) in a study of text entry errors, found that operators detect and correct about eleven errors per thousand characters typed. These corrections occur, on the average, about every nineteen seconds. The majority (78 percent) are performed on the word typed. Ninety-five percent existed in the last five characters. Overall, 89 percent of all errors are detected and corrected immediately. Neal and Emmons conclude that an easy-to-use error correction is a necessity, and a small keyboard/display buffer may be desirable.

For existing text, change and manipulation is easier if the user can identify target areas larger than one character. The ability to specify a word, sentence, paragraph, page, or combination thereof provides greater flexibility and facility than one-character identification. Possible ways to accomplish this are through cursor manipulations, function key depressions, the keying of commands, or combinations of these.

Common text processing tasks which are extremely time consuming are merging lists of variable data into standard formats (such as form letter generation) and locating and replacing defined character strings. Automated assistance in these tasks is most desirable.

A person should be able to see an exact image of the text to be printed so that errors, inconsistencies, and problems are obvious. Miller and Thomas (1977), Morgan (1976), and Jong (1982) present fuller discussions of text editors.

Screen Formats

Human/machine dialogue is often carried out through a series of screen displays that capture or display information in an alphanumeric or graphic format. Displays may be monochromatic or include various colors.

A display screen must be structured to avoid perceptual confusions of those using them. Good screen design is a clean design—without irrelevancies. A cluttered screen can create the impression of being too complex to understand, or users may feel that understanding it will require more time than they are willing to commit.

While usable, many screens today lack visual clarity, and this lengthens visual search times and increases errors. The importance of this fact has been illustrated by a recent review of the consequences of inefficient screen design in a system that was to process about 4.8 million screens per year. The review established that if poor clarity forced users to spend one extra second per screen, almost one additional person-year would be required to process all the screens. A twenty-second degradation in screen processing would cost an additional fourteen person-years. Table 6-2 summarizes the findings of this review.

Dunsmore (1982) attempted to improve screen clarity and readability by making them less crowded. Separate items, which had been combined on the same display line to conserve space, were placed on separate lines instead. The results were that subjects were about twenty percent more productive with the less-crowded version. Failure to achieve visual clarity, then, can have an enormous impact on time and people costs.

Most Wanted Features of Screen

What are people looking for in the design of screens? One organization asked this of a group of users. Their response is summarized below.

- An orderly, clean, clutter-free appearance;
- An obvious indication of what is being shown and what should be done with it;
- Expected information where it should be;
- A clear indication of what relates to what (headings, captions, data, instructions, options, and so on.)
- Plain, simple English;
- A simple way of finding what is in the system and how to get it out;
- A clear indication of when an action could make a permanent change in the data or system operation.

The desired direction is toward simplicity, clarity, and understandability, qualities lacking in many of today's screens.

The Test for Good Screen Design

Visual clarity is influenced by a number of factors, including information organization, grouping, legibility, and relevancy. Clarity is achieved when display elements are grouped in meaningful and understandable ways, rather

Table 6-2. Impact of Inefficient Screen Design on Processing Time

Additional Seconds Required per Screen in Seconds	Additional Person-Years Required to Process 4.8 Million Screens per Year
1	0.7
5	3.6
10	7.1
20	14.2

than in random and confusing patterns. A simple test for good screen design does exist. A screen that passes this test will have surmounted the first hurdle on the road to effectiveness.

The Test. Can all screen elements (captions, data, title, command field, messages, and so on) be identified without reading the words that make them up? That is, can all components of a screen be identified through cues independent of their content? If this is so, a person's attention can quickly be drawn to that part of the screen that is relevant at the moment. Visual search times will be greatly reduced and confusion minimized. Try this test on the front page of your morning newspaper. Where is the headline? A story heading? The weather report? How did you find them? The headlines are probably identified by their visually large and bold type size. Story headings are generally found by a type size noticeably different from other page components. The weather report is found by its location (bottom right or top left, for example).

All the tools available to the creator of the newspaper's front page are not yet available to the screen designer. An effective solution can be achieved, however, with the array of tools that are at hand. It simply involves the thoughtful application of the display techniques that exist, consistent locations, and the proper use of white space.

Screen Design Considerations

Screen design must consider a number of factors. A well-designed screen format should:

- reflect the needs and idiosyncracies of its users;
- be developed within the physical constraints imposed by the terminal;
- fully utilize the capabilities of its software;
- if used for data entry, be developed within the constraints imposed by related source materials, such as worksheets, forms, or manuals;
- be consistent within itself, with related screen formats, and with other screens within the application and the organization.

How, then, can screens be structured to make them more acceptable to people? Obviously, the final answers are task specific, but general rules for where to place information on a screen, what information to include, and how to place it on the screen can help. The guidelines that follow provide general rules addressing these questions of *where, what,* and *how.* They will be followed by guidelines unique to specific types of screens, such as data entry, inquiry, and menu. Although these guidelines are not exhaustive, they provide a solid foundation for most screen design activities. The reader desiring a more detailed discussion of screen design considerations and processes is referred to Galitz (1981).

Where to Put Information on a Screen

- Provide an obvious starting point in the upper-left corner of the screen.
- Reserve specific areas of the screen for certain kinds of information, such as commands, status messages, and input fields, and maintain these areas consistently on all screens.
- Provide cohesive groupings of screen elements by using blank spaces, surrounding lines, different intensity levels, and so on.

    - If blank spaces are used, keep three to five rows or columns blank.
    - Do not, however, break the screen into many small windows.

- Provide symmetrical balance by:

    - centering titles and illustrations on the vertical axis;
    - placing like elements on both sides of the axis;
    - placing lighter elements further from the vertical axis and larger elements closer to it.

- Instructions on how to use a screen or process information on it should precede the screen text or be at the top of the text.
- Instructions concerning the disposition of a completed screen should be at the bottom of the screen.

Eyeball fixation studies indicate that initially the human eye usually moves to the upper-left center of a display. The eyes then move in a clockwise direction. During and following this movement, people are influenced by the display's symmetrical balance and the weight of its titles, graphics, and text. The human information processing system also tries to impose structure when confronted with uncertainty. It seeks order and meaning and will quickly discern whether a screen has a meaningful form or is cluttered.

Screens should provide cohesive groupings of screen elements so that people perceive large screens to have identifiable pieces. People prefer viewing groups or chunks of data. Use of contrasting elements is an excellent way to call attention to differing display elements, since contrast is the source of all human understanding. Screens should also be structured to provide symmetrical balance to help viewers establish a meaningful form. Also, by reserving specific areas for certain items, users know where to look.

Screens should provide only relevant information because the more information, the greater the competition among screen components for a person's attention. Visual search times will be longer and meaningful patterns more difficult to perceive if the screen floods the user with too much information.

What Information to Put on a Screen

- Provide only information that is essential to making a decision or performing an action. Do not flood the user with information.
- Provide all data related to one task on a single screen. Users should not have to remember data from one screen to the next.

How much display information is too much has not been determined. An ultimate answer must undoubtedly reflect, among other things, the requirements of the application and how the screen is formatted. Vitz (1966) has found that people have subjective preferences for the amount of information presented on a display, and that subjective ratings decline as the amount of information displayed deviates, either way, from the preferred amount. Danchak (1976) reports that a well-designed page of printed material has a density loading of only 40 percent and that screens qualitatively judged *good* possessed loadings of about 15 percent. Another study found that search time on a inquiry screen rapidly increased as screen density exceeded 60 percent.

These values should not be construed as absolute guidelines, however, but are presented for illustrative purposes only. The ultimate determination of guideline values will depend upon many complicated factors, many of which are yet poorly understood.

How to Place Information on a Screen

The following guidelines for determining how to put data on screens address general considerations, word and text arrangement, illustrations, fonts, field captions, data display and organization, and menu screens.

General

- Present information in a directly usable form. Do not require reference to documentation, translations, transpositions, interpolations, and so on.
- Use contrasting display features (different intensities and character sizes, underlining, reverse images, and so on) to call attention to:

    - different screen components;
    - items being operated upon; and
    - urgent items.

- Guide the user through the screen with implicit or explicit lines formed by display elements.
- Visual appearance and procedural usage should be consistent.

Screens can guide eye movement horizontally or vertically with lines formed by the display elements. More complex movements, however, must be aided by display contrasts.

Fonts

- For text, use lower case with the initial sentence letter capitalized.
- For captions, labels, and visual search tasks, use upper case (capitals).

Tinker (1955) found that lower-case text is read significantly faster than text all in capitals. Not being able to perceive word shapes (which is harder in all upper case) may slow reading rate as much as 13 percent (Rehe, 1974). Labels, however, are read faster in upper case than in lower or mixed cases. Vartabedian (1971) established that screens with upper-case headings are visually read faster than those using lower-case characters.

Words

- Use standard alphabetic characters to form words or captions. Do not use restricted alphabetic sets.
- Use complete words, not contractions or short forms.

  INVALID   NOT VALID
  WON'T   WILL NOT
- Do not stack words. Text is more readable if the entire statement is on one line.

  AMOUNT
  PAID   AMOUNT PAID
- Do not hyphenate words.
- Abbreviations, mnemonics, and acronyms should not include punctuations.

  CRT.   CRT

Text

- Use short sentences composed of familiar, personal words.
- Place a period at the end of each sentence.
- Include no more than 50 to 60 characters on each line. A double column of 30 to 35 characters separated by five spaces is also acceptable.
- Separate paragraphs by at least one blank line.

Illustrations

- Use line drawings to illustrate or supplement text whenever possible.

Development of words and text for use on screens should follow the message construction guidelines listed. These guidelines describe how the selected words and text should be displayed. They are intended to minimize ambiguity and confusion and to yield faster, more accurate performance.

Text. Rehe (1974) recommends that a text line should contain no more than about forty to sixty characters. He has also found that unjustified (of unequal length) text lines are just as legible as justified text. Large spaces in justified text may interrupt eye movement and impede reading.

Field Captions

- Identify fields with captions or labels. Do not assume that users will identify individual information items from past experience. Context plays a significant role.

    215-584-6320 ~~(crossed out)~~   TEL: 215-584-6320

- Choose distinct and meaningful caption names that can be easily distinguished from other captions. Minimal differences (one letter or word) cause confusion.
- Differentiate field captions from field data by using:

    - contrasting features, such as different intensities, separating colons, and so forth.

        SEX FEMALE ~~(crossed out)~~   SEX: FEMALE
        RELATION DAUGHTER ~~(crossed out)~~   RELATION: DAUGHTER

    - consistent positional relationships:

        SEX: ~~(crossed out)~~
        FEMALE ~~(crossed out)~~   SEX: FEMALE
        RELATION: DAUGHTER ~~(crossed out)~~   RELATION: DAUGHTER

- Separate captions from data fields by at least one blank space.

    CITY CHICAGO ~~(crossed out)~~   CITY: CHICAGO

- Identify input fields with underscores.

Many screens contain data that must be identified by a caption or label. The preceding guidelines aim at producing captions that are complete, clear, easy to identify, and distinguishable from other captions and input fields.

A common failing of many screens is that their captions and data have the same general appearance and tend to blend into one another when the screen is filled. This makes discrimination difficult. Another common failing is that related captions often repeat the same word or words over and over again. This increases the potential for confusion and often adds to screen clutter.

There are two ways to establish a relationship between captions and associated data fields. As Figure 6–2 shows, the caption may immediately precede the associated data field (A), or it may be above the associated field (B). The horizontal relationship (A) is recommended because it allows a better compromise between caption clarity and space utilization than the vertical relationship (B).

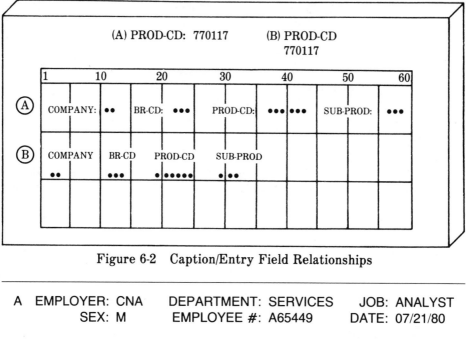

Figure 6-2 Caption/Entry Field Relationships

A EMPLOYER: CNA   DEPARTMENT: SERVICES   JOB: ANALYST
          SEX: M   EMPLOYEE #: A65449   DATE: 07/21/80

        EMPLOYER DEPARTMENT   JOB
        CNA   SERVICES   ANALYST
  B   SEX   EMPLOYER #   DATE
        M   A65449   07/21/80

Figure 6-3.   Visual Discrimination of Captions/Entry Fields

The A relationship consumes 59 character positions, while B consumes 74. Space usage in B can be reduced only by reducing some caption sizes. This is a solution often implemented, thus affecting screen clarity. B allows only 12 lines of data on a 24-line screen, while A accommodates 24 lines of data. Viewed in relation to source document design, the good fit between 8½ inch × 11 inch documents and 80-character-wide screens occurs with the horizontal (A) orientation. On completely filled screens, a horizontal format (with colons) provides better visual discrimination between captions and keyed data, as shown in Figure 6-3. On large or crowded screens, the caption-above alternative can cause captions and data to visually merge.

For fields that are repeated two or more times, captions should be placed above a stack of entry fields.

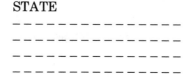

Horizontal caption formats for single fields will also provide better discrimination between single and repeating fields. The single-field caption will always precede the data, and captions for repeating columnar fields will always be above the top data field.

Monochromatic Display Features

Blinking

- has excellent attention-getting capability;
- reduces legibility;
- is distracting;
- limit to situations where a person must respond quickly;
- should be capable of being turned off when the person has responded.

High Brightness

- has good attention-getting capability;
- is the least disturbing feature;
- may be used to call attention to errors or differing screen components.

Reverse Video

- has good attention-getting capability;
- may reduce character legibility;
- should be used in moderation;
- may be used to call attention to errors or important screen components.

Lower Case

- has moderate attention-getting capability;
- should be used for textual information.

Upper Case

- has moderate attention-getting capability;
- should be used for captions and labels.

Underlining

- has poor attention-getting capability;
- may reduce legibility.

Double-Size Characters

- has moderate attention-getting capability;
- should be used for titles and headings.

Thin/Thick/Double Rulings

- Use rules to break the screen into pieces; guide the eye through the screen.

Scrolling

- Use smooth as opposed to jump movement.

Today's monochromatic displays provide a wide range of techniques to aid the screen design process. Few terminals will have all the features described. The more there are, the more flexibility the designer will have. Effective screen design can be accomplished, however, with only a small number of features available.

Before beginning screen design, the designer must be aware of the capabilities of the terminal on which the screen will be displayed. It is important to note whether the various features are available on an individual-field basis, or whether they must be incorporated on a screenwide basis. (For example, can any one caption be displayed at high intensity or must all captions be displayed at high intensity?) The latter will, of course, allow less flexibility in design.

Often these features are used to call attention to various items on the display. The attraction capability of a mechanism is directly related to how well it stands out from its surroundings. Its maximum value is achieved when it is used in moderation. Overuse will be self-defeating, since contrast with the surroundings is reduced and distraction may even result.

Not all display features are ideal for all situations. Following are some recommended uses, and limitations that currently exist.

Blinking is very distracting. Its use should be reserved for situations where a person must respond quickly. A person should have the capability of turning off the blinking when attention has been captured.

High brightness has a good attention-getting capability and no disturbing features. If it has a fault, it is that terminals with improperly set manual screen-contrast controls can diminish its effectiveness, even causing it to disappear.

Reverse video has been looked upon as the feature which permits the display screen to resemble the normal printed page (that is, black letters on a white background). Unfortunately, the white background light is subject to the phenomenon of bright light tending to bleed into dark. A reverse video display, therefore, finds the background bleeding into the characters, thus possibly reducing their legibility.

Lower case should be used for the display of textual information, and *upper case* for captions and labels. *Double-size* characters can be used for titles and headings, and where emphasis is needed. *Underlining* may reduce legibility and should be used with caution.

Scrolling is a technique used to move data across or through the display screen. This movement should be smooth, as opposed to the jump method whose movement bothers most people.

Data Entry Screens

Data entry screens are designed primarily to collect information quickly and accurately. Quite often the data are edited on line so that errors can be quickly corrected. System specifications frequently require large numbers of data elements. Several screens may be required for one transaction, and a system may comprise many transactions.

The most important variable in data entry screen design is the availability of a specially designed source document from which data are keyed. If such a document is used, and if it has been designed in conjunction with the screen, the primary visual focus of the user will be toward the document, with the screen assuming a secondary role in the keying process. If a special source document is not developed, the user's primary visual focus is usually the screen, and the data source assumes a less important role in the overall design.

This distinction is important because it determines whether keying aids are built into the screens or into source documents. With a dedicated source document, the document itself can include keying aids. But without a dedicated source document, the screen format must incorporate such aids. The resulting screens will have fundamental conceptual differences in data organization, content, and structure. The guidelines described below reflect these differences when appropriate. The discussion that follows reviews the most important points. The reader who needs more detailed information on all aspects of data entry screen design is again referred to Galitz (1981).

Manual Tabbing and Auto Skip

Auto skip is a display terminal feature that causes a cursor to automatically move to the beginning of the next entry field once a field is completely filled. Auto skip obviates manual tabbing and requires fewer keystrokes to complete a screen. Theoretically, keying speeds should increase with auto skip. In practice, however, they don't always do so.

Many entry screen fields are never or rarely completely filled with data. When an entry field is not full, the user must still depress the tab key to move the cursor to the next entry field. Figure 6-4 illustrates the functions required when using auto skip.

Auto skip, therefore, imposes decision-making and learning requirements. After keying data in each field, one must determine where the cursor is and whether to depress the manual tab key. Only then can the next keying action be performed. With manual tabbing, which Figure 6-5 illustrates, extra key strokes are required, but no decisions need be made. The data entry task is rhythmic and consistent. Galitz (1972) summarizes operator performance data from a study of both auto skip and manual tabbing. In that study, manual tabbing resulted in faster performance and fewer keying errors.

Auto skip can delay detection of one particular human error. If an extra character is inadvertently keyed into a field, the cursor will still move automatically to the next entry field and keying can continue. The error will not be immediately detected, and the spacing in subsequent fields may also be one position off, at least until the tab key is depressed. If this situation were to occur while using manual tabbing, the keyboard would lock as soon as the

General

- Information grouping should be logical, orderly, and meaningful to the user.
- Keying procedures should have:

  - manual tabbing for large volume and many screen tasks:
  - no recoding, including, omitting, or changing data based on special rules or logical transformations.

- Character entry should:
  - be accomplished by direct character replacement;
  - have keyed entries always visible (except for secure entries such as passwords);
  - have data keyed without separators, delimiters, or dimensional units;
  - have data keyed without leading zeros;
  - not require right or left justification;
  - not require removal of unused underscores.

- Screen transmission should be accomplished by a single explicit action when all entries are completed.

With Source Document

- Screen organization should be in the image of source document.

- Field captions and labels should have abbreviations and contractions separated by hyphens.

- Data fields should optimally have field identified by characters such as underscores; minimally have the starting point of field identified.

Without Source Document

- Screen organization should be columnized for optimum visual clarity.

- Field captions and labels should be fully spelled out in natural language.

- Data fields should optimally have field identified by characters such as underscores; minimally have the starting point of field identified.

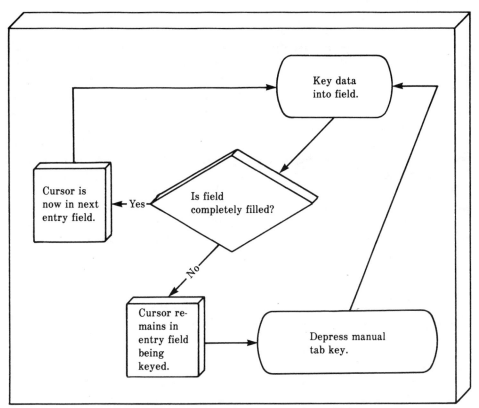

Figure 6-4. Data Entry Using Auto Skip

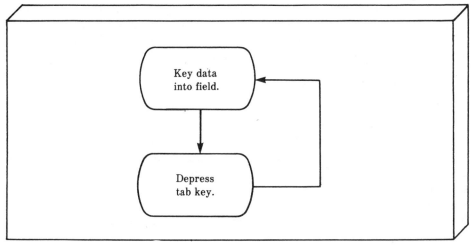

Figure 6-5. Data Entry Using Manual Tabbing

entry field was full or when an attempt was made to key the extra character. The error would immediately be obvious.

But auto skip, despite its limitations, can be useful if a system's screens are easily learned or if all screen fields are always completely filled. Most larger data entry applications would not appear to meet the criteria, however.

While using manual tab control, and when an entry field is completely filled, the cursor will move to the first character position of the next protected field to await a manual tab command. This command will direct the cursor to the first character position of the next entry field. After a line of data is keyed, the user can also depress the return key to direct the cursor to the first entry field of the next line. If an entry field extends into the next-to-last or last column in a line, however, depression of the return key can put the cursor in the wrong location. Figure 6-6 illustrates how this happens. Restricting the endpoint of an entry field to the second-to-last column in a line will prevent the situation in example B, thus eliminating a potential error and establishing a consistent data-entry procedure.

Keying Rules

Data entry keying speeds will be slowed and error probability increased if users must make such decisions as:

- Should this datum always be keyed?
- If that field is keyed, should this one be keyed?
- If the datum is "X," then should "I" be keyed in the field?
- If a "4" goes here, where should other figures be keyed?

Such keying decisions impose learning requirements on users. Except in the most simple systems, this learning will never reach a satisfactory level. The fewer rules and decisions involved in keying, the faster and more accurate data entry will be. Coding, omitting, changing, or including data by special rules or transformations are probably the greatest obstacles to data entry speed.

Data Entry Screens with Source Documents

A data entry screen used with a source document must be organized in the image of the source document. Skipping around a source document to locate data adds time to the data entry process. It also imposes learning requirements on users since they must master the order and location of fields. Having the source document and screen in the same sequence can eliminate these problems. Cursor location on the screen is then always known because it corresponds with one's position on the source document. Proper sequence also allows a person's eyes to move easily ahead of one's hands—another design objective of data entry.

Ideally, keying should never require moving one's eyes from the source document to the screen. Theoretically (and frequently, if the design is proper),

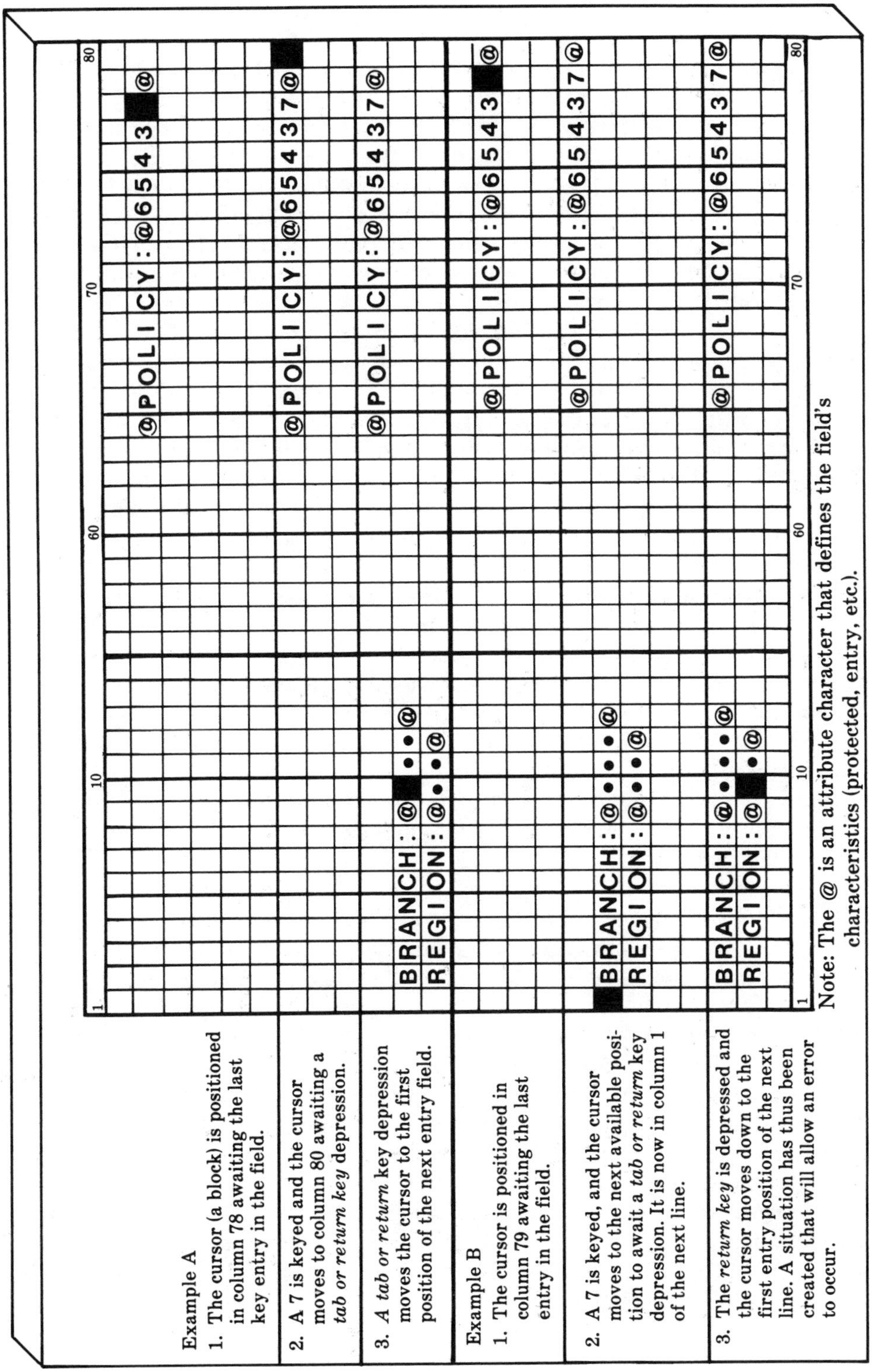

Example A

1. The cursor (a block) is positioned in column 78 awaiting the last key entry in the field.

2. A 7 is keyed and the cursor moves to column 80 awaiting a *tab or return key* depression.

3. A *tab or return* key depression moves the cursor to the first position of the next entry field.

Example B

1. The cursor is positioned in column 79 awaiting the last entry in the field.

2. A 7 is keyed, and the cursor moves to the next available position to await a *tab or return* key depression. It is now in column 1 of the next line.

3. The *return key* is depressed and the cursor moves down to the first entry position of the next line. A situation has thus been created that will allow an error to occur.

Note: The @ is an attribute character that defines the field's characteristics (protected, entry, etc.).

Figure 6-6.   The Need for a Cursor-Rest Position

113

a person should be able to key an entire screen without glancing at it. Often, however, eye movements between document and screen are necessary to check for possible keying errors and to correct edit-detected errors. This eye movement will be most efficient (and natural) if fields on the screen and the document are in the same relative position. The considerations lead to this cardinal rule for developing data entry systems: *Develop screens that are exact images of source documents*. Fields on a screen should be located on the same line and in the same order as fields on the source document. This factor is more important than absolute visual clarity.

The rule should not be interpreted literally, however. Differing caption sizes and the number of fields included on one line can cause minor distortions. The goal, then, should be relative positioning since the eye will not detect minor distortions in the exact image relationship.

If a source document contains non-entry fields, ink screening techniques can maintain the image relationship. If a source document contains a large number of these fields, the positioning of data entry fields on the screen may appear awkward. For consistency, however, the relative positioning rule must be maintained. The only exception would be a revised scheme that could eliminate the awkwardness while maintaining consistency within the application and the ability to easily locate specific fields.

Screens of this kind and their associated source documents, then, cannot be developed separately. Constraints imposed by source document design considerations must be reflected in screen format design, and vice versa.

When a dedicated source document is used for keying, field *captions* are normally needed only for error detection or correction, or to find one's exact place on the screen when momentarily confused. Thus, captions are a supportive rather than primary function in the data entry process, and abbreviations and contractions should be used.

The caption size limit is eight characters. This is a compromise between screen space utilization and clarity. It results in a good fit between standard (8½ inches × 11 inches) documents and 80-character-wide screens (Galitz 1975), while maintaining an exact image relationship. Learning requirements do exist, but they are minimal. Since screen captions are derived from associated fields on the source document, the document provides a constant reference to aid in caption interpretation and learning.

The eight-character limitation should not be considered an absolute since a longer caption may occasionally be needed to achieve clarity. Since caption pieces are small, hyphens should be used to visually tie them together. This will minimize misinterpretations and erroneous associations.

Data fields should always be obvious, ideally through the use of underscores to define field size, as in example A below. But if underscores are not possible, an acceptable alternative is the use of colons to signify the starting point of an entry field, as example B illustrates.

(A) NAME: – – – – – – – –   (B) NAME:
        ZIP   ZIP
        – – – – – – – –   :
        – – – – – – – –   :
        – – – – – – – –   :

The entry field will usually start immediately after the colon and one blank space. Absolute identification of field length is not essential if the system is operating with manual tabbing because the terminal will identify the end by locking the keyboard.

When using a dedicated source document, the document/screen image relationship is maintained through placement of entry fields on the screen, as illustrated in Figure 6-7. Captions need not be aligned. Note that the third field in the second line of the form (F. Medical Payments—Each Accident) is a nonentry field. It is shaded on the form and does not appear on the screen. Leave a blank line on the screen where breaks or spaces occur on the source document. The objective, again, is to maintain an identical image relationship between document and screen.

Data Entry Screens without Source Documents

If data entry screens must be developed without dedicated source documents, the screen organization should be based on the organization of the manuals, other documents, or the environment from which the data are keyed. But since these variables cannot always be controlled, an exact correspondence

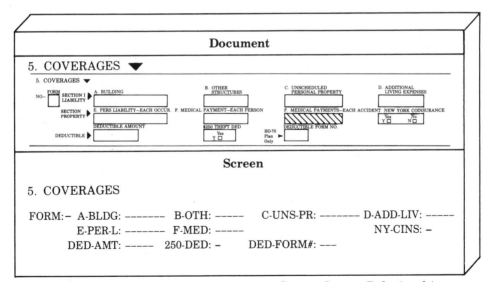

Figure 6–7. Maintaining a Document/Screen Image Relationship

between source and screen isn't usually achievable. Thus the screen format must be the controlling force in the development. A person usually identifies a field on the screen and then seeks data for keying from appropriate materials. The rules for optimizing screen visual clarity should be applied here. Data entry will be enhanced, however, to the extent that required visual references to the screen can be minimized. Every attempt should be made to reflect in the screen format the organization of the world from which the entry data are taken.

When a dedicated source document is not used, screens need captions to identify what data must be keyed into a field. Normal data entry requires that the user read the caption, find the data in the source materials, and then key. If data to be keyed must instead be identified from the screen, captions must clearly and concisely describe the information required.

Captions that are ambiguous, imprecise, or unclear will impair data entry until they are learned. Abbreviations and contractions should be used in such captions only if they are common to the everyday language of the application, or if they can be easily and quickly associated with data fields on source materials.

Data fields should be obvious, ideally through the use of underscores. Identifying the structure of data fields on screens is necessary only if a source document is not available. With a dedicated source document, the structure is obvious from the design of the form. Data keyed are simply those coded on the document. Without a dedicated source document, field completion aids may be included on the screen, as in these examples:

(1)		(or)		(2)
DATE (MMDDYY): _ _ _ _ _ _			DATE:	MMDDYY
*RATE (NN.N): _ _ _ _			*RATE:	NN.N
AMOUNT ($¢): _ _ _ _ _ _ _ _			AMOUNT:	$¢

In alternative 2, data are keyed over the field completion aid. Required fields may be indicated by a special character, such as the asterisk in the rate field.

Justification without a dedicated source document, if caption sizes are relatively equal, involves left justifying both captions and entry fields. Leave one space between the longest caption and the column of entry fields.

> POLICY NUMBER: _ _ _ _ _ _ _ _ _ _
> ACCOUNT NUMBER: _ _ _ _ _ _ _ _
> EFFECTIVE DATE: _ _ _ _ _ _
> EXPIRATION DATE: _ _ _ _ _ _
> POLICY STATUS: _ _ _ _ _ _ _ _ _

If caption sizes are quite variable, left justify entry fields and right justify captions one space from entry fields, again leaving one space between captions and the start of entry fields.

```
        CORPORATION:  _ _ _ _ _ _ _ _ _ _
              TITLE:  _ _ _ _ _ _ _ _ _ _ _ _ _
SOCIAL SECURITY NUMBER:  _ _ _ _ _ _ _ _ _
```

The second approach often gives a more balanced look to a screen.

To improve readability of groups of elements, leave a blank line at logical breaks or after every fifth row (if space permits, after every third row). For example:

```
POLICY NUMBER:     _ _ _ _ _ _ _ _ _ _
ACCOUNT NUMBER:    _ _ _ _ _ _ _ _
EFFECTIVE DATE:    _ _ _ _ _ _
EXPIRATION DATE:   _ _ _ _ _ _
POLICY STATUS:     _ _ _ _ _ _ _ _ _

POLICY FORM:       _ _
PROPERTY:          _ _ _ _ _ _ _ _
LIABILITY:         _ _ _ _ _ _ _ _
DEDUCTIBLE:        _ _ _ _ _
ENDORSEMENT:       _ _ _ _ _ _ _ _ _ _
```

Inquiry Screens

- *Screen organization should:*

  - be logical, orderly, and meaningful to the user;
  - have most frequently requested information on earliest screens;
  - have most frequently requested information on a screen in the upper left portion;
  - be perceptually organized in a balanced manner;
  - be columnized for optimum visual clarity;
  - not be packed with information;

- *Field captions/labels should be fully spelled out in natural language.*

- *Data fields should:*

  - have natural split or breaks included;
  - have recognizable orders;
  - have accepted organizations and formats;
  - be justified for ease in scanning;
  - be visually emphasized.

Inquiry screens are those developed for displaying the contents of computer files. Data on these screens are permanent, and the screens are structured for ease in locating information and for visual clarity.

Screen organization should be logical, orderly, and meaningful to the user. When information is structured in a manner that is consistent with a person's organizational view of the topic, more information is comprehended (Kintish 1978).

Field captions should be fully spelled out in the user's natural language. Abbreviations and contractions should be used only if they are common to the application.

Data fields should be emphasized since this is what the user is scanning, usually by context. In looking for a date, for instance, the user's visual search usually involves scanning for numeric characters in a certain structure (such as 09/21/63), while a name search might involve scanning for a recognizable combination of alphabetic characters of an approximate size and format (such as "Johnson, Carl"). Actual captions are only occasionally needed on these screens—perhaps in looking for seldom-used data or data with similar content.

Data displays should also be compatible with the human tendency to break things into groups. People handle information more easily when it is in chunks.

Justification of fields on an inquiry screen will be similar to that on a data entry screen without source document. If caption sizes are relatively equal, left justify both captions and data fields, leaving one space between the longest caption and the column of data fields, as previously illustrated. If caption sizes are quite variable, left justify data fields and right justify captions one space from the column of the data fields. To improve readability of groups of elements, again leave a blank line at logical breaks or after every third or fifth row. More information on inquiry screen design can again be found in Galitz (1981).

An office system contains a great deal of data and performs a wide variety of functions. Regardless of its purpose, some means must be provided to tell users about the information the system possesses and the things it can do. A commonly employed technique is the use of a menu screen that displays alternatives one has at appropriate points while using the system.

Menu screens are useful to new users of systems because they rely on our more powerful capability of recognition rather than recall. Working with menus reminds people of available options and information that they might not be aware of or may have forgotten. Menu screens are not without their problems for new system users, however. Learning is often made difficult because people must integrate information across a series of displays (Engel and Granda 1975; Dray et al. 1981). Words and phrases with multiple meanings may be interpreted incorrectly because they are not seen in proper context or in relation to other choices (Bower et al. 1969). Ambiguities may be resolved on the basis of assumptions of hierarchical structure that are incorrect (Cuff 1980; Durding

Menu Screens

Structure of screens should include:

- hierarchical groupings of logically-related elements;
- a minimum number of levels within limits of clarity;
- Immediate access to critical or frequently chosen alternatives.

Components of screens should include:

- all relevant alternatives;
- only relevant alternatives;
- an escape mechanism;
- location in hierarchy.

Ordering of screens should have:

- distinctive groupings;
- a small number of options - order by sequence or frequency of use;
- a large number of options - order alphabetically

Organization of screens should be:

- in columns;
- perceptually balanced;
- with selections keyed in a fixed location.

Item Identification should be either numerical or mnemonical.

et al. 1977). The frequent result is that people make mistakes and quite often get lost in the hierarchical structure.

Experienced users of systems, while finding menus helpful in the beginning, soon find them tedious. Not all functions may be available from all menus, thus greatly increasing the effort and time to get something accomplished. The design of a menu, then, must try to balance the conflicting needs of users with differing experience levels.

Structure. Menus should consist of hierarchical groupings of logically related elements, not an undifferentiated string of alternatives. All too often menu structures are arbitrary or have been based on the characteristics of the controlling software or developed to maximize use of available memory. Liebelt et al. (1982) have demonstrated that logically organized menus are easier to learn and yield faster and more accurate performance.

To assist learning of the structure of a hierarchical series of menus, a graphic representation or map of the structure is an invaluable aid. People utilize spatial structure in learning hierarchically organized information. Billingsley (1982) has experimentally found an overall improvement in information retrieval across time through presentation of a menu map. Access to a pictorial representation of a menu's structure facilitates the development of a mental mode of that structure.

A menu hierarchical structure should be comprised of a minimum number of levels within limits of clarity. Miller (1981) studied the depth/breadth tradeoff for a list of 64 alternatives. He compared speed and accuracy in locating one of 64 alternatives in menu hierarchies ranging from one to six levels. He found that eight items at a depth of two levels yielded fastest performance, fewest errors, and was easiest to learn.

Components. Display *all* relevant alternatives and *only* relevant alternatives. If choices that are not relevant at the moment are displayed, performance is degraded (Baker and Goldstein 1966) and user learning requirements are increased. Provide an *escape mechanism* on each menu screen. This permits the experienced user who knows the system to bypass interim menus and go directly to the desired choice or alternative. Include, also, a menu-addressing scheme so that a user will know their location in the hierarchy.

Ordering. Segment menus into distinctive groupings where possible. Avoid using the same words repeatedly. For menus with a *small* number of options, sequence or frequency of use is the best ordering scheme. A small number would generally be less than seven or eight items. For a *large* number of options, alphabetic ordering of alternatives is desirable. Alphabetic ordering is also recommended for small lists where no sequence or frequency pattern is obvious.

Card (1982) compared scanning times for alphabetic, functional, and randomly organized 18-item menus. The fastest was alphabetic. The random organization was one-fourth as fast as the alphabetic. Search time was a function of saccadic eye movements through the display. Search patterns were random, but fewer eye movements were required with the alphabetic arrangement. After twenty trials, however, only one eye movement was required for all conditions and search time was the same. Learning does take place but is aided by the ordering scheme.

Organization. Menu alternatives should be columnized and perceptually balanced on the screen. Selections should be keyed in a fixed location. The recommended position for a single selection field is at the bottom of the column of choices. It should be labeled for novice users.

Item identification. If an ordinal identification scheme is chosen to identify alternatives, use numbers starting with number 1. Always place a period after each number. A mnemonic identification scheme, however, is recommended. Mnemonics are easier to recall, thus providing an easier transition to a command language. Touch typists find letters easier to type, and the reordering of menus to accommodate new alternatives can be accomplished without relearning.

Color in Screen Design

The addition of color to screens can add a new dimension to usability. As a formatting aid, color can assist a person in understanding the logical structure of the data on the screen. As a coding aid it can aid in establishing meaning to the data or information displayed.

There is little concrete research data currently available about using color in screen design. An excellent general summary of the use of color in displays is that of Krebs (1978). The most thorough review of research on the effects of color in displays is that of Christ (1975), although it includes little concerning CRT-generated displays. A more detailed discussion of some practical guidelines based upon experience using color alphanumeric screens can be found in Robertson (1979). While these references are short on experimental validation, they do provide useful guidance on how color may be used in screens, and form the basis for the guidelines to follow.

First we shall review how color may be used as either a formatting aid or as a coding vehicle. Next, how categories of data may be chosen for color will be discussed, and then what colors to choose.

Some Cautions on Using Color

- Color's high attention-getting quality may be distracting, causing a person to:

  - notice differences in color, regardless of whether they have task-related meaning;
  - visually group items of the same color in a way that is unrelated to the task, or in conflict with another task-related group of items.

- Indiscriminate or poor use of color on one display may interfere with color's attention-getting power on another display.

First, here are some cautions on using color. When color is used improperly, performance will show little improvement or may even suffer. On an uncluttered, highly structured display, color will be of little value. Inappropriate color usage in complex displays may distract users and interfere with their handling of information. Another disadvantage of color is that about 8 percent of the male population and 0.4 percent of all women have some form of color vision deficiency.

Color as a Formatting Aid

- Use color as a formatting aid to:

  - relate or tie fields into groupings;
  - differentiate groupings of fields from one another;
  - relate fields that are spatially separated;
  - emphasize or call attention to important fields;
  - assist reading of long lines of text or data.

As a formatting aid, color can be used to provide better structure and meaning to a screen. It is especially useful when large amounts of data must be included on a screen, and spacing to differentiate components is difficult to employ.

For example, differentiation of logical groupings of fields can be enhanced by displaying related groupings in different colors. Spatially separated but related fields can also be tied together through a color scheme.

Color can also replace highlighting as a means of calling attention to a field or fields. Color is much more flexible in this manner because of the number that are available. Color as an attention-getting mechanism must be chosen in light of the psychological and physiological considerations to be described shortly.

Wide blocks of data or text can be made more legible by breaking it up into three-row groupings of alternate colors (similar to printout paper). This guides the eye in jumping from one line to the next.

Color as a Visual Code

- Use color as a visual code to identify:

  - kinds of data;
  - sources of data;
  - status of data;
  - order of operations.

- The color coding scheme must be:

  - relevant; and
  - known.

A color code will show what category the data being displayed fall into. It will have meaning to the screen's user. A properly selected color-coding scheme will permit a person to identify a relevant category quickly without first having to read the contents of the data. This permits focusing of concentration on this category while the remaining data are excluded from attention.

One common color-coding scheme used to differentiate kinds of data is to display captions and data fields in different colors. Another is to identify data from different sources—data added to a transaction from different locations or text added to a message from different departments may be colored differently. An application of color coding to convey status might involve displaying data that passed or failed system edits in a different color. Color can also be used as a prompt, guiding a person through a complex transaction.

Color as a visual code must be relevant and known. Relevance is achieved when the code enables a person to attend selectively only to the data needed. It must attract a person's attention to the particular class of data that is desired at the moment. A relevant code, however, will be useless unless it is also known to the person who must use it. Not knowing a code's meaning only distracts and degrades performance.

Choosing Categories of Data for Color

- Choosing categories of data for color requires a clear understanding of how a person uses information. For example:

    - If different sets of data are attended to separately:
        - color-code the sets to help selective attention to each in turn.
    - If decisions are made based on the status of certain data:
        - color code the types of status the data may possess.
    - If display searching is performed to locate data possessing a particular status or quality:
        - color code such data to contrast with the rest of the data.
    - If certain kinds of data are not used frequently:
        - use an unobtrusive color for display.
    - If the sequence of using data is constrained:
        - use color to identify the sequence.

Color chosen to classify data on a screen must aid the transfer of information from the display to the user. This requires a clear understanding of how the information is selected from a screen and used. The examples above describe some common ways of classifying data for color-coding purposes.

It is important to remember, however, that data on one screen may be used in more than one way. What is useful in one context may not be in another and may only cause interference. Therefore, when developing a color-coding strategy, consider how spatial formatting, highlighting, and messages may also be useful.

Choosing Colors to Display

Having chosen the categories of display data to receive different colors, the final step is to assign colors to each of the different categories. Color assignment should be based on the above considerations of:

- terminal color capabilities;
- consistency;
- compatibility with expectancies;
- discriminability;
- frequency of use and importance;
- relevance and confusion.

Terminal Color Capabilities

- Design must occur within the population of colors available for display on the terminal.

Colors assigned must be those that are available on the display terminal to be used. The exact colors (chromaticities) must be known because they will affect their identifiability, distinguishability, and legibility. Since the population of measurable colors is about 7.5 million (Geldard 1953), the handful displayed on any one device provides an extremely wide margin for variation.

From a practical standpoint the basic colors on most displays can be identified as a variation of what is perceived as red, green, blue, and white. Colors selected from other points along the visual spectrum provide greater opportunities for between-terminal variability.

In the guidelines that follow, color will be described in terms of general characteristics and readers must extrapolate based upon the exact qualities of their own terminal.

Table 6-3. The Visible Spectrum

Color	Approximate Wavelength in Millimicrons
Red	700
Orange	600
Yellow	570
Yellow-green	535
Green	500
Blue-green	493
Blue	470
Violet	400

Consistency

- There should be consistency within a screen, an application, and a set of applications used by a person.
- Broad definitions of color meaning provide less chance for confusion.

Colors used as codes are expected to have some meaning. Changing meanings between displays will lead to difficulties in interpretation, confusion, and errors. The degree of consistency required at the detail level will depend upon the application. In general, broadly defined meanings (such as red indicates there is a problem) permits more scope for variations without inconsistency.

Compatibility with Expectancies

- Use color meanings that already exist in a person's job.
- Use color associations that exist in the world at large, such as:

Status:

- Red   = Stop or danger
- Amber   = Caution
- Green   = Go or normal

Ordering:

• Red	• Blue
• Orange	• Indigo
• Yellow	• Violet
• Green	• White

Color meanings consistent with traditional color expectancies are also easier to use (for example, red equals danger). They are well ingrained in human behavior and difficult to unlearn.

Color meanings are more easily learned if color codes conform to color meanings that already exist in a person's job. Color codes employing different meanings will be much more difficult to use.

Discriminability

In spite of the millions of measurable colors, the human eye cannot effectively distinguish more than eight at one time. If color discrimination is important, this number should not be exceeded.

To aid discrimination, any set of colors selected for a display should be as widely spaced along the visible spectrum as possible. Table 6-3 summarizes the visible spectrum for the most common colors.

- If color discrimination is required, do not use more than eight colors.
- For normal discrimination, select colors that are widely spaced along the visual spectrum (see Table 6-3).

  - The most generally useful colors are red, green, yellow, and blue.
  - Other acceptable colors include orange, yellow-green, blue-green, and violet.

- For emphasis and separation, use contrasting colors such as:

  - Red and green
  - Blue and yellow
  - Red, green, and blue
  - Red, green, blue, and white

- To convey similarity, use similar colors such as:

  - Orange and yellow
  - Blue and violet

Assuming a reasonable level of ambient illumination, displays can effectively use these eight colors, which are also mentioned in the preceding guidelines (Krebs 1978). But as the number of colors in a display increases, the following will also increase:

- the time required to respond to a specific color;
- the probability of confusion among colors;
- the demands on hardware for reliably reproducing each color.

In a color application, to emphasize and convey separation use contrasting colors. To convey similarity use similar, but differentiable colors.

Frequency of Use and Importance.

Emphasis of data may also be achieved by using colors of differing intensities. Frequently used information, such as inquiry screen data fields, may be displayed in a bright color while less frequently used information, such as captions, can be displayed in a less bright color.

When a single color must be selected for a display, an important consideration is character or symbol visibility. Visibility depends on character or symbol luminance and luminance contrast. The preceding guidelines give visibility characteristics of several colors at various luminance and illumination levels.

- Use bright colors to emphasize data and colors lacking brightness to de-emphasize data. The brightness of colors, from most to least is:

  - white;
  - yellow;
  - green;
  - blue;
  - red.

- Character visibility considerations:

  - Red provides good visibility under high ambient lighting, but poor visibility at low symbol luminance.
  - Blue provides good visibility at low symbol luminance, but provides the poorest visual acuity.
  - Green provides good general visibility over a broad range of intermediate luminances.
  - Yellow provides good general visibility over a broad range of luminances.

Under levels of high ambient illumination, colors frequently seem washed out or unsaturated. If some means of light attenuation is not possible, or character luminance is not bright enough to counter the illumination, color should be used with caution.

Relevance and Confusion

- Do not overuse color. Use of too many colors may make a screen confusing or unpleasant to look at.
- Use only enough colors to fulfill the needs of the application.
- Alphanumeric screens should display no more than four colors at one time.

Color as a coding mechanism has such attention-getting power that its use must be carefully planned and controlled. It is particularly important not to overuse color. A display containing a glittering hodgepodge of colors will probably only confuse a person (especially during high workloads or at critical points) and will negate color's value as an attention-getting mechanism.

Overuse of colors will not occur if colors are selected in terms of usefulness to the display user. If six colors enhance a screen's usability, then use six. If only three are useful, then use only three. The issue is relevance to the task.

In general, graphic displays can employ more colors than alphanumeric displays. It is a subjective finding that too many colors on an alphanumeric display varies from screen to screen, but using more than four colors generally elicits this comment. (This does not mean that an alphanumeric screen application must be restricted to four colors, but only that no more than four colors should be displayed at one time.)

In a graphic application, Miller (1979) reports some interactions among various colors. Perception of area sizes, such as a bar graph, may depend on the foreground and surrounding colors. Tedford et al. (1977), in a review of several studies of this phenomenon, conclude that warm colors (red and yellow) usually appear larger than cooler colors (green and blue).

Table 6–4. Maximum Number of Codes for Effective Human Differentiation

Encoding Method	Recommended Maximum	Comments
Size	3	Considerable space required; location time longer than for colors and shapes.
Line length	3–4	Will clutter display with many signals.
Line width	2–3	
Solid and broken lines	3–4	
Brightness	2–3	Creates problems on screens with poor contrast.
Flashing	2–3	Confusing for general encoding but the best way to attract attention; interacts poorly with other codes.
Number of dots or marks	5	Minimum number best for quick assimilation.
Geometric shapes	10	High mnemonic value.
Color	6–8	No extra space required; short location time.
Orientation (location on display surface)	4–8	

Graphics

Graphics opens up new vistas in screen format design, offering the ability to:

- duplicate the real world of forms, documents, and so on;
- pack more information into a smaller space;
- allow comparisons that free people from short-term memory limitations;
- simplify perceptions of structure (by using bar graphs instead of numeric tables, for example).

The use of graphics must, however, consider human differentiation limits. Table 6-4 summarizes the maximum number of codes for different coding methods that permit effective (rapid and error-free) human differentiation. This was derived from Martin (1973) and Barmack and Sinaiko (1966). How many methods can be used on one display is not known. Interaction effects are also probable, but more experience in developing computer graphic displays will be required to understand them.

The first incorporation of graphic geometric shapes into what is essentially an alphanumeric display occurred with the advent of Xerox's STAR. Using representations (called *icons*) of tools, storage locations, and optional actions, people achieve the same visual access to tools that they have always had. These pictorial descriptions result in easier and faster identification than do alphanumeric descriptions or arbitrary designations. The result is also faster learning times. This approach has been continued by Apple's *Lisa* and will continue to evolve as an extremely effective interface between people and computers.

Form Design

In spite of the move toward the paperless office, paper forms will continue to be ingredients in a variety of applications. Source documents for data-entry applications are but one example. Design criteria for forms are similar to those of a data-entry screen. Money spent on creating a form that accurately and completely collects and transmits data will be returned to its user manyfold. Currently it is estimated that the processing cost for a form is 50–100 times its production cost. That is, a form that costs one penny to create will cost fifty cents to a dollar to process.

Lack of sufficient writing space for encoding information is a failing of many forms. Information legibility can be severely impaired if the size of fill-in areas is reduced to squeeze too many elements onto one piece of paper. In a study by a large insurance company, adequate spacing for form completion or encoding was ranked by insurance agents as the most important factor in simplifying forms (Galitz 1973).

Information arrangement on forms should be based on sequence and frequency of use, function, and importance.

A set of guidelines for form design includes the following items.

- Provide sufficient writing space.
- Maximize visibility of fill-in fields.
- Provide intelligent and clearly stated captions.
- Clearly associate captions with fill-in fields.
- Incorporate coding aids.
- Use preprinted codes wherever possible.
- Arrange information according to an acceptable combination of:

  - sequence of use;
  - frequency of use;
  - function; and
  - importance.

- Provide clear design and clean reproduction by using perceptual groupings.
- Minimize irrelevant information.
- Use orderly and logical data sequence (top to bottom, and left to right).
- Locate instructions at the top or beginning of the form.
- Develop for completion by handwriting, typewriter, or both.

Sequence-of-use grouping involves arranging information items in the order in which they are commonly received or transmitted, or in natural groups. A person's address, for example, is normally given by street, city, state, and zip code. Another example of natural grouping is the league standings of football teams, appearing in order from best to worst records.

Frequency of use is a design technique based on the principle that information items used most frequently should be grouped at the beginning of the form. The second most frequently used items are grouped next, and so forth.

Function involves grouping information items according to their purpose. All items pertaining to insurance coverages, for example, may be placed in one location. Such grouping also allows convenient group identification for both preparer and user.

Importance grouping is based on the information's importance to the task being performed. Important items are placed in the most prominent positions.

Form design normally reflects a combination of these techniques. Information may be organized functionally, but within each function individual items may be arranged by sequence or importance. Numerous permutations are possible.

Wright and Barnard (1975) discuss problems associated with form language. In a later (1978) reference, Wright and Barnard also make recommendations concerning matrix designs on forms. For a general overview of form design, see Galitz (1979b), and for examples of thorough form design standards, CNA (1978 and 1979).

Summing Up

In spite of the rhetoric and the proliferation of buzzwords like *user-friendly* to describe software products, true ease-of-use remains far down the road. One problem is that the human-interface design remains an art rather than a science. While numerous principles for interface engineering exist, many are not supported by statistical evidence. Therefore, instead of a broad theory, numerous and sometimes conflicting guidelines prevail. The issues also have great depth and subtlety. Even straightforward considerations such as consistency and simplicity soon run up against roadblocks in widespread implementation. Too often the designer is forced to rely upon intuition and experience in making the final decision. Intuition, however, is error prone, no matter how good or bad the designer. Experience covering the wide diversity of considerations rarely exists.

A second problem is that many software designers still do not recognize poorly designed interfaces. The evaluative criteria applied are often far removed from the realities of human needs and the business office.

What is obviously needed is a much stronger foundation. A body of work rich in hypotheses and couched in observable aspects of human behavior and performance is a necessity. Also needed are more trained practitioners in the field of human interface engineering. The gap between people and computers will never be closed without the proper professional attention.

Perhaps some lessons can also be learned by understanding what makes computer games so popular. Malone (1982) describes these games as having the following qualities:

- *Challenge.* A clear goal exists and players are advised about how close they are to achieving the goal. Whether the goal will be achieved is uncertain, however.
- *Fantasy.* Computer games appeal to emotional fantasies. They embody metaphors with physical or other systems players already understand.
- *Curiosity.* Games capitalize on players' desires to have well-formed knowledge structures. They introduce new information when players feel their existing knowledge is incomplete, inconsistent, and unparsimonious. They provide an optimal level of informational complexity. They also add randomness in a way that adds variety without creating unreliability.

Challenge, fantasy, and curiosity. The goals of business system design do not seem incompatible with these qualities.

References

Baker, J. D., and Goldstein, I. "Batch vs. Sequential Displays: Effects on Human Problem Solving." *Human Factors* 8 (1966): 225–235.

Barmack, J. E., and Sinaiko, H. W. *Human Factors Problems in Computer-Generated Graphic Displays*. Inst. for Defense Analysis. AD-636170. 1966.

Barnard, P. "Presuppositions in Active and Passive Questions." Paper read to the Experimental Psychology Society, 1974.

Barnard, P.; Hammond, N.; MacLean, A.; and Morton, J. "Learning and Remembering Interactive Commands." *Proceedings: Human Factors in Computer Systems*. Gaithersburg, Md., March 15–17, 1982.

Barnard, P.; Hammond, N.; Morton, J.; Long, J.; and Clark, I. "Consistency and Compatibility in Human-Computer Dialogue." Internation Journal of Man-Machine Studies 15 (1981): 87–134.

Black, J. B., and Moran, T. P. "Learning and Remembering Command Names." *Proceedings: Human Factors in Computer Systems*. Gaithersburg, Md., March 15-17, 1982.

Billingsley, P. A. "Navigation Through Hierarchical Menu Structures: Does It Help to Have a Map?" *Proceedings of the Human Factors Society—26th Annual Meeting (1982)*. Santa Monica, Calif., 1982.

Boies, S. J. "User Behavior in an Interactive Computer System." *IBM Systems Journal* 13 (1974): 1–18.

Bower, G. H.; Clark, M. C.; Lesgold, A. M.; and Winenz, D. "Hierarchical Retrieval Schemes in Recall of Categorical Word Lists." *Journal of Verbal Learning and Verbal Behavior* 8 (1969): 323–343.

Carbonell, J. R.; Elkind, J. I.; and Nickerson, R. S. "On the Psychological Importance of Time in a Time-Sharing System." *Human Factors* 10 (1969): 135–142.

Card, S. K. "User Perceptual Mechanisms in the Search of Computer Command Menus." *Proceedings: Human Factors in Computer Systems*. Gaithersburg, Md., March 15– 17, 1982.

Carroll, J. M. "Learning, Using and Designing Command Paradigms." *IBM Research Report RC 8141*. 1980.

Chafin, R., and Martin, T. *DSN Human Factors Project Final Report*. Los Angeles, Calif.: University of Southern California. Contract No. 955013m RD–142. 1980.

Chapanis, A.; Parrish, R. N.; Ochsman, R. B. and Weeks, G. D. "Studies in Interactive Communication: II. The Effects of Four Communication Modes on the Linguistic Performance of Teams During Cooperative Problem Solving." *Human Factors* 19, No. 2 (1977): 101–126.

Christ, R. E. "Review and Analysis of Color Coding Research for Visual Displays." *Human Factors* 17, No. 6 (1975): 542–570.

CNA. *Design Standards for Producer Completed Forms*, 1 May 1978, pp. 1–22.

CNA. "Standards for Display Terminal Source Documents." *Systems and Data Processing Manual*, 5 January 1979, HB13-3207, pp. 1–18.

Cuff, R. N. "On Casual Users." *International Journal of Man-Machine Studies* 12 (1980): 163–187.

Danchak, M. M. "CRT Displays for Power Plants." *Instrumentation Technology* 23, No. 10 (1976): 29–36.

Doherty, W. J. "The Commercial Significance of Man-Computer Interaction." *Man/Computer Communication*. Vol. 2. Maidenhead, Berkshire, England: Infotech International, 1979, pp. 81–94.

Dray, S. M.; Ogden, W. G.; and Vestewig, R. E. "Measuring Performance with a Menu-Selection Human-Computer Interface." *Proceedings of the Human Factors Society-25th Annual Meeting (1981).* Santa Monica, Calif, 1981, pp. 746–748.

Dunsmore, H. E. "Using Formal Grammars to Predict the Most Useful Characteristics of Interactive Systems." *Office Automation Conference Digest.* San Francisco, April 5–7, 1982, pp. 53–56.

Durding, B. M.; Becker, C. A. and Gould, J. D. "Data Organization." *Human Factors* 19, No. 1 (1977): 1–14.

Eason, K. "Man-Computer Communication in Public and Private Computing." *HUSAT Memo 173.* Loughborough, Leics., 1979.

Elam, P. G. "Considering Human Needs Can Boost Network Efficiency." *Data Communications,* October 1978, pp. 50–60.

Engel, S. E., and Granda, R. E. "Guidelines for Man/Display Interfaces." *IBM Technical Report,* 19 December 1975. TR 00.2720.

Foley, J., and Wallace, V. "The Art of Natural Graphic Man-Machine Conversation." *Proceedings of the IEEE* 62, No. 4 (April 1974).

Furnas, G. W.; Gomez, L. M.; Landauer, T. K.; and Dumais, S. T. "Statistical Semantics: How Can a Computer Use What People Name Things to Guess What Things People Mean When They Name Things?" *Proceedings: Human Factors in Computer Sytems.* Gaithersburg, Md., March 15–17, 1982.

Galitz, W. O. "IBM 3270 On-Line Evaluation." *INA Technical Report,* 20 January 1972. E5320-A02/M72-0001.

Galitz, W. O. "DEBUT II—The CNA Data Entry Utility." *Proceedings of the 23rd Annual Meeting of the Human Factors Society (1979a),* pp. 50–54. Santa Monica, Calif., 1979.

Galitz, W. O. "An Evaluation of the Impact of Mnemonic CRT Labels on the Design and Use of EIS Forms and Screens." *INA Technical Report,* March 1975.

Galitz, W. O. *Form and Screen Design—Why?* Chicago, Ill.: CNA, October 1979b.

Galitz, W. O. *"Handbook of Screen Format Design,* 2nd ed. Wellesley, Mass.: Q.E.D. Information Sciences, 1984.

Galitz, W. O. "Summary Report of the Personal Lines Form Questionnaire and Agency Visits." *INA Technical Report,* 20 September 1973. E5710-A05/N73-0001.

Geldard, F. A. *The Human Senses.* New York: John Wiley, 1953.

Gilfoil, D. M. "Warming Up to Computers: A Study of Cognitive and Affective Interactions Over Time." *Proceedings: Human Factors in Computer Systems.* Gaithersburg, Md., March 15–17, 1982.

Goodwin, N. C. "Effect of Interface Design on Usability of Message Handling Systems." *Proceedings of the Human Factors Society—26th Annual Meeting (1982).* Santa Monica, Calif., 1982.

Gould, J. D.; Lewis, C.; and Becker, A. *Writing and Following Procedural, Descriptive and Restricted Syntax Language Instructions.* Yorktown Heights, N.Y.: IBM, 1976.

Greene, J. M. *Psycholinguistics: Chomsky and Psychology.* Harmondsworth, Middlesex, U.K.: Penguin, 1972.

Hammond, N.; Barnard, P.; Clark, I.; Morton, J,; and Long, J. "Structure and Content in Interactive Dialogue." *Paper presented at APA Montreal,* September 1980, and *IBM Human Factors Report HFO 34,* October 1980.

Hammond, N.; Long, J.; Clark, I.; Barnard, P.; and Morton, J. "Documenting Human-Computer Mismatch in Interactive Systems." *Proceedings of the Ninth Annual Symposium on Human Factors in Telecommunications,* 1980b.

Hansen, J. "Man-Machine Communication." *IEEE Transactions on Man, Systems and Cybernetics*. Vol. SMC-6, No. 11, November 1976.

Herriot, P. *An Introduction to the Psychology of Language*. London: Methuen, 1970.

Hicks, K. I., and Keller, A. "Editing with Contextual and Screen-Oriented Cursors." *Proceedings of the Human Factors Society-26th Annual Meeting (1982).*, pp. 703–707. Santa Monica, Calif., 1982.

Jones, P. F. "Four Principles of Man-Computer Dialogue." *Computer Aided Design* 10 (1978): 197–202.

Jong, S. "Designing a Text Editor? The User Comes First." *BYTE*, April 1982, pp. 284–300.

Kaplow, R., and Molnar, M. "A Computer Terminal Hardware/Software System With Enhanced User Input Capabilities." *Computer Graphics*. New York: ACM, 1976.

Kelly, M. J., and Chapanis, A. "Limited Vocabulary Natural Language Dialogue." *International Journal of Man-Machine Studies* 9 (1977): 479–501.

Kintish, W. "Comprehension and Memory of Text." *Handbook of Learning and Cognitive Processes*, Vol. 6, edited by W. K. Estes. Hillsdale, N. J.: Lawrence Erlbaum Associates, 1978.

Krebs, M. J. "Design Principles for the Use of Color in Displays." *1978 SID International Symposium Digest of Technical Papers*. Los Angeles, CA: Society for Information Display, 1978, pp. 28–29.

Ledgard, H.; Whiteside, J. A.; Singer, A.; and Seymour, W. "The Natural Language of Interactive Systems." *Communications of the ACM* 23, No. 10 (October 1980): 556–563.

Liebelt, L. S.; McDonald, J. E.; Stone, J. D.; and Karat, J. "The Effect of Organization on Learning Menu Access." *Proceedings of the Human Factors Society—26th Annual Meeting (1982)*. Santa Monica, Calif., 1982.

Loftus, E. F.; Freedman, J. L.; and Loftus, G. R. "Retrieval of Words from Subordinate and Supraordinate Categories in Semantic Hierarchies." *Psychonomic Science*, 1970, pp. 235–236.

Malone, T. W. "Heuristics for Designing Enjoyable Human Interfaces: Lessons from Computer Games." *Proceedings: Human Factors in Computer Systems*. Gaithersburg, Md., March 15–17, 1982.

Martin, J. *Design of Man-Computer Dialogues*. Englewood Cliffs, N. J.: Prentice-Hall, 1973.

Miller, D. P. "The Depth/Breadth Tradeoff in Hierarchical Computer Menus." *Proceedings of the Human Factors Society—25th Annual Meeting (1981)*. Santa Monica, Calif., 1981.

Miller, I. M. "A Tutorial in Computer Graphics. "*Proceedings of the Human Factors Society—23rd Annual Meeting (1979)*. Santa Monica, Calif., 1979.

Miller, L. A., and Thomas, J. C. "Behaviorial Issues in the Use of Interactive Systems." *International Journal of Man-Machine Studies* 9, No. 5 (September 1977): 509–536.

Miller, R. B. *Human Ease-of-Use Criteria and Their Trade-offs*. TR 00.2185. Poughkeepsie, N. Y.: IBM Corp., 12 April 1971.

Morgan, H. L. "Office Automation Project—A Research Prospective." *Proceedings of the National Computer Conference*, 1976, pp. 605–610.

Neal, A. S., and Emmons, W. H. "Operator Corrections during Text Entry with Word Processing Systems." *Proceedings of the Human Factors Society—26th Annual Meeting (1982)*. Santa Monica, Calif., 1982, pp. 625–628.

Nemeth, C. *User-Oriented Computer Input Devices.* Masters Thesis. Chicago, Ill.: The Institute of Design, Illinois Institute of Technology, 1982.

Nickerson, R. S. "Man-Computer Interaction: A Challenge for Human Factors Research." *IEEE Transactions on Man-Machine Systems*, MSS-10, No. 4 (December 1969).

Reed, A. V. "Error-Correcting Strategies and Human Interaction with Computer Systems." *Proceedings: Human Factors in Computer Systems.* Gaithersburg, Md., March 15–17, 1982.

Rehe, R. F. "Typography: How to Make It More Legible." Carmel, In: Design Research International, 1974.

Robertson, P. J. "A Guide to Using Color on Alphanumeric Displays." *IBM Technical Report*, TR 12.183. December 1979.

Roemer, J., and Chapanis, A. "Learning Performance and Attitudes as a Function of the Reading Grade Level of a Computer-presented Tutorial." *Proceedings: Human Factors in Computer Systems.* Gaithersburg, Md., March 15–17, 1982.

Rosenberg, J. "Evaluating the Suggestiveness of Command Names." *Proceedings: Human Factors in Computer Systems.* Gaithersburg, Md., March 15–17, 1982.

Scapin, D. L. "Computer Commands Labelled by Users versus Imposed Commands and Their Effect of Structuring Rules on Recall." *Proceedings: Human Factors in Computer Systems.* Gaithersburg, Md., March 15–17, 1982.

Schneiderman, R. *Software Psychology.* Cambridge, Mass.: Winthrop Publishers, 1980.

Schoonard, J. W., and Boies, S. J. "Short-Type: A Behavioral Analysis of Typing and Text Entry." *Human Factors* 17, No. 2 (1975): 203–214.

Smith, D. "Faster Is Better—A Business Case for Subsecond Response Time."*Computerworld*, 1983.

Stewart, T. F. M. "Displays and the Software Interface," *Applied Ergonomics*, September 1976.

Tedford, W. H.; Berquist, S. L.; and Flynn, W. E. "The Size-Color Illusion." *Journal of General Psychology* 97, No. 1 (July 1977): 145–149.

Tinker, M. A. "Prolonged Reading Tasks in Visual Research." *Journal of Applied Psychology* 39 (1955): 444–446.

Treu, S., ed. "User-Oriented Design of Interactive Graphics Systems." *Proceedings of the ACM. SIGGRAPH Workshop,* October 14–15, 1976, Pittsburgh, Pa. New York: ACM, 1977.

Vartabedian, A. G. "The Effects of Letter Size, Case and Generation Method on CRT Display Search Time." *Human Factors* 13, No. 4 (1971): 363–368.

Vitz, P. C. "Preference for Different Amounts of Visual Complexity." *Behavioral Science* Vol. II, 1966, pp. 105–114.

Wason, P. C., and Johnson-Laird, P. N. *Psychology of Reasoning: Structure and Content.* London: Batsford, 1972.

Watson, R. W. "User Interface Design Issues for a Large Interactive System." *AFIPS Conference Proceedings* 45 (1976): 357–364.

Weinberg, G. M. *The Psychology of Computer Programming.* New York: Van Nostrand Reinhold, 1971.

Wright, P., and Barnard, P. "Just Fill in This Form: A Review for Designers." *Applied Ergonomics* 6 (1975): 213–220.

Wright, P., and Bernard, P. "Asking Multiple Questions About Several Items: The Design of Matrix Structures on Application Forms." *Applied Ergonomics* 9, No. 1 (1978): 7–14.

7

Electronic Meetings and Other New Communication Technologies

Today's office and society are dependent upon communications. Office automation technologies are opening whole new vistas in our abilities to communicate with one another. They are freeing people from joint presence in time and space. But they are also limiting the physical manner the communication may take.

Human communication is characterized by a lot of things. One is the variety of human senses applied to the process. Spoken words, for example, are only 30 percent of the communication process. The remainder are the unspoken: gestures, facial expressions, the proximity sensed, and touches felt. Person-to-person communication also satisfies a basic social need. Being around others is stimulating and provides needed feedback.

The limitations imposed by the new technologies are causing behaviorists to ask a variety of questions. These questions include:

- Are the new communication methods a psychologically acceptable substitute for face-to-face communication?
- Are the results obtained worse, equal to, or better than those yielded by face-to-face communication?
- Will use over an extended period of time eventually have behavioral or social consequences?

The new technologies take many forms. The commonality is a physical communication medium of some form. One variable is the breadth of human senses that can be applied to the process. Another is the physical proximity of one person to another. This section will discuss these new technologies in terms of their behavioral implications. It begins with a look at the human sensing mechanisms and their relationship to communications. It next describes some alternative behavioral roads that may be followed (either consciously or unconsciously chosen), some broad implications imposed by the technology, and the criteria by which the new communication media will be judged—the face-to-face conference. Finally the new technologies themselves are considered. These include:

- audio teleconferencing;
- audiographic teleconferencing;
- video teleconferencing;
- computer conferencing;
- electronic message systems;
- voice message systems;
- telecommuting and working alone.

Human Senses and Communication

The major human senses are sight, hearing, and touch, with smell and taste playing smaller roles. The more senses that are utilized the greater the amount of information that can be absorbed and processed by the human information-processing system. As more senses are applied, however, the chances for information overload are increased. As fewer senses are utilized, the variety of communication cues are reduced. The information available to make decisions and take action is also reduced. The quality and diversity of data available for processing is greatest in the face-to-face meeting, as all five senses are utilized. In a video system only two receptors are available (sight and hearing), and in an audio system, one.

Certain senses are better equipped to handle certain kinds of information. The eye is most sensitive to the spatial arrangement of things, the ear to sequentially ordered auditory signals. The eye can make extremely fine discriminations of spatial arrangements while the ear's spatial sensitivity is poor. The eye, however, has sluggish time sensitivity.

Information communicated over a medium must be compatible with the capabilities of the sensing mechanisms of the receiver. Complex or unfamiliar spatial concepts, for example, would be difficult to communicate in an audio teleconferencing situation.

It is interesting to note that the skin has the ability to distinguish time nearly as well as the ear, and its spatial discrimination is superior to that of the eye. Its use in communications may be underused. For a good discussion of teleconferencing and information theory, see Ryan (1981).

The New Communication Technologies: Promises and Pitfalls

The new communication technologies offer much promise: improved communications, greater independence and freedom of choice, an enlarged social sphere, and greatly increased human productivity. Like anything, however, there is an opposite side, a darker and more frightening one. This negative aspect is characterized by enhanced miscommunication, technology dependence and addiction, social illiteracy, and, ultimately, accelerated human burnout. In addition to all the promises, the pitfalls must also be considered. The path to be followed, and the ultimate results, must be in the direction we wish it to lead. The end must be worthwhile in terms of human values. If not, what will we have achieved? And why? The choices the new communication technologies are leading to are discussed in the following sections.

Improved Communication or Miscommunication?

The electronic speeds at which information can be widely dispersed can inform an entire population almost instantly. In 1788, when Captain Cook discovered Australia, the folks back home heard of it two months later. Today, a world leader dies and everyone knows within hours. What if Cook had sent the flagship home with the good news of Australia's discovery and instructions to collect colonists and return, then realized he was not in Australia at all, but in the Antarctic? He had the recourse of sending after the flagship: "Row harder boys, we'll catch her before she hits the channel!" The time for reflection and to take action to prevent a chilling problem that was available to Cook does not exist for us.

The speed and breadth of information dissemination through today's technologies is awesome. But what if the information is incorrect or objectionable in some way? The time to undo the harm is greatly diminished. The reaction of the recipients may also be hasty. Their responses may not be tempered by time to reflect and undo. Problems quickly escalate. Bad information abounds and expands. Others join the fray. Is this improved communication or miscommunication? Can we have one without the other? How do we build in the necessary controls to achieve accelerated communication while minimizing the effects of miscommunication?

Greater Independence and Freedom of Choice or Dependence and Electronic Addiction?

The physical links to the office are being unshackled. The sphere of contacts is no longer limited to those who share the same floor or building. The freedom to work when we want, where we want, and with whom we want, is becoming a reality. A 3 AM conference from one's bedroom with colleagues in Norway, Japan, and New Zealand is not unusual today. Greater independence and freedom of choice is an important communication by-product.

Now consider these instances:

- The system goes down and you feel helpless and frustrated.
- You feel ineffectual using the typewriter or telephone.
- Someone calls you on the telephone and you are annoyed.
- Someone walks into your office and you are annoyed.
- Computer metaphors such as "message you" and "clear buffer" creep into your spoken words.

Unlikely? Not so, say Hiltz and Turoff (1982). Twenty percent of the 500 scientific users of an electronic information exchange system showed these behavioral characteristics. Hiltz and Turoff characterize these people as suffering "network addiction."

What will be the result of the new technologies? Will it be greater independence and freedom of choice—or terminal dependence and network addiction? How do we maintain the proper human perspective in our lives?

An Enlarged Social Sphere or Social Illiteracy?

Expanding one's communication capabilities opens up possibilities for a greatly enlarged social sphere. These expanded contacts can foster personal gatherings and relationships, yielding a greater variety and richness in one's social experiences. On the other hand, the addictive nature of technology can cause a person to shun all human contacts, ultimately leading to social illiteracy. Witness the behavior characteristics exhibited by those studied by Hiltz and Turoff (1982). Also, witness the increasing number of young people walking the streets of our American cities shutting out the din and clatter, and fellow human beings, with the beat of loud music produced by the technology of the earphones clasping their heads.

Greater Human Productivity or Faster Burn-out?

The goal of the new communication technologies—and of automation in general—is greater human productivity. It promises freedom from the mundane, routine, and time-consuming, permitting energies to be focused on that which is creative, difficult, and demanding. The assumption is that hitherto wasted time will be used in a much more efficient and effective manner.

The human body, however, is not like a machine, capable of steady and continuous performance. It ebbs and flows, alternating periods of sustained activity with relaxed intervals while batteries are recharged. Often this recharging occurs simultaneously with the mundane or routine task. An occasional trip to the photocopy machine provides a restful interval from a period of intense concentration. It also results in a change in one's sensory environment which could conceivably trigger a new chain of mental associations, thus releasing new ideas. Elimination of opportunities for needed rest breaks and their replacement with more intense activities could lead to faster burnout as the sustained activities telescope into one another. Forty years of work activities compressed into twenty-five may not, from a health standpoint, be a desirable achievement.

The new communication technologies, then, require us to walk carefully along the path toward the promised land at the end. The challenge will be to avoid the pitfalls that lie in wait. Otherwise, the price for mankind is immense.

Electronic Meetings

Communication is a complex phenomenon. While electronic meetings ease the task of making contact, they do not reduce the complexity of group communication. Actually, the opposite occurs. Communication is influenced by a variety of assumptions, perceptions, and rules. Many are unconscious and have been derived from *in-person* meetings. So when electronic meetings are held, the old rules for meetings need to be revised. Unfortunately, few new rules exist. They are now being developed both on a trial-and-error and experimental basis as we slowly move ahead. Electronic meetings, also called teleconferencing, are changing the nature of the business meeting in a number of ways. These changes can influence the possibilities for both good and bad outcomes. They are linked to the following fundamental characteristics of electronic meetings that all the media possess (Johansen et al. 1979):

Physical separation. The most obvious characteristic is the physical separation of meeting members. Meetings may cross time zones or even days. Communication is affected in several obvious ways:

- Objects cannot be exchanged.
- The sense of touch disappears.
- Interpersonal distance cues are lost.
- The fear of violence is eliminated.
- The cultural context is eliminated.

There can be no coffee break chit-chat, luncheon discussions, or dinner socializing. Distance also precludes the sense of social presence within a meeting. Short et al. (1976) believe that social presence is an important key to understanding person-to-person telecommunications. All meetings are also out of context in the sense that they do not take place within a single culture or place. There is no home team and little understanding of how one's culture may influence other meeting participants. Words spoken may be the primary focus of attention with little understanding of the context within which they are said.

Access to remote resources. Because of convenience, cost, and accessibility, many people are routinely excluded from face-to-face meetings. Geographic distance remains a major barrier. Teleconferencing opens up meetings to a wider group of participants, and the increased knowledge that these people possess.

Simple increases in the number of inputs do not guarantee increased effectiveness, however. A wider diversity in views may make agreement more difficult. Information overload may also develop. Easy accessibility to experts may work in other ways. Dialogue may be stifled as expert opinion is relied upon to solve all problems, even though the experts' view of the problem may be narrow or limited.

Limited communication channels. Teleconferencing will, to varying degrees, filter out body language and the nonverbal cues supporting the communication process. The information accepted into the decision-making process could become limited to that which easily fits into the communication channels.

The narrowness of the communication channel might foster a false sense of consensus, encouraging *groupthink* (Janis 1972). Instead of pulling in all directions, participants may produce too much cohesiveness, screening out divergent ideas. The result could well be lower quality group decisions or conclusions.

While limited communication channels may result in intentions not being perceived accurately, they may also filter out unnecessary and distracting signals. The result of this may well be increased effectiveness.

Control of group interaction. Electronic meetings are more easily controlled. Someone must determine who can be seen, who can speak, and how loud they will come across (as volumes are turned down to reduce shouting). Rigidly controlled interaction inhibits the informal interpersonal communication needed to foster consensus and feelings of trust. Sequential information exchanges can oversimplify complex problems, resulting in failure to address the real issues.

On the positive side, control should assist in focusing attention on the task at hand. It would result in greater equality of participation and better adherence to topics and time schedules.

Dependence on technology. Electronic meetings are much more vulnerable to failures in technology. At best, they could slow the whole communication process as a restart occurs. At worst, a system failure could be interpreted as an intentional cutoff, undermining or destroying group trust.

Technology also places restrictions on the physical behavior of participants. Objects like cameras and microphones necessitate more fixed locations, preventing such things as moving chairs about, or walking, and talking. More fixed body postures may also result.

Johansen et al. (1979) feel that the sensitive zones in electronic meetings are the following:

- building and maintaining group trust;
- the recognition and reconciliation of diverse perspectives; particularly those imposed by culture differences;
- the resolution of group conflict;
- the use of outside resources, especially those of experts.

Our review of electronic meetings will follow a standardized format. Based upon research findings and reported experiences with the various media, the perceived behavioral strengths, weaknesses, and implementation usefulness of each will first be summarized. A fuller description will then follow. It begins with a review of the meeting considered the standard by which the remainder will be judged, the face-to-face meeting. This review is an extension of the data and format first presented by Johansen et al. (1979). More detailed descriptions of the research and references will be found in their book.

Face-to-Face Meetings

Strengths

- Protocol and etiquette are well established.
- Permit employment of all sensory communication channels.
- Permit greater information exchange.
- Considered more friendly.
- Perceived as more commanding.
- Generally preferred.

Weaknesses

- Not always necessary.
- Not always convenient.
- May inhibit communication.

Usefulness

- Permit person-oriented discussion.
- Establish acquaintance with strangers.
- Encourage negotiation.
- Conducive to persuasion.
- Help resolve conflict.

Strengths. The etiquette of face-to-face meetings is well established in the behavioral repertoire of its participants. Whether conscious or unconscious, this etiquette governs meeting conduct and behavior toward others. Since there is physical presence, all sensory communication channels are available to participants.

Face-to-face meetings promote greater exchange of information than other types. There is less time spent maintaining group organization and the spoken word is an efficient mode of transmitting information. Therefore, there are more messages exchanged and more solutions discussed than there can be in other media.

These meetings are friendly in the sense that there is less tendency for a person to inflict pain on a visible victim than one that is invisible. In face-to-face meetings people tend to address their remarks to the group as a whole, while in electronic meetings there is a greater tendency to address individuals or a subgroup. More commanding occurs in the sense that people are more likely to obey commands issued face-to-face than those issued remotely.

Face-to-face meetings are generally rated more favorably than audio or video meetings. People tend to be more confident in their perception of others.

Weaknesses. Face-to-face meetings may not always be necessary. It is variously estimated that 30–40 percent of all business meetings may be satisfactorily concluded without the physical coming together of the participants. Face-to-face meetings are not always convenient, especially if the participants are widely dispersed geographically.

Communications may be inhibited by visual distractions that impede concentration on the tasks at hand. Meetings may also be dominated by one or a few people, thereby limiting the range of ideas and quality of decisions. Participants may also be more influenced by emotional factors.

Usefulness. Face-to-face meetings are particularly useful for intense, interpersonal tasks. The most important aspects of social interaction are transmitted by the visual channel. Thus meetings dealing with conflict, negotiation, persuasion, establishing acquaintance, and other people-oriented discussions, are best held face-to-face.

An audio teleconference is the traditional telephone conference call. Compared to other electronic conferencing modes, telephoning is easy, well understood, less costly, and accessible to most people. A major advantage is that it employs a simple and primary communication medium, the spoken word. Its major disadvantage is that the communication recipient is able to employ only one sensory mechanism, hearing.

Strengths. The telephone is a familiar and easily used technology. It permits rapid point-to-point communication anywhere in the world. Media that employ voice communication are much faster than writing and typing, in both number of words transmitted and speed of problem solution. Audio promotes accurate communication. Accuracy in the transmission and reception of information is not affected by the absence of vision. Participants feel they pay more attention to what is said, and the assessment of other people is at least as effective as that occurring face-to-face. More controlled participation results because meetings are more orderly or businesslike, and individuals who dominate face-to-face meetings have less opportunity to do so.

Audio Teleconferencing

Strengths

- Familiar technology.
- Rapid communication.
- Accurate communication.
- Controlled participation.

Weaknesses

- Personally demanding.
- User expectations negative.
- Less personal.
- Less productive.
- Unsatisfactory for interpersonal commmunication or complex tasks.
- Order of speaking difficult to determine.
- Identity of speaker difficult to determine.

Usefulness

- Information exchange.
- Simple problem-solving.
- Idea discussion.
- Giving orders.
- Holding briefings.
- Maintaining contact with others.
- Interviewing.
- Promotes short, regular meetings.
- Short cut among people who already know each other.

Weaknesses. Audio meetings are personally demanding. They are more tiring and require more time to organize and control. Varied speech accents are also more difficult to understand over the telephone. People typically have negative expectations about audio meetings. People are skeptical about them and most often prefer modes containing video as well.

Audio meetings are perceived as less personal. Important nonverbal cues are missing and more hostility may be evident, as participants cannot be seen. *We* and *they* tendencies are more likely to develop between participating groups. Audio may also be less productive than other media. Audio groups spend less time on task-related discussion, fewer words are spoken in a given time period than in video and face-to-face, and fewer and less complex recommendations result.

Audio meetings are not satisfactory for tasks stressing interpersonal communication or dealing with complexities. Examples include resolving conflicts, persuading others, resolving disagreements, negotiating, forming impressions of others, and getting to know others. In some intense communication situations, however, subtle advantages may exist for the side with the strongest case, or where visual images are distracting to more important substantive considerations. Participants also feel it is easier to get a point across without lengthy debate than in face-to-face meetings.

Audio conferences do not always afford clear indications of who is to speak next, whether a statement has been understood, or which voice belongs to whose body. In face-to-face meetings, regulators of information flow include facial expressions and gestures. They regulate speech rate and provide feedback indicating comprehension or agreement. Information flow regulators increase significantly in audio conferencing as the number of participants increases. Such issues as identity and location of participants, getting the floor, assuring understanding, sticking to the topic, and obtaining agreement require their heavy use (Ryan 1981). Nutall (1973), in a study of telephone behavior, found that 33 percent of the utterances were of the information flow regulation type.

Usefulness. In general, audio conferencing is most useful when meetings are short and regular, and among people who know one another. As mentioned, they are not useful for tasks stressing interpersonal communications or those that are complex. Effective use has been found for those situations described above.

Audiographic Teleconferencing

Audiographic teleconferencing adds to the voice a limited amount of visual aids including electronic blackboards, remotely controlled projectors, slow-scan television, and facsimile equipment. As such, it blends most of the characteristics of a pure audio conference with some of the video version.

The strengths of audioelectronic meetings remain the same. The basic weakness that is addressed is the capability of dealing with more complex issues. Addition of a non-person-oriented visual dimension enables participants to deal with spatial relationships in a much more satisfactory manner.

A video teleconference adds the dimension of human sight. Information is presented and shared in television format, either on a standard television monitor or on a large-screen wall display. Video teleconferencing has been in experimental use since the mid-1960s; one of the earliest applications was American Telephone and Telegraph's *Picturephone.*

Strengths. The addition of seeing greatly expands the complexity of what can be handled. The more complicated the task, the more visual channel is likely to make a contribution and to be perceived as necessary. A person's detection, information processing, and retention are greater when both the

Video Teleconferencing

Strengths

- Adds sensory dimension of seeing.
- Satisfactory for a wider range of business talks than audio teleconferencing.
- More effective than audio for such interpersonal communication situations as forming impressions of others, providing feelings of social contact, noting reactions.
- Promotes orderly meetings.
- Promotes faster meetings.
- Promotes polite relations.
- Positive new user reactions.

Weaknesses

- Precludes total sensory awareness.
- Less satisfactory for communicating with strangers or people of differing ranks.
- Less effective than face-to-face communication for tasks stressing interpersonal relations.
- Lacks sense of personal contact.
- Physical movements may be misinterpreted.
- Uncomfortable for some participants.
- Susceptible to the *Hollywood syndrome.*
- May inhibit personal communication style.
- Requires more rigid control.
- Studio distance can diminish incentive.

Usefulness

- Information dissemination.
- Information or opinion exchange.
- Status reporting.
- Asking questions.
- Generating ideas.
- Training.
- Coordination.

auditory and visual senses are used. Eye contact is an important part of the communication process, providing cues for feedback and synchronization of speech. There is also less uncertainty when participants in a meeting can be seen.

In general, video teleconferencing is found to be much more satisfactory than audio for a wide range of business tasks. Among them are interpersonal communication situations, such as forming impressions of others, establishing feelings of personal contact, and noting reactions. It has also been found to be as useful as face-to-face meetings for information exchange tasks.

Video conferencing promotes more orderly and faster meetings than face-to-face conferencing. People also tend to be more polite when others can be seen. New users typically have positive attitudes toward its use.

Weaknesses. Since a video teleconferencing link can only represent the auditory and visual dimensions of sensory awareness, it precludes activities involving other senses, which are normally associated with face-to-face meetings. Nonverbal communication theory indicates that the absence of these other dimensions explains some of the difficulty experienced in getting to know someone over a telecommunications link (Argyle 1967). This is why participants are more likely to prefer a face-to-face meeting if they have not known each other previously.

While better than audio communication for some interpersonal tasks, video teleconferencing is less effective than face-to-face meetings for many interpersonal communication situations. Questionable uses include bargaining, persuasion, and solving conflicts. Video conferencing is sometimes perceived as lacking a sense of personal contact with others and lacking a feeling of presence.

Duncanson and Williams (1973) rated the productivity, efficiency, and enjoyability of video as opposed to face-to-face conferences. Figure 7-1 summarizes their findings. Face-to-face conferences slightly exceeded video teleconferencing for all criteria, but video was considered an acceptable alternative for many kinds of meetings.

One critical video teleconferencing problem is that some people feel uncomfortable on camera, probably because of the studio atmosphere of some systems. Johansen et al. (1979) speculate that such an atmosphere may cause a *Hollywood syndrome* that emphasizes the presentation, not communication. In the extreme, deliberate deception is possible, complete with makeup kits and hired actors. The physical arrangement of studios could also cause resentment or discomfort if one studio seems more imposing or glamorous than another.

Another potential problem with video teleconferencing is that seeing physical activities out of context may cause errors in interpretation. A dramatic arm movement may appear as a shaken fist. Off-camera conversations among those sharing a studio could raise the suspicions and hostilities of those operating alone.

Video meetings are also perceived as less private than audio or face-to-face meetings. Personal communication styles, such as referring to notes while talking, may also be limited. A video teleconference must also be controlled to a much greater degree than a face-to-face meeting. Orders of speaking and time limits must be more firmly orchestrated imposing studio-like techniques that may be bothersome or poorly understood. Rigid programming aimed at

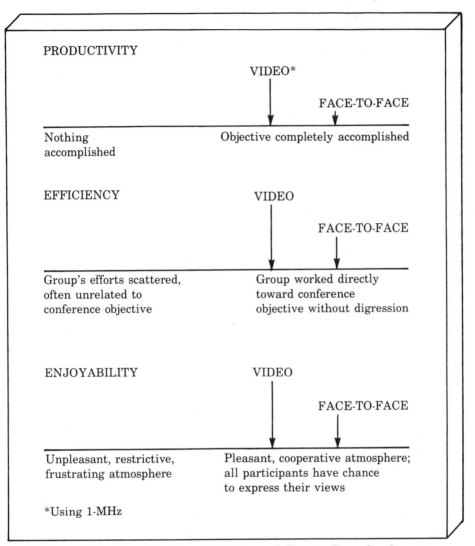

Figure 7–1. Mean Ratings of Video and Face-to-Face Conferences

creating more orderly meetings, may stifle creative and more free-form discussion. Lastly, even a small distance to a video studio can inhibit the use of video teleconferencing systems.

Usefulness. Video teleconferencing is perceived as satisfactory for a wide range of tasks, including exchanging information or opinions, asking questions, solving problems, coordinating, and generating ideas. Many business meetings can and will be satisfactorily completed using teleconferencing. As the depth of the meeting increases, and interpersonal relations fulfill an important role, the usefulness of teleconferencing diminishes. This leads Albertson (1974) to conclude that video communications will never equal face-to-face communications and that there may be an optimum point beyond which technological improvement is self-defeating.

Computer Teleconferencing

Strengths

- May be asynchronous.
- Improves continuity of communication.
- Provides written record.
- Permits time for reflection.
- Inhibits verbosity.
- Promotes equality of participation.
- Enhances candor of opinion.
- Focuses on communication content.
- Does not require highly specialized skills.

Weaknesses

- Less efficient.
- Self-activated nature can inhibit use.
- Demanding: training needed; poor design and/or information overload possible.
- Vulnerable to position and status stereotypes.
- Vulnerable to poor human interface design.
- Vulnerable to information overload.
- Cannot satisfy need for immediate verbal communication.
- Requires strong leadership.
- Weak sense of interpersonal interaction.
- Unsatisfactory for interpersonal relations tasks.

Usefulness

- Information or opinion exchange.
- Asking questions.
- Generating ideas.
- Staying in touch.
- Coordination of activities.

Computer teleconferencing (also called simply computer conferencing) utilizes the power of the computer and a communication network to enable people to interact with one another. It most commonly employs the capabilities of a visual display terminal on which messages may be created and distributed to one, some, or all participants in a conference setting. While all participants may confer at the same time, a computer conference, unlike other teleconferences, does not require this. Conferees may come and go, safe in the knowledge that all communications will be available for perusal as time and situations permit. Thus synchronization is not a condition for successful computer teleconferencing.

Strengths. The asynchronous nature of a computer teleconference does away with the big headache associated with getting the attention of a large number of people at the same time. Other workday activities need not suffer because of requirements imposed by the conference. Similarly, the conference need not suffer for the opposite reason. Continuity of communication can be maintained in spite of other pressures as time and space dependencies are eliminated. And problems can be dealt with as they arise.

A significant advantage of computer conferencing is that it leaves a written record, thus supporting faltering memories. An electronic library is at one's fingertips. There is some evidence that written requests are more persuasive than those issued verbally. (A counter argument holds, however, that people may hesitate to put everything in writing, therefore inhibiting free and open communication.) Computer conferencing also permits time for reflection on topics under consideration. People can unobtrusively drop out of the conference to do research and gather background information, then rejoin with a better-prepared response.

Computer teleconference communication is also less verbose. Spoken communications are characterized by a greater number of words and unruliness, hand-drafted communications are much more efficient in terms of number and focus of words. Equality of participation is also fostered. The amount of participation is more nearly equal for keyboard-constructed communication than it is for spoken communication. (This equality may also be construed as a weakness if one considers the quality of the communication as well.)

Eliminating the ability to see other participants enhances candor of expression and focuses attention on the content of the communication. Sometimes, disturbing visible facial features or behavioral mannerisms of individuals may impair concentration on the topic at hand. While computer conferencing does require interacting with a computer, lack of typing ability is not a barrier to effective participation. Typing skill has not been found to be an advantage. Unlike video teleconferencing, no acting or performing skills are required.

Weaknesses. Written communication is less efficient than other media. Many more spoken than typed messages can be exchanged in the same period of time, and problems take longer to solve in the written mode. It has also been found that it is often more difficult to focus discussions in computer conferencing. Weeks et al. (1974) compared the problem-solving speed of collaborators communicating through voice and hearing as opposed to that of individuals using typewriters. They found the following:

- Conversing face to face solved problems three and a half times faster than communicating through typewriters.
- Subjects sent two to eight times more messages when speaking than when typing.
- Speaking subjects communicated six times as many words per minute as typing subjects.

Chapanis et al. (1977) compared three modes of communication in problem solving: oral (with and without being face to face), handwriting, and typing. They found that:

- Face-to-face conversing solves problems requiring exchange of factual information about twice as fast as communicating by typing or handwriting.
- The oral mode is fast, but wordy. It uses about thirteen times as many words as other modes.
- Simple voice communication is about as good as face-to-face voice communication.
- Sentences in hard copy (that is written, typed, or printed) tend to be longer than oral sentences. Perhaps this is because a visible record of the communication frees the communicator from the restrictions of short-term memory, making it easier to construct longer sentences.

Also, as previously mentioned, people may sometimes be reluctant to say certain things in writing. Finally, typing forces a person to focus attention on the keying task, whereas other things can be done while one is talking.

Computer conferencing can also be demanding. Training is necessary, some new skills must be learned, and there is susceptibility to visual and postural problems associated with the use of visual display terminals. There may also be vulnerability to poor design of the human-machine interface. Bad design can cause inefficient or ineffective use and even discourage participation entirely. Information overload for conferees is also a potential problem. The volume of information generated can be overwhelming, resulting in confusion rather than clarification. Since the nature of the computer conference often requires voluntary participation, regular participation may be difficult to encourage and enforce. Pressures for participation evident in a group setting may dissolve in the privacy of one's own office. Therefore strong leadership is required. Computer conferencing also does not satisfy the strong preference that managers and executives have for immediate verbal communication.

There may also be vulnerability to stereotypes associated with one's status and position within an organization. Typing at a computer may be regarded as something done by underlings. Imperfections, of course, do not exist. Typing may expose imperfections (such as a spelling weakness) whose existence might better remain submerged.

Computer teleconferences sometimes promote a weak sense of interpersonal interaction. Immediate feedback is not always received and this may be frustrating. Questions or requests may go completely unanswered. A lack of group interaction may be felt. Feelings of trust and security can be weakened if surrogates or stand-ins have access to communications. No guarantee exists that you are talking to who you think you are talking to. A careless word or comment may have destructive consequences.

Usefulness. Computer conferencing, like other teleconferencing modes, is not satisfactory for tasks needing inputs from the broad range of human senses. Activities focusing on interpersonal relations, bargaining, resolving disagreements, persuasion, and getting to know someone would best be handled face to face. It is, however, well suited to activities involving management of technical information. Information exchange, staying in touch, and coordinating technical projects are a few tasks that may be well handled by this medium.

Travel and Electronic Meetings

A significant perceived advantage of teleconferencing is its ability to reduce or eliminate costly and time-consuming travel. Various estimates indicate that 30–40 percent of all business meetings can be satisfactorily replaced by one electronic medium or another. Whether or not travel is actually reduced is difficult to assess, however.

To many workers travel is a desirable perquisite. A meeting in a distant city followed by a leisurely dinner with colleagues is a strong enticement for getting away for a few days. A Bell Canada study (Livingston 1983) found that for frequent business travelers (fifteen or more trips a year) only 45 percent preferred to reduce their travel. For the infrequent traveler (five or less trips per year) those preferring to reduce travel numbered only 16 percent. Some studies report a general decrease in travel expenses (Pomerantz 1982) or savings of 15–29 percent (*Computerworld* 1983), while others indicate that sufficient data are not yet available to reach a conclusion.

In her summary of teleconferencing as a replacement for travel, Albertson (1974) concludes that teleconferencing:

- does replace some travel;
- prompts more meetings than would otherwise have occurred;
- directly involves many more people in the communication process than traveling does;
- does not completely eliminate face-to-face meetings;
- makes long-distance communication more feasible, thus resulting in more communication, which itself generates travel.

What we may conclude is that, in general, not enough is yet known about the complex relationships between the transportation and communication sectors of modern society.

Teleconferencing Guidelines

General

- People should know each other or have a peer group relationship.
- There must be a strong leader or chairperson.
- The meeting topic should be compatible with the medium employed.
- The group should be cohesive and share a sense of common purpose.
- A clear written agenda should be provided before the meeting.
- The meeting site should be free from noise and distractions.
- The meeting should start on time, run on time, and end on time.

Audio

- Audio meetings should include no more than eight to ten people.
- Each person should introduce himself or herself (in order to anchor the sound of each voice).
- There should be frequent pauses to allow interruptions.

Design guidelines for electronic meetings remain few, since experience with the various media is limited and experimental research is not extensive. Based on what is known so far, however, the guidelines summarized above provide a good starting foundation.

General. Since it is difficult to get to know one another electronically, meeting participants should know each other or have a peer group relationship. If meeting participants do not know each other, a face-to-face meeting prior to the electronic meeting would be desirable. If this is not possible, an exchange of personal fact sheets and photos should at least be carried out.

A strong leader or chairperson is essential. This person should prepare the meeting plan, assure that it is implemented, introduce participants, take up the slack in the conversation, and stimulate participation by all. The leader should also maintain continuing commitment to the electronic meeting. (If the meeting is a computer conference, however, between-meeting commitments should be by telephone, not by the computer.) The leader should also foster the sense of sharing a common purpose. Addressing each participant by name will help do this.

Meeting topics should also be compatible with the medium employed. Tasks stressing interpersonal relations are not suitable for all media and the materials to be discussed may not suit all communication channels.

Before the meeting a clear written agenda should be provided to all participants. The agenda should describe the meeting's objectives, topics, and time schedule. Meeting locations should also be free of noise and other distractions. Electronic meetings are more susceptible to jamming and noise interference than the face-to-face variety. Finally, meeting schedules should be adhered to, starting and ending promptly.

Audio conferences. Stockbridge (1980) provides some useful additional guidelines for audio meetings. He first suggests that they should include no more than eight to ten people. He then suggests that people should introduce themselves to familiarize participants with the sounds of their voices, and that speakers should also pause frequently to allow for interruptions. He further suggests that speakers should talk for no more than ten to fifteen minutes, that interruptions should be encouraged, and the layout of the room should be in an arc, rather than in rows as in classrooms. An arc encourages greater participation.

Electronic Meetings: A Conclusion

Since the path of teleconferencing still remains relatively uncharted, one's approach must be cautious. We still know very little about this technology. Based upon our review, however, the following tentative conclusions appear warranted:

- Teleconferencing is appropriate for the exchange of information and factual materials.
- Meetings requiring interpersonal skills and where nonverbal expression and reaction visibility are important do not appear to be good candidates for teleconferencing.
- The level of information complexity at which a teleconferencing system becomes undesirable is not known.
- The possibility of substituting teleconferencing for face-to-face meetings is ultimately affected by user willingness to forego the peripheral advantages of face-to-face exchange.
- The impact of teleconferencing on meetings may depend more upon changing human perceptions of what is socially acceptable than measurable characteristics of the communication device itself. Learning to use the device in the technical sense is usually not difficult. But behavioral adaptation may take time.

Electronic message systems (also called electronic mail) enable a person to create, edit, address, and transmit messages in electronic format. They also permit incoming messages to be read, forwarded, filed, and so on. Using an electronic message system is similar to using a computer conferencing system. The vehicle and methods may, in fact, be identical. The distinguishing feature

Electronic Message Systems

Strengths

- Fast.
- Asynchronous.
- Prevent interruptions.
- Provide written record.
- Facilitate wide message distribution.
- Do not require highly specialized skills.
- User reaction positive.

Weaknesses

- Not suited to lengthy communications.
- Foster breakdown of institutional hierarchies.
- Etiquette not established.
- Message receipt and reply not guaranteed.
- Do not alleviate poor communication habits.
- Vulnerable to participant communication needs.
- Can foster escalating problems.
- Invite information overload.
- May violate privacy.
- Susceptible to entrapment.
- Standardization issues unresolved.

is more one of intent than definition. A computer conference implies a group of people exchanging messages pertaining to a common topic or objective. An electronic message is simply a substitute for a telephone call or letter.

The focus of attention in this section is the electronic message system itself. Many organizations have installed these systems for practical or experimental use, and the behavioral implications are just beginning to surface.

Strengths. Electronic message systems improve communication by eliminating the time-dependent nature of traditional forms of message exchange. Neither sender nor recipient need be immediately available in order to successfully complete the communication. Furthermore, these systems neutralize the intrusive nature of phone calls which so often come at inopportune times.

Since there is a written record, human memory fallibility is less of a problem. Communications are taken more seriously because a written audit trail is established. Electronic message systems also facilitate wide distribution of communications since a few keystrokes can cause things to go in many directions, up and down, as well as sideways in the corporate structure.

Electronic message systems do not require highly specialized skills. As mentioned earlier, several studies have concluded that typing ability does not influence problem-solving abilities. Johansen et al. (1980), in describing another study, indicated that the message patterns (their numbers and lengths) of nontypists do not differ significantly from those of more practiced typists.

Finally, user reactions to these systems are usually positive.

Weaknesses. Memos and letters are better suited to electronic messaging than reports or large documents. Panko (1981) estimates that 70 percent of the messages will be one page in length and the remainder between two and five pages. Document lengths will be limited until easier scanability is achieved.

Some tendency for institutional hierarchies to break down in using electronic communications has been noted. It is easier for electronic communication to go farther than it should without proper approval than paper communication. Palace guards can find it difficult to control who gets to the boss. In addition, people can easily send copies of electronic messages to innumerable individuals, thus demanding the attention of many more people than a paper message would have required. Junk mail can more easily proliferate with electronic media.

To solve these problems of direction, vigilance can be built directly into system software. A difficulty with this solution, however, is that needed communication should not be impeded, and the line between needed and unneeded communication is thin and often changing.

Electronic messaging is championed as a replacement for the telephone call and the business letter, both of which are steeped in usage etiquette, either conscious or unconscious. Telephone etiquette tends to be informal, warm, and personal, while the business memo is more formal and impersonal. Electronic messaging, a cross-fertilization of both, is now developing its own etiquette.

The inhibiting factor in using telephone etiquette in electronic messaging is keying constraints. A kind word or   phrase requires some effort, and voice inflections cannot be simulated. On the other hand, the more stilted language of the business letter may seem redundant, due to the greater immediacy of responses and freedom from the need of memory joggers. In many cases a simple *yes* or *no* is all that is required, but such brief responses may imply a coldness that is easily misinterpreted.

As the medium strives for its own etiquette, situations requiring delicate interpersonal diplomacy can become a straitjacket. This has led Johansen et al. (1979) to conclude that electronic messaging " . . . provides potentially effective technical structures for controlling group interaction, but few of the familiar social structures. Training people to use the system will be technically easy but socially difficult."

Feedback on the receipt of an electronic message does not always exist. A message may go unread because it is not retrieved, is lost, or the recipient is on vacation. With a telephone message, feedback such as *not here* or *on vacation* will probably occur. The system also will not alleviate poor communication habits. Those who don't return phone calls probably won't return electronic calls, but they are more likely to read messages. Messages that were previously piled on desks, in baskets, or in dog-eared file folders will probably accumulate, safely out of sight and mind, on a disk. Worthless information may abound.

Electronic message systems are also vulnerable to the communication needs of participants and to poor human/machine interface design. If system participants have no need to communicate, system disuse will result. If the system is not easy to use, its usage will be discouraged.

A participant's failure to properly understand a message can cause quickly escalating problems. The volume of information the system can generate easily and maintain may overload the user. Extensive communication to higher management can place pressure on lower management. Bosses know all the problems in the area. Pressures on subordinates can also increase because now the boss never forgets.

Electronic messaging also raises privacy issues by exposing participants to new kinds of scrutiny. At a personal level, it can expose weaknesses in grammar and spelling that were previously masked by secretaries. Will fear of such exposure discourage a person from using a system? Will the exposed weaknesses influence performance appraisals?

On a broader scale, electronic mail can monitor mailboxes and determine when messages are read. The problem, however, is whether it is anyone else's business when people read their mail. Another concern is sender control—whether senders should be able to erase a letter after a recipient has read it. This amounts to keeping one's hands in the envelope after the letter is sent.

Privacy of the communication itself must also be considered. It has been found that people will not use a system if management can review their messages. Corporate policies, then, must consider privacy controls that will ensure effective system usage.

Some people may never get over a negative attitude toward typing, and require an intermediary to perform typing chores. These intermediaries may not be able to participate in friendly chats on behalf of the people they represent. Their inappropriate responses or lack of response can cause hard feelings (since recipients may not know with whom they are actually communicating), and eventually impede communication.

An electronic messaging system may entrap or addict some people. A terminal might become too much a part of their life. In the extreme, it becomes a twenty-four-hour companion that never goes away and that could make a person a slave to the machine. There is no place to hide from one's job or one's boss.

Finally, standardization issues have not been resolved. Modern systems only work with small user populations, and addressing large populations is a problem. Inconsistencies in message structure, the user interface, and message delivery impose a wide range of severe usability constraints.

Other concerns. One concern about electronic messaging systems is whether users will use soft copy displays in lieu of hard copies of memos and letters. The only evidence to answer this question is provided by an experimental study by Engel et al. (1979), which found that soft copy fulfilled both informational and personal security needs of system users in most cases.

Still another expressed concern is that electronic messaging seems to put good speakers at a disadvantage—they lose out to good writers, fast typists, and bad listeners. This remains to be seen.

Electronic Messaging Guidelines

Design

- Verify that there is a need to communicate.
- Involve at least eight to fifteen people.
- Encourage informal usage.
- Design for individual differences in system use and personality characteristics.

Usage

- Be careful of message tone. Err on the side of formality and courtesy.
- Maintain the proper perspective. The person in your office comes first, the one on the telephone second, and the electronic message last.
- If comments are solicited on a long document, follow up with a paper copy.
- Retain copies of messages you send.
- Immediately acknowledge all messages received.
- Respect other people's privacy by:

  - exercising care and control in sending messages;
  - resisting the temptation to read the screen of the person you are visiting.

- Never try to weasel into another's office electronically.
- Occasionally send pleasant messages.

Design. Electronic message systems are most successful when there is a genuine need to communicate. If participants have no need to communicate, they will reject the system (Bair 1979). Communication traffic generators include common goals, tasks, management, and interests. And usage generates more usage (Morgan 1979). Morgan also recommends that for a system to have a chance of succeeding, eight to fifteen users must participate.

Informal applications of electronic messaging systems have also been successfully developed, including communication of social events and gossip (Driscoll 1979). These help establish familiarity with the technology in an enjoyable and relaxed manner, rather than being a formidable electronic barrier to formal tasks. Initial electronic mail usage for such communication has been found to be wordy and nonproductive, but when the novelty wears off, communication diminishes.

Electronic messaging systems should also reflect the needs of the user. Usage amounts and kinds may require access to differing components. The needs of the casual user will not be the same as those of the heavy user. The system should be flexible enough to handle both easily. A system's personality can also be structured to match the varying needs of people.

One system developer has created three distinct personalities. Users select the one they prefer:

- Assertive: It calls you with messages.
- Interrogative: It calls to ask if you want messages.
- Passive: It waits for you to call.

Usage. The etiquette for electronic messaging will slowly evolve. Until it does, we shall have to cope as best we can. Known characteristics of electronic message systems and the implications they have for human behavior, lead one to suggest some basic usage guidelines to make the medium as comfortable as possible for all, at least until we know better. Most of the following guidelines were first put forth by Windt (1983).

Err on the side of formality and courtesy in message tone. Reserve informality for those you know well. Treat guests in your office with the importance they deserve. Avoid nervous eye darts between them and the terminal. Refrain from furtive glances and longing gazes. Avoid swivelling away to answer each message that leaps to the screen. In terms of priorities, the visitor comes first.

If comments are solicited on a long document, follow up with a paper copy. Few people can edit someone else's material on the screen. A red pencil is still a satisfying tool for many. Retain copies of messages sent, especially those needing a reply. It may save embarrassment weeks later when the answer returns and you have forgotten the question. Immediately acknowledge all messages received, even if you are unable to provide a full answer. The sender's mind will rest a little easier.

Respect other people's privacy. Send only that which is needed and relevant. Don't send messages to the company president unless he or she asks you to. When in another's office, resist the temptation to look at that person's screen. What is there may be personal or sensitive, thereby creating an awkward or embarrassing situation. Never try to weasel into another's office electronically. The closed door or telephone busy signal should be respected. Be satisfied just to line up in the queue.

Finally, occasionally say something nice. A pleasant greeting or words of praise are appreciated by all. This is a reminder that *high touch* is compatible with *high tech*.

Voice messaging systems are computer-based methods of recording and transmitting spoken messages. The message is spoken using a standard tele-

Voice Message Systems

Strengths

- Familiar and common technology.
- Fast.
- Asynchronous.
- Prevents interruptions.
- Provides spoken record.
- Assures message integrity.
- Facilitates wide message distribution.

Weaknesses

- Unsuited to long communications.
- Accessed separately from telephone.
- Message arrival not always evident.
- Vulnerable to information overload.

---

phone handset and stored in digital form. It is then forwarded to one or more recipients. In essence it is the auditory twin of the electronic message system.

Strengths. Voice messaging systems share many of the advantages of electronic message systems, including being asynchronous, preventing interruptions, and facilitating wide message distribution. They do, however, have two significant advantages over their twin: speed and technology familiarity. Speaking is much faster than keying. There is a terminal in most offices, hotel rooms, airports, and on many street corners. This terminal contains no mysteries. People are not afraid of it and have mastered its use.

The recorded spoken word, when compared to traditional handwritten notes for phone calls that miss their intended recipient, offers other advantages. Voice recordings are protection against garbled messages due to misunderstandings or poor handwriting. Moreover, a tone of voice (of urgency or anger) is a clue that is often lost in a written or keyed note.

Weaknesses. Voice messages, like electronic messages, are not suited to long communications. Voice message scanning, while it can be accomplished, is not performed as efficiently as visual scanning of keyed messages.

Many voice systems have to be addressed separately from the telephone. If a call is made and the line is busy, instead of being switched automatically to the voice mailbox, the caller will have to redial in order to leave a message. This is costly and time consuming. Another common problem is that the user cannot always be notified that a message is waiting. The person must call to see if any are there. Frequent calls to discover that there are no messages can be frustrating.

Finally, voice mail systems are also subject to information overload. A proliferation of stored messages can create *junk voice*, the verbal version of junk mail. Systems that automatically purge files after certain time periods, however, may erase messages before they are heard by all recipients.

For a good review of voice messaging systems, see Shea (1983).

Telecommuting

A centralized place of work is a relatively recent phenomenon. For 10,000 years people labored in their own cottages and fields, moving to the factory only when the division of labor promised increased productivity. Cheap energy, a relatively low value on personal time, and difficulties in moving and storing information, sustained this direction for more than two centuries. Today, however, all this is rapidly changing. Energy is no longer cheap, personal time has greater human value, and paper as a medium of information exchange and storage is being replaced by electronics. Coupled with the high cost of workspace, and its inefficient use (the typical office is fully staffed only one-third of the time), the necessity and desirability of a centralized office is greatly reduced. Why not move the workplace to the home? (After all, many homes remain empty precisely the same hours the office is full.) Thus was born the concept of telecommuting—extending the traditional office into the confines of one's personal living space. It really is not such a radical idea at all—many professional workers have blended home and work for years as have those who have surrounded themselves at the kitchen table in the evening with "…a few things brought home from the office."

Estimates of the percentage of office workers who could effectively telecommute range as high as 50 percent. Telecommuting has awesome benefits. But it has frightening sociological and behavioral implications as well.

Advantages of Telecommuting

Increased productivity. Telecommuting frees one from the tyranny of time, transportation, and location. The workday can begin only minutes after leaving one's bed, and end just minutes before retiring. It is common in many large metropolitan areas to spend up to two hours commuting each way to the office. Work can be accomplished when one is inspired, even at 2:00 AM. The disruptions and distractions of the busy office disappear. People are available when they previously couldn't be, such as while commuting, after hours, or during business trips.

Expanded available workforce. The ability to hire and retain employees in many of today's highly competitive office jobs is increased. Eliminating geographical restrictions and providing work flexibility are important factors to many potential and existing workers. The home-bound labor force is also made available. Mothers of young children, the aged, or the handicapped are readily utilized.

Advantages of Telecommuting

- Increases productivity by:

    - creating a longer work day;
    - permitting activities when inspiration strikes;
    - eliminating disruptions and distractions;
    - reducing nonavailability times.

- Expands available work force by:

    - removing geographical restrictions in employment;
    - providing flexibility;
    - tapping the home-bound labor force.

- It reduces operating and overhead costs.
- It conserves energy.
- It provides more personal time.

Disadvantages of Telecommuting

- Isolation, which includes

    - lack of social contacts;
    - absence of feedback;
    - absence of idea fertilization.

- Professional anonymity.
- Blurring of distinction between home and work.
- Lack of management acceptance.
- Difficulties in measuring productivity.
- Legal, logistical, and personnel problems.

Reduced overhead and operating costs. Office space, and the costs associated with it, are reduced. So are those dealing with employee relocations.

Conserving energy. Fuel consumption for transportation and for heating and cooling the office are greatly reduced. The impact on automobile gasoline consumption could be dramatic—saving of more than 300,000 barrels a day. A person reducing driving by 500 miles a month could save from $50 to $100 a month.

More personal time. The worker benefits from having more personal time. Commuting times eliminated can be used to fulfill personal needs, including leisure, recreation, hobbies, or just being with one's family.

Disadvantages of Telecommuting

Isolation. People are social creatures and to many the work experience is a social outlet. The coffee klatch, or just plain gossip, can be stimulating and refreshing. For many workers, the social organization of the workplace is a means of enhancing self-esteem and of satisfying needs for companionship, affiliation, and belonging (Harvey 1967). The social atmosphere of the office satisfies a real need for those looking for a mate. We also need the physical presence of others to share in the nonverbal forms of communication which make us human, visible, and real to each other. The spontaneity and richness of human-to-human communication is missing for the isolated worker. The presence of others is reassuring, and feedback is a much-needed commodity.

One implementor of an electronic mail system found that messages from remote workers demonstrated gradually increasing anxiety and misunderstanding. Their messages eventually became paranoid. The company found that when workers reached that point, it was best to bring them back temporarily to the work society. Thus, it appears that eliminating social feedback may have a critical impact on some people. Imagine sitting in the office for weeks and never seeing another soul!

Cross-fertilization of ideas is also lacking. We learn from each other, and isolation inhibits professional development. For some, visibility around the office is the key to getting ahead.

Blurring of distinction between home and work. Home to many is the refuge from the trials and tribulations of work. The work personality is formal and less personal, that in the home less formal and warmer. What are the implications of carrying the work personality home? of continuous proximity to one's spouse? of continuing visibility in one's office? Will domestic roles—as parents, wives, or husbands—interfere with jobs? Will jobs interfere with domestic roles? Some suggest that the result will be increased stress, and a strain on marriages. Forced proximity may not guarantee happiness. Spillover of work-related issues into the home may not be healthy.

Interruptions and distractions of a different sort may also occur. Schedules may have to be shuffled to meet family demands. (The garbage collector always comes on Thursday afternoon!) Interruptions of well-meaning people under three feet tall, and shaggy critters with wagging tails, may have to be fended off, thereby pleasing neither the concept of work life or of family life. Powers of self-discipline may be severely tested.

Management acceptance. Managers see their presence in the office as necessary for direction, motivation, and morale (Carne 1972). Many are accustomed to having armies of people under observation and control. They are trained to supervise people who sit at desks and look as if they are working hard. Eight hours at one's desk equates to eight hours of work. Often the attitude exists that people who work at home are not really working.

The work of many executives, managers, and workers is directly concerned with interpersonal communication, most of it face to face. Evidence already presented indicates that many of these interpersonal relationships are not conducive to technologically-mediated communications.

Difficulties in measuring productivity. How can the telecommuting worker be monitored? How can productivity be measured? Are specific outputs and deliverables a desirable criterion? Is invisible monitoring through the terminal acceptable? This, of course, conjures up images of *Big Brother*.

Legal, logistical, and personnel problems. Telecommuting includes its share of legal, logistical, and other personnel problems. Manning (1981), in describing the Control Data Corporation working-at-home program, mentions several.

Legal questions are associated with state and federal regulations as well as corporate policies and procedures. They include:

- security of equipment;
- privacy of customer information;
- municipal ordinances and neighborhood businesses;
- insurance—both theft and liability;
- eligibility and selection criteria as related to home accommodations;
- tax matters;
- worker's compensation insurance limitations.

Logistical problems include:

- space scheduling and long-range facility requirements;
- selection of equipment to support remote employees;
- supply of office supplies, telephones, and so on;
- distribution of internal and external communication, mail, job postings, and so on;
- provision of clerical and secretarial support.

Additional personnel problems to be considered include:

- providing satisfactory formal meetings and informal communication;
- eligibility and selection criteria for homework assignments;
- education and training of staff;
- employee/labor relations issues.

These are but a few of a wide range of problems that must be addressed.

Experimental Telecommuting Programs

Many organizations—among them Control Data Corporation, Mountain Bell of Colorado, and the Continental Illinois National Bank of Chicago—have installed pilot telecommuting projects. The results, so far, are mixed. Control Data Corporation (Manning 1981) found self-rated increases in productivity of from 12 to 20 percent. Telecommuting workers' supervisors agreed with these self-ratings. They reported that one-day increases as high as 200 to 300 percent in some jobs are possible. Mountain Bell reported increases anywhere from 50 to 150 percent (Rifkin 1982). A study conducted at Cornell University (McClintock 1982) found that telecommuting resulted in an overall increase in the output of complex, nonroutine work.

On the other hand, Continental Illinois Bank's program, begun in 1978, was terminated in 1982. The reason given was that it was not cost effective. Too many people were involved in getting information to the home and back to bank officials who had to see it.

In interpreting the results of these studies it must be kept in mind that the participants were selected people performing selected jobs. The issues are complicated and situations specific to each employer. A great deal remains to be learned.

Telecommuting Guidelines

- The worker must want to telecommute.
- The work must be conducive to telecommuting.
- The manager must understand and actively support the concept.
- Others in the organization must understand and support the concept.
- There must be plenty of easy communication.

Control Data Corporation has found a number of factors influencing the success of telecommuting projects. First, the worker must want to telecommute. People who have the option of choosing the work location that best suits their personal or work needs will be more motivated at whatever location they choose. One problem, however, is that people often do not know if they will like working at a remote site. Furthermore, the task must be conducive to being performed outside of the regular office. Enough is still not known, however, about which tasks and jobs best fit telecommuting. Finally, management and those who do not choose to telecommute must understand and support the concept.

Plenty of ready communication to telecommuters is also necessary. The worker must be made to feel a part of the group.

Satellite Offices

Satellite offices—neighborhood offices scattered about the metropolitan area where the main office is located—may yield the best of both worlds for the telecommuting worker. While maintaining many of the advantages of the home (shorter commute, more free time, and so forth), it eliminates some of the more severe disadvantages—such as isolation and the blurring of distinction between work and home. Some feel, however, that this approach would be too costly unless the facility is shared among other organizations (Manning 1981). If this is the case, it may still limit the learning experiences that availability of a lot of professional peers provides.

Long-Term Implications of Telecommuting

These include:
- loosening of the 9–5 workday structure;
- lessened employee affiliation with work;
- greater flexibility in living location;
- more fluid employment situation;
- more flexible organizations; ·
- restructuring of personal relationships and life styles;
- restructuring of the home.

On a longer-term basis, telecommuting has implications which can impact the structure of work, the business organization, life styles, and society as a whole. Some of these were first presented by Albertson (1977). They include the following.

Loosening of the 9–5 workday structure. Work will no longer be confined to traditional working hours. Work and leisure pursuits will provide a more balanced week. Queuing and crowding currently associated with weekend activities like skiing will diminish as leveling throughout the week occurs.

Lessened employee affiliation with work. The corporate logo above the office entrance will no longer be visible, nor will the obvious visual reminders scattered throughout the building of who pays the check. Because job changes will not require physical moves, higher turnover may very well result.

Greater flexibility in living location. Physical proximity of one's home to one's job will no longer be important. Convenience to public transportation or good roads will no longer be necessary. Replacing these will be convenience for personal, recreational, or avocational reasons. Small towns, rural locations, and fair-weather areas will be in much greater demand.

More fluid employment situation. Using hours of work as a basis of payment will be difficult, and people may have to work under short-term contracts, with payment predicated on project completion. Changing jobs will be as easy as dialing a new telephone number on Monday morning.

More flexible organizations. Without having to provide accommodations, employers can adjust employee numbers to changing needs and can easily form ad hoc organizations and task forces.

Restructuring of personal relationships and life styles. Compatibility of husbands and wives will be tested and possibly reshaped by continuing proximity. Continuous exposure to each other's job interests and work circumstances, however, can create a greater bond, making it less likely that spouses will grow apart. The sharing of both job-work and housekeeping would be possible. A husband and wife could even split a full-time job. The criteria for marriage could expand beyond the traditional love attachment to include a variety of work-related issues such as responsibility and self-discipline. Children will be able to observe work-day role models instead of hearing vague descriptions.

Restructuring of the Home. Houses will get larger as population densities decrease due to decentralization. Storage needs will increase as fewer trips into town occur. Work areas may become independently accessible from the outside, and less accessible from the living area, so as to provide a better balance between the two.

1990 and Beyond

Electronic meetings and the other new communication technologies that we have discussed are here to stay. It is a lot easier to move information than it is to move people. As we have seen, the potential benefits to the individual, to the organization, and to society, are immense. We have also seen, however, that innumerable dangers and traps lie in wait. We must not lose sight of what the new communication technologies are for: to increase the productivity of ourselves and our organizations while at the same time expanding our human potential and creating a more fulfilling life. Let us hope that when we look back from our vantage point in the 1990s we will feel that the decisions we made in the 1980s were wise.

References

Albertson, L. A. *A Preliminary Report on the Teleconference User Opinion Questionnaire.* Melbourne: Australian Post Office, 1974. Mimeographed.

Albertson, L. A. "Telecommunications as a Travel Substitute: Some Psychological, Organizational and Social Aspects," *Journal of Communications* 27, No. 2 (Spring 1977): 32–43.

Argyle, M. *The Psychology of Interpersonal Behavior.* Harmondsworth: Penguin, 1967.

Bair, J. H. "Planning for Office Automation." *The Automated Office,* American Inst. for Industrial Engr., 1979, pp. 449–462.

Carne, E. B. "Telecommunications: Its Impact on Business." *Harvard Business Review* 50, No. 4 (1972): 925–933.

Chapanis, A.; Parrish, R. N.; Ochsman, R. B.; and Weeks, G. D. "Studies in Interactive Communication: II. The Effects of Four Communication Modes on the Linguistic Performance of Teams During Cooperative Problem Solving." *Human Factors* 19, No. 2 (1977): 101–126.

Driscoll, J. W. "People and the Automated Office." *Datamation* Nov. 1979, pp. 106–112.

Duncanson, J. P., and Williams, A. D. "Video Conferencing: Reaction of Users." *Human Factors* 15, No. 5 (1973): 471–485.

Engel, G. H.; Groppuso, J.; Lowenstein, R. A.; and Traub, W. G. "An Office Communications System." *IBM Systems Journal* 18, No. 3 (1979): 402–431.

Harvey, L. V. *Interpersonal Communication*, Paper Presented at the Annual Conference of the Australian Psychological Soc., 1967.

Hiltz, S. R., and Turoff, M. "Users Found Suffering 'Network Addiction'." *Computerworld*, 3 May 1982, p. 4.

Janis, I. *Victims of Groupthink*. Boston: Houghton-Mifflin, 1972.

Johansen, R., Vallee, J.; and Spangler, K. *Electronic Meetings: Technical Alternatives and Social Choices*. Reading, Mass.: Addison-Wesley, 1979.

Johansen, R.; Vallee, J.; and Spangler, K. "Electronic Meetings: Alternatives to Face-to-Face Interaction." *Automated Office Solutions*, A20-675. Delran, N.J.: Datapro Research Corp., January 1980.

Livingston, D. "Teleconferencing." *Computerworld OA*, 1983.

Manning, R. A. "Alternate Work Site Programs." *Proceedings, Office Technology Research Group (1981 Fall Meeting)*, Williamsburg, Va., Nov. 1981.

McClintock, C. G. "Study: No Rush to Board Telecommuting Express." *Computerworld*, 11 January 1982, pp. 61–62.

Morgan, H. L. "Office Automation Project—A Research Prospective." *Proceedings of the National Computer Conference*, 1979, pp. 605—610.

Nuttall, E. C. "Analysis of Business Telephone Calls." *Report prepared for the XEROX Corporation*. Norman: University of Oklahoma, 1973.

Panko, R. R. "The EMS Revolution." *Computerworld*, 1981.

Pomerantz, D. "The Ins and Outs of Teleconferencing." *TODAY'S OFFICE*, July 1982, pp.66–70.

Rifkin, G. "Working Remotely: Where Will Your Office Be?" *Computerworld OA*, 1982.

Ryan, M. G. "Telematics, Teleconferencing, and Education." *Telecommunications Policy*, Vol. 5, No. 4, December 1981.

Shea, E. "Voice Mail Delivers the Message." *Office Administration and Automation*, March 1983, pp. 43–47.

Short, J. A.; Williams, E. and Christie, B. *The Social Psychology of Telecommunications*. London: John Wiley, 1976.

Stockbridge, C. "Multilocation Audiographic Conferencing." *Telecommunications Policy*, Vol. 4, No. 2, June 1980.

"Videoconferencing Attracts Growing Interest." *Computerworld*, 4 April 1983, p. 31.

Weeks, G. D.; Kelly, M. J.; and Chapanis, A. "Studies in Interactive Communication: V. Cooperative Problem Solving by Skilled and Unskilled Typists in a Teletypewriter Mode." *Journal of Applied Psychology* 59, No. 6 (1974): 665–674.

Windt, J. H. "Forum." *Computerworld OA*, 1983.

8

Equipment

Early Kinds of Equipment

The visible symbol of office automation is the equipment or hardware itself. In the early days of computing, the standard typewriter style keyboard was selected as the mechanism by which people could communicate their needs and desires to the computer. This keyboard was familiar, contained all the necessary keys and characters to construct inputs, and was flexible and versatile. Paired with this keyboard was a hard-copy printer. This printer enabled a user to view the inputs as they were keyed and was also a mechanism on which computer outputs could be written. While slow and frequently requiring highly structured inputs, these devices satisfied many of the needs of the technicians who were the most common computer users.

A significant advancement in the coupling of people and computers occurred when the typewriter keyboard was combined with the cathode ray tube (CRT). Mechanical restrictions were removed and the speed of interaction was dramatically increased as alphanumeric information, lines, and graphics were displayed at electronic speeds. User inputs were greatly simplified and accelerated as electronic editing became possible. The earliest users of these new devices, today commonly called the visual display terminal (VDT), were mostly military personnel. In the early 1960s commercial applications began to appear. Early users included the nation's airlines. There was a certain amount of human engineering of these devices as attempts were made to make the displays more readable and comfortable, and the keyboard touch characteristics compatible with human needs.

In the 1970s new generations of display terminals appeared with more sophisticated capabilities. Resolution improved and techniques for displaying information greatly expanded. Whereas older alphanumeric terminals simply displayed a character of one size and brightness, newer terminals possessed such techniques as two levels of character brightness, upper- and lower-case characters, and dark characters on light backgrounds as well as the reverse. The 1970s also saw a movement toward better human engineering as keyboards were detached from the display tube.

The terminal of the 1980s has been the beneficiary of even greater human engineering as the problems and concerns with their use have escalated. Rotatable and variable-tilt display screens and improved glare-reducing filters are some of these innovations. If the VDT of today does not greatly resemble in many ways its earlier brothers and sisters, it does so in one respect. It is still quite a large device, consuming a significant amount of desk space.

It is expected that CRT display technology will remain the dominant person/computer interface method at least through the remainder of this decade. Capabilities will continue to increase through improved electronic support. Advancements will occur in greatly improved resolution, color, split-screen capabilities, and three-dimensional perspectives.

A significant reduction in terminal size will eventually occur as flat-panel electronic displays with superior resolution become more widely available. Beginning to appear now, these devices may become dominant by the end of the 1980s.

The present style of alphanumeric terminal keyboard has been viewed as the ideal way to communicate with a system for a variety of users. Arranged like the original typewriter keyboard designed by Sholes in the 1870s, it requires a certain amount of learning and practice to achieve skillful performance. Performance levels are limited by the existing arrangement of keys, however, and a variety of other arrangements are perceived as being better for skillful typists or even for hunt-and-peck typists.

It has also been suggested that the alphanumeric keyboard should be replaced by more natural communication methods such as pointing or talking. Screens sensitive to human touch, either by one's finger, a light pen, or a *mouse* on one's desk, are common methods of accomplishing this. These have been implemented with varying levels of success. Actually talking to a computer, and being talked back to by it, is increasing as costs rapidly decline. Limitations in computer recognition of spoken commands and directions, however, will limit widespread application before the end of the century.

The equipment itself has received more attention than most other office design factors because it generally deals with measurable characteristics such as key pressure, phosphor regeneration rates, and display character sizes. Broadly speaking, equipment must be designed within the limits of human sensory awareness, human anthropometrics, and acceptable human behavior.

Visual Display Terminals

Our survey of equipment will begin with a look at the components of the VDT: the unit itself, the keyboard, and the display screen.

Comfort. Critical comfort considerations include a detachable keyboard and adjustable display screen tilt, swivel, and height. These capabilities are

The Visual Display Terminal Unit

A VDT unit must be looked at in terms of comfort, safety, and appearance.

Comfort

- It should have a detachable keyboard.
- The display screen should have a variable tilt and be rotatable.
- The height of the display screen should be adjustable.
- Wires and cables should be positioned for least interference.
- Wires and cables should be flexible enough to avoid entangling.
- There should be no sharp edges.
- There should be no snag, nip, or pinch points.
- There should be no drafts for cooling and it should be well ventilated.
- There should be no cold or warm edges or surfaces.
- It should have a light-diffusing or semi-gloss surface.
- The unit should produce no excessive noise (over 65db) during operation.
- It should make no annoying sounds during operation.
- There should be no vibration during operation.

Safety

- Heat sources should not be accessible.
- Voltage sources should not be accessible.
- Interlocks and safety devices should not be easily defeated.
- The unit must be maintained regularly.

Appearance

- The unit should have sealed surfaces.
- It should not have any collection points for debris.
- It should be free of smudging and smearing.
- It should have a clean and pleasing appearance.
- It should be maintained regularly.

important to permit all users to establish comfortable operating and viewing conditions. Cords and cables should neither interfere with manual tasks nor entangle with one another. Sharp edges, snag points, drafts, cold or warm surfaces, surface light reflections, noises, and vibrations must be avoided.

Safety. Dangerous sources of heat and voltage must not be accessible. Regular maintenance is necessary to keep all elements within acceptable ranges for human use.

Appearance. The unit must convey and maintain a neat, clean, and professional appearance. Sealed surfaces and an absence of debris-collection points will aid this objective. So will surfaces that do not easily smudge and smear. Regular housekeeping maintenance will eliminate problems of appearance as they develop.

The Keyboard

The VDT keyboard is a much-maligned entity. It is accused of being inefficient for the skilled typist and intimidating for the executive. There is some truth to each accusation. It may not always be efficient, and it can be intimidating. Stone (1983) argues that most executives are not intimidated by keyboards as such, but they become irritated with system designers who produce user-hostile and user-unforgiving interfaces for business systems. This argument certainly is justifiable. It can also be argued that, just because we have created badly designed keyboards in the past, the future must continue to produce them. This need not be the case. Keyboards can be well designed, as is being evidenced today. They can also be advantageous. Keyboards can support failing human memories and with simple actions can cause many good things to happen.

The keyboard, then, will surely be around for awhile. What can we do to make it more responsive to our needs and desires?

Components

Keyboards generally contain up to five kinds of keys: standard typewriter, numeric pad, function/transmit, cursor control, and edit keys. The essential kinds of keys are illustrated in Table 8-1. The numeric pad is not essential since numeric keys exist in the typewriter configuration. Any one application may find a numeric pad essential, however.

Usage characteristics of keys also depend upon the application. Generally speaking, however, usage frequencies are as follows:

- HIGH usage:
  - typewriter keys;
  - tab, back tab, back space, return, cursor-control keys.
- MEDIUM usage:
  - numeric pad;
  - up/down left/right cursor-control keys;
  - edit keys.
- LOW usage:
  - function/transmission keys.

The organization of a keyboard should reflect all of these characteristics:

All essential keys. Table 8-1 outlines the essential keys. Keyboards that require simultaneous depression of two or more keys to achieve a result are unacceptable.

Table 8-1. Essential Keyboard Keys

Typewriter
- Standard alphanumeric symbols and punctuation

Edit
- Insert (character and line)
- Delete (character, field, line, and screen)

Function
- At least 10 to 15 that perform common application functions

Cursor Control
- Up/down/left/right
- Tab
- Back tab
- Back space
- Return
- Home

Keyboard Organization

A keyboard should have:

- all essential keys;
- logical groupings;
- discernible groupings;
- priority keys in prominent locations;
- individual control differentiation;
- minimum potential for accidental activation of critical keys;
- no irrelevant keys;
- positions that reflect human habit patterns;
- obvious key states.

Logical grouping. Keys should be grouped by the functions they perform. Those that through long usage have gained standard positions, however, should maintain those positions. For example, tab, back tab, back space, and return are commonly located next to the touch positions.

Discernible groupings. Keys performing different functions should be easily and immediately discernible from one another through separations, colors, lines, or combinations of these.

Prominent location of frequently used keys. Proximity to touch positioning is a prerequisite for the most frequently used keys. Locations should be based on the usage frequency estimations. The most desirable areas for keys, based on their frequency of use, are illustrated in Figure 8-1. This distribution assumes that the keyboard user is right handed, which is the case for seventy-five percent of the population. Also, frequently used single-action keys, such as tab and return, should be larger than other keys.

Individual control differentiation. A key's function must be clearly identified by its label, size, shape, or color.

Minimum potential for accidental activation of critical keys. The *clear* key, for example, must be located where the potential for accidental activation is minimized.

No irrelevant keys. Keys not required for use in an office system should not be on the keyboard. If unnecessary keys are on the keyboard, they should be deactivated and covered with a blank cap.

*Positions that reflect human habit patterns.*Keys within the touch area of the standard typewriter should maintain their normal positions. Up/down/left/right and cursor-control keys should be positioned according to popular stereotypes—up on top, down on bottom, left on left, and right on right.

Obvious key states. Keys that when activated cause the status of the key or keyboard to change (such as shift for upper and lower case) must provide a visual indication of the key's current state, such as an indicator light or a key remaining depressed.

Alphanumeric Keyboards

Most display terminals have alphanumeric keyboards, as designed by Sholes, with the standard typewriter layout (called QWERTY, after the first six characters on the second row). Many studies have shown this arrangement

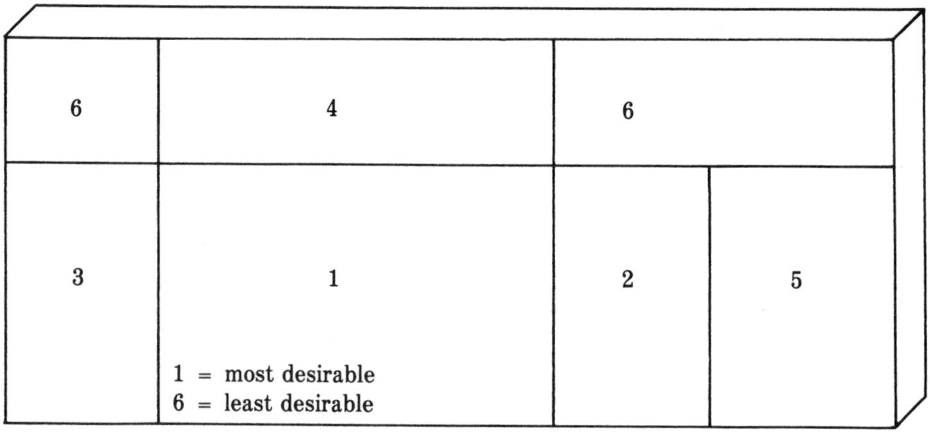

6	4	6	
3	1	2	5

1 = most desirable
6 = least desirable

Figure 8-1.   Desired Key Locations

to be inefficient for skilled typists in terms of speed and error rates. In fact, it was originally designed in 1873 to slow typists down in order to allow time for the keys to fall back into place by gravity. Its common failings as found by Griffith (1949) include:

- Forty-eight percent of the lateral finger repositioning movements are slower one-handed movements.
- Sixty-eight percent of the finger movements necessitate leaving the home row.
- Fifty-six percent of the keystrokes are with the left hand.
- The distribution of keystrokes between fingers is not equitable.

A more efficient layout would meet the following criteria (Cakir et al. 1980):

- Have hand changes between consecutive keystrokes.
- Have the most frequently used letters in the home row and the least frequent in the bottom row.
- Slightly favor the right hand in the distribution of keystrokes between hands.
- Use the little and ring fingers least.
- Avoid wide and awkward spans of fingers.
- Avoid repeated use of the same finger.

The past is littered with keyboards designed more logically, or more efficiently. One of early vintage is the Dvorak simplified keyboard (Dvorak et al. 1936), which rearranged the characters based on frequency of character usage. The Dvorak layout reduces the distance typists' fingers must move from approximately ten miles per day to one mile per day, and its proponents have frequently demonstrated its superiority in learning time and typing speed. While it is well engineered for human use, the enormous retraining program it would require has prevented its acceptance. This may change, however. In early 1983, after twelve years of subcommittee debate, The American National Standards Institute's (ANSI) Board of Standards Review endorsed the Dvorak keyboard as an alternative to the QWERTY design (*Computerworld* 1983a). The state government of New Jersey is also testing this keyboard to see whether it should be implemented. Dvorak died in 1975 at the age of 81, never having achieved success with a product that was available a decade before the first computer. His time may yet come.

Another early alternative keyboard design was that of a German named Klockenberg in 1926. He felt that the one-piece keyboard forced a typist to assume a posture that was unnatural and fatiguing. His solution was to separate the left and right hand components, and angle the bottoms away from one another, as in an inverted V (Λ). Kroemer (1972) found better performance using this keyboard.

A more recent innovation is the Maltron keyboard (*Computerworld* 1983b).

This keyboard is split and places the special function keys, numbers, and the letter *E*, in the middle of a keyboard tilted toward normal hand and body positions. It saves time and motion by dividing keys into more efficient groups.

The keying problems of nontouch typists have also been considered. Since a casual user must often visually scan the keyboard to locate the proper keys, it has frequently been suggested that a systematic alphabetic layout may be preferable for such people. Alas, a number of studies of various alphabetic layouts (Hirsch 1970; Michaels 1971; and Norman and Fisher 1982) have found no advantages for alphabetic layouts over the QWERTY layout for unskilled people. In many cases the QWERTY was actually better. The reasons are only speculative. In spite of ourselves, we all have some familiarity with the QWERTY layout. Perhaps this layout does permit easy visual scanning after all.

Using a computer simulation model, Norman and Fisher (1982) estimated that the Dvorak layout will yield an improvement of about five percent over the QWERTY, and the various horizontal alphabetic layouts will result in a decrement of performance ranging from two to nine percent. They conclude that the expert typist has little reason to choose one over the other based on typing speed.

Numeric Pads

Even the organization of the ten keys on the numeric pad cannot be resolved in a consistent manner. There is the accounting arrangement (reading from left to right, top to bottom–987 654 321 0) and the push-button telephone arrangement (123 456 789 0). Studies have shown that the telephone arrangement is preferred in terms of speed and accuracy (Conrad and Hull 1968). It appears that this arrangement is more compatible with our reading expectancy of left to right and top to bottom.

Function Keys

Terminal keyboard layouts are complicated because of the proliferation of functions they must communicate. In building a computer keyboard, the primary design consideration is whether it should include unique keys that can accomplish requests with one simple keystroke, or whether standard typewriter keys should be used. The standard keys keep their normal identity and often require more than one keystroke to communicate functions. There is no simple answer to this question since both approaches have advantages and disadvantages.

Because they rely on human recognition (which is more efficient than recall) keyboards containing a large number of function keys are easier to learn and use than alphanumeric keyboards. But since they are less familiar than standard keyboards, they can be initially threatening. Also, they are more expensive than standard keyboards and are less flexible for making changes. Many manufacturers have taken a middle road by including some special-purpose function keys with a standard layout. Such keys may have a dedicated function, or change meanings, as defined either by user or system.

Some specific guidelines for defining and using function keys were discussed in chapter 6. Some important reminders are:

- Require only single actions to activate.
- Provide informative descriptions of purpose and, if multifunctional, describe current function.
- Provide logical and systematic arrangements.

An excellent solution to defining current functions for multifunction keys exists in terminals that use the bottom line of the display itself to identify and dynamically change the function-key label as its meaning changes. Care must be taken, however, that the label is correctly related to the key it represents. This is usually achieved through groupings and spacings.

Cursor Control Keys

A cursor is a pointer on the screen. It informs the system and the user where an action is to be taken. It may take the form of a rectangle, underscore, or other similar symbol. Alternative display methods will be discussed in the following section. As a pointer, the cursor must be freely and easily moved about the display screen. A variety of keys may be used to accomplish this, including the tab key, the back tab key, and a group of keys that simply move the cursor left or right, up or down. This latter group of keys can be arranged in a variety of patterns. The significant concern is that they be arranged in a manner that is compatible with expectancies. Desired arrangements, from best to worst, are illustrated in Table 8–2.

Table 8-2. Cursor Control Key Arrangements

Cross	U L R D	Easiest, fewest mistakes for heavy cursor movement situations
Triangle	U L D R	Best compromise between square and cross
Square	U D L R	Use only for infrequent cur- sor movement situations
Straight Line	U D L R	Poorest, last resource

Mice and other crawling creatures. A cursor can also be manipulated by a device on the work surface itself. Called a *mouse* because of the obvious similarities, it propels the cursor in the same directions as it is pushed. Although this device has been around since 1967, (English et al. 1967) it has been a *Star* and *Apple* that have made it popular. Its significant advantage is that it eliminates keystrokes as the driving mechanism.

The principle issue is how many buttons should the mouse possess, one or two? The *Lisa* mouse has a single button used for various functions such as selecting. Some functions require double clicks to be performed. The *two-button* mouse uses one button for scrolling material on the screen and the other for horizontal selection.

While evidence on the mouse's effectiveness and optimum use is still scarce, its ease of use as a position control is obvious. That it requires a suitable flat surface on which to roam is also obvious. Encounters with full cups of coffee and stray paperclips are hazards to be considered. The general consensus is that, in spite of its promise, the jury is still out.

To window or to scroll. Often data on display must be moved. Two choices exist, to *scroll* the data up or down behind a fixed window, or to move the *window* up or down over the fixed data. An astronomer searching the sky through a moving telescope illustrates the window approach. A biologist looking through a fixed microscope moves the slide as he studies bacteria; this illustrates the scrolling approach. In the display of information on a VDT, which is the better approach? Should the scroll key move the window or the data?

Bury et al. (1982) found that the window approach resulted in fewer movements and faster actions. Subjects also preferred the window approach. The answer, then, is to *window.*

Desirable Key Characteristics

Force and travel. Important operating characteristics of keyboards include key force, displacement, activation, and activation feedback. The keyboards of many early computers were built for solidarity, not speed. Early attempts to incorporate these keyboards into display terminals resulted in high error rates when used by touch typists. Experimental studies (Galitz 1965, 1966a, 1966b; Alden et al. 1972) have helped refine keyboard designs to enhance operator performance and eliminate many causes of error.

An important ingredient in keying is the feedback indicating that the key activation has occurred. Feedback enables users to detect errors—mainly omitted keystrokes or duplicate keystrokes. With an increase in the key resistance as the key is pressed and then a decrease as activation occurs, the resulting tactile cue is usually sufficient acknowledgement, especially if it is accompanied by an audible sound as the key hits the bottom. Some manufacturers reinforce the tactile feedback through a mechanically generated click or other sound.

Force and Travel

- The key force range should be between one and three ounces.
- The key travel range should be between .125 and .187 inches
- The key should have a steadily increasing force for 65 to 75 percent of its downward travel, then a noticeable decrease in force.
- Consecutive key entries of 100 microseconds or less should be possible.

Character Display

- Characters should be displayed within 0.2 second of key activation.

Keytops

- The keys should be one-half inch across the top.
- There should be three-quarters of an inch separation between adjacent key centers.
- The keys should be either square or slightly rounded in shape.
- They should have a slightly concave surface.
- They should have a matte surface.
- They should have a nonreflective surface.

Labels

- The labels should be clear, familiar, and unambiguous.
- They should be clearly associated with relevant keys.
- They should be readable from all expected usage positions.
- They should be readable in all expected usage conditions.
- They should be durable and resistant to dirt and discoloration.

As some people find audible feedback assists objectionable, they should be made adjustable.

Character display. Reaction to a depressed key must occur almost immediately on the display. Lags of more than one-fifth second can be very distracting.

Keytops. A matte, slightly concave, keytop surface increases friction and minimizes the chances of fingers slipping off. Nonreflective surfaces make reading easier.

Labels. Many users will visually search the keyboard looking for the proper key. Key labels should be readable from all expected usage positions (on the lap, for example) and in all expected usage conditions (in a dimly lighted room, for instance).

Membrane touch keys. Membrane-switch technology has become increasingly popular in consumer-oriented products. Membrane keys, however, lack any key movement and the corresponding tactile feedback that key activation has occurred. As a result, their use in typing tasks has been restricted. Cohen (1982) has found that for nontouch typists there was little difference in performance between conventional full-travel switches and membrane switches. Touch typists, while initially performing poorly on membrane keyboards, quickly closed the gap with practice. The conventional keyboard, however, still maintains some advantages for the touch typist.

Keyboard Height and Slope

- For adjustable-slope keyboards, the range should be from 10 to 25 degrees.
- For fixed-slope keyboards, the range should be within 10 to 18 degrees.

Various worldwide ergonomic standards recommend that the height of a keyboard's home row should not exceed 1.2 inches (30 mm) above the keyboard's supporting surface. The rationale is that instead of lowering the desk, the keyboard should be lowered to allow a more comfortable operating position. The effective result of this regulation is that the keyboard slope be reduced to five degrees.

Keyboard slope has been the subject of studies by Scales and Chapanis (1954), Galitz (1965), and more recently Miller and Suther (1981), Emmons and Hirsch (1982), and Suther and McTyre (1982). A variety of slopes have been investigated, ranging from the recommended 5 degrees up to 25 degrees. In general, operator performance and preference point to the middle ranges as being best. People with small hands tend to dislike the flat keyboard. The heels of the palm have to be raised and the reach is longer to the back row. Conversely, people with long hands tend to dislike the steeper-angled keyboard.

The results of this research point to the need for adjustability in keyboard slope. An acceptable range to most people would be from 5 to 25 degrees. If a fixed slope is necessary, a point within a range of 10 to 18 degrees would be most desirable.

Palm Rest

- Keyboards should provide an optional two-inch-high palm rest.

To reduce strain, it is recommended that the wrist should maintain an angle of less than 10 degrees while involved in heavy keying. If the design of the keyboard and its height above the floor cause this angle to be exceeded, a palm rest should be provided. As reported earlier, the majority of users in the Grandjean et al. (1982) study found that palm rests increase comfort.

Other Controls

- The power control should be at the front of the terminal, away from keyboard controls.
- Separate display brightness and contrast controls should be at the front of the terminal, away from keyboard controls.

Power controls at the back of the terminal are inaccessible when the terminal is against a wall. And power controls placed near the keyboard controls are prone to accidental activation.

Summing up Keyboards

The operating characteristics of keyboards have improved tremendously in the past twenty years. Current designs allow fast and accurate key entry within limits of keyboard structure by both skilled and unskilled typists. Keyboard layout has, in general, moved past the primitive stage and has significantly improved in the past five years. Logical groupings are more evident, and dynamic labeling of function keys has been a significant advancement. Greater consistency among keyboards is still much needed.

There does seem to be room for substantial revision of the typewriter structure. Litterick (1981) and Norman and Fisher (1982) point out that there is little justification for its present overall size, the staggered arrangement of its keys, and the size of its space bar. They argue for a separation of the left and right sides (as per Klockenberg), a mirror image configuration of keys on both sides, and a smaller space bar.

In short, the keyboard will be with us for many years to come. Its simplicity and accuracy, the richness and variety it permits, the power it unleashes, will make it a useful tool as long as people communicate with computers.

The Display Screen

The display screen, which is the window between a user and the computer system, must permit fast, accurate, and fatigue-free viewing of its contents. Because it generates emitted light, not reflected light as does a piece of paper, its characteristics and design considerations are somewhat different. Some important design parameters are character resolution, phosphor persistence and color, and regeneration frequency.

In the earlier years of computers, poor display characteristics were compensated for by the shorter time periods that they were used and inherent human adaptability. It is only in recent years, as usage frequencies have increased, that their shortcomings have become evident. That is not to say that physical problems experienced by users have gone unnoticed. Some noticeable but harmless visual aftereffects were noted in the 1960s (Galitz 1968).

Display Characteristics

Characters

- A luminance-contrast ratio of from 5:1 to 10:1 between display character and display background should be maintained.
- There should be a minimum 7 × 9 dot matrix construction.
- Character height should be 1/200 of viewing distance.
- Character width should be 50 to 100 percent of character height.
- Character stroke width should be 1/8 to 1/10 of character height.

Character Spacing

- Spacing between characters should be 20 to 50 percent of character height.
- Spacing between lines should be equal to character height.

Stability

- Displays should be free of flicker.
- They should be free of jitter or movement.

Phosphor Color

- The color should be in the yellow-green portion of the visual spectrum.

Display characters must be visible and legible. Visibility is the measure of the ability to differentiate the characters from the background. Can they be seen? Legibility is a measure of the ability to differentiate the characters from one another. What are they? Display design must reflect both of these human needs within the limits of technology.

Characters and character spacing. Visual acuity—the eye's ability to discern and resolve detail—is enhanced if display screens have sharp and clear images. A sharp and clear image is a function of an element's brightness, construction, size, and color. It is generally recommended that luminance-contrast ratio of character and display background be in the range of 5:1 to 10:1 for light characters on dark background displays. This contrast ratio can be affected, however, by the illumination level in the room in which the terminal is used. Thus the measured contrast ratio must be that obtained in the working environment. For dark character on light background displays, the recommended luminance-contrast ratio is 1:3.

A common method of generating characters is through a dot matrix block containing cells. Each cell (or *pixel*) position is capable of being independently illuminated to form the character shape desired. The overall size of the cell block is described by the outer dimensions of the largest character that can be produced within it. This is referred to as *resolution*. The higher the resolution the finer the detail. The smallest size deemed acceptable is 5 × 7. It is felt that a 7 × 9 block is better, yielding larger, well-formed characters, however. McTyre (1982) found no significant difference in legibility between 7 × 7 and 7 × 9 blocks, though. Simple character fonts with no serifs or slanting (italics) are best.

Character size should be at least 1/200 of its viewing distance. Character width, stroke width, and spacing should be as described above for maximum legibility and minimum confusion.

Flicker and jitter. Display characters must be free of flicker and jitter. Flicker is the eye's perception of a change in the brightness level of the displayed characters as the screen's phosphor is refreshed and decays. Flicker can be irritating and cause visual fatigue. The perception of flicker is a function of the phosphor's regeneration rate, persistence, and color, and the size of the display element. For screens displaying light characters on a dark background, a 60-cycle-per-second refresh rate is sufficient to make the eye see the pulsed images as continuous. For displays of dark characters on a light background, however, a 90-100 cycle refresh rate may be necessary.

Jitter is the perception of movement or shaking of the characters. Jitter is also irritating and fatiguing and must not exist.

Phosphor color. Controversy still exists over the best phosphor color for a display screen. It is generally agreed, however, that colors in the amber–green–white portion of the visual spectrum are best. Some researchers have concluded that orange-phosphor CRT terminals are the most soothing to the eye (Dooley 1980). Orange-phosphor display screens that display a yellow character on the amber background offer the following advantages:

- The generally brighter amber background brightens the primary viewing area, counterbalancing somewhat the light entering the periphery of the field of vision. Contrast glare and the need for eye adaptations are thus reduced.
- Because yellow is at the top of the visual sensitivity curve, less brightness is needed to perceive it. This reduces contrast glare problems created by excessively bright characters.
- Yellow is in the middle of the visual spectrum and thus minimizes problems with dual-source light.

Sweden has mandated that all terminal screens be orange (Dooley 1980). In an insurance company study that asked users to compare orange and gray phosphor displays, the orange was preferred by a large margin (Galitz 1980).

Green is also at the peak of the visual sensitivity curve and is preferred by a number of users as well. If green has a disadvantage it is in areas of high illumination where amber is better (Sanders 1981). Green can also leave a pink afterimage in some people's vision. This afterimage is not harmful and will disappear in a short time (Galitz 1968). The safest bet seems to be to choose either the yellow or green range of the visual color spectrum.

Display Cursors

- Display cursors must have distinctive visual features. Acceptable styles are:

  - the box or rectangle;
  - diamond;
  - cross;
  - underline blinking.

- They should not obscure the characters they mark.
- They must be stable.
- They must permit fast and accurate movement.

The display pointer, or cursor, should possess distinctive visual features so that it is easy to find. In general, nonblinking cursors give inferior search performance, but blinking can be distracting. Best overall search performance is with a box blinking at three to four hertz (Vartabedian 1970). The best compromise is a cursor as visually distinct from the background as possible, but not blinking. If the cursor is superimposed over a display character, the character must still be legible. Cursor repositioning should be accomplished quickly and accurately. Cursor movements should be in consistent incremental distances except on displays that have variable character sizes. Then incremental movements should be from character to character.

Antireflection Treatments

Reflections of light from the glass surface of the VDT screen reduce contrast between character and background luminance and make the information more difficult to read. Such reflections also contribute to the visual problems associated with extended VDT use. A variety of treatments are available to reduce reflections. These are summarized in Table 8-3.

Treatments directed at the screen face are all less than optimum. This is because the nature of the display requires that light exit the CRT so that the display images may be read. This exiting light is also affected by the antireflection treatments, resulting in a deterioration of the image quality.

Habinek et al. (1982) studied the effects of the three kinds of treatments (etched glass, micromesh filter, and optical coating) on performance and found all methods superior to untreated glass. Differences in effectiveness between the three, however, were not appreciable. User preferences yielded the same results. The researchers concluded that the choice of a treatment might more

Table 8-3. VDT Antireflection Treatments

Treatment	Effect	Disadvantages
Etched or roughened glass display surface	Scatters and defocuses light from ambient sources	Diffuses character image also, reducing image focus and clarity
Mesh filters on display	Absorbs a large percentage of the light passing through spaces in the mesh	Reduces character brightness and sharpness. Causes image to jump or vanish if viewed from the side
Thin-film optical coating on display surface	Changes physics of the way light reacts on glass, reducing reflectance to as little as 0.5 percent with minimal loss in image clarity	Extremely susceptible to smudging and smearing from fingerprints and dust, reducing image clarity
Terminal hood	Blocks out light sources	Cannot block light sources that cause the greatest problems

properly be based on economic, reliability, and maintenance factors. Their conclusion reinforces the point that efforts might better be directed toward making the environment more compatible with VDT use.

Voice Input/Output

The most common and natural human communication mechanism is speech. Utopia would consist of a computer that understands spoken language as well as a human does and responds accordingly. Or it may be a speech typewriter, into which a person speaks and then receives a perfectly typed manuscript. The technical problems associated with such objectives are not within the scope of this book, but behavioral conditions within today's state of the art are summarized in Table 8-4.

Among the advantages of the voice input are that it is natural, fast, easy to learn, and requires no special skills or tools to accomplish. It is particularly well suited to the executive who spends a great deal of time communicating. Among the disadvantages are the need to control one's speech by pausing—and having to be deliberate can be frustrating. The human voice is also a major contributor to the noise level in offices. A lot of people speaking to their computers could have drastic acoustic implications. Another disadvantage is that effective communication also includes body language. It is estimated that the spoken word is only 30 percent of the process, with gestures, facial expressions,

Table 8–4. Voice Input

Advantages	Disadvantages
Natural	Carefully controlled voice required
Fast	Vocabulary limited
Easy to learn	Ambient noise may reduce accuracy and reliability
No special skills or tools needed	
Allows hands and eyes to do other things	May interfere with other operations or people
	Good communication includes body language as well

and so forth comprising the remainder. The ultimate solution may require an *eye*, or lens, watching us as we speak.

Research indicates the following conclusions. The number of errors expected with hand printing and voice input is about the same. When entering text, speech tends to be a little faster than keying while keying is faster than hand printing. Welch (1980) found that users with some experience could key numbers almost twice as fast as they could read them.

In general, voice input is useful in the following situations:

- when eye-hand coordination is needed;
- when people move around a lot;
- for the handicapped;
- for nontypists.

When using voice input the following points should be observed:

- Keep commands simple and in a conventional language.
- Avoid rhyming commands and one-syllable words.
- Provide feedback to assure accuracy.
- Eliminate background noise as much as possible.
- Provide a reject capability so that inadvertent sounds (such as a cough) can be eliminated.

Speech output, or computer-generated speech, is a more advanced science than speech input. Computers now create output signals sounding like words produced by a human voice. It comes at us over the telephone or if we leave our car door open. Where it is useful and when it is useful is still open to question. The environment is now saturated with voices coming at us from all directions. These voices are often tuned out. A tone or bell may still be a more effective attention getter.

Natural-sounding, continuous discourse requires a lot more work, however. As an interface medium, computer-generated speech has the advantage of being nondirectional. A person's attention need not be directed toward the interface mechanism. But the approach has drawbacks, too. Besides being disturbing to other users, it does not permit:

- graphic displays;
- browsing or skimming of displayed material at one's own pace;
- simultaneous display of multiple alternatives for selection;
- convenient memory aids in the display medium.

Speech output will never entirely replace visual displays, but it may be a useful complementing vehicle, say, for providing spoken directions to interpret a complex display. And for simple or attention-getting communications, stand-alone use may be quite satisfactory. For a more thorough review of voice input/output, see Funk and McDowell (1982).

Touch-Screen Devices

Instead of (1) using the finger to (2) press a key to (3) move a cursor to a desired spot on the display screen, why not eliminate the middle element, the keyboard, and go right to the screen itself? The finger as a pointer is a simple, natural, and direct movement. Consider a speaker explaining a flowchart or graph to a group.

The advantages and disadvantages of the finger are summarized in Table 8-5. The biggest drawbacks are concerned with fatigue issues. Beringer and Maxwell (1982) report that in a study of touch at varying display screen angles, shoulder and arm fatigue was a problem with a display angled at 90 degrees from line of sight, and wrist fatigue was a problem at a 35-degree angle. Other declination angles also created fatigue and use problems.

Touch-screen devices would seem potentially useful for:

- infrequent users;
- naive users;
- short-duration tasks;
- high-stress environments;
- limited workspace environments.

Table 8-5. Touch-Screen Devices

Advantages	*Disadvantages*
Direct visual to tactile control	Less flexible than a keyboard
Minimal eye/hand coordination	Parallax affects touch locations
Symbolic/graphical representation possible	Screen glare
Minimal learning requirements	Physical fatigue from reaching to screen
Minimal errors	Finger obstructs screen view
High acceptance	

Light Pens

Light pens also seem to have distinct advantages as control mechanisms. First, since they too replicate common human activities (such as pointing and writing), they appear simple to use. They are fast for simple input and highly efficient for several successive selections. In addition, they require minimal perceptual-motor skills and no visual scanning to locate a cursor. If properly implemented, they maintain low error rates.

But the use of light pens has never blossomed as earlier predicted, due to several disadvantages (Engel and Granda 1975), mainly because light pens:

- do not feel as natural as real pens or pencils.
- lack precision because of pen aperture, distance from screen surface, and parallax.
- frequently require simultaneous button depression, which can cause slipping and inaccuracy.
- must be attached to terminals, which may be inconvenient.
- cause glare problems if the tube is tilted at a certain angle.
- cause fatigue if the tube is ninety degrees to the work surface.
- are cumbersome to use with an alternate, incompatible method, such as a keyboard.
- are awkward or difficult for left-handed users.
- obstruct portions of the screen when in use.
- are often used for unintended purposes, such as key depression.
- are slow in making multiple, logical, scattered choices.

These disadvantages preclude the effective and effortless use of light pens in many applications.

The Telephone

The telephone is assuming greater importance as a terminal in today's office. With the ability to speak to computers, and the escalating implementation of voice mail, the telephone is assuming other roles than just as a facilitator of long-distance conversations. Its advantages are speed and range (anyone in the world with another telephone is almost immediately available), ease of use (simple key entry or dialing a short combination of numbers), accessibility (it fits on a desk), and acceptability (holding a telephone handset to one's ear during conversation is an established behavior pattern).

But, as Reid (1973) describes, the telephone has disadvantages as well. The first is its storage characteristics. The printed word can be scanned quickly without the aid of special equipment, but extracting information from an audio recording is, by comparison, quite tedious. Another disadvantage is fatigue. Holding a handset to one's ear for an extended period of time can be uncomfortable.

Conclusion

The hardware in today's electronic office is rich and varied. While much recent progress has been made, some formidable problems still exist. First is the viewing difficulties with the VDT. This must be alleviated if an effective, efficient, and comfortable interface is to be found. Second is the large size of many pieces of electronic technology. Their bulk is preventing an effective integration into the workstation. Third, a much better understanding must be achieved of how the various components may be most effectively used and integrated to achieve overall human objectives. If our vision of the future at first appears overwhelming, it seems manageable when we turn around and look at the accomplishments of the recent past.

References

Alden, D. G.; Daniels, R. W.; and Kanarick, A. F. "Keyboard Design and Operations: A Review of the Major Issues." *Human Factors* 14, No. 4 (1972): 275–294.

"ANSI Endorses a Different Keyboard Design." *Computerworld*, 7 March 1983.

Beringer, D. B., and Maxwell, S. R. "The Use of Touch-Sensitive Human-Computer Interfaces: Behavioral and Design Implications." *Proceedings of the Human Factors Society—26th Annual Meeting (1982)*. Santa Monica, Calif., 1982.

Bury, K. F.; Boyle, J. M.; Evey, R. J.; and Neal, A. S. "Windowing versus Scrolling on a Visual Display Terminal." *Human Factors* 24 (4) (1982): 385–394.

Cakir, A.; Hart, D. J.; and Stewart, T. *Visual Display Terminals*. New York: John Wiley, 1980.

Cohen, K. M. "Membrane Keyboards and Human Performance." *Proceedings of the Human Factors Society—26th Annual Meeting (1982)*. Santa Monica, Calif., 1982.

Conrad, R., and Hull, A. J. "The Preferred Layout for Numerical Data-entry Keysets." *Ergonomics* 11, No. 2 (1968) 165–173.

Dooley, A. "Human Factors Challenging Terminal Vendors." *Computerworld*, 11 August 1980, p. 4

Dvorak, A.; Merrick, N. F.; Dealey, W. L.; and Ford, G. C. *Typewriting Behavior: Psychology Applied to Teaching and Learning Typewriting*. New York: American Book Company, 1936.

Emmons, W. H., and Hirsch, R. S. "Thirty Millimeter Keyboards—How Good Are They?" *Proceedings of the Human Factors Society—26th Annual Meeting (1982)*. Santa Monica, Calif., 1982.

Engel, S. E., and Granda, R. E. *Guidelines for Man/Display Interfaces*. IBM Technical Report, 19 December 1975. TR 00.2720.

English, W. K.; Engelbart, D. C.; and Berman, M. L. "Display—Selection Techniques for Text Manipulation." *IRE Transactions on Human Factors in Electronics. HFE-8*, 1967, pp. 5–15.

Funk, K., and McDowell, E. "Voice Input/Output in Perspective." *Proceedings of the Human Factors Society—26th Annual Meeting (1982)*. Santa Monica, Calif., 1982, pp. 218–222.

Galitz, W. O. "CRT Keyboard Human Factors Evaluation." *UNIVAC Technical Report.* Roseville, Minn.: DPD, March 1965.

Galitz, W. O. "CRT Keyboard Human Factors Evaluation: Study II." *UNIVAC Technical Report.* Roseville, Minn.: DPD, February 1966a.

Galitz, W. O. "CRT Keyboard Human Factors Evaluation: Study III." *UNIVAC Technical Report.* Roseville, Minn.: DPD, June 1966b.

Galitz, W. O. "CRT Viewing and Visual Aftereffects." *UNIVAC Internal Report.* Roseville, Minn., 1 August 1968.

Grandjean, E.; Hunting, W.; and Piderman, M. *A Field Study of Preferred Settings on an Adjustable VDT Workstation and Their Effects on Body Postures and Subjective Feelings."* Department of Hygiene and Ergonomics of the Swiss Federal Institute of Technology. Zurich, Switzerland, 22 June 1982.

Griffith, R. T. "The Minimotion Typewriter Keyboard." *Journal of Franklin Institute,* 1949, pp. 399–436.

Habinek, J.; Jacobson, P. M.; Miller, W.; and Suther, T. W. III. "A Comparison of VDT Antireflection Treatments." *Proceedings of the Human Factors Society—26th Annual Meeting (1982).* Santa Monica, Calif., 1982, pp. 285–289.

Hirsch, R. S. "Effects of Standard Alphabetical Keyboard on Typing Performance." *Journal of Applied Psychology* 54 No. 6 (1970): 484–490.

Kroemer, K. H. E. "Human Engineering the Keyboard." *Human Factors* 14 No. 1 (1972): 51–63.

Litterick, I. "QWERTYUIOP—Dinosaur in a Computer Age." *New Scientist,* 8 January 1981, pp. 66–68.

McTyre, J. H. "Legibility Comparison of 7 by 7 and 7 by 9 Dot Character Matrices." *Proceedings of the Human Factors Society—26th Annual Meeting (1982).* Santa Monica, Calif., 1982.

Michaels, S. E. "QWERTY versus Alphabetic Keyboards as a Function of Typing Skill." *Human Factors* 13 No. 5 (1971): 419–426.

Miller, I., and Suther, T. "Preferred Height and Angle Settings of CRT and Keyboard for a Display Station Input Task." *Proceedings of the Human Factors Society—25th Annual Meeting (1981).* Santa Monica, Calif., 1981.

Norman, D. A., and Fisher, D. "Why Alphabetic Keyboards Are Not Easy to Use: Keyboard Layout Doesn't Matter Much." *Human Factors* 24 No. 5 (1982): 509–519.

"Other Keyboards Proposed Over the Years," *Computerworld,* 7 March 1983.

Reid, A. A. L. "Channel Versus System Innovation Person/Person Telecommunications." *Human Factors* 15, No. 5 (1973): 449–457.

Sanders, M. "Executives Consider the Human Side of Computer Systems." *Modern Office Procedures,* December 1981, pp. 56–64.

Scales, E. M., and Chapanis, A. "The Effect on Performance of Tilting the Toll Operator's Keyset." *Journal of Applied Psychology* 38, No. 6 (1954): 452–456.

Stone, J. "Forum." *Computerworld OA,* 1983.

Suther, T. W. III, and McTyre, J. H. "Effect on Operator Performance at Thin Profile Keyboard Slopes of 5°, 10°, 15° and 25°." *Proceedings of the Human Factors Society—26th Annual Meeting (1982).* Santa Monica, Calif., 1982.

Vartabedian, A. G. "Effects of Parameters of Symbol Formation on Legibility. *Information Display* 7, No. 5 (May 1970): 23–26.

Welch, J. R. "Automated Speech Recognition—Putting It to Work in Industry." *Computer,* May 1980.

9

The Office Environment

Most of us spend nearly one-third of our adult lives at work. The workplace can be friendly, comfortable, and aesthetically attractive; or it can be inhospitable to various physical and psychological needs. The experience of most office workers has more often been the latter than the former. The result is that poor environmental design has robbed them of the chance to use their full potential.

Major Considerations of the Working Environment

The roots of the problem are not hard to trace. While human productivity is difficult to measure, the costs of walls and desks is not. Cost-effectiveness formulas for workspace design have traditionally emphasized the cost and paid little attention to human effectiveness. Status or rank in an organization has been a key factor in the design process.

Early in the evolution of office automation some experts were recognizing that office environments must be improved if we were to take maximum advantage of automation (for example, Driscoll 1979). They felt that environmental design might be the Achilles' heel of the office automation movement unless a conscientious effort was made to bring it into step with the new technologies. The environmental problems that have surfaced in recent years are mute testimony to their foresightedness.

Office workers have long been saying that not everything is all right. The results of a Steelcase/Louis Harris survey (*Contract* 1979), summarized in Table 9-1, show the environmental factors some office workers felt were most important to doing a job well. The first item, "ability to concentrate without noise and other distractions" leads a list of many concerns. Seventy-four percent of the respondents felt they could accomplish more work if their working environment were improved.

Table 9-1. The Office Environment

Items workers choose as most important to doing their jobs well:	*Total*	*Percent*
Ability to concentrate without noise and other distractions	429	41
Heat, air conditioning, and ventilation	272	26
Access to the tools, equipment, and materials to work with	261	25
Conversational privacy	240	23
Lighting required for the work to be done	199	19
Ability to adjust the work surface, chair, and storage space to suit the work requirements	157	15
Access to other areas and departments	157	15
Overall lighting	136	13
Storage space for working materials	115	11
Comfort of one's chair	115	11
Working surfaces	115	11
Size	83	8
Visual privacy	83	8
Back support of one's chair	43	4
Safety	31	3

There were 1,047 respondents. The greater totals are due to multiple responses.

A second Steelcase/Louis Harris survey (*Contract* 1980) found that 80 percent of the office workers surveyed felt that their job performance had been adversely affected by environmental discomforts. Also, encouragingly, 84 percent of executives surveyed felt that an improved environment would improve the office workers' productivity.

Fortunately, these feelings are now being translated into actual measured increases in productivity. Springer (1982) found that a properly designed workstation from a human usage perspective yielded performance improvements of 10–15 percent. Dainoff et al. (1982) found a 20–25 percent improvement in performance and a decrease in physical complaints when comparing well and poorly designed workstations.

The importance of environmental influences on the productive use of new technologies is now clear. Following is a review of critical environmental considerations and guidelines to assist in the design of office environments. The topics considered include lighting, acoustics, workstations, office layout, and climate control.

Lighting

A vital component of any office environment is lighting. Poor or improper lighting can cause eyestrain or headaches, while good lighting can increase a person's productivity. In recent years, as office environments have moved toward open landscapes and specially designed workstations and as office energy consumption has become increasingly important, office lighting has become a highly technical and somewhat controversial topic. There are many divergent opinions on the quantity, quality, and type of lighting needed to perform tasks in today's office.

Basically, good lighting is that which fulfills the needs of the worker and causes minimal glare. These rather broad statements have many implications.

Illumination Levels

Ambient light levels in general office work areas have steadily increased since the introduction of electric lighting. Today, lighting levels in many modern office buildings are in the 90 to 150 footcandle range. High levels of illumination are preferable for paper-based operations because, generally speaking, more light results in easier reading of paper documents. A life insurance company found, for example, that substituting 100 footcandle lighting for 50 footcandle lighting improved productivity by 2.8 percent. Productivity improved by 8.1 percent using 150 footcandles. In an office of 100 workers, improvements in worker accuracy resulted in savings of $17,000 using 100 footcandles and $52,000 using 150 footcandles (*Fortune* 1979). As a consequence, many offices are generally over-illuminated. Areas where reading of documents is not important bathe in light supplied for that purpose.

VDTs and office illumination, however, have an adversary relationship. Higher levels of lighting make it more difficult to read the VDT by reducing the contrast of its luminous characters with the display background. The whole concept of office illumination, therefore, is being restructured to confront the problems imposed by the VDT. Illumination level is becoming a more technical and complicated consideration as new technologies emerge.

The following general statements can be made about illumination levels:

- In terms of light direction, the central part of one's field of vision should receive the most light, for both attention-getting and physiological reasons. The eyes have a distinct tendency to turn towards light.
- Once one reaches the age of forty, the amount of illumination needed for seeing increases. For people of age fifty, 50 percent more light is

needed than was required when they were young, and for those over sixty, 100 percent more light is needed.

- The level of illumination should correspond with the needs of the task being performed.

Glare

Another critical factor in office lighting is the amount of glare it causes one to perceive. Glare results when the difference in brightness in one's field of vision is greater than that to which the eye is adapted, thereby causing annoyance. Lesser amounts of glare reduce the ability to discern objects while absolute glare may completely block sight. To be considered good, lighting must be free of glare. Since glare increases faster than the illumination level (doubling illumination at least triples the risk of glare) some glare cannot be avoided at high illumination levels.

The most important factor in reducing glare is providing well balanced luminance contrast between adjacent work areas. Low luminance contrasts cause difficulty in distinguishing fine details, but sharp contrasts can themselves cause glare. To reduce glare, a luminance/contrast ratio of 3:1 between adjacent workstation surfaces is desirable. Positioning light sources so that they are not directly visible and so that light does not reflect directly into the eyes can also reduce glare.

Natural Light

A vital ingredient of the earth's life-support system is light from the sun, or full-spectrum light. For years, people have substituted artificial light for sunlight when the sun is blocked or of insufficient intensity. Recently, photobiologists (those who study light's effects on living creatures) have determined that the wrong kind of artificial lighting can increase fatigue and stress and impair human visual acuity. Often, the consequence is lower worker productivity.

The light these scientists consider proper is full-spectrum sunlight or light from specially designed fluorescent bulbs that closely simulate sunlight. Incandescent bulbs and most fluorescent bulbs are a less-than-optimum light source since they do not produce full-spectrum light. Yet they are commonly used in today's offices.

At Cornell University, students working in a class with full-spectrum fluorescent light experienced a significant increase in visual acuity and less overall fatigue, compared to performance under regular fluorescent light. Russian scientific reports show that full-spectrum lighting in schools helps academic performance, improves student behavior, and lessens fatigue. And in Russian industry it has been demonstrated that, with full-spectrum light, production goes up and absenteeism drops. As a result, many Russian workplaces have mandated this kind of lighting (McCormack 1980).

It has also been found that people favor work environments with windows. Workers frequently indicate that they think daylight is better for eyes than artificial light, and they markedly overestimate the amount of daylight present at their workstations (Wells 1965).

Full-spectrum light can also lessen depression. Scientists at the National Institute of Mental Health report that exposure to this kind of light during the predawn and after-dusk hours effectively lengthens the period of daylight and dramatically buoys people's moods. (Morton 1982).

Light is rated to determine its spectral qualities by the color-rendering index (CRI). Natural outdoor light has a CRI of 100, while the CRI of full-spectrum, fluorescent light is 91. That of standard, cool-white fluorescent light is 68, and other fluorescents are 56. This is a relatively new field of illumination, and further understanding of lighting needs and effects is expected in the future.

Visual Display Terminals and Illumination

The illumination environment in which a VDT is used can never be considered independently of the characteristics of the device itself and the task being performed. Hardware considerations, such as the brightness of the display screen, the use of glare-reducing filters, and rotatable and tiltable display screens, also play an integral role in any solutions. So do such characteristics as whether a person will be using a VDT exclusively or part time, whether or not paper-based materials must be read, and so forth. Environmental solutions should also not be viewed as the solution to problems caused by poor system design. Situations that force a person to look many thousands of times a day between the display screen and source materials are better addressed by improving the system. Lighting solutions will only alleviate a symptom, not address a cause.

Maintain proper luminance-contrast ratios. The luminance-contrast ratio is the difference in brightness of the light emitted from different surfaces. Large contrasts in brightness can cause the eye to adapt to the brighter light and pose difficulties in seeing things that have a much lower luminance. VDTs containing dark display screens and used in bright offices are susceptible to this problem. Sharp contrasts can also cause glare. For best viewing, luminance-contrast ratios in the work area should not exceed 1:3 between the focus of the visual task and immediately adjacent seeing areas (near field), and 1:5 for visual tasks and objects in the peripheral field of vision (far field).

The proper brightness of a room's light in terms of footcandles cannot really be specified without considering luminance-contrast ratios. From a practical standpoint, however, the typical VDT used in today's office would probably find light levels in the 45–65 footcandle range satisfactory for jobs requiring both VDT and paper reading. For jobs involving VDT reading only, 10–15

- Maintain proper luminance-contrast ratios in the field of vision:

  - 1:3 for near field;
  - 1:5 for far field.

- Minimize direct and reflected glare.

  - Position light sources outside of the direct line of sight or screen off those in the direct line of sight.
  - Position light sources so that their emitted light is not reflected from the screen back toward one's eyes.
  - Use many small light sources instead of a few large ones, or use indirect lighting or diffused lighting.
  - Position lights away from work surfaces.
  - Minimize reflectance levels of surrounding room and furniture surfaces. Recommended reflectances are:

    - floors: 20%–40%;
    - furniture: 25%–45%;
    - business machines: 25%–45%;
    - desk tops: 25%–45%;
    - walls: 40%–60%;
    - window blinds: 40%–60%
    - ceiling: 80%–90%.

- Position VDTs so that the display screen is perpendicular to windows.
- Provide window blinds that are horizontal, adjustable, full-length, and off-white or grey in color.
- Surround windows with a light-colored surface.
- Set windows a good distance above the floor.
- Construct outdoor window overhangs.

footcandles would be appropriate. Ways of reducing background luminances, in addition to altering the office lighting, include such measures as changing the terminal's location and repainting the walls. These and other factors are described in the following paragraphs.

Position light sources outside of the direct line of sight. A VDT should never be positioned so that while it is in use a light source is in the user's line of sight. Either eliminate the light source or reposition the VDT so that the light is above and slightly in front of the user. If neither of these is possible, screen off the offending light source through the use of a shield, hood, or visor.

***Position light sources so that their emitted light is not reflected from
the screen back toward one's eyes.*** Overhead fluorescent lights common in
many offices often appear as white bars reflected on the screen's face. These
reflections are frequently responsible for the perception of glare. Desk lights
at adjacent workstations may also be offenders. When locating VDT's in the
office, the positions of existing lights, and their potential for creating reflections
and glare, must be considered. Ideally, the plane of the display screen surface
should be perpendicular to all visible light sources.

***Use many small light sources instead of a few large ones, or use
indirect lighting or diffused lighting.*** Bright artificial light sources can be
subdued by using a variety of techniques, such as by diffusing emitted light
from standard ceiling-mounted fixtures, by replacing ceiling fixtures with
workstation-mounted ambient light, and by providing task lighting either
mounted on the ceiling or directly on the workstation. Advantages and disadvantages of these different approaches will be discussed shortly.

Position lights away from work surfaces. Lights positioned close to
work surfaces are another potential source of glare.

***Minimize reflectance levels of surrounding room and furniture sur-
faces.*** In addition to artificial and natural light sources, a host of other factors
may contribute to glare. These include shiny workstation walls, pieces of paper
or photos attached to workstation walls, and a white shirt or blouse worn by
the VDT user. Anything that causes a contrast in the terminal's viewing
surface must be considered a potential source of glare. To minimize these
potentials for glare, the reflectance levels of surfaces of walls and objects in
the workstation and office should not exceed 20–45 percent for horizontal
surfaces, 40–60 percent for vertical surfaces, and 80–90 percent for ceilings.
Some typical reflectance values for common office wall colors are illustrated
in Table 9-2. Bright objects such as wall graphics and pinups should also be
carefully positioned so that no disturbing reflections are created.

***Position VDTs so that the display screen is perpendicular to win-
dows.*** To avoid window glare, position the display screen surface perpendicular
to windows so that the light strikes the working surface at a right angle. For
particularly bright windows it may also be necessary to place a panel between
the terminal operator and the window.

***Provide window blinds that are horizontal, adjustable, full-length,
and off-white or grey in color.*** The amount of light entering a room may be
controlled through the use of window blinds. Horizontal, adjustable, full-length
blinds permit easy adjustability to compensate for differing conditions of outside

Table 9-2. Representative Color-Reflectance Values

Color Name	Description	Reflectance Percent
Eggshell	White	85
Neutral	Off-white	60
Buttercup	Bright yellow	52
Mushroom	Light tan	44
Pumpkin	Medium orange	31
Apple	Medium red	16
Sky	Light blue	14
Wine	Dark red	4
Eggplant	Purplish-black	3

brightness caused by the sun's position and clouds. An off-white or grey color minimizes the likelihood of the blind becoming a source of reflection and glare.

Surround windows with a light-colored surface. A light-colored surface surrounding the windows will minimize the luminance-contrast ratio between the window itself and the wall.

Set windows a good distance above the floor. Buildings whose architectural design permits locating windows well above the floor will eliminate some of the problems caused by waist-high or lower windows. Other remedial measures may still be necessary, however.

Construct outdoor window overhangs. Bright outdoor light can be reduced by providing outdoor window overhangs. Again, further remedial measures may still have to be taken, however.

The above glare-reduction guidelines are found in McCormick (1976), the *Illuminating Engineering Society (IES) Lighting Handbook* (1972), and a number of other sources. In addition, the IES has adopted a standard procedure for computing the *discomfort glare rating* (DGR) for luminaries and interior lighting (Illuminating Engineering Society 1966). The calculation of DGR ratings for a specific lighting layout takes into account most of the factors that affect visual comfort. A derived DGR can then be converted into a *visual comfort probability* (VCP) for any situation. The scheme for estimating a DGR is complex and beyond the scope of this book. The IES handbook gives a full description.

Task/Ambient Lighting

The ceiling-mounted fluorescent lighting fixtures commonly found in today's offices contain standard refractors which present to the VDT display screen a very bright surface. These bright surfaces are a primary source of the reflections and glare seen by VDT users. What is more, studies have shown that only 20 percent of traditional overhead lighting is directed toward work surfaces. The remaining 80 percent is devoted to lighting for occasional conferences and circulation of people. Since vision is improved when light is directed toward the primary work area, it makes sense to direct more light toward this area, where it is most needed. These factors of increased visual comfort and improved economy have created an interest in task/ambient lighting as a viable concept in the automated office.

Task Lighting

Task lighting provides light only where it is needed. It is accomplished by directing light from ceiling sources toward the workstation, building light sources into the workstation, or providing free-standing or attachable desktop lamps. Task lighting at the workstation consists of fluorescent or high-intensity unidirectional lamps directed at the work surface from a position below seated eye level. Task lighting of this kind, while achieving the aim of directing light where it is needed, has been known to cause the following problems (*Canadian Office* 1978; Brandston 1978):

- Producing bright pools of light that cause eyestrain for individuals who alternate between light and dark areas.
- Producing direct or reflected glare if task lighting is positioned too close to work surfaces.
- Causing eye irritation due to the 60-cycle blink of fluorescent task lamps. (Overhead fluorescent lamps flicker too, although not as noticeably as from a distance.)
- Causing fluorescing (glow effects) of papers and office materials under halide lamps.
- Producing general discomfort for some people in spaces using stroboscopic (noncontinuous) illumination.

The typical under-cabinet-mounted fluorescent task light is often not acceptable for VDTs positioned on the work surface because the light is too far behind the keyboard and annoying hot spots are generated on the terminal enclosure. There is the added disadvantage of ceiling lights used in task lighting having to be redesigned whenever office layouts change.

In general, it appears that permanently affixed workstation task lighting is more appropriately located to the left or right side of the VDT work surface. Ideally, flexible positioned task lighting is the choice since the light can be moved to meet changing needs. The traditional architect's arm lamp illustrates this kind of flexibility (although sometimes the arm may get in the way).

Task lighting should possess the following general qualities:

- The light level should be continuously variable and adjustable by the workstation user. The amount of light can then be matched to the exact needs of each person.
- The position of the light should be flexible on both horizontal and vertical planes. The light can then be exactly matched to the task being performed.
- The illumination pattern should be rectangular or elliptical rather than round. Most documents are rectangular in shape.
- Desk space needed for manual activities should not be taken up by the task light.

The greatest problem with task lighting comes from its complexity. It must be developed in conjunction with many factors, such as: the size and location of the work surface; the size, location, and color of adjacent walls, ceilings, and desk surfaces; and a person's work positions. Light sources located closer to these variables will be more influenced by their design. Subtle design changes may cause enormous lighting changes and problems. Some problems have apparently been created by well-meaning workstation designers who did not understand the complexity of the subject.

If there is a single message about task lighting it is that it possesses significant advantages if applied properly and under the right circumstances. But achieving its benefits requires the help of a lighting professional.

Ambient Lighting

Ambient lighting is the general level of illumination provided in the office or work area. When combined with task lighting, ambient lighting should achieve an overall low-level lighting environment punctuated by brighter task lighting where needed. It is felt that this approach is aesthetically pleasing, more economical, and more truly satisfies the visual needs of office people. Ambient lighting may be provided by lights directed upward toward the ceiling or by the ceiling fixtures themselves.

Upward-directed ambient lighting. Ambient lighting of this kind is affixed to furnishings or pillars above standing eye height and pointed toward the ceiling. It then bounces off the ceiling as indirect light and provides a diffuse low-level general illumination. For low ceilings (eight to ten feet) fluorescent lights are satisfactory. For higher ceilings, mercury vapor, metal halide, or high-pressure sodium vapor lamps may be necessary.

The advantages and disadvantages of upward-directed and ceiling-mounted lighting schemes are summarized in Table 9-3. Nuckolls (1981) reports that studies indicate that this kind of ambient lighting is not energy efficient because of light loss occurring when the light travels upward, is partially absorbed by the 80 percent reflective ceiling, and then travels downward again. Ceiling-mounted lighting has only the direct path to travel.

Table 9-3. Advantages and Disadvantages of Various Kinds of Ambient Lighting

Upward-Directed Lighting
    Advantages
    Moves with furniture and should always be in the proper position.

    Disadvantages
    Some component may still end up within the terminal's offending zone, appearing as a light hazy reflection
    Not energy efficient

Ceiling-Mounted Lighting
1. *Small-Cell (Half-Inch) Parabolic Louvers*
    Advantages
    Low brightness

    Disadvantages
    Ages poorly
    Difficult to maintain
    Not efficient
2. *Large-Cell Parabolic Louvers*
    Advantages
    More efficient
    Easier to maintain

    Disadvantages
    Lamp image visible from directly beneath
    Brighter than small-cell parabolic louvers
    Greater recessing depth necessary
3. *Low-Brightness Lenses*
    Advantages
    Easier to maintain
    Shallower recessing depth necessary

    Disadvantages
    Few suppliers
    Not efficient
4. *Polarizing Lenses*
    Advantages
    Reduces glare

    Disadvantages
    Uneven brightness
    Few suppliers
    Costly

Adapted from Nuckolls, 1981

Ceiling-mounted ambient lighting. Alternatives to the bright standard refractors on ceiling lights include parabolic louvers of varying sizes, low-brightness lenses, and polarizing lenses.

Small-cell parabolic louvers or half-inch parabolic reflectors can be placed between the lamp and the room to reduce the angle of light spread by about 95 percent. Diffuser lenses can be positioned between the lamps and the parabolic reflectors to reduce glare from overhead lights, particularly for workstations located directly beneath the light. Advantages and disadvantages to this design are summarized in Table 9-3. While achieving low brightness, these louvers age poorly, are difficult to maintain, and are not very efficient. Dust and cigarette smoke may build up and affect their brightness and quality, and cleaning is difficult. Light output may drop by 25–40 percent. Efficiency is in the 50–60 percent range.

Large-cell parabolic louvers may have cell openings as large as eleven inches square and eight inches deep. Light brightness is greater than for the small-cell louver, but maintenance is easier and efficiency is improved. Light output will drop only about 15 percent and efficiency may approach 80 percent.

Low-brightness lenses, though not as dark as the small parabolic louver or as efficient as the large parabolic louver, provide a solid enclosure with comparatively low brightness. Since they require a recessing depth of only five inches they may be useful where recessing depth is restricted.

Polarizing lenses produce results similar to those seen when looking through polarized dark glasses.

In sum, task/ambient lighting can help solve office lighting problems posed by VDTs. Extreme care must be taken, however, to provide a quality solution. It is important to avoid shadows, as well as bright and dim spots, poorly directed light, and so forth.

Conclusion

Attention to the lighting needs of workers in office systems is now extremely important. Serious attention to it is warranted by the impact it can have on worker productivity and health. The increasing complexity of office lighting also requires greater involvement of lighting consultants, since proceeding in ignorance may cause more harm than good. More detailed discussions of general lighting and task/ambient lighting may be found in Shellko and Williams (1976), Brandston (1978), LeFort (1978), Shemitz (1978), Marquard (1977), *Canadian Office* (1978), and Nuckolls (1981).

Acoustics

Technology has roared into the modern office with a clatter and a bang. In the Steelcase/Harris survey mentioned earlier, office workers indicated that their ability to concentrate without noise and other distractions has a strong effect on how well they do their jobs. But there is inconclusive evidence as to whether moderate noise levels affect general work performance. There is no concrete evidence to date concerning the adverse effects of general noise levels on reaction time, or the learning of simple tasks, or on the results of intelligence and coordination tests. There are, however, indications that certain noises may affect performance on such complex tasks as those calling for: (1) vigilance (Broadbent 1958; Jerison 1959); (2) skill and speed (Roth 1968); (3) a high level of perceptual capacity (Boggs and Simon 1968); and (4) complex psychomotor tasks (Eschenbrenner 1971).

Recent research also indicates that how we perceive noise depends upon our attitudes as well as on decibel level. The degree of irritation people feel appears to vary greatly depending upon how predictable the noise is and how necessary it seems to be. Evidence also suggests that noise can reduce a person's sociability and sensitivity to the needs of others (Cohen 1981).

While the effects on work performance are not fully established, the annoyance characteristics of some sounds and their ability to disturb concentration are well known to anyone working in today's offices. Figure 9-1 (Kaplan 1978b) illustrates typical office sound levels. The sound generated by human speech approaches 80 decibels. Most teleprinters, word processors, and typewriters produce sounds in the 60–80 decibel range. Each doubling of a noise source increases the noise level by 3 decibels. A collection of office machinery operating in a single office can quickly raise the noise level to unsatisfactory limits. Relaxed conversation is usually possible below 45 decibels. Telephone conversations become difficult around 55 decibels, and one has to shout to be heard at 80 decibels.

To prevent health hazards, the government has established upper limits for acoustic noise, as Table 9-4 summarizes. These standards are much too high for an office, however.

Sound levels above 60 decibels in offices are generally considered noisy. According to Kaplan (1978a) high noise levels in offices can cause such physiological and psychological effects as: increased blood pressure, accelerated

Table 9-4. Government Standards for Exposure to Sound

Maximum Hours Exposure per Day	*Sound Level (Decibels)*
8	90
6	92
4	95
3	97
2	100
1.5	102
1	105
0.5	110
0.25 or less	115

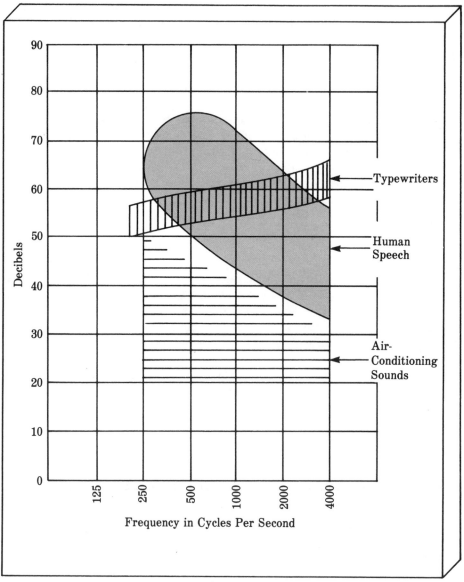

Figure 9-1. Sounds of the Office

heart rate, increased metabolic rate and muscular tension, decreased digestive activity, tension, mental stress, irritability, and inability to think and work efficiently.

Sound has an attention-getting quality and usually competes for a person's attention. It may be perceived as either pleasant, neutral, or unpleasant. Unpleasant sounds are generally considered to be noise, but defining sound quality is difficult and is more an aesthetic problem than an objective science. For humans, sound possesses the characteristics of absence, frequency, adaptation, and variety.

Absence. A total lack of sound is disturbing to most people, and can have adverse psychological effects.

Frequency. People react more favorably to continual, steady, and rhythmical sounds rather than to irregular patterns. The irregular timing of some sounds can be distressing.

Adaptation. Because the hearing mechanism adapts to sound levels, people condition themselves to an existing acoustical environment, be it good or bad. Several degrees of change for better or worse can be accepted, but radical change in either direction can be psychologically upsetting.

Variety. A variety of sounds are necessary to maintain sensory alertness and interest.

Acoustical Privacy

A major sound source in the office is people. The distracting effects of overheard conversations can be devastating to concentration. In office design, the ability to hear coworkers' conversations at adjacent workstations is not as important as whether the conversation is understood. Awareness of the conversation may exist, but its content should not be discernible.

Freedom from the distracting influences of noise and overheard conversations is called acoustical privacy. A measure of acoustical privacy is the articulation index, which indicates the percentage of words coming from an adjacent workstation that can be understood when the speaker is using a conversational voice. Figure 9-2 illustrates the articulation index. Confidential privacy in

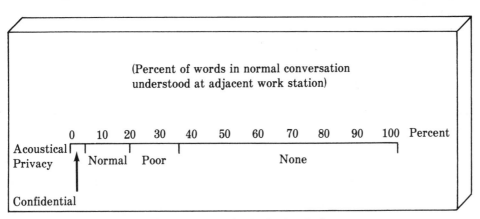

Figure 9-2.   Articulation Index

offices generally requires an articulation index of five percent or less, while normal privacy requires at least 20 percent.

Noise Control

The objective of an office acoustics program is to keep sound and noise levels within a range that is comfortable for performing human office activities. Those levels should eliminate distractions, allow good hearing, and provide speech privacy.

In planning a noise-control program, the primary consideration is the source of unwanted sound. Sound radiates in an expanding spherical wave. As waves hit various objects (ceilings, walls, furniture, people), they may be absorbed or reflected, depending on the kind of material they encounter. The objective of acoustical design should be to minimize sound-reflective surfaces so that sounds diminish quickly, according to the laws of physics (five to six decibels per doubling of distance).

Some sounds, like the human voice, are directional in nature—when people speak, the sound waves travel mainly in front. A design objective should be to channel these sounds in directions that cause the least disturbance.

An effective noise-control program focuses on three areas: the use of sound-absorbent materials, a sound-masking system, and office layout.

Sound-absorbent materials. Such materials are used on walls and furniture, and it is critical that they be used on ceilings.

Sound-masking systems. These eliminate the startling effects of sporadic noise. When a correctly adjusted sound-masking system is first installed, people are usually aware not of the new sound, but of a quieter work space (Turley 1978). Music or nature sounds combined with random-pattern noise, however, can exacerbate undesirable noise (Young and Berry 1979).

Office layout. Barriers and desks should be located so that workers are not in the path of voice or machine sounds. People walking past workstations are major sources of disturbance.

Specific guidelines for noise control are included in the following discussion of workstations. For more detailed discussions of acoustics, see Herbert (1978) and Turley (1978). Like lighting, acoustics is extremely complex and technical, and an extensive sound-control program should not be undertaken without expert guidance.

Workstations

Integration of the physical components that enable a person to perform a job comfortably, quickly, accurately, and with a sense of satisfaction begins with the design of the workstation. A workstation may be simple, including only a desk, some storage facilities, and a chair. Or it may be complex, incorporating extensive storage facilities, visual display units, large working areas, and much more.

In recent years the term *executive workstation* has achieved wide usage within the office automation movement. As it is used, however, this term encompasses nothing more than a terminal and its associated software. The true definition of workstation is much broader than this, since the terminal is but one ingredient.

Workstation Problems Caused by the VDT

The VDT is a large device. It has often been treated like a typewriter, being placed on a convenient desk or table where it will physically fit. Whether this location matches the requirements of the job or the person using it has escaped attention. As a result, many VDT users have been forced to cope with three critical problems: awkward terminal operating positions, lost workspace, and inefficient workspace organization.

Awkward operating positions. Problems caused by placing VDTs on standard desks include:

- keyboards too high or low;
- display screen too high or low;
- display screen too near or far away.

Being forced to maintain an awkward operating position has led to the problems associated with the neck, shoulder, arm, and hand described in Chapter 3.

Springer (1980) describes the results of a survey of insurance company employees which demonstrates the kind of problems that can result from improper work environment design. The company surveyed 384 office personnel ninety days before and after installing a computer-inquiry system. The survey assessed worker attitudes on a variety of work environment factors related to the new system. Sixty-two percent of the respondents reported some physical discomfort while using display terminals with traditional furniture, and 74 percent of those said that back problems were the primary discomfort.

Lack of workspace. VDTs crowd desk tops. Their large size consumes anywhere from 20 to 40 percent of the available work surface. If the amount of paper handled at the newly automated job does not decrease (which is often the case), or if all manual tasks are not eliminated (which is also often the case), a workspace crisis develops. The workers are usually left to solve the problem themselves. The result is a constant layering, shuffling, and losing of important materials. Signs of this condition are:

- materials stored off the desk;
- materials piled on top of the VDT;
- items taped to the front of the VDT;
- things stacked on other things;
- laps being used to hold manuals or other materials;
- excessive opening and closing of drawers.

Inefficient workspace organization. Lack of workspace leads to inefficient workstations. Papers and tools are poorly organized. Desk components are not displayed to best advantage, and reshuffling makes it difficult to remember their location. Time-consuming visual searches must be made. Economy of motion problems also occur. Things are positioned not in the best sequence but wherever space is available. Manual transition times are greatly increased. An analysis of one organization's workstation revealed five different locations for input/output materials and four different locations for storage of manuals.

Such workstation problems rob the system and the worker of effectiveness. The VDT can no longer be viewed simply as an entity in and of itself. It is but one component in a much larger complex.

Workstation Design

Good workstation design depends upon proper construction and arrangement of the parts so that they work well together. As we have seen, a poor design can cause fatigue and cumulative discomfort and seriously impair human performance. Springer (1982) asked office workers what characteristics of workstations were of greatest importance to them. Their answers are summarized in Table 9-5. The most important were comfort, the ability to adjust furniture themselves, and the ability to adjust the writing surface, terminal screen surface, and keyboard surface.

A workstation is a collection of many ingredients whose shape is formed by technology, the task to be performed, and the various human needs. The design structure and process is illustrated in Figure 9-3. Design will always follow a systems approach and be directed toward maximum human effectiveness.

A Shaping Influence: Technology

A workstation will reflect the demands of technology. We are now witnessing a revolution in workstation design brought about by the VDT. Technology has not yet, however, been totally integrated into the workstation. Workstations are still structured around the technology. Technology remains, for the most part, a stand-alone device absorbed into the workstation as best as possible. This is sure to change as terminals become smaller and less expensive. The use of VDTs as work-display surfaces are on the horizon.

Another technology that has a profound influence on workstation design is voice recognition and talking computers. An electron gun is quiet, a keyswitch

Table 9-5. Characteristics of Workstations of Greatest Importance to Office Workers

General Features	Average Valence	Rank
Comfort	7.0	1
Amount of work space	6.2	2
Ability to adjust furniture oneself	5.2	3
Amount of storage space	4.3	4
Ease of adjustment	4.3	4
Amount of light available	4.2	6
Privacy	3.3	7
Noise control	2.7	8
Desk Characteristics		
Writing surface height adjustment	8.1	1
Terminal screen height adjustment	7.9	2
Terminal keyboard height adjustment	7.9	2
Separate heights for terminal screen and keyboard	7.9	2
Terminal screen tilt	6.9	5
File drawer storage	6.5	6
Shelves	6.2	7
Terminal keyboard tilt	5.6	8
Terminal viewing distance adjustment	5.6	8
Locking storage area for personal items	5.1	10
Chair Characteristics		
Seat height adjustment	8.9	1
Backrest height adjustment	8.2	2
Ability to swivel while seated	7.8	3
Back tilt adjustment	6.6	4
Arms	5.6	5
Seat tilt adjustment	5.2	6
Ability to lean back	5.2	6
Carpet casters	4.8	8
Footrest	2.8	9

almost so. But large numbers of people speaking at, or listening to, their computers will generate acoustical problems that today's office and workstations are poorly prepared to confront.

A Shaping Influence: Tasks

A workstation also reflects the tasks to be performed. A thorough analysis of the user's tasks must precede design. Designers must clearly define and understand both emergency and routine functions, specific operational require-

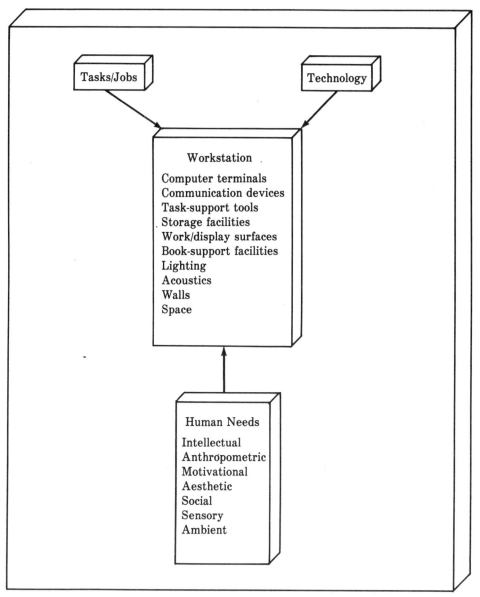

Figure 9-3.   Workstation Design

ments (how much, how fast, and how frequent), the sequence of operations, and the information flow necessary to efficiently accomplish the tasks. The product of this analysis should be a set of specifications that describe workstation components and how those components interrelate. If designers fail to perform good task analyses, important components could be forgotten or a poorly integrated collection of parts could be created. The result would be a workstation unsuitable for the human tasks to be performed there.

The task, the VDT, and the workstation. The per capita ratio of white-collar workers to display terminals in today's offices is rapidly diminishing. Ratios of ten to one and lower are common in many organizations. By 1990, the estimated nationwide ratio will be about two to three workers to every terminal.

While it is clear that the VDT has not yet been successfully integrated into the workstation, it is also clear that the ultimate solution will be more than one simple set of specifications. The characteristics of the task and frequency of terminal use will yield a series of alternatives.

Until recently, terminal use environments were poorly understood. The relationship between frequency of terminal use, terminal location, the kinds of task done, and human effectiveness may have been in our awareness but had never been fully defined and described. This is rapidly changing as a result of a research effort started by the Facility Management Institute (Ryburg 1982). By studying a number of large companies, the Institute has identified four basic ways terminals are typically employed in organizations. They have also related these employment profiles to usage characteristics, tasks, and the impact on worker effectiveness.

Regional terminals are groups of terminals in one location which support large groups of mostly professional or technical people. A walking distance of fifty to a hundred feet from the workstation to the terminal area is common, as are frequent return trips. One community terminal can support from ten to twenty workers as long as each worker's tasks demand terminal use only about five percent of the time.

Regional terminals are placed in standardized environments with little concern given to varying human needs. Varying requirements for differing amounts of workspace, privacy, screen viewing distance, and body comfort can seldom be fulfilled. Since the users are usually high-salaried professionals, the dollar cost of these inefficiencies can be high.

Satellite terminals consist of terminals placed closer to where people do their work. The processing needs of four to six users may be satisfied by one terminal located just a few feet away from their workstations. Usage characteristics and terminal workstation design deficiencies are similar to those of the regional variety.

Cluster terminals consist of one or more terminals placed in a fixed position within equal reach of two to four people. No one person has optimum access to such a terminal, but all are within seated arms' reach. Cluster use normally evolves when time requirements for using the VDT are in the 10–15 percent range. Usage may increase to 20–30 percent of each one's time, at which point contention develops for access, and queuing results if four people are sharing. Since clustering results in terminals being placed outside of the primary work zone, optimal use relationships do not exist for anyone. Long and fatiguing reaches to the keyboard may be required and viewing distance and angle may be unsatisfactory.

Dedicated terminals are those placed in a workstation for the use of only one primary worker. They can be optimally located for this purpose and are normally found when 20 percent or more of a worker's tasks require terminal usage. Dedicated terminals are, of course, the largest and fastest-growing kind of terminal environment. Their impact on the worker (lost space, comfort problems) have already been described.

In these environments, and for different kinds of terminal users (such as senior management, middle management, professional, technical, and clerical), and considering the different kinds of tasks (decision support, teleconferencing, data entry, and so on), the Facility Management Institute has defined more than sixty different potential workstations that may be needed to support the automated office. The implications of the task will have a great impact on the workstation's structure and the structure of the office itself.

A Shaping Influence: Human Needs

Workstation design must also reflect human needs, including biological (anthropometric, sensory, and ambient) and psychological (intellectual, social, motivational, and aesthetic).

Anthropometric factors refer to body dimensions and physical capabilities, such as seated or standing heights, reach lengths, arm angles in keying, and viewing angles. These greatly affect personal comfort in performing office tasks. The ideal design is one that enables a person to achieve economy of effort. Designs insensitive to anthropometrics cause fatigue, and a fatigued person will make more errors and will not perform tasks as quickly.

Sensory factors are the characteristics of human senses, such as sight and hearing, which have a decided impact on the effectiveness of design. Designers should consider the directional nature of sight in locating displays and the limits imposed by legibility and eye convergence requirements in positioning source documents and display screens. Similarly, the nondirectional nature of hearing will influence the location of auditory signals. The design must also try to minimize distractions within the workstation and from external sources.

Ambient factors are the ambient conditions affecting workstation design—light, sound, temperature, and humidity. Light and sound have already been reviewed. Temperature and humidity ranges are also important at workstations, and station design should not inhibit the establishment of their optimum ranges.

Intellectual factors include the informational requirements needed to support one's memory and information processing capabilities. These may vary among different tasks for one person, or they may vary among different people for the same task. Informational needs may be supported by the system through use of prompts and help facilities, or they may be supported by various hard-copy materials such as procedure manuals, job aids, checklists, or training documents. In either case, the need for informational support must be satisfied by the workstation design.

Social factors refer to the interpersonal relationships (either face-to-face or electronic) that the workstation design must facilitate. Face-to-face requirements may range from conference privacy to direct visual and physical access among members of the same work group or related work groups. The design must also reflect the workers' interactions with communications devices, such as telephones, visual display units, and teleconferencing facilities.

Motivational factors are important in workstation design since it is now recognized that workstations can have a significant impact on attitudes toward work. A design that permits fulfillment of basic human motivational needs will contribute to effective performance. Some important basic needs identified by behaviorists are *privacy, individuality, status,* and *belonging*.

Privacy is the ability to regulate or control social interaction and interruptions. It means being able to engage in conversations that require confidentiality and security, freedom from interruptions to concentrate on creative work, security from the discomfort of people standing nearby, and protection from noise and other distracting sounds. People attempt to maintain privacy by defining the following conditions (Kaplan 1978a; Hunsaker 1981):

- *Territoriality:* An area with boundaries that is under the control of workers and designed for their exclusive use. When fixed boundaries do not exist, people create a semifixed territory by establishing boundaries with such objects as notebooks, coffee cups, or jackets over the backs of chairs. While legal right to the territory is not granted, proprietary right is assumed and territory violation may lead to feelings of loss, anger, and a desire to regain the space.
- *Personal Space:* An immediate space or *bubble* that is constantly around a worker and is inviolate.
- *Interpersonal Space:* The distance people regulate between themselves and others. Research has found that adult American business people interact in the following four zones:

  - *Intimate zone:* ranges from actual physical contact to a two-foot distance.
  - *Personal zone:* ranges from about two to four feet.
  - *Social zone:* extends from about four to twelve feet.
  - *Public zone:* Stretches from about twelve feet to the limits of sight and hearing.

The importance of these zones is rarely recognized until a violation occurs. Then tension and distrust may occur and effective communication may be hindered. Tactics used to prevent intrusion into personal space include stepping back, avoiding eye contact, or separating the intruder with an object such as a chair or one's elbow or leg.

- *Crowding:* Perception and reaction to the number of people within an area, not as a population density, but as a subjective and changing experience.

Privacy does not necessarily mean aloneness. It simply means controlling interpersonal situations by controlling the physical environment. Privacy requirements may change as activities and feelings change.

Individuality is the mechanism by which people control and own their environment. People typically try to put a personal stamp on what is theirs. Something initially strange and hostile then becomes something uniquely theirs with which they are comfortable. Bomberg (1979) provides an interesting paper on this topic.

Status involves possession of a workstation that is commensurate with one's title and experience. Status in the office is reflected in greater privacy, preferred locations, and the kinds of objects that comprise the workstation. Hunsaker (1981) provides the following generalizations:

Privacy and location—related indicators of status:

- More personal territory is better than less.
- Private is better than public.
- Higher is better than lower.
- Close to the top executive is better than far away.
- *In* is better than *out.*

Object-related indicators of status:

- Big is better than small.
- Many is better than few.
- Clean is better than dirty.
- Neat is better than messy.
- Expensive is better than cheap.
- Very old or very new is better than recent.
- Personal is better than public or company-issued.

A sense of *belonging* is also important to people. Workstation design should foster identification with or belonging to a group.

Aesthetic factors are the final component of workstation design. The workstation configuration should be pleasing to the eye. But a danger to be avoided and a mistake made innumerable times is the subverting of performance criteria to aesthetic considerations. Any design trade-off must be a function of human performance. Making the workstation attractive instead of making it efficient is self-defeating.

Workstation Design Guidelines

A well-designed workstation, then, must reflect the needs of technology, the task to be done, and its human occupant. Its ultimate objective is to foster effective human performance. Following is a series of design guidelines directed toward achieving a properly structured workstation. First the concept of adjustability is discussed. Then the individual components of the workstation are examined in greater detail.

Adjustability

The postural and visual problems associated with using display terminals are being solved by providing easily adjustable workstation work surfaces, display surfaces, and chairs. Arguments in favor of adjustability are summarized in Table 9-6. The installation of a VDT on a traditional desk of fixed height suggests that:

- Work posture is not important.
- People adapt easily to awkward arrangements.
- VDT users are about the 99th percentile in seated elbow height.
- VDT users are about the 1st percentile in seated eye height.
- Workstation costs are more important than human costs.

The concept of adjustability is now being studied experimentally with positive results. Springer (1982), as reported earlier, found a 10–15 percent performance improvement for adjustable workstations when compared to conventional workstations. Dainoff et al. (1982) found a 20–25 percent improvement in performance when comparing well and poorly adjusted workstations.

Table 9-6. Reasons for Adjustable Workstations

- People vary in all dimensions
- Body proportions vary widely within any group
- Different tasks may require different work layouts
- People vary their postures and positions frequently
- Medical problems, aches, and pains may require temporary changes for comfort
- Experience may change a person's preference for position
- Older people may require up to ten times more light
- Temperature, humidity, air flow, and angle of sunlight may require position shifts
- Fatigue may make frequent condition changes desirable
- Different people may occupy the workstation over short periods of time
- A feeling of control over the work situation is fostered

The latter also found a decrease in musculoskeletal complaints resulted from properly designed workstations. A Louis Harris survey sponsored by the New England Life Insurance Company found that productivity increased by as much as 17 percent when workstations were designed to meet the needs of people using them (Emmanuel and Saunders 1983).

A number of research efforts have also reported means and ranges of setting levels for a variety of adjustable workstation components. A compilation based on the results of studies by Grandjean et al. (1982), Miller and Suther (1981), and Springer (1982) is described in Table 9-7. The second column (*Low*) indicates the lowest value reported in any of the studies, the third column (*Mean*) provides the mean setting for each study, and the fourth column (*High*) indicates the highest value reported in any of the studies. The wide variety of settings in each of the dimensions is noteworthy. Further comments on the study results are included in the sections discussing each component.

Adjustable working surface heights, then, are recommended because, when properly adjusted, they permit a correct working posture for all workers. No compromises are necessary for workers whose size varies greatly from the average (such as footrests for shorter people). Correct work posture does not normally mean a single fixed posture, but a relaxed, natural one that enables a person to assume a number of alternative postures. Correct work posture is variable, not fixed.

Work Surfaces

Workstation work surfaces include the desk top, keyboard, and keyboard support surface, display-screen support surface, the display-screen image surface, and source document or other material support surfaces. Critical dimensions include heights above the floor, sizes (length and width), and viewing distances, and viewing angles.

Working surface heights are based on the premise that when a worker is correctly seated, the upper arm should be nearly vertical and the lower arm nearly horizontal. For tasks requiring heavy manual effort, the surface should be a little lower to get the help of body weight. For fine work a slightly higher surface may be desirable. Work surfaces that require the upper arm to be raised above the relaxed elbow height increase the metabolic costs of work (Tichauer 1967).

Bex (1971) reported on a European survey that found that the most common work surface heights have decreased from about 30 inches in 1958 to about 28½ inches in 1970. Mandal (1982) reports that, while desk tops have been getting lower, people have been getting taller (almost four inches over the past century). This divergence in distances between desk-top height and human height leads to increased flexion and loading of the lumbar region of the back as a person is forced to assume a more bent over position to work. Lower desks, he concludes, are a contributing factor to back problems and have no obvious advantage. He argues for higher tilting chairs and higher sloping work surfaces.

Table 9-7. Preferred Adjustments of Keyboard Display, Support Surface, and Seat

	Low	Mean	High
Keyboard			
Support Surface Height	22.0" (Miller)	24.8" (Miller) 28.1" (Grandjean)	34.7" (Grandjean)
Home Row Height	25.1" (Miller)	27.8" (Miller) 31.2" (Grandjean)	37.8" (Grandjean)
Angle	14° (Miller)	18° (Miller)	25° (Miller)
Display			
Screen Height (Center)	30.8" (Miller)	36.4" (Miller)	45.2" (Grandjean)
Support Surface Height	24.0" (Springer)	40.2" (Grandjean)	32.0" (Springer)
Distance from Front of Support Surface	19.5" (Grandjean)	25.0" (Grandjean)	30.8" (Grandjean)
Screen Inclination (Degrees Back from Vertical)	-2° (Grandjean)	4° (Grandjean) 3° (Miller)	13° (Grandjean)
Viewing Angle (Degrees Down from Horizontal)	-2° (Grandjean)	9° (Grandjean)	26° (Grandjean)
Viewing Distance	16.0" (Springer)	20.0" (Springer) 29.6" (Grandjean)	36.3" (Grandjean)
Seat			
Height	12.6" (Miller)	16.0" (Miller) 18.7" (Grandjean)	24.0" (Springer)
Sample Standing Height	58" (Springer)	66" (Grandjean) 67" (Miller)	76" (Springer)

Adapted from Grandjean et al. (1982), Miller and Suther (1981), and Springer (1982).

Working Surface

Height

- Should be independently adjustable within a range of 23–32 inches above the floor.
- If a fixed height is necessary, it should be 28½ or 29 inches above the floor.

Size

- The work surface should be large enough to allow tasks to be completed in an efficient and effective manner.

Structure

- It should have a thin top.
- There should be no skirting drawers to obstruct free movement.
- It should have rounded corners.

The adjustable range recommended for work surfaces is 23–32 inches above the floor. Bex (1971) suggests 23–30 inches. The Grandjean et al. (1982) data suggest a higher upper limit. A 23–32-inch range should cover the majority of desk users. For those cases where adjustability is not possible, a fixed height of 28½ or 29 inches above the floor appears to be the most practical.

The size of the working surface is very task dependent. It is obvious that larger working surfaces are needed to compensate for the space consumed by the VDT. Springer (1982) concluded that a minimum working area of 30 × 48 inches was needed for data entry and inquiry tasks. The minimum depth of the working surface should be at least 32 inches to permit proper viewing distances of desk-standing display screens. Optimum working surface configurations are discussed in a following section.

Working surfaces should be thin and should not possess drawers that can hinder one's movement. All corners should be rounded, not sharp.

The keyboard support surface should be adjustable within a range of 23–32 inches. This height adjustment should be independent of that for other working surfaces and the display screen support. The keyboard support surface should allow the keyboard to be positioned up to 12 inches from the front of the table top. This will permit placing source documents or forearm/wrist supports in front of the keyboard, if desired. While the distance between the front of the keyboard and the desk edge should not exceed 2–4 inches, Grandjean et al. (1982) found a mean distance of over 6 inches, with some measurements exceeding 12 inches. Increased depth will therefore meet a variety of needs.

Grandjean et al. collected some data on the use of forearm/wrist supports. They found that 80 percent of the people studied rested their forearms and

Keyboard Support Surfaces

Height

- The height shoud be independently adjustable within a range of 23–32 inches above the floor.

Depth

- The depth should permit positioning the keyboard up to 12 inches from the front edge of the desk to allow for:

  - source documents;
  - forearm wrist supports.

wrists on a support if one was provided. Without one, however, only 50 percent used the desk surface for this purpose. Forearm/wrist supports were judged as comfortable by 80 percent of their subjects and as uncomfortable by only 3 percent. The desk itself as a resting place was found to be comfortable by 52 percent and uncomfortable by 21 percent.

Display Screen Surfaces

Height

- The height should be independently adjustable with the screen centerline within a range of 10–16 inches above the keyboard support surface.

Viewing Distance

- This should be within a range of 13–24 inches.

Screen Inclination

- This should be adjustable within a tilt range of -5 degrees forward to 45 degrees backward from a vertical display screen.

Proper display height is a function of eye position. A person's normal line of sight is about 10 degrees below the horizontal. The primary display area should be within a 30-degree cone, lowered 10 degrees from the horizontal. So a precise display height above desk level is a function of actual viewing distance. In recommending location for the center of the display area (about 10–16 inches above the keyboard support surface), then, we must also consider viewing distance.

An optimum screen height will permit a person to read the whole screen without neck bending or stooping. Comfortable viewing angles for reading paper materials in a sitting posture have been established by Lehmann and Stier (1961). The mean angle is 38 degrees below horizontal, with a significant majority falling within a range of 26–50 degrees. Grandjean et al. (1982) found the mean angle for viewing a VDT screen was 9 degrees with a range of -2 to 26 degrees. This smaller angle shown by VDT viewers must be caused primarily by the physical size of the display screen itself and the reflective characteristics of its screen surface.

Normally recommended viewing distances for VDT display screens is about 13–24 inches. IBM (1979) recommends a display viewing distance of 20 inches as best for lessening the probability of visual fatigue from eye convergence and accommodation. Eyeglass wearers, however, will find a shorter distance more comfortable. Reading lenses optimize focusing at about 13 inches (Oestberg 1976). Springer (1982) found that the range of viewing distances for a variety of people (with monofocal, bifocal, and trifocal glasses, contact lenses, and no eyeglasses) ranged from 16 to 26 inches with means in the 18–20 inch range. Grandjean et al. (1982) however, found significantly greater viewing distances in their study. The range was about 23 to 36 inches, with a mean close to 30 inches. A major contributing factor to this increase was that the VDT users they studied generally assumed more reclined postures than the upright postures of those who had been measured in laboratory settings. As a result their heads were further from the table edge and the display screen. The results of all this research leads one to believe that adjustability of the display screen distance on a horizontal plane is also desirable.

All viewing surfaces should also be located to achieve uniform viewing distances and thus minimize the need to constantly refocus the eye. Since the normal viewing angle of a VDT is a number of degrees downward, to get the display surface perpendicular to one's line of sight normally requires tilting the display screen an equal number of degrees backward from a vertical line. Ideally this inclination should be adjustable to coincide with differing viewing angles. The mean preferred inclination found by Grandjean et al. (1982) was 4 degrees and by Miller and Suther (1981) it was 3 degrees. As the screen is tilted backward, the chances of picking up reflections from overhead lighting is increased, however. Direct reflections of overhead light can be minimized by tilting the display screen downward several degrees from the normal line of sight. Several degrees of tilt has a minor effect on the angular size of the characters but may have a significant effect on the glare problem. Those in the Grandjean et al. and Miller and Suther studies were apparently tilting their display screens slightly forward from line of sight to minimize reflected glare. The screen inclination range found by Grandjean et al. was from -2 degrees to 13 degrees. The lower the height of the screen the greater the preferred backward inclination. An adjustable screen inclination within a range of -5 degrees to 45 degrees would satisfy most all viewing requirements considering room lighting conditions and preferred viewing angles.

A display screen surface which can be rotated several degrees to the left and right would also serve as a means of reducing undesirable reflections.

Source Documents

Location

• Source documents should be positioned close to the keyboard and display screen.

Viewing Distance

• This should provide a viewing distance similar to the display screen (16–24 inches).

Viewing Angle

• Position documents perpendicular to one's line of sight.

Documents and manuscripts being processed should be positioned as close to the keyboard and display screen as possible in order to minimize eye transition movements. Wide separations will slow down keying and writing. They should also be positioned at uniform viewing distances with other display components. Document holders should also be utilized to achieve uniform viewing planes.

A well-designed chair is one of the most important parts of the workstation. It affects posture, circulation, the amount of effort required to maintain a position, and the amount of pressure on the spine.

The German orthopedic surgeon Staffel constructed the forerunner of the modern office chair in 1884. He stressed the importance of lumbar back support and designed a chair which produced a right-angled, upright position. This posture has been uncritically accepted by experts all over the world and forms the basis of correct sitting posture in many references and texts. This posture has been coming under increasing attack in recent years, however. Mandal (1982) argues that the lumbar support carries only about 5 percent of the body weight as opposed to the seat pan that carries 80–95 percent. He further argues that studies of actual workers almost always shows them leaning forward with maximal flexion of their backs. Patkin (1983) calls attention to how often people fidget and move about in their chairs and how constrained postures yield stiff and lame bodies as free blood circulation is impeded. Grandjean et al. (1982) describe the postures of their VDT users as often being characterized by:

• leaning backwards;
• extended legs;

Chair

Seat Pan

- The seat should be easily adjustable within a range of 14–24 inches above the floor.
- The size should be approximately 16 × 16 inches.
- It should be parallel to the floor.
- It should conform to the shape of the buttocks.
- The seat edge should be rounded at the front.
- It should be neither too firm nor too soft (with about a two-inch sink).
- It should be able to rotate 360 degrees without changing its height.

Backrest

- The backrest should support the back of the waist.
- It should be easily adjustable in height and angle.
- It should conform to the shape of the lumbar (lower back) region.

Armrest

- This should be large enough to support a resting elbow in different positions but small enough so as not to interfere with pulling the chair up close to the work surface.

Base

- The chair should have five legs for stability.
- There should be casters for ease of motion.

- a forward bending of the head.
- no support for the lower spine;
- lifted arms.

Adjustability in chair dimensions and providing adequate support for a variety of seated postures is a compelling direction if the evidence is to be believed. (Think for a moment how many times you change your seated posture as you read this book.) Perhaps the back problems of the world are more easily solved than we had thought. (It is estimated that half of the population of the industrialized world suffers from some sort of back complaint.)

Seat pan. A correctly adjusted seat height allows the feet to rest comfortably on the floor without pressure on the undersides of the legs above the knees. The knees should be bent at a 90–100 degree angle, with 80–150 degree angles permissible. The arm, when bent, should form a right angle at the elbow when the hand is resting on the keyboard (or desk top). The seat height should be easy to adjust. One modern way to accomplish this is a *gas action* mechanism controlled by a lever under the seat pan (*Administrative Management* 1982). The older kind of adjustment where the seat has to be screwed up or down on its base is tedious, and many people just won't use it. The overall size of the seat pan should be no more than necessary to support a person comfortably. It should conform to the shape of the human buttocks and have a rounded edge at the front to prevent constriction of muscles and blood vessels of the thigh. There must also be a one-inch clearance from the front edge of the pan to the lower leg or calf. It is often recommended that the seat slope backward between 4 and 8 degrees, but some experts claim this causes or increases backaches. Mandal (1981) argues for a forward slope to straighten out the lumbar curve as in standing. A forward slope brings into play the forces of gravity, however, causing a person to slide forward. The best answer may be an adjustable slope mechanism.

Too hard a seat is uncomfortable, while too soft a seat will not relieve pressures with changes in position. Patkin (1983) makes a "firm" recommendation that the seat should sink in about two inches under average body weight. The seat pan should also be able to rotate 360 degrees without changing height.

Backrest. It is important that the back have support. This support should fit into the small of the back, be padded, and be adjustable both fore and aft and up and down. A correctly adjusted backrest is positioned at the back of the waist, about one inch higher than the top of the hip bone. High backrests are also desirable as they provide support to the upper back muscles and muscles along the spine. High backrests also enable the body to assume a variety of good resting positions.

Armrest. Armrests provide needed support for the arm from the elbow to the center of the forearm. They should be broad (about four inches), well-padded, but not long enough to bump against the desk when sitting up close.

Base. The chair should have five legs for stability and casters or wheels for ease of motion. Wheels enable a person to move about from one part of a desk to another, providing both physical and psychological freedom. They must be well built, however, or they will be an irritation.

A well-organized workstation will minimize stretching, aid memorization of component locations and minimize transition distances between various elements. Stretching results in a greater reach but increases muscle loads which can be fatiguing. Memorization of element locations will make them easy to find without a lot of searching. Minimizing transition distances allows economy of motion and results in more efficient performance.

Desktop Logistics

Hierarchical Positioning

• Position workstation components hierarchically, based upon frequency, sequence, and duration of use.

> • For writing, keying, and reading, use the primary zone, which is the front area of the workspace within bent arms' reach.
> • For supporting materials and equipment only occasionally used or waiting to be used, use the secondary zone, which is the area of extended arm's reach.
> • For storage purposes use the remainder of the workspace.

• Provide uniform viewing distances for frequently viewed material.

Standardized Locations

• Provide standardized locations for workstation elements.

Visual Access

• Provide visual access to all frequently used workstation elements.

Hierarchical positioning. The overall configuration of each workstation should be based on a task analysis, and final positioning of components depends on the frequency, sequence, and duration of tasks. A basic rule is that the most frequently used components of the workstation be located within a person's convenient reach, with the elbow resting on the desk top. Writing, reading, and keying tasks will normally occur in this zone, called the primary zone. Elements not frequently used, such as *in* and *out* baskets and equipment only occasionally used or waiting to be used, should be located in the secondary zone of the workstation. This zone normally encompasses the area of extended arm's reach. The remaining workstation elements, such as materials and manuals, may be positioned outside of these zones. An analysis of several kinds of workstations in a financial organization found that proper organization of workstation elements could reduce transition distances by about 50 percent, and increase productivity by an estimated 4–7 percent (Ryburg 1981).

Standardized locations. Standardized locations of elements will aid memorizing where they are located in the work area. Therefore they will be accessed more quickly as visual searches are reduced.

Visual access. Workstation elements should be displayed to good advantage. Where memorization of exact locations is not possible, a visual search must be able to locate them quickly. Opening and closing drawers greatly contributes to wasted time, as does shuffling through piles of materials. Elements being searched for should be identified clearly and simply. This includes manuals, job aids, forms, and keyboard keys. The necessity of using drawers or files to complete processing tasks should be eliminated or minimized. The size of storage units should be appropriate to the size of their contents. The dimensions of the storage unit should not impinge on the workspace needed for manual tasks.

Integrating VDTs

- Only use VDTs with detachable keyboards.
- Permit source documents and materials to be located:

  - between the person and the keyboard;
  - to either side of the keyboard;
  - between the keyboard and the display screen.

- Provide for moving the VDT across the working surface:

  - forward and backward;
  - laterally.

Since VDTs are not truly integrated into workstations in the sense that they are not built into it, proper integration requires that they be considered as one of the elements in the desktop logistics. Location flexibility is a prime consideration. Therefore, only use display terminals that have detachable keyboards. In addition to the differing height adjustment advantages, the keyboard may be positioned to reflect different tasks and differing individual preferences. Large-volume data-entry tasks will require the keyboard to be positioned directly in front of a person, while manual activities with occasional dialogues might find the keyboard better positioned to the side. Either right- or left-handed preferences may be supported equally as well. Detachable keyboards also permit flexibility in positioning source materials in relation to the keyboard and display screen as eye movements are minimized.

Providing for lateral movement of the VDT across the working surface by placing it on wheels or casters permits proper location based on the needs of the task. Forward and backward positioning enables a person to control viewing distances.

Arrangement. Springer (1982) solicited preferences for a variety of workstation arrangements incorporating VDTs and found that the most preferred was an L-shaped configuration, one arm possessing the writing surface and the other containing the terminal. An arrangement like this will keep arm

Configuration

Arrangement

- Provide an L-shaped workstation arrangement that enhances efficiency of motion between the two sections.

Walls

- Provide a minimum of three walls or sides, with a slightly widened opening.

Size

- For normal privacy, allow at least 80 square feet per workstation.
- For confidential privacy, allow a minimum of 200 square feet per workstation.

---

reaches to a minimum and maximize the amount of available workspace in the major work zones.

Walls. Robert Propst of Herman Miller Inc., designer of the "Action Office," recommends a three-sided enclosure as the best approach to designing workstation walls. Propst feels this is best because it provides good definition of territory and allows both privacy and the ability to participate. A four-sided enclosure, he feels, is "bad for the wide-awake, activity-oriented person who is isolated, insulated, and remote." Another advantage of enclosures is that they give workers the opportunity to personalize their work spaces (*Rough Notes* 1978).

Other writers have suggested a two-sided enclosure, which may be satisfactory if the layout of the stations minimizes eye contact and other visual and sound distractions. Such distractions are discussed more fully later in this chapter.

Size. In general, the greater the space between workstations, the more privacy a person will have. These guidelines assume, however, that a noise-control program is in effect in the work area. Without such a program, 3,000 square feet per workstation might not guarantee privacy. Under good acoustical conditions, an area smaller than 200 square feet may be quite satisfactory.

Workstation Visual and Acoustic Distraction Control

- Use workstation walls to block sound transmission and to prevent visual distractions. Walls should be at least five feet high, preferably six feet high.
- Position workstations so that people are not facing other people.
- Have workstations open to zones where there is little movement.

Acoustic control is accomplished at the workstation by using sound-absorbing materials on the workstation walls. Acoustic and distraction control is accomplished by orienting workstations so that they do not face other people and opening them into zones where little movement occurs.

Conclusion

The office furniture industry has recognized present furniture shortcomings and is moving toward a systems approach to workstation design. Task/ambient lighting, component furniture systems, modular storage, and easily adjustable component heights illustrate this approach. The dramatic increase in the variety of considerations and services that support a VDT (such as lighting, telephone and data communication cables) will in the future make workstations more built-in and fixed in location.

The next major restructuring of the workstation will occur as the components of the computer interface system are included within the working surfaces. Terminals will cease to be instruments supported by a surface, but will become part of the work surface. In some ways the workstation may become one large terminal. Another technology on the horizon will soon have a large impact on workstation design—talking computers. Voice communications between people and systems will usher in a whole new era of acoustical concerns and solutions as the office din increases while workstation size decreases as a result of more costly office space. The creative worker, while being freed from the mechanics of interfacing with a keyboard, will be exposed to the distractions caused by an escalating major noise source in the office—the human voice.

Ultimately, an effective workstation design is going to require even closer cooperation among all interested parties—furniture manufacturers, terminal manufacturers, facility managers, and computer users. Those who are not yet talking to each other had better start quickly.

Office Design

Workstations must ultimately be integrated into the total office environment. The way this is done can have a significant impact on human performance. A variety of factors are involved, ranging from office layout, distraction control, color, and climate to some unique considerations imposed by the use of VDTs.

The Open Office

The trend today is toward the open office—a large room usually containing twenty or more people that is functionally organized and landscaped with temporary walls, dividers, or plants. The primary advantages postulated for this approach are:

- economy (more usable floor space, Schmid 1967);
- a more favorable work environment (light, acoustics, and climate, Einbrodt and Beckmann 1969);
- organizational benefits (increased flexibility in reorganization, quicker communications, and easier information exchange, Kyburz 1968).

Strong arguments against the open office include psychosocial factors, such as decreased personal interest in the working sphere and difficulty in integrating into large groups (Heusser 1968), and susceptibility to visual and auditory distractions.

There is little evidence to indicate whether the open office improves or impairs productivity. Most current data focus on attitudes toward the concept. McCarrey et al. (1974) found that the open approach resulted in positive attitudes toward job satisfaction, communication effectiveness, and high productivity. Negative attitudes were directed toward the lack of visual and auditory privacy, inability to communicate confidentially, poor territorial definitions, and reduced freedom.

Nemecek and Grandjean (1973), in a study of Swiss offices, found that perceived advantages of the open office included: better communication (40 percent of responses); personal contacts (28 percent); and workflow, supervision, and discipline (15 percent). Primary disadvantages were: disturbance in concentration (69 percent) and impossibility of confidential conversations (11 percent). Acoustical distractions were the most frequent cause of disturbed concentration. Other relevant findings were that almost two-thirds (63 percent) of the workers thought the large office space more efficient and more practical, and almost the same proportion (62 percent) of those initially disagreeable to the open office concept later indicated they had adjusted to it.

Turley (1978) has attributed the failure of many open office plans to hard ceilings that increase the spread of sound and reflect it over the tops of partial-height barriers. Others argue that neither the open office nor the traditional office has yet solved the problem of the person who needs both high levels of personal interaction and high levels of privacy.

It is still being debated whether or not the trend toward the open office is continuing. Trade associations report that open office furniture sales have grown at twice the rate of conventional furniture in recent years and that about 50 percent of the white-collar force is in open offices. They estimate that the open office utilization ratio will widen to 3:1 in the next decade. Other experts (space planners, environmental psychologists, and others) claim that the trend is swinging back to offices with walls and drawers.

Whichever is correct, it appears that the open office is here to stay, and office automation will have to settle comfortably into it.

The open office, if it is to truly reflect the changing needs of people, must be placed in a building that is technically capable of handling it. Adams et al. (1979) described the building-related characteristics listed above as those

Building Requirements of the Open Office

The open office requires a building with these characteristics:

- It should have an open block not constrained or inhibited by fixed architectural elements.
- It should be rectangular and not excessively irregular, elongated, or subject to odd geometrics.
- It should have fixed architectural elements (such as toilets, elevators, and stairs) consolidated on the perimeter.
- It should include easily accessible chases, raceways, and cavities as an integral part of the building shell.

needed to permit the most effective implementation of the open office concept. They state that while interior open office systems can adapt well to most kinds of spaces, too often they are placed in buildings that are poorly designed to accommodate changing requirements. The result is that the building shell and services become a limiting factor in the ideal application of open office systems. Ultimately, they believe, the evolution toward the open office will determine the form of building envelopes.

Office Layout

The following principles should determine office layouts:
- Keep people close to those with whom they must frequently communicate.
- Keep files and other references close to the people who use them.
- Keep people who have many outside visitors close to the work area entrance.
- Common destinations (toilets, elevators, photocopy machines, and so on) should be close together and accessible by direct routes.
- Workstations should be away from sources of intermittent sounds and areas of frequent conversations.

An office layout should accomplish two things. It should optimize the flow of work between various departments and people, and it should minimize movement and sound distractions caused by people going about their activities.

Terminal Location

- Terminals must be conveniently located and immediately accessible to users.
- For professional and managerial use, terminal placement should permit visual and auditory privacy.

If a terminal is not located on a person's desk (and is of the regional or satellite variety) its location can greatly affect its usage. Evidence indicates that the distance between a device and its users is a critical factor in its utilization, particularly when it must be shared or reserved in advance (Reid 1973).

Care must be taken in terminal placement so as not to disrupt the social patterns of the office. Systems have failed in the past because terminal operators were isolated from their colleagues (Heffernan 1979).

Terminals should also permit visual and auditory privacy because many people, especially those in more prestigious positions, do not want to feel foolish in front of their peers or subordinates. They are prepared to use a terminal only if their mistakes will not be observed. Managers and other untrained users must not be put in a position in which someone else is looking over their shoulder. Even a skilled user would find it difficult to think creatively under such circumstances.

Controlling Visual and Acoustic Distractions

• Use barriers to block sound transmissions and prevent visual distractions. Barriers should be at least five feet (preferably six feet) high and should go to the floor.
• Use efficient sound-absorbent materials with high absorption coefficients for ceilings (most important) and for barriers and walls. For walls, the most important area is from desk-top height to six feet above the floor.
• Position overhead lights so as to minimize sound reflected from the lens material to workstations.
• Angle windows slightly outward at the top so that sound energy is reflected toward the sound-absorbent ceiling.
• Consider using supplemental sound-absorbing baffles.
• Use a noise-masking system so that there is a continuous, unobtrusive, and indistinguishable murmur throughout the work space.

Even an ideal office layout cannot eliminate distracting influences in the work environment since people must communicate and occasionally move about. Control of the distracting influence of these activities is best accomplished through treatment of the office environment.

Acoustical planning is a complicated subject involving many factors, such as the materials composing ceilings, walls, floors, and barriers; where people are located; and how far apart people are. The guidelines here are simply intended to point out possible distraction problems and to suggest ways of controlling them. Herbert (1978), Kaplan (1978a), and Turley (1978) provide thorough discussions of acoustic programs.

Effective sound-absorbent material must be at least one-half inch thick and have a porous surface. It should also have a high absorption coefficient (the percent of sound absorbed).

Barriers are one good method of blocking sound transmission and preventing visual distractions. Turley (1978) found that the optimum barrier height is six feet. A four-foot barrier was found to be useless, while a five-foot one was twice as effective as the four-foot barrier for many applications. Optimum barrier lengths depend on the needs of the work area.

A highly sound-absorbent ceiling is the most important component of an open office plan. A ceiling's absorption coefficient at important speech frequencies should be 0.85 or higher. Ceilings rated below 0.8 are inferior. Ceiling height should be at least nine feet.

Vertical surfaces adjacent to workstations can be as important as ceilings. Sound-absorbent panels can be placed on these walls or columns. The most critical area is from desk-top height to six feet above the floor.

A major sound reflector is the large flat lens covering many ceiling light fixtures. Louvered or egg-crate diffusers can sometimes help eliminate strong reflections.

In office layout, the position of overhead lighting fixtures in relation to workstations should be coordinated to avoid annoying sound reflections. Task lighting can alleviate these problems.

Most carpets are acoustically ineffective since they are thin and, on the average, absorb only abut 10 to 30 percent of the sound energy hitting them. Their major advantage is that they reduce impact noise caused by footsteps, scraping chairs, and falling objects.

Plants offer no acoustical advantage at all, but they do make the work area more pleasant.

Windows create difficult acoustical problems. The desire to see outside and the need to control sound reflections are usually not compatible. An effective compromise is to angle windows slightly outward at the top so that the sound energy is reflected toward a sound-absorbent ceiling. Other less effective solutions for stopping window sound reflections include vertical venetian blinds with adjustable angles.

Climate

Temperature and Humidity

- Maintain room temperatures between 68 and 76 degrees.
- Maintain relative humidity between 40 and 60 percent.

Ventilation

- Eliminate drafts from fans and ventilators.

Climate conditions can influence performance, depending on an individual's stress and energy levels and the time period over which work is performed. Table 9-8 describes some general temperature and ventilation considerations.

Table 9-8. Climate Considerations

Temperature

Personal preferences may vary up to 15° for the same job and conditions

Females often prefer higher skin temperatures than males

The comfort range is often only about 8° F between too cool and too warm

Higher humidity (above 80%) requires 3° to 5° F lower temperature for comfort than lower humidity

High muscle activity can reduce the preferred air temperature by 30° F

Short sleeves and light clothing require 5° to 10° F higher temperature than long sleeves and medium clothing for comfort

Preferred temperatures vary slightly with outdoor temperatures: cooler in winter and warmer in summer

Still air feels warmer than moving air

Warm or cold areas (walls, floors, etc.) can affect comfort, even if air temperature is ideal

Ventilation

Drafts from fans and ventilators can be very annoying and even intolerable to some people

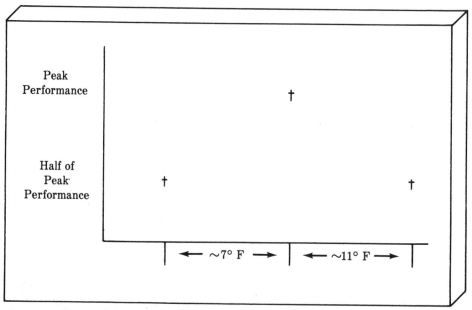

Figure 9-4. Performance as a Function of Temperature

No absolute or simple rules exist. Wing (1965) analyzed the results of a number of studies concerning mental performance and heat, and identified temperatures which, with different exposure times, caused decreased performance. The upper limit for unimpaired mental performance began in the mid-80s (Fahrenheit) for exposure periods from four to five hours, and reached the following approximate points: 90° F for two hours exposure, and 95° F for one hour. Generally speaking, comfort levels are lower than those at which performance begins to deteriorate (McCormick 1976).

Carlton-Foss (1982) reports that performance drops about 50 percent when the temperature increases 11 degrees, or decreases 7 degrees, from the central temperature at which a person performs best. This relationship is illustrated in Figure 9-4. The temperature for best performance is not identified here because it varies from one person to another and from one task to another.

The best that can be done is to keep temperatures within desirable ranges. The electrical components of VDTs generally produce a certain amount of waste heat. It is estimated that the heat generated by one VDT is equivalent to that generated by one person. Thus in an office where each worker has a VDT at his or her workstation, the additional heat created is equal to that of doubling the workforce in the room.

Office ventilation is becoming an increasingly volatile topic. In addition to eliminating drafts from fans and ventilators, cigarette smoke should be effectively removed, not just recirculated. Cigar smoking should be confined to sealed offices or to places with direct outside air. Many who object to cigar smoke will simply not get used to it. For a thorough discussion of energy engineering, see Carlton-Foss (1982).

Color

Color is everywhere. It affects our moods, our attitudes, and our feelings of comfort. If used properly it can enhance our performance, creating a positive, satisfying environment. It is one of the softer aspects of design called *High-Touch* that John Naisbitt defined in his book *Megatrends* as countermeasures to *High-Tech*. These countermeasures are adopted to balance the pervasive effects of technology on our lives.

The psychological and physiological effects of color on people are described in Table 9-9 (from Digerness 1982) and Table 9-10 (from Beach 1973).

Bright colors are fatiguing because the human eye reacts to the volume of light entering it. Bright colors make the pupil contract, and since the action is muscular, the eyes tire when a shift is made from this brightness to surrounding dull colors.

Human response-time to color signals has been measured from fastest to slowest as: red, green, yellow, and white. Any bright signal that has a good contrast ratio against a dark background, however, has good attention-getting qualities (Reynolds et al. 1972).

Selecting a color or colors for use in an office depends upon a variety of factors. Included are:

Table 9-9. Effects of Color

Red

Overstimulates and increases blood pressure

Creates feelings of warmth

Black and Brown

Create feelings of fatigue

Decrease perception of light

White

Produces no strong reactions

Increases perception of light and space

Blue

Relaxing—reduces blood pressure and the effects of stress

Overuse can cause sluggish behavior

Perceived as cold

Yellow

No effect on blood pressure

Can cause eyestrain if too bright or overused

Perceived as warm

Can stimulate a cheerful mood

Highest retention rating of all colors

Green

Considered the most normal color

No abnormal reactions

Can have a sedative effect

May be perceived as cool or cold

- What work functions will take place in the office? Formal? Informal?
- Where is the area located in relation to the rest of the building? In sunlight? Exposed to outdoor light? Under artificial light?
- What effect is to be achieved? To stimulate? To relax?

Digerness (1982) provides an interesting discussion of the use of color in today's offices. The understanding and proper use of colors can contribute greatly to

Table 9-10. Physiological and Psychological Effects of Color

Condition	Worst	Best
Fatiguing	Red Orange Yellow	Light tints (buff, ivory, cream, pale yellow, pale green)
Reading Speed	Red and blue backgrounds	Black on white Black on yellow
Preferences		Blue Red Green
Emotional Reactions:		
• Stimulating		Red Orange
• Restful/depressing		Blue Violet Blue-green

the subjective quality of the office environment as well as alleviating reported eye discomforts associated with using VDTs.

Other Office Environmental Considerations

- The restroom facilities should:

  - be restfully decorated;
  - be well lighted;
  - have no strong contrasts of:
        lightness and shade;
        stillness and movement;
  - have horizons encouraging the eyes to focus at a distance different from work.

- The workspace should offer an outlook beyond the VDT for the eyes to focus on a nonmoving, tranquil background.

To provide relief for the eyes of one who has to spend a large part of the day in close work with a VDT and source materials, a restroom facility with the above qualities is suggested. This will provide a restful diversion for the eye mechanism. Workstation design should also permit, where possible, a horizon beyond the VDT where the eyes can focus on a tranquilizing background.

The effect of background music on the office worker is conflicting. For creative, mentally challenging tasks, it does not appear to be beneficial. For repetitive tasks, positive results have been reported.

Conclusion

The office environment is becoming increasingly important as technology settles into it. Office lighting is critical, and increasing demands for privacy will require much greater visual and acoustic distraction control.

The flow of work, the movement of people, and the location of office components must be studied more thoroughly, and solutions to problems developed more scientifically. Galitz and Laska (1970) provide a methodological example. Based on an analysis of computer operator activities and movements, this study derived a computer center layout that optimized the operator's visual environment and minimized required physical movements.

The benefits of technology will fail to be achieved if it is not properly assimilated into the office. A tangible benefit of increased attention to the environment will be increased worker productivity. Intangible benefits include decreased absenteeism, improved job satisfaction and morale (see Seal and Sylvester 1982), and lowered workers' compensation claims and costs. Humanizing the workplace can also serve as a proactive response to charges by interest groups and organized labor about the health and safety of working with VDTs.

References

Adams, J.; Nuttall, C.; and Propst, R. *The Integrated Office Facility.* Ann Arbor, Mich.: Herman Miller Research Corp., June 1979.

Beach, T. "Color in Paperwork." *The Office,* May 1973, pp. 80–86.

Bex, F. H. A. "Desk Heights." *Applied Ergonomics* 2, No. 3 (1971): 138–140.

Boggs, D. H., and Simon, J. R. "Differential Effect of Noise on Tasks of Varying Complexity." *Journal of Applied Psychology* 52, No. 2 (1968): 148–153.

Bomberg, H. "Workflow/Workspace, People vs. the Process: The Case for Personal Space." *IMPACT,* Jan. 1979. Report in *Space Planning,* Office of the Future, Pasadena, Calif.: Office Technology Research Group.

Brandston, H. "Furniture-Integrated Task/Ambient Lighting." *Interior Design,* Feb. 1978. Report in *Space Planning,* Office of the Future, Pasadena, Calif.: Office Technology Research Group.

Broadbent, D. E. "Effect of Noise on an 'Intellectual' Task." *Journal of the Acoustical Society of America* 30 (1958): 824–827,

Carlton-Foss, J. A., "Energy Engineering for Occupied Places." *Ashrae Journal,* October 1982, pp. 35–39.

Cohen, S. "Sound Effects on Behavior." *Psychology Today,* October 1981.

Contract, June 1980 issue. New York: Gralla Publications.

Dainoff, M. J.; Fraser, L.; and Taylor, B.J. "Visual, Musculoskeletal, and Performance Differences Between Good and Poor VDT Workstations: Preliminary Findings," *Proceedings of the Human Factors Society 26th Annual Meeting (1982).* Santa Monica, Calif., 1982.

Digerness, B. "Color It Productive." *Administrative Management,* December 1982, pp. 46–49.

Driscoll, J. W. "People and the Automated Office." *Datamation* November 1979, pp. 106–112.

Einbrodt, H. J., and Beckmann, H. "Luft-, Licht- und Lärmproblem in Klein- und Grossraumbüros." *Arbeitsmedizin Sozialmedizin Arbeitshygiene* 2 (1969): 49–52.

Emanuel, H. M., and Saunders, S. "Plugging into the Open Office." *Today's Office*, June 1983, pp. 29–31.

Eschenbrenner, A. J., Jr. "Effects of Intermittent Noise on the Performance of a Complex Psychomotor Task." *Human Factors* 13, No. 1 (1971): 59–63.

Galitz, W. O., and Laska, T. J. "The Computer Operator and His Environment." *Human Factors* 12, No. 6 (1970): 563–573.

Grandjean, E.; Hunting, W., and Piderman, M. *A Field Study of Preferred Settings on an Adjustable VDT Workstation and their Effects on Body Postures and Subjective Feelings.* Zurich, Switzerland: Department of Hygiene and Ergonomics of the Swiss Federal Institute of Technology, 22 June 1982.

Heffernan, J. of American Mutual Insurance Companies, Wakefield, Mass. Personal conversation, October 1979.

Herbert, R. K. "Planning Acoustics." *The Office*, Mar. 1978. Report in *Space Planning*, Office of the Future, Pasadena, Calif.: Office Technology Research Group.

Heusser, M. *"Psychologische Aspekte des Grossraumbüros." Büro und Verkauf* 37 (1968): 452–457.

Hunsaker, P. L., "Proxemics Set Guidelines for Territoriality in Planning Office Spaces." *Contract*, March 1981.

IBM. *Human Factors of Workstations With Display Terminals.* San Jose, Calif., September 1979. G320-6102-1.

IES Lighting Handbook. 5th ed. New York: Illuminating Engineering Society., 1972.

Illuminating Engineering Society. "Visual Discomfort Ratings for Interior Lighting: Report 2." Prepared by Sub-Committee on Direct Glare, Committee on Recommendations for Quality and Quantity of Illumination, IES. *Illuminating Engineering* 61, No. 10 (1966): 643–666.

Jerison, H. J. "Effects of Noise on Human Performance." *Journal of Applied Psychology* 43 (1959): 96–101.

Kaplan, A. "An Ergonomic Approach to Acoustics." *Modern Office Procedures,* Mar. 1978a. Report in *Space Planning,* Office of the Future, Pasadena, Calif.: Office Technology Research Group.

Kaplan, A. "Ergonomics of Open Planning Workstations." *Modern Office Procedures,* Apr. 1978b. Report in *Space Planning,* Office of the Future, Pasadena, Calif.: Office Technology Research Group.

Kyburz, W. *"Der Grossraum als Organisatorisches Ideal." Büro und Verkauf* 37 (1968): 433–435.

LeFort, R. J. "Furniture-Integrated Task/Ambient Lighting." *Interior Design,* Feb. 1978. Report in *Space Planning,* Office of Future, Pasadena, Calif.: Office Technology Research Group.

Lehman, G., and Stier, F. "Mensch and Gerät," *Handbuch Der Gesamten Arbeitsmedizin,* Band 1, pp. 718–788, Urbana and Schwarzenberg, Berlin, 1961.

Mandal, A. C., "The Seated Man. Theories and Realities." *Proceedings of the Human Factors Society—26th Annual Meeting (1982).* Santa Monica, Calif., 1982.

McCormack, P. "Take It Straight from the Sun: Get More Light in Your Diet." *Extra,* Continental Airlines, May 1980, pp. 28–32.

McCormick, E. J. *Human Factors in Engineering and Design.* 4th ed. New York: McGraw-Hill, 1976.

Marquard, R. J. "Energy-Efficient Office Lighting." *The Office,* Sep. 1977. Report in *Space Planning,* Office of the Future, Pasadena, Calif.: Office Technology Research Group.

McCarrey, M. W.; Peterson, L.; Edwards, S.; and Von Kulmiz, P. "Landscape Office Attitudes: Reflections of Perceived Degree of Control Over Transactions With the Environment." *Journal of Applied Psychology* 59 (1974): 401–403.

Miller, I., and Suther, T. W. "Preferred Height and Angle Settings of CRT and Keyboard for Display Station Input Task," *Proceedings, Human Factors Society—25th Annual Meeting (1981).* Santa Monica, Calif., 1981.

Morton, A. H., *Administrative Management,* November 1982, p. 41.

Nemecek, J., and Grandjean, E. "Results of an Ergonomics Investigation of Large-Space Offices." *Human Factors* 15, No. 2 (1973): 111–124.

"New Concepts in Lighting Offer Big Energy Savings." *Canadian Office,* Report in *Space Planning,* Office of the Future, Pasadena, Calif.: Office Technology Research Group, March 1978.

Nuckolls, J. L. "Illuminations." *Interiors,* June 1981.

"Office Chair." *Administrative Management,* May 1982.

Oestberg, O. *Office Computerization in Sweden: Worker Participation, Workplace Considerations and the Reduction of Visual Strain.* Paper Presented at the NATO Advanced Study Inst. on Man-Computer Interaction, Mati, Greece, September 1976.

Patkin, Michael *Problems of Body Dimensions and Eyesight in the V.D.U. Workplace,* Whyalla, Australia; Ergon House Publishing, 1983.

"Productivity and the Total Office Environment."; *Fortune,* 21 May 1979. Report in *Space Planning,* Office of the Future, Pasadena, Calif.: Office Technology Research Group.

Reid, A. A. L. "Channel Versus System Innovation Person/Person Telecommunications." *Human Factors* 15, No. 5 (1973): 449–457.

Reynolds, R. E.; White, R. M., Jr. and Hilgendorf, R. L. "Detection and Recognition of Colored Signal Lights." *Human Factors* 14, No. 3 (1972): 227–236.

Roth. E. M., ed. *Compendium of Human Responses to the Aerospace Environment.* 5 vols. November 1968. NASA CR-1205.

Ryburg, J. B., "The Facility Management Implications of Office Automation." *Proceedings, Office Automation Conference.* San Francisco, Calif.: AFIPS, April 1982.

Ryburg, J., Personal conversation. Ann Arbor, Michigan, December, 1981.

Schmid, R. *"Der Mittelgrosse Büroraum." Industrielle Organisation,* 36 (1967): 348–356.

Seal, D. J., and Sylvester, G. E. "Design Applications for Optimizing the Working Environment of the Software Employee: A Case Study," *Proceedings of the Human Factors Society—26th Annual Meeting (1982).* Santa Monica, Calif., 1982, pp. 150–154.

Shellko, P. L., and Williams, H. G. "Integration of Task and Ambient Lighting in Furniture." *Lighting Design and Application,* September 1976. Report in *Space Planning,* Office of the Future, Pasadena, Calif.: Office Technology Research Group.

Shemitz, S. R. "Furniture-Integrated Task/Ambient Lighting." *Interior Design,* February 1978. Report in *Space Planning,* Office of the Future, Pasadena, Calif.: Office Technology Research Group.

"Special Report—Steelcase/Louis Harris Survey: Study Reveals More Open Plan in Office Future." *Contract*, Jan. 1979. Report in *Space Planning,* Office of the Future, Pasadena, Calif.: Office Technology Research Group.

Springer, T. J. "VDT Workstations: A Comparative Evaluation of Alternatives." *Applied Ergonomics* 13, No. 3 (1982): 211–212.

Springer, T. J. *Visual Display Units in the Office Environment: Blessings or Curses?* Paper Presented at Human Factors in Industrial Design in Consumer Products, Tufts Univ., May 28–30, 1980.

Tichauer, E. R. "Industrial Engineering in the Rehabilitation of the Handicapped." *Proceedings of the 18th Annual Institute Conference and Convention,* May 1967, pp. 171–177. American Inst. of Industrial Engr.

Turley, A. M. "Acoustical Privacy for the Open Office." *The Office,* May 1978. Report in *Space Planning,* Office of the Future, Pasadena, Calif.: Office Technology Research Group.

"Weighing the Pros and Cons of Open Plan Office Layout." *Rough Notes,* August 1978. Report in *Space Planning,* Office of the Future, Pasadena, Calif.: Office Technology Research Group.

Wells, B. W. P. "Subjective Responses to the Lighting Installation in a Modern Office Building and Their Design Implications." *Building Science,* 1, SFB:Ab7:UDC 628.9777 (1965): 57–68.

Wing, J. F. *A Review of the Effects of High Ambient Temperature on Mental Performance.* USAF. AMRL. TR65-102. September 1965.

Young, H. H., and Berry, G. L. "The Impact of Environment on the Productivity Attitudes of Intellectually Challenged Office Workers." *Human Factors* 21, No. 4 (1979): 399–407.

10

Documentation

No matter how well equipment and systems are designed, people will still need clear, accurate, and complete instructions as well as reference materials to use them effectively. This documentation may be printed on paper or stored electronically within the system.

The purpose of documentation is to inform. Much documentation of office systems has failed to accomplish this objective because of the documentation itself. Wakerman and Gleason (1983) point out that people do not like documentation that:

- has too much information or detail;
- has a demeaning or childish tone;
- is formal, stiff-sounding, or full of jargon;
- has poor printing quality;
- is poorly organized so that information is hard to find;
- is inaccurate.

Others point out that much documentation tends to be written at an expert level that incorrectly assumes the reader possesses as much knowledge as the writer. (Lieberman et al. 1982; Bailey 1982).

Documentation also fails to achieve its objective because of the characteristics of its human reader. People often do not read, preferring instead to simply try things. When reading is done it often is not sequential but involves skipping around (Thomas 1982). Furthermore, that which is read is misunderstood one third of the time (Kammann 1975). Finally, the University of Texas Adult Performance Level Project estimates that 22 percent of the United States' population is functionally incompetent at reading (Dalton 1982), and is incapable of reading even if the desire were there. Good documentation must overcome a variety of problems, not all of its own making. It must satisfy the need to be informed quickly and accurately and yet impose only a light reading burden.

Kinds of Documentation

Documentation needed for an office system consists of at least three kinds, each with a different purpose:

- Training Guide;
- Reference Manual;
- Quick-Reference Guide.

Training guide. The training guide is a manual that goes step-by-step through the uses and functions of the equipment or system. It usually contains practice exercises as well. Wakerman and Gleason (1983) suggest that it should contain only what a person needs to know to perform the required tasks. Therefore it should contain only brief, concise, step-by-step operations in a structured format. For systems with a large number of functions, it may not be necessary to cover all functions in the training guide. Users can learn omitted functions through familiarity with the reference manual and experimentation.

Reference manual. The reference manual should thoroughly describe the system's capabilities and how to use them. It should also contain information to aid in identifying and solving problems or errors. It should provide greater detail by being organized in a more traditional sense around system features and functions.

Quick-reference guide. The quick-reference guide is used for momentarily forgotten information. It may summarize keys, functions, and possibly the most common procedures.

Documentation Qualities

Good documentation possesses good communicative and technical qualities (Pakin 1980). Communicative quality refers to the ease of assimilation of the document's content. Affecting communicative quality are the documentation's components of clarity, legibility, scanability, and appearance. Technical quality refers to the effectiveness with which the technical information is presented. Affecting technical quality is the applicability to the audience, completeness, and organization.

Creating documentation requires a great deal of planning. Good documentation usually requires about eighty percent of one's time to be devoted to research and planning and only twenty percent to actual writing.

Communicative Quality: Components

Table of Contents

- The table of contents is a complete listing of all topics.
- It is ordered in the same sequence as the topics appear in the book.
- Major and subordinate components must be easily distinguishable.
- It contains page numbers for all of the components, including:

  - parts (if any);
  - chapters;
  - sections;
  - subsections (if any).

- Manual segments separated by tabs should have a separate table of contents for materials following each tab.
- A separate listing of examples and illustrations should immediately follow the table of contents.

Introduction

- The following aspects of the manual or documentation should be described in the introduction:

  - its purpose;
  - how it is organized;
  - the expected knowledge level of the reader at the start.

- The manual's subject matter should be described, including:

  - the purpose of the system documented;
  - a system processing flow to indicate how the system is used;
  - the system's relationship to other systems.

- Descriptions should be organized according to a logical flow of ideas.
- Introductions or overviews may also be provided for each chapter or major section.

Body of Text

- Use of illustrations to reduce or eliminate extensive narration.

  - Illustrations must be clearly referenced in the text.
  - They must be properly labeled.

- Use summary lists as reference aids.
- Use examples to show what to do.

  - Examples may be either detailed or general.
  - They should use actual data.

Sample Problems/Practice Exercises

- Problems and exercises should illustrate how a system or application operates in a real-life environment.
- They should be brief and interspersed thoughout the manual.
- They should also provide feedback to what has been done right or wrong.

Troubleshooting Guides

- These guides describe possible problem conditions.
- They provide steps for problem diagnosis.
- They also explain causes of the problems.
- And they detail corrective actions.

Glossary

- The glossary defines special terms as they apply to a system or its applications.
- Definitions should be brief.
- For common terms that have differing meanings, define how the term is used in the manual.

Index

- The index appears at the end of the manual.
- It should be as complete and precise as possible.
- Entries should be arranged in alphabetical order by topic.
- Entries should be included from various directions such as:

  - features of the equipment;
  - functions of the keys;
  - tasks to be performed.

- For separate manuals related to a single subject, provide an integrated index covering all the manuals.

Bibliographical References

- Locate references just before the index.
- Arrange them in alphabetical order by author.

The components of good documentation include all those described above. The principal reference aids are the table of contents, index, and glossary. All three should be found in every manual. The introduction orients the manual's reader, provides needed information about the system, such as its information flow and the relationship of the various components. Sample problems tie the documentation to the real-world environment. They bridge the gap between where the information or data reside in the office environment and how the system collects and uses this information. Troubleshooting guides make the user independent. They enable one to diagnose and solve problems without assistance.

Communicative Quality: Clarity

Use Words That Are:

- meaningful;
- familiar and with few syllables;
- simple;
- correct;
- consistent;
- not abbreviated.

Use Sentences That Are:

- short (less than twenty words);
- complete;
- well organized;
- not ambiguous;
- concise;
- grammatically correct;
- positive;
- active;
- readable at the eighth-grade level;
- descriptive.

General

- Describe the central ideas or purpose in each section.
- Emphasize graphic and pictorial formats.
- If abbreviations, acronyms, and symbols are used, define them the first time they are encountered.

The documentation must be clearly understandable. Ambiguity and confusion must be minimized so that fast and easy interpretation may result. This is accomplished through the proper structure of words and sentences and by the use of illustrations where possible.

Words. Meaningful words have a high associative value. They generally evoke greater imagery and understanding than less meaningful words. The result is faster learning. Words containing few syllables are also preferred. Do, however, use multisyllable words if the intended meaning is conveyed more readily with them than with shorter words. Use words correctly and consistently, and avoid jargon, abbreviations, and acronyms.

Sentences. Sentence style and structure also influence clarity. Ideally, sentences should be short—twenty words or less. An occasional long sentence will break up the choppiness and monotony, however. Sentences should also be complete, well organized, unambiguous, concise, and grammatically correct. Safire (1980) cleverly illustrates some good rules of composition in his *Fumberules of Grammar*, repeated in Table 10-1. Additional sets of guidelines may be found in Strunk and White (1972).

As a general rule, positive and active sentences are easier to understand than negative and passive sentences. A number of researchers have confirmed this, including Slobin (1966) and Broadbent (1977).

Readability measures. To enhance understanding, it is wise to write at a readability level below the intended audiences' reading skills. Reading skills are normally defined as one's score on a standard reading test which equates to a school grade level. Roemer and Chapanis (1982), in a study described in Chapter 6, compared fifth, tenth, and fifteenth grade reading levels for computer system messages. The fifth grade version was found to be best for people of all education levels. Wakerman and Gleason (1983) recommend an eighth grade reading level for all documentation. Brighter people, they state, are not offended by simply written material. They just read it faster.

To determine readability levels, a number of measures have been developed. Bailey (1982), based upon an evaluation by Coke (1978), recommends the measures of Kincaid et al. (1975) or Smith and Kincaid (1970). The Kincaid et al. measure is described in Table 10-2. In applying this formula keep in mind that it does not address whether or not the material makes sense. Format, organization, structure, and grammar are also important.

General. Use as many graphic and pictorial formats as practicable. They eliminate the need for extensive narrative explanations and can make the presentation of dull material more lively. Illustrations should not be used if all they do is repeat in graphical form something already conveyed in words, unless it is to make an important point. Captions and labels on illustrations should be kept to a minimum, and symbols should be few, familiar, and precise. Illustrations must be kept close to the related narrative.

Table 10-1. Fumberules of Grammar (Safire, 1980)

- Never split an infinitive.
- The passive voice should never be used.
- Avoid run-on sentences they are hard to read.
- Don't use no double negatives.
- Use the semicolon properly, always use it where it is appropriate; and never where it isn't.
- Reserve the apostrophe for it's proper use and omit it when its not needed.
- Do not put statements in the negative form.
- Verbs has to agree with their subjects.
- No sentence fragments.
- Proofread carefully to see if you any words out.
- Avoid commas, that are not necessary.
- If you reread your work, you will find on rereading that a great deal of repetition can be avoided by rereading and editing.
- A writer must not shift your point of view.
- And don't start a sentence with a conjunction.
- Don't overuse exclamation marks!!!
- Place pronouns as close as possible, especially in long sentences, as of 10 or more words, to their antecedents.
- Hyphenate between syllables and avoid un-neccessary hyphens.
- Write all adverbial forms correct.
- Don't use contractions in normal writing.
- Writing carefully, dangling participles must be avoided.
- It is incumbent on us to avoid archaisms.
- If any word is improper at the end of a sentence, a linking verb is.
- Steer clear of incorrect forms of verbs that have snuck in the language.
- Take the bull by the hand and avoid mixed metaphors.
- Avoid trendy locutions that sound flaky.
- Never, ever use repetitive redundancies.
- Everyone should be careful to use a singular pronoun with singular nouns in their writing.
- If I've told you once, I've told you a thousand times, resist hyperbole.
- Don't string too many prepositional phrases together unless you are walking through the valley of the shadow of death.
- Always pick on the correct idiom.
- "Avoid overuse of 'quotation "marks" ' "
- The adverb always follows the verb.
- Last but not least, avoid cliches like the plague; seek viable alternatives.

Table 10-2. Readability Formula

- Select five or more 100- to 150-word samples
- Determine the average number of syllables per word in each sample
- Determine the average number of words per sentence in each sample
- Determine the reading grade level of each sample by the following calculation:

$$(11.8 \times \text{average syllables/word}) + (0.39 \times \text{average words/sentence}) - 15.59 = \text{reading grade level}$$

- Determine the reading grade level of the material as a whole by computing the average of the reading grade levels calculated for each sample.

Source: Kincaid et al 1975.

Communicative Quality: Legibility

Typeface

- Size to within a 9–11 point range.
- Use a clean simple style.
- Set in lower case using capital letters as necessary.
- Keep line width down to 1½–2 alphabets (about 4½–5½ inches).

Color

- Use black ink on white, ivory, or buff paper.

Justification

- Use right justification in conjunction with proper hyphenation and equal distribution of white space.

Margins

- Inside margins should be wide enough to:

  - prevent words and illustrations from being lost in the curvature of the page;
  - prevent holes for ring binders from obliterating words or illustrations.

Legibility is greatly affected by such typographical factors as type size and style, paper and ink colors, line widths and margins. Legibility has an important impact on reading ease and speed.

Typeface. Type size is measured in units called points. One point equals 0.01384 inch. One inch approximates 72 points. The point size of a type is estimated by measuring the distance from the top of its tallest letter to the bottom of its lowest letter. This is the distance between the top of capital letters (A–Z) and the bottom of lower-case letters with descenders (g, j, p, q, y). Tinker (1963) found the optimum point range to be 9–11 points. Smaller or larger sizes lowered reading speeds. The type size in books and magazines usually ranges from 7 to 14 points.

Most type styles in common use are about equally legible. Italic (slanted) print does slow reading, however, as does a wide assortment of type styles printed in the same documentation. Lower-case text is read faster than upper case. Readers generally prefer line widths of moderate lengths, about 2½–6 inches, depending on type size (Tinker 1963). A line length of 1½–2 alphabets (39–52 characters or 4½–5½ inches) will achieve a good fit between type size and line width (Pakin 1980).

Color. Black print on a white background is much more legible than the reverse. Black on white is also preferred by readers. Black print on tinted paper is acceptable if the reflectance of the paper is at least 70 percent and the type size at least 10 point (Bailey 1982). Colored ink on colored paper often results in poor legibility.

Justification. Justify text at the right only if the type is proportionally spaced and properly hyphenated. Large gaps between words to create right justification or excessively short lines (ragged right) impair reading speed.

Margins. Inside margins should be wide enough to prevent words or illustrations from being lost in the curvature of the page. This depends greatly on the type of binding which must be considered when designing the pages of the body. Holes for ring binders should also not obliterate information.

Communicative Quality: Scannability

For maximum scannability the document should:

- Provide meaningful headings easily distinguishable from the text.
- Provide running heads on each page to identify chapter or section.
- Justify running heads to the outer margins of both left and right pages.
- Provide a structured format.
- Provide such other aids to scanning as:

  - easily distinguishable figure captions;
  - highlighted lists of key information.

Documentation is more often used for reference than for straight reading. Therefore, the ability to scan the material is particularly important. Scanning is facilitated if easily distinguishable headings are included on each page. Running heads on each page that identify chapter or section are particularly important if the format being followed results in similar section or subsection heads within chapters. A structured format is beneficial in that it aids skipping the sections a person knows are not needed. Other documentation scanning aids are highlighted lists of key information, checklists, and summary tables.

Technical Quality: Audience Applicability

* Write in a manner that suits the audiences' vocabulary, interest, and needs.
* Provide relevant and needed information only.
* Complement and be consistent with existing documentation.

Documentation should be prepared for the people who will use it. Therefore the characteristics of the reader must be established before starting to write. Decisions on style, organization, and simplicity should not be made as the writing proceeds. Relevant and needed information is all that should be presented. Following a structured format will aid this process, as only information that fits the format can be provided, thus discouraging rambling and excessive detail.

Technical Quality: Completeness and Organization

Completeness

* All content expectations raised in the introduction should be satisfied.
* Depth of discussion should answer all of the readers' common questions and most of their other questions.
* The main points should be properly stressed.
* The glossary should contain all important terms.
* All visual aids should be introduced and properly interpreted in the text.

Organization

* Provide a structured format.
* Emphasis on each section should be appropriate to its significance.
* References to other sections should be avoided or at least minimized.

Documentation should be complete, providing a person all that is needed to take proper actions. Documentation should be organized in a manner best suited to its purpose.

Technical Quality: Appearance

General

The documentation should be:
- attractive;
- small.

Cover

- The title and author should be identifiable by both spine and cover markings.
- Binding and cover should be durable but not awkward.
- It should lie flat when open or folded under.

Pages

- There should be plenty of white space.
- Provide adequate margins.
- Include variable line spacings between paragraphs, subsections, and sections.

A document's appearance greatly affects the reader's desire to use it. Something that is attractive creates a stronger desire to use it than something that is dull. Attractiveness results from a number of factors, including color, novelty, simplicity, typography, and layout. Creativity is important in good packaging of documentation.

A 6 × 9-inch size is recommended by Wakerman and Gleason (1983) instead of the traditional 8½ × 11-inch size. They feel it is less intimidating

Testing and Evaluation

Testing

- Read the documentation out loud.
- Frequently test it out on representative users.

Evaluation

- Evaluate the documentation after it is implemented.

Updating

- Continually and efficiently update all documentation.
- Ensure that the documentation is used.

and easier to hold on one's lap when sitting at a piece of equipment. A large manual can also be made smaller and more manageable by breaking it into several smaller booklets.

The layout of documentation should be clean and simple. Plenty of white space on a page helps to achieve this.

Documentation must undergo a continuous testing process. Frequent try-outs on prospective readers are needed to establish whether or not it is clearly fulfilling its purpose. Reading the materials aloud to oneself also aids in achieving the right tone. Demeaning or patronizing language becomes more obvious.

Systems are dynamic entities that are continually changing. People are also dynamic and documentation, although thorough and complete when issued, soon loses its value if it is not continually updated. Documentation is also of no value if its use is not enforced. Systems soon lose their effectiveness if the documentation is merely filed away in a drawer and forgotten.

References

Bailey, R. W. *Human Performance Engineering: A Guide for System Designers*. Englewood Cliffs, N.J.: Prentice-Hall, 1982.

Broadbent, D. E. "Language and Ergonomics" *Applied Ergonomics* 8 No. 1 (1977): 15–18,

Coke, E. U. "Readability and the Evaluation of Technical Documents," October 1978. (Reported in Bailey, above).

Dalton, R. "Is Seriousness an Overrated Virtue?" *Open Systems* 3, No. 6 (June 1982): 2.

Kammann, R. "The Comprehensibility of Printed Instructions." *Human Factors* 17, No. 2 (1975): 183–191.

Kincaid, J. P.; Fishburne, R. P.; Rogers, R. L.; and Chissom, B. S. "Derivation of New Readability Formulas (Automated Readability Index, Fog Count, and Flesch Reading Ease Formula) for Navy enlisted personnel. *Naval Training Command Research Branch Report 8-75*, February 1975.

Lieberman, M.; Selig, G.; and Walsh, J. *Office Automation: A Managers Guide for Improved Productivity*. New York: John Wiley, 1982.

Pakin, S. "Evaluate User Documentation Before You Buy the Software." *Infosystems*, October 1980, pp. 91–96.

Roemer, J., and Chapanis, A. "Learning Performance and Attitudes as a Function of the Reading Grade Level of a Computer-presented Tutorial." *Proceedings: Human Factors in Computer Systems*. Gaithersburg, Md., March 15–17, 1982.

Safire, W. *On Language*. New York: Time Books, 1980.

Slobin, D. "Grammatical Transformations and Sentence Comprehension in Childhood and Adulthood." *Journal of Verbal Learning and Verbal Behavior*. 5 (1966): 219–227.

Smith, E. A., and Kincaid, P. "Derivation and Validation of the Automated Readability Index for Use with Technical Materials." *Human Factors* 12 (1970): 457–464.

Strunk, W., and White, E. B. *The Elements of Style*. New York: MacMillan, 1972.

Thomas, J. C. "Ergonomics Takes Many Types of Experts: IBMer." *Computerworld,* 7 June 1982, p. 22.

Tinker, M. A. *Legibility of Print*. Ames, Iowa: Iowa State University Press, 1963.

Wakerman, J. and Gleason, J. "Manual Dexterity—What Makes Instructional Manuals Usable?" *Computerworld*, 1983.

11

Training

The following three points sum up the basic principles that apply to training:

- Provide adequate formal training with valid and measurable objectives that effectively teach what must be done and how to do it.
- Provide performance criteria that workers must achieve before they can perform on the job.
- Make the materials used on the job an integral part of the training session.

Training is the process by which people acquire the skills, knowledge, and attitudes that enable them to effectively use office systems and equipment. A system may be well designed and properly documented, but if people are not taught what to do and how to do it, the system will never fully achieve its objectives. A sloppy introduction of a system can quickly destroy any existing enthusiasm.

Many still do not realize the importance of training, however. As a result, office systems training often suffers from a variety of problems ranging from benign neglect to being viewed as a device to mask poor design. Some designers feel that the training responsibility is completed once the training materials are prepared. The objective of effecting a change in a person is frequently forgotten. In addition, this important principle is often disregarded: Human performance can be greatly accelerated if design minimizes learning time. Others sometimes view training as the bandage to cover up design decisions aimed at making the designer's job easier. These latter points contribute significantly to the staggering amount of office systems training that is deemed necessary.

The neglect of training is apparent when one looks at the amount of money devoted to it. McConnel (1981) reports that, of the estimated $500 billion spent each year on information processing, only about 0.5 percent is applied to the training of technically skilled data-processing personnel. An even smaller share goes into end-user training.

Principles of Training Program Development

- Provide meaningful materials.
- Keep the learner active.
- Provide immediate feedback on performance.
- Make use of reinforcement.
- Make use of repetition.
- Provide distributed practice.
- Provide practice in a variety of situations.
- Encourage divergent thinking.
- Provide early guidance.
- Consider the learner's ability to learn.
- Maintain accurate records of the learner's progress.

For many years a great deal of research has been directed toward determining the conditions that enhance the learning process. While much still remains unknown, the following learning principles have been established and are now commonly accepted (Gagne 1966; Hilgard and Bower 1975).

Provide meaningful materials. Meaningful materials, and meaningfully organized programs, have higher associative value. Greater imagery and understanding will result.

Keep the learner active. Skills are best developed by doing, not just by reading and listening.

Provide immediate feedback on performance. Behavior can only be modified through knowledge of the results of one's actions. Feedback is the ultimate shaper of human performance.

Make use of reinforcement. Reward correct responses or actions. Rewards may be psychological or physical, and include praise, attention or status, privileges, prizes, awards, or more money. Reinforcement should be immediate and should recognize all desired behavior, even if overall or final performance is not adequate. Punishment is almost always undesirable. Ignoring undesirable performance is usually sufficient to prevent the unwanted response from being repeated.

Make use of repetition. Practice makes perfect.

Provide distributed practice. Practice over a longer period of time with frequent breaks is better than concentrated or massed practice. Material taught in a distributed mode will also be retained longer than that taught in a massed mode.

Practice in a wide variety of situations. Generalization to a wide variety of situations is thereby enhanced.

Encourage divergent thinking. The development of creative solutions and the exploration of alternative solutions should be fostered.

Provide early guidance. Guidance early in the training helps to weed out improper responses before they become reinforced.

Consider the learner's ability to learn. Individual differences are bound to exist. Some people learn faster than others.

Maintain accurate records of the learner's progress. Maintaining good records permits an assessment of how the learner is progressing toward achieving the established performance objectives.

Kinds of Training

Training may take a variety of forms. An important distinction is between group-paced and self-paced forms. Group-paced methods include lectures, movies, videotapes, discussions, and panels. Their most obvious characteristic is that the trainees constitute a group and move at the same pace. Self-paced methods include videotapes with various supplemental materials including workbooks and examinations, audiotapes with supplements, slides and tapes, and computer-based training. The self-paced mode permits moving at each trainee's own pace, reflecting the individual learning differences in people. Self-paced methods also eliminate the logistical problems associated with bringing a large number of people together at one time, but they also require more thorough and careful development. An instructor in a group-paced course can overcome omissions or deficiencies that may spell disaster in a self-paced course. Table 11-1 summarizes the strengths and weaknesses of the two approaches.

Computer-Based Training

The same computer used as a tool in the automated office can also serve as the vehicle by which training is accomplished. Its strengths as a teacher include the ability to keep the learner active, to provide frequent feedback, to provide practice in a realistic situation, and to ascertain learner performance level. It also permits centralized development and control of the training program as well as easy scheduling and delivery of the training. Disadvantages

Table 11-1. Two Types of Training.

Self-Paced Training

    Strengths
- Learner works at own pace
- Yields more consistent results
- Fewer logistical problems
- Eliminates scheduling and location problems

    Weaknesses
- Difficult to handle volatile and changing subject matter
- Less economical
- Requires careful development
- Not conducive to group learning exercises
- More vulnerable to learner motivation level

Group-Paced Training

    Strengths
- Easier to handle volatile and changing subject matter
- Permits group learning exercises
- Less expensive
- Instructor can overcome program development omissions and deficiencies

    Weaknesses
- Little individual attention
- Less time for questions
- Difficult to ascertain learner understanding level
- Greater logistical problems

include the high costs associated with its use and the care and thoroughness with which training programs must be developed. Training programs that simply "turn pages" are not representative of well-designed computer-based training programs. A good course may require up to 200–300 hours of development per hour of instruction (Bailey 1982).

Computer-based training is not desirable in all situations. Table 11-2 summarizes its applicability, or lack of applicability, depending on the conditions that exist. Whether it is significantly more effective than other training methods remains an open question. Many studies to date have found no significant differences between it and a variety of other methods in a variety of settings (Jamison et al. 1974; Gilbert 1979). Others, however, have reported more effective and less expensive training (Trollip 1979).

Table 11-2. Application of Computer-Based Training

Desirable if:

- Measurable objectives must be mastered
- Frequent practice is needed
- Constant and predictable job conditions exist
- Long development time is acceptable
- The subject matter is fairly stable
- A large number of people will take the training
- Flexible training scheduling is desired
- Instructors are expensive or hard to find

Not desirable if:

- The subject matter rapidly changes
- Job conditions rapidly change
- The subject requires interpersonal skills
- Short development time is needed
- Resources are limited
- The program will have a short life span

On-the-Job Training

On-the-job training as part of a formal training program has a distinct advantage: It is realistic and minimizes the problem of transfer from the training environment to the real world. Informal on-the-job training, however, has drawbacks. It results in experienced workers passing on their habits—both good and bad—to trainees. Since training objectives are seldom stated and materials infrequently used, this kind of training is not thorough. It emphasizes frequent occurrences and rarely covers unusual situations. The obvious is sometimes forgotten, and basic concepts, which give workers an understanding of their role in the system, receive little attention. The usual result is that people know only part of what should be known, and some of that is erroneous. The Galitz (1979) field audit study illustrates these kinds of deficiencies.

Training Evaluation and Follow-up

Skills developed during a training program will be forgotten if not used. Furthermore, inefficiencies may creep in and gradually become accepted behavior. Usually workers are unaware of these deviations from correct and efficient performance, and only an effective follow-up program can detect them.

Training must also be ongoing as people and methods change. Too often, systematically developed formal programs deteriorate into informal on-the-job training.

- Provide on-the-job follow-up to ensure that skills are effectively developed.
- Provide periodic refresher training.
- Provide new training on updates or changes.
- Ensure that local supervisors are capable of conducting follow-up training and can clearly explain procedures.

The Trainer and the Training Climate

The training climate is an important influence in the learning process. For instructor-led training sessions, the instructor can greatly influence this climate through attitude and demeanor. Sandburg (1983) has put together a list of instructor actions that can turn off the class on the instructor and the entire training session. These undesirable actions are summarized in Table 11-3.

Table 11-3. How to Turn Off Training Class

- Arrive late without a reasonable excuse or apology
- Suggest that a manual be read and then leave the room
- Receive or make telephone calls during class
- Do not follow up on answers to questions
- Be vague or evasive in answering questions about confusing issues or complicated problems
- Talk negatively about others
- Be amused at the learners' problems
- Talk down to the group
- Be condescending
- Talk over the learners' heads
- Lecture without observing reactions, interest, comprehension, or asking for feedback
- Never return telephone calls
- Constantly look at the clock or a watch
- Be unprepared or disorganized
- Play favorites with class members
- Be uninformed about the learners' business
- Forget names after repeated prompts or corrections
- Be impatient
- Treat the class like children
- Be sarcastic
- Be unpleasant
- Be discourteous

So, if an otherwise well-designed training program must be sabotaged, mimic the actions described in the table. If, however, the proper climate and learning conditions are important, an occasional look in the mirror may be necessary to verify that none of these disturbing behaviors have raised their ugly heads. Even the most experienced instructor is not immune.

References

Bailey, R. W. *Human Performance Engineering: A Guide for System Designers*. Englewood Cliffs, N.J.: Prentice-Hall, 1982.

Gagne, R. M., ed. *Psychological Principles in System Development*. New York: Holt, Reinhart, and Winston, 1966.

Galitz, W. O. *Field Audit of DEBUT II*. Chicago, IL.: CNA, January 1979.

Gilbert, W. "CAI Notes." *Use Inc Newsletter*, 1979.

Hilgard, E. R., and Bower, G. H. *Theories of Learning*. Englewood Cliffs, N.J.: Prentice-Hall, 1975.

Jamison, D.; Suppes, P.; and Wells, S. "The Effectiveness of Alternative Instructional Media: A Survey." *Review of Educational Research* 44, No. 1 (1974): 1–67.

McConnell, V. "Training of Non-tech End Users Seen Vital to High Productivity." *Computerworld*, 16 November 1981.

Sandburg, D. "Attitude Creates the Training Climate." *Office Administration and Automation,* June 1983, p. 96.

Trollip, S. R. "The Evaluation of Complex Computer-based Flight Procedure Trainer." *Human Factors* 21, No. 1 (1979): 47–54.

12

Managing Change

New technologies present dramatic changes to office personnel. People's roles, functions, responsibilities, and relations with each other change, as does their working environment and how they accomplish work. Managing and coping with this change will require more than simply adapting to a new status quo. It calls for adapting to a continuing pattern of change. No meaningful precedents exist for the changeover process. It is filled with uncertainty.

Introducing change in any organization is delicate, frustrating, potentially disruptive, time-consuming, and costly. Many changes collide with established, familiar behavior patterns that are grounded in the strong, deep-seated habits and social relationships of people and organizations. There is always resistance to change whether the change is right or wrong.

Many systems that require change have failed to live up to their expectations because too little attention was given to the change process (Diran 1978; Johnson et al. 1978). Hackman (1976) estimates that as many job-redesign programs fail due to the way changes are implemented as fail due to the intrinsic merit (or lack thereof) of the changes themselves.

The key considerations in planning for change are not technological, but behavioral. This chapter briefly explores the variables affecting attitudes toward change and presents some guidelines for confronting resistance to it.

Attitudes toward Change

Attitudes toward change stem from many things. The following are among the more important.

Feelings of inadequacy. Change often threatens one's self-esteem or image in the eyes of others. Often low self-images are brought to work and confrontation with machines threatens to reveal a person's own worst fear of incompetence. Levitt (1972) concludes that many people are far behind technology and already feel badly bruised by their failure to comprehend even simple technologies. For them, sophisticated new technologies do not solve problems, they create them.

Fear of being replaced by a machine. The computer may be perceived as an instrument that actually replaces the worker. One's own value in the workplace may be totally undermined with disastrous monetary and psychological consequences.

Fear of failure. Many workers have spent years developing the skills that have made them proficient at their jobs. Why change? Should workers give up jobs that afford a relatively high degree of security for jobs that are new and strange and that require learning new skills, adjusting to unfamiliar methods and operating procedures, and establishing new working relationships? What happens if they are unable to handle the pressures of working with the new technologies? Will job performance suffer and if things move too swiftly will they be able to hang on?

Fear of the unknown. People need to be able to predict what they will face in the future. Established patterns are known factors, while new systems pose the threat of ambiguity and uncertainty.

Psychological habit. Established rules, policies, and procedures frequently become habits, and people rely on them for both guidance and protection. These habits are their security blanket. Change frequently disrupts this security by making established habits inapplicable.

Loss of control. Computers are frequently perceived as a threat to one's power or influence. Computer systems are also commonly perceived as things over which one has no control. If a person perceives a loss of control or feels ignored or helpless, pathological symptoms (such as anxiety, depression, depersonalization, or even violence) may develop.

Disturbed relationships. People have a strong need to interact with others. Changes that disrupt existing social patterns or result in isolation are unbearable. Change can also disturb worker relationships with superiors. Because highly proficient workers require little direct supervision they can achieve a satisfying sense of freedom and independence. Change requires closer and more frequent supervision, especially if training to master new skills is involved. Going from a state of independence to even a temporary state of dependence may not be welcome.

Lack of understanding. Resistance to change is likely if workers don't understand its purpose. Rumor, which tends to distort facts, is one of the most common methods of acquiring information about change. Mumford and Banks (1967) found that workers who heard about changes from an official source were more likely to approve of them than those who heard unofficially.

Lack of identification. A system should not be perceived as imposed. If the change is not initially sought by workers and if the consequences of the change do not appear directly beneficial to them, their resistance is likely. The result will be a lack of identification with and alienation from the system. Diran (1978) and Johnson et al. (1978) provide good illustrations of this phenomenon.

Addressing Change

A significant portion of the time and money devoted to an office system must be used to prepare the organization for the change. Preparation should begin in the planning phase and continue through the development, installation, and evaluation stages. The recommendations that follow incorporate a wide variety of strategies for easing the transition to office systems. Table 12-1 provides a checklist of these strategies. Their implications go beyond the few words that describe them here, and few of them can be achieved without substantial effort. If new technologies are ever to fulfill their highest expectations, people must accept them. Millions of dollars will have been spent for nothing if this last obstacle is not overcome.

Planning for Change

Planning is the foundation of the whole change process. If change is to be successful, its base of support must be firm. The planning process is directed toward deciding:

- when change is necessary or appropriate;
- what has to be changed;
- the development of a blueprint of the organization's desired state;
- how to implement the change, including solution of the technological and behavioral problems it poses.

Planning strategies for easing the transition to new technologies include all of the following:

Get top management support. Office automation spans traditional organization boundaries. Systematic change programs that affect several organizational levels are often prey to political strategies seeking to block them. Middle managers can stall and deenergize to avoid a loss of power (Schein 1977). Because bottom-up change will never work (Reddin 1977), complete top management support is mandatory. Driscoll (1979) concludes that the logical

Table 12-1. Addressing Change

Planning for Change

- Get top management support
- Encourage innovation in affected organizations
- Move slowly
- Limit technological advances
- Proceed in small steps
- Focus on high-potential-for-success changes
- Focus on systems that guarantee adequate usage
- Develop a solid research foundation
- Encourage resistance

Designing for Change

- Worker participation
- Ease of use
- Within user capabilities
- Acceptable job design
- Hospitable work environment
- Thorough documentation

Implementing Change

- Communicate:

  - the goals and objectives of the new system
  - benefits
  - people's roles
  - a road map and timetable

- Instill reasonable expectations
- Work through facilitators
- Provide thorough training
- Consider proper timing
- Allow a nonevaluative period
- Provide extra controls and early responses to problems
- Provide formal avenues of appeal

vehicle for the careful management of change is a high-level, interdepartmental task force that combines all the disciplines affected by the new technology.

Encourage innovation. Employers should encourage local user organizations to initiate new ideas (Driscoll 1979). This will foster a diffusion of positive attitudes toward the change. Rigid organizations are least receptive to change.

Move slowly. User commitment and innovation requires a slow-paced transition. The very nature of office work is, after all, being changed (Driscoll 1979).

Limit technological advances. Technological advances should also proceed slowly. The greater the advancement, the higher the probability that it will exceed the workers' adaptive capabilities (Mealiea 1978).

Proceed in small steps. Change should be implemented in small modules, steps, or stages (Diran 1978; Mealiea 1978). This approach reduces the perception that the change is radical.

Focus on changes with high success potential. The changes that yield the most obvious benefits to an organization should be implemented first (Lodahl et al. 1979). Resistance to these changes will be lower, and implementing them will condition the organization toward future change offering less obvious benefits.

Focus on systems that guarantee frequent usage. If no effort is made to maintain an adequate level of usage of a new office system, the system will fall into disuse as skills and procedures are forgotten. If workers can deal with some people through an office system but not with others, they will be frustrated by the resulting inefficiencies. People will also be frustrated if the system is not available when they need it. Resistance to both current systems and new systems will increase. The first systems to implement are those whose business objectives guarantee high levels of usage.

Develop a solid research foundation. A change agent must not be perceived as an interloper or rabble-rouser who knows nothing about the tasks or organization being changed (Schein 1977). Research, familiarization with the job being changed and the technologies involved, and expertise achieved through applied studies will all give the change agent credibility and legitimacy. Other things being equal, beliefs and attitudes are more amenable to change if the change agent is perceived as credible, attractive, or powerful (Morgan and King 1971).

Encourage resistance. Resistance to change, whether the change is reasonable or unreasonable, occasionally results in overt or covert counterimplementation actions to sabotage the change. Counterimplementation strategies include measures like failing to support an automation project by doing nothing or unnecessarily complicating the project. Keen (1982) feels that counterimplementation strategies can best be met by providing genuine opportunities for expressing resistance. Unfeasible designs or unwise directions may be identified and corrected early, and it will then be more difficult or even illegitimate to resist later.

Designing for Change

Strategies for achieving the acceptance of automation can also be built into the design process itself. Most of these strategies are nothing more than conscientious application of *human factors* to design.

Worker participation. In general, worker participation in the design (and implementation) of new sytems should be permitted. Selection of workers to participate should be based on their familiarity with tasks and functions, not their authority or position. A participative strategy should be implemented only after a study has verified that high resistance to change does not exist; that employees will not sense their jobs are at stake or otherwise be adversely affected by the change; and that there is a perceived need among workers to participate.

Ease of use. People will use something if it is easy and convenient, but will reject something more complicated than what they are already using. Office system users will not make enormous changes in their accustomed ways of doing things, nor employ a formidable piece of equipment that requires special training. Great ease also compensates for low motivation.

Within user capabilities. Office systems must be designed within the limits of user capabilities. Designs insensitive to this factor will be rejected.

Acceptable job design. Another key factor in the acceptance of a system is the characteristics of the new jobs. Job design must permit perceived job satisfaction, skill, originality, and status.

Hospitable work environment. Office system design must take into account the social needs that the organizational structure is expected to satisfy. A comfortable work environment must also be provided. Designs insensitive to these factors will be rejected.

Thorough documentation. If workers do not know what to do and cannot easily find out, the office system is doomed.

Implementing Change

No matter how well an office system is designed, an employer cannot simply present it to workers and assume it will be effectively used, or even used at all. An installation strategy must be carried out.

Communication. The most common office communications are informal. Informal communications (such as rumor) can distort facts, create misunderstanding, and cause resentments that result in a system's rejection even before its arrival. The best way to confront rumor is to ensure that formal communication is plentiful and continual so that it anticipates and guides information passing through the informal channels. Communicated information should be relevant and reassuring and should begin as early as possible. It should include such things as goals, benefits, role definitions, and projected schedules.

Clear goals and objectives are important. People must understand the rationale behind a new system and what it is supposed to accomplish. Lack of understanding often leads to lack of acceptance (Carlisle 1976).

Demonstrated benefits are critical, too. People must perceive that the system is operating in their interest. Systems have failed because it was mistakenly assumed that their benefits would be obvious to everyone (Diran 1978; Johnson et al. 1978). If the benefits to the individual are truly obvious, new technologies will be used (Engel et al. 1979; Lodahl et al. 1979). Inexperienced users have consistently more negative attitudes than do experienced users (Zoltan 1982).

How people fit into the system, their responsibilities and the roles of others, should be explained. People need such role definitions to be able to predict what they will face in the future.

Employees should receive *a road map and a timetable*—again, to enable them to predict their futures. Employers should communicate their implementation strategy and the projected time frame.

Instill reasonable expectations. The expectations of system users must be realistic and accurate. Raising expectations beyond what is possible will only cause dissatisfaction, rejection of the system, and a negative attitude toward future change.

Work through facilitators. Change can be expedited by working through informal leaders (Mealiea 1978). Involvement of such people can give a change program credibility.

Provide thorough training. Provide heavy and continuous training in the use of the new system both during and after the introductory phase. If a person cannot use a system (effectively or at all) because of training deficiencies, its benefits will never be achieved. Again, rejection of the system and negative attitudes toward future systems will result.

Consider proper timing. An organization should not install a new office system during busy time periods. When people are busy and pressured by deadlines, they would rather remain under known pressures than risk losing time with new, unfamiliar approaches.

Allow a nonevaluative period. Allow each person to adjust to the new system at his or her own pace. The learning process cannot be rushed. When implementing change, allow a system stabilization period, during which performance will not have a negative impact on a worker's review, income, or other perceived benefits. Failure to allow this trial period can also increase resistance to future change.

Provide extra controls and early responses. One's first experiences with an office system can crystallize attitudes toward it and toward future office systems. System implementors must respond quickly and satisfactorily to unforeseen problems early on so that unfavorable attitudes do not develop.

Provide formal avenues of appeal. Do not force anyone to use equipment he or she does not want to use. A few people in any office will be unable to cope with change. People do care about their futures, and the company must care as well. Formal avenues of appeal should be established for these individuals so that they may be identified and their talents and skills redirected into other channels more suitable to themselves and the company.

References

Carlisle, J. H. "Evaluating the Impact of Office Automation on Top Management Communication." *AFIPS Conference Proceedings* 45 (1976): 611–616.

Diran, K. M. "Management Information Systems: The Human Factor." *Journal of Higher Education* 49, No. 3 (May/June 1978): 273–282.

Driscoll, J. W. "People and the Automated Office." *Datamation,* November 1979, 106–112·

Engel, G. H.; Groppuso, J.; Lowenstein, R. A.; and Traub, W. G. "An Office Communications System." *IBM Systems Journal* 18, No.. 3 (1979): 402–431.

Hackman, J. R. "Work Design." *Improving Life at Work: Behavioral Science Approach to Organized Change,* edited by J. R. Hackman and J. L. Suttle. Pacific Palisades, Calif.: Goodyear, 1976.

Johnson, J. H.; Williams, T.A.; Giannetti, R. A.; Klinger, D. E.; and Nakashima, S. R. "Organizational Preparedness for Change: Staff Acceptance of an On-Line Computer-Assisted Assessment System." *Behavioral Research Methods and Instrumentation* 10, No. 2 (April 1978): 186–190.

Keen, P. G. W. "Introducing Change." *Computerworld OA,* 1982.

Levitt, T. "Production-Line Approach to Service." *Harvard Business Review,* September/October 1972, pp. 41–52.

Lodahl, T. M.; Williams, L. K.; and Williams, P. "Providing Management Support in the Automated Office." *Corporate Systems,* June 1979, pp. 43–46.

Mealiea, L. W. "Learned Behavior: The Key to Understanding and Preventing Employee Resistance to Change." *Group and Organization Studies* 3, No. 2 (June 1978): 211–223.

Morgan, C. T., and King, R. A. *Introduction to Psychology.* New York: McGraw-Hill, 1971.

Mumford, E., and Banks, O. *The Computer and the Clerk.* London: Routledge and Kegan Paul, 1967.

Reddin, W. J. "Confessions of an Organizational Change Report." *Group and Organizational Studies* 2, No. 1 (March 1977): 33–41.

Schein, V. E. "Political Strategies for Implementing Organizational Change." *Group and Organizational Studies* 2, No. 1 (March 1977): 42–48.

Zoltan, E. "How Acceptable Are Computers to Professional Persons?" *Proceedings: Human Factors in Computer Systems*. Gaithersburg, Md., March 15–17, 1982, pp. 74–77.

13

Another Look Back—And Ahead

Looking back over this exploration of the role of human factors in office automation provides an opportunity to add some overall perspective. In doing so, it may be worthwhile to compare today's perspective with that in the book that served as the foundation for the materials contained on the preceding pages, *Human Factors in Office Automation* (Galitz 1980). That perspective is restated below.

The 1979–1980 Perspective

The exploration started in late 1979 with the following hypotheses:

- The number of voices expressing concern about human factors in office automation greatly exceed the useful design information available.
- Many of those concerned voices do not fully understand what human factors really encompasses.
- Equipment manufacturers, system designers, and users have a long way to go in achieving a real marriage of people and office systems.

Now, a year later, how have those hypotheses fared? First, much more design information was found than expected. A variety of information exists that should be useful to office system designers and implementors. Buried in journals, technical documents, and periodicals is a wealth of applicable information. This book taps only a portion of it. Getting to this information and then structuring it in a usable format presents problems, however. Perhaps office system technologies themselves will eventually provide a solution to this. The more one knows, however, the less one really knows, and concerns in this area will probably always exceed useful design information because of the nature of the entity with which it deals—the human being.

This review did nothing to change the second hypothesis concerning popular understanding of human factors. Literature tends to be general and focus on conditions that are under the user's immediate control, such as the environment. Computer system design information is often buried in less accessible publications, and this not only makes applying human factors difficult, but also prevents full understanding of the true scope of human factors. Professional conferences tend to reflect these shortcomings, too.

The blame for this knowledge gap may be at least partially attributed to human factors practitioners themselves (the writer included), who have failed to adequately communicate their interests, methods, and findings to the growing number of people thirsting for this knowledge.

Personal experience and comments in literature continue to reinforce the hypothesis that we still have a long way to go to achieve a real marriage of people and office systems. Though we have come a long way, much more remains to be done. These guidelines should provide a more effective criterion by which to make judgments. Readers must, however, evaluate their own situations and reach their own specific conclusions.

The View Today

The first hypothesis—that the number of voices of concern greatly exceeds the useful design information—remains true today. While we do possess much more design information, (as evidenced by the increased size of this book and others beginning to appear), the number of voices of concern is also growing. The crescendo, once confined to the experts, has been joined by those being asked to use the new equipment and systems. The result has been increasing efforts toward legislation and unionization.

Why this greater concern among users of systems? A variety of reasons probably contribute, including:

- more accurate diagnoses of injuries and problems that were previously considered minor (sprains, arthritis, etc.);
- increased education and awareness of system users;
- decreased job opportunities that reduce seeking alternative employment when problems develop;
- poor ergonomic climates in offices.

Some of the guidelines identified in this book have already been incorporated into legislation in a number of European countries. Several state legislatures, including those of Illinois and Massachusetts, have had similar bills introduced. Is this a healthy trend? Many experts (among them Ketchel 1982 and Hirsch 1982), as well as this writer, do not think so.

The research base for many of the guidelines is not yet adequate. While many solutions are straightforward and well established, the tendency for legislation is to fill in our many knowledge gaps with mandated requirements based upon tenuous research. Inconsistencies in requirements often result. This is evidenced in the review by Rupp (1981) and the disagreements between experts that surfaced at the International Scientific Conference on Ergonomic and

Health Aspects in Modern Offices (1983). Even the blind application of reasonably straightforward rules can be dangerous. Many factors, as we have shown, interact with one another. We must get a much better grasp of all the issues before allowing office automation to enter the legislative arena.

Legislation may also give us a false sense of security, since it implies that the problem is solved—leading to two undesirable outcomes. One is that much-needed research will be stifled. Another is that research will head in trivial or nonproductive directions, deflecting valuable resources from exploration of the meaningful issues.

Lastly, legislation may impose an unnecessary financial burden on the occasional users of VDTs. Occasional users are not subjected to all the problems described here; to impose solutions to nonproblems is not cost effective. Furthermore, state or federally mandated requirements necessitate monitoring mechanisms to assure company compliance with the law. This results in tax dollars being spent for solutions of dubious long-term value to companies and society. This creates a double whammy for users of office computer technology: unnecessary pitfalls and attenuated payoffs.

Efforts toward unionization often serve to polarize the adversaries. Critical issues may be submerged and noncritical issues escalated, all becoming pawns in a game of political chess. Most often the victim is not management or the union, but the individual worker. True and proper solutions to problems will only be achieved through a meaningful dialogue between all affected parties.

Concerning hypothesis two, while an understanding of human factors in office automation has greatly increased in the past several years, the previous criticisms also still apply. Systematic dissemination of design information, while getting better, can still be greatly improved by the professionals and professional organizations charged with producing it. A good example of what is needed is the guideline concerning the user interface produced by Smith and Aucella (1983).

Many system developers and users also still possess too narrow a view of all that human factors encompasses. For too many practitioners it is still *the environment, the hardware, the system,* or *managing change.* Until there is an awareness among all that the issues cannot be viewed separately, meaningful complete solutions will be difficult to accomplish.

Regarding the third hypothesis, while great strides have been made in achieving a beneficial marriage between people and office systems, there is still much to be done. Significant remaining problems include the failure of many to recognize what is good and bad in design, and the willy-nilly application of terms like *user friendly* and *ergonomically designed* to products regardless of their actual qualities.

1984 and Beyond

The objective of an office system is to effectively support people who have jobs to do. Developing an office of the future that succeeds in this will require a number of things. First, we must continue in our efforts to achieve a better understanding of the office of today. We must continue to expand our knowledge about the office work process, how to improve office tasks, and how technology can be used to improve the wellbeing of the worker and the organization.

Second, we must expand our research efforts to achieve a clearer understanding of the cause-and-effect relationships of the problems that have been reported. Specific questions that must be addressed include these:

- What proportions of the problems are attitudinal or psychological as opposed to physical?
- Are the reported fatigue effects cumulative or completely reversible?
- What are the behavioral effects of visual fatigue?
- What are the interactive relationships between the equipment, the job, and the environment?

Third, management and office workers must work together to address the real problems. The goals of each are really not very different; the harmonization of people, the organization, and technology will yield the greatest benefits for all.

Fourth, the path to successful office automation will require massive effort and some expense. Those who seek benefits without effort and expense are sure to fail.

Finally, we must continue to learn from our past triumphs and failures. For, as the philosopher Santayana once said: *Those who cannot remember the past are condemned to repeat it.*

References

Galitz, W. O. *Human Factors in Office Automation.* Atlanta, Georgia: Life Office Management Association, 1980.

Hirsch, R. S. "National Standards for the Design of Visual Display Terminals." *Proceedings of the Human Factors Society—26th Annual Meeting (1982)*, pp. 290–293. Santa Monica, CA, 1982.

International Scientific Conference on Ergonomic and Health Aspects in Modern Offices, Turin, Italy, November 7–9, 1983.

Ketchel, J. "Human Factors Issues in the Design and Use of Visual Display Terminals (VDTs)." *Office Automation Conference Digest.* San Francisco, Calif., April 5–7, 1982.

Rupp, B. A. "Visual Display Terminals: A Review of the Issues." *Proceedings of the SID.* Vol. 22, No. 1, 1981.

Smith, S. L., and Aucella, A. F. *"Design Guidelines for the User Interface to Computer-Based Information Systems.* The MITRE Corporation, March 1983.